Physician Assistant Review Guide

Edited by

David Paulk, EdD, PA-C

Academic Coordinator and Associate Professor
Department of Medical Science and Community Health
Arcadia University
Glenside, Pennsylvania

Donna M. Agnew, MT (ASCP), MSPAS, PA-C

Associate Director and Assistant Professor
Department of Medical Science and Community Health
Arcadia University
Glenside, Pennsylvania

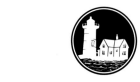

JONES AND BARTLETT PUBLISHERS

Sudbury, Massachusetts

BOSTON   TORONTO   LONDON   SINGAPORE

World Headquarters

Jones and Bartlett Publishers
40 Tall Pine Drive
Sudbury, MA 01776
978-443-5000
info@jbpub.com
www.jbpub.com

Jones and Bartlett Publishers Canada
6339 Ormindale Way
Mississauga, Ontario L5V 1J2
Canada

Jones and Bartlett Publishers International
Barb House, Barb Mews
London W6 7PA
United Kingdom

Jones and Bartlett's books and products are available through most bookstores and online booksellers. To contact Jones and Bartlett Publishers directly, call 800-832-0034, fax 978-443-8000, or visit our website, www.jbpub.com.

Substantial discounts on bulk quantities of Jones and Bartlett's publications are available to corporations, professional associations, and other qualified organizations. For details and specific discount information, contact the special sales department at Jones and Bartlett via the above contact information or send an email to specialsales@jbpub.com.

The authors, editor, and publisher have made every effort to provide accurate information. However, they are not responsible for errors, omissions, or for any outcomes related to the use of the contents of this book and take no responsibility for the use of the products and procedures described. Treatments and side effects described in this book may not be applicable to all people; likewise, some people may require a dose or experience a side effect that is not described herein. Drugs and medical devices are discussed that may have limited availability controlled by the Food and Drug Administration (FDA) for use only in a research study or clinical trial. Research, clinical practice, and government regulations often change the accepted standard in this field. When consideration is being given to use of any drug in the clinical setting, the health care provider or reader is responsible for determining FDA status of the drug, reading the package insert, and reviewing prescribing information for the most up-to-date recommendations on dose, precautions, and contraindications, and determining the appropriate usage for the product. This is especially important in the case of drugs that are new or seldom used.

Production Credits

Publisher: David Cella
Associate Editor: Maro Gartside
Production Manager: Julie Champagne Bolduc
Production Assistant: Jessica Steele Newfell
Senior Marketing Manager: Barb Bartoszek
Manufacturing and Inventory Control Supervisor: Amy Bacus
Composition and Interior Design: Publishers' Design and Production Services, Inc.
Cover Design: Kristin E. Parker/Brian Moore
Assistant Photo Researcher: Jessica Elias
Cover Image: © Photodisc
Printing and Binding: Replika Press PVT LTD
Cover Printing: Replika Press PVT LTD

Library of Congress Cataloging-in-Publication Data

Physician assistant review guide / [edited] by David Paulk and Donna Agnew.
      p. ; cm.
  Includes bibliographical references.
  ISBN-13: 978-0-7637-5266-8
  ISBN-10: 0-7637-5266-5
  1. Physicians' assistants—Examinations, questions, etc.   I. Paulk, David.   II. Agnew, Donna.
  [DNLM: 1. Physician Assistants--Examination Questions. 2. Certification--Examination Questions.
W 18.2 P5787 2009]
  R697.P45P486 2009
  610.76--dc22

                        2008043400

6048

Printed in India

13 12 11 10 09   10 9 8 7 6 5 4 3 2 1

DEDICATION

To the students we have the privilege of teaching and to the patients entrusted to our care. We have learned volumes from you—more than we could ever teach.

ACKNOWLEDGMENTS

We would especially like to thank our families—specifically our spouses, Sarah and Michael— for their unfailing love, support, and encouragement.

Contents

Preface   *vii*

Introduction:
Test-Taking Strategies   *ix*

> Christopher R. A. Sim, MPAS, PA-C
> David Paulk, EdD, PA-C

Contributors   *xvii*

Chapter 1

Dermatology   **1**

> Pamela L. Meyer, DO

Chapter 2

Ophthalmology   **34**

> Gwenn Amos, OD

Chapter 3

Ear, Nose, and Throat   **49**

> Douglas Nadel, MD (ASCP)
> Donna M. Agnew, MT (ASCP), MSPAS, PA-C

Chapter 4

Pulmonology   **61**

> Les A. Szekely, MD, FCCP, DABSM
> Donna M. Agnew, MT (ASCP), MSPAS, PA-C

Chapter 5

Cardiology   **77**

> Jennifer L. Arnold, MHS, PA-C
> Jill M. Cowen, MSPAS, PA-C
> Wendy Eaton, MSPAS, PA-C

Chapter 6

Electrocardiography   **99**

> Charles D. Bortle, MEd, RRTNPS, NREMT-P

Chapter 7

Gastroenterology   **114**

> Jon Shapiro, MD

Chapter 8

Orthopedics   **131**

> Jonathan T. Hirsch, PA-C
> Robert Howard, PT, MD
> David Paulk, EdD, PA-C

Chapter 9

Rheumatology   **154**

> Nicole M. Orzechowski, DO

Chapter 10

Neurology   **168**

> Barry Korn, DO, DPM, DAAPM

Chapter 11

General Practice   **185**

> Tabassum Salam, MD, FACP
> Irwin Wolfert, MD

Contents

Chapter 12

Infectious Disease   200

Robert Bettiker, MD

Chapter 13

Pharmacology   218

Tep Kang, PharmD, BCPS

Chapter 14

Physical Diagnosis   224

Donna M. Agnew, MT (ASCP), MSPAS, PA-C

Chapter 15

Radiology   247

Melissa Kohler Justice, PA-C, MHS

Chapter 16

Laboratory Medicine   271

Donna M. Agnew, MT (ASCP), MSPAS, PA-C

Chapter 17

Obstetrics and Gynecology   289

Rachel Catanzaro Ditoro, MSPAS, PA-C
Donna M. Agnew, MT (ASCP), MSPAS, PA-C

Chapter 18

Pediatrics   310

Keith Herzog, MD

Chapter 19

General Urology   327

Irvin H. Hirsch, MD
Mark L. Pe, MD
Eleanor Davis, PA-C

Chapter 20

Renal Medicine   339

Barry Korn, DO, DPM, DAAPM

Chapter 21

Emergency Medicine   346

Michael Lucca, MD, FACEP, FAAEM
Henry D. Unger, MD, FACEP

Chapter 22

Endocrinology   363

Renee E. Amori, MD
Richard D. Siegel, MD

Chapter 23

Hematology/Oncology   378

Dale Bryansmith, MD
Donna M. Agnew, MT (ASCP), MSPAS, PA-C

Chapter 24

Surgery   396

Jennifer L. Arnold, MHS, PA-C
Richard L. Commaille, PA-C

Chapter 25

Mental Health and Illness   413

Mary Puckett, PhD, PA-C

Chapter 26

Geriatrics   434

John A. Batsis, MD
Paul Y. Takahashi, MD, FACP, AGSF

Figure Captions   455

Preface

The practice of medicine affords no room for complacency. It is a dynamic force. Over time, this force humbles each of us. Diagnosis and standards of care are often moving targets as technology affords new insights into the pathophysiology of disease. We frequently find ourselves teasing through patient histories for relevant and crucial data. We navigate through a myriad of diagnostic studies to develop an assessment and treatment plan for our patients, all the while juggling constraints of time and an ever-changing health care arena. Even when patients present classically in textbook fashion, we question, "What else might I be missing?" Additionally, who of us has not spent those hours just before sleep replaying the patients seen earlier in the day?

This need for self-improvement and refinement is what fuels us to survive the rigors of physician assistant school in the first place and challenges us to remain current in practice. Although we belong to a profession that allows us the luxury of turning to our supervising physicians to discuss a perplexing patient's case, we are always mindful of the gravity of serving patients entrusted to our care. It is for this reason that we should welcome the certifying examinations.

So, how did we find ourselves compiling a review book for the Physician Assistant National Certifying Examination (PANCE) and the Physician Assistant National Recertifying Examination (PANRE)? Over the past few years, various publishers have afforded us the privilege to review journal articles and various book chapters. After such a review, Jones and Bartlett Publishers proposed that we consider writing our own board review text. Once the initial flattery faded, we gave it earnest consideration. We can both candidly say that neither one of us appreciated the amount of work involved in writing and editing a review book. Soliciting specialists, editing a wide range of questions, securing complementary images, and researching and providing adequate explanations of answers far exceeded our anticipated expectations of the time required. Even after exhaustive efforts, once again we found ourselves asking, "What else might I be missing?" Every reread of the text compelled us to alter questions or elucidate a corresponding answer.

Writing this review reinforced what we guess we already knew—that medicine is not a black-and-white set of absolutes, but rather a holistic gray zone. Respected authors or practitioners may have a difference of opinion or approach to the same clinical scenario and, as long as they maintain altruistic care of their patients, they would both be "correct." We have attempted to explain such discrepancies to the best of our abilities in this book. We also recognize that this review book serves only as one of many tools in preparing you for the examination. We hope that it will refresh your memory regarding some topics and identify some weaknesses in your knowledge base to further direct your self-study. The ultimate responsibility rests with you. Of course, every board examination presents with some trepidation. Our desire is that this book reduces yours in some fashion. We wish you the best of success on the examination and in clinical practice.

Introduction

Test-Taking Strategies

Christopher R. A. Sim, MPAS, PA-C
David Paulk, EdD, PA-C

Although it may be apparent that this book has been written with the practicing clinician in mind, if history holds true, both practicing clinicians and newly graduated physician assistants (PAs) will use this book as one of the many tools available to help them prepare for the board examinations. Many of the test-taking strategies presented in this introduction should seem familiar, and indeed simplistic, to those who have already taken the Physician Assistant National Recertifying Examination (PANRE). For those preparing to take the Physician Assistant National Certifying Examination (PANCE), perhaps the techniques will be new to you. In either case, we believe that a little review goes a long way (otherwise why write a review book in the first place?). To those experienced test-takers, bear with us—use what you need, just as in practice. To those just graduating, memorize these tips as though your life depends on it, or, better yet, relax and, just like an experienced clinician, use what you can as you need it.

OUR GOAL

In this introduction, we will deal primarily with the techniques and strategies the PANCE or PANRE candidate should utilize in preparing for these examinations. We hope this introduction will assist you in preparing for successful performance on these examinations, helping you confidently approach your new profession or to reinforce the basic core knowledge required of all physician assistants.

SETTING GOALS AND PREPARATION

By the time you are reading this, you probably already have a great deal invested in the outcome of the PANCE or PANRE. If you are about to graduate from a PA program or have recently graduated, you spent a considerable sum of money on your education. Likewise, you logged countless hours of lectures, study, and clinical rotations in your quest to become a physician assistant. You skipped meals, stood for hours in an operating room, waited on laboring mothers, and sutured squirming children.

If you are an experienced PA with at least 5 years of practice, you may not have taken an examination since your PANCE or last PANRE. Not surprisingly, you also may have skipped meals, stood for hours in an operating room, waited on laboring mothers, and sutured squirming children. You, too, have much invested. In the case of the PANRE, much continues to be reinvested each year, culminating in the retaking of a certifying examination.

In either case, we suspect there will be some anxiety—how much depends on your personality and/or how much you may have put into preparation. There are those who see the examination as a potential roadblock in their careers, but we hope they will take it as one of the many speed bumps we all encounter as we journey through our careers.

SETTING SPECIFIC GOALS

Any time we set out to do something, we set a goal or series of goals. This may involve something as simple as going to the grocery store to buy the food necessary to prepare dinner. Alternatively, it can also be a complicated set of goals leading to an ultimate, or final, goal. How you completed your PA program best describes these principles. First, you attended a series of lectures, seminars, and other formalized educational programming, which allowed you to accumulate a body of specialized knowledge. Next, you participated in clinical rotations, which by nature were more freeform than your didactic year. This type of learning was more experiential in that you were applying the knowledge you accumulated in the didactic phase and learning new skills and information as you saw patients on a daily basis during the clinical phase, and, of course, in your practice.

Interestingly enough, the preceding paragraph roughly describes how most adults tend to learn best. Essentially, there is a period of *memorization* during which students literally "fill the tank" with information, so that they can progress to the next step. In other words, we are cognitive learners, and cognitive learning is key to the diagnostic reasoning process.

The next step in the process of adult learning is *comprehension*. This occurs throughout formalized education. Comprehension represents the student's ability to catalyze raw information into a usable product. Learning to perform a complete history and physical examination, for instance, is a good example of using raw data and then assembling them into a product. During this stage, written, oral, and practical examinations assess the student's comprehension of the subject matter. These measures serve to reinforce and validate student learning.

Finally, the student combines memorization and comprehension into the final step—*application*. Application is the *goal* we set before we begin the memorization or comprehension processes. After all, would we want to go through all this if there was not an ultimate goal?

Although all of us (presumably) utilize the diagnostic reasoning process with a strong basis in evidence-based medicine, sometimes this is not always true. Anecdotal evidence exists that we all do what we are comfortable doing. For example, your instincts may tell you something is "wrong" with a patient's condition in spite of the fact that very little, if any, evidence exists to confirm or rule out a diagnosis. Yet, our experiences have shown us sometimes patients present in different ways, so part of our diagnostic reasoning process may involve parts of evidence-based medicine and instinctual response, which ultimately leads to our own personal brand of cognitive reasoning.

Interestingly enough, the diagnostic reasoning process follows this closely. Theoretically, it is almost indistinguishable from what psychologists and theorists identify as the *cognitive reasoning process*. That is, we retrieve information from our various experiences (educational and otherwise) and apply it based on experiences (evidentiary and otherwise).

Setting goals—whatever they are—essentially establishes a standard that confirms our efforts and a reference point that defines success. You have committed yourself to the care of patients (and of course, to do this, the passing of your board examinations). This commitment gives you a starting point for establishing your goal. One assumes that you bought this book in order to help you achieve a goal—to pass the PANRE or PANCE. Perhaps you wish to expand that goal not only to pass, but also to excel. Success here validates your efforts toward taking an exam. Additionally, and perhaps more importantly, this aids you in your motivation to serve patients well. When we begin with our goal of passing the PANCE/PANRE, we must break that larger goal down into smaller goals, which facilitate our pursuit. That is to say, we must view that large goal in terms of a series of smaller goals that will help us to succeed.

WRITE IT DOWN

Many people find it helpful to keep a journal of activities related to an important achievement in their life. Graduate study, buying a house, starting a family, or dealing with an illness are all important stressors in life, and these events have both positive and negative aspects.

Keeping a small journal of your thoughts and feelings during this process can help you to maintain perspective, allowing you to see the progress you have made, even when there may be a slow or not-so-positive period in this quest. Additionally, a journal can help you "stay on track" toward achieving your goal. We also suggest for those not inclined to journal their experiences that you use the time to study—to "journal" what you know and do not know—and use this as a guide to help you study.

SUGGESTED STUDY TECHNIQUES

We know that it is important to establish a series of facilitative goals in order to achieve the larger goal. Techniques you might consider could include:

- Study notes from basic sciences and clinical medicine courses from PA school 12 hours a week
- Take part in study group 4 hours a week (if possible)
- Read and study the review book at least 1 hour nightly
- Identify weaknesses and review these areas until your confidence level improves
- Perform all of the above until you actually take the PANCE/PANRE

Giving your goal structure and devising a plan make it easier to stay with the plan when you are juggling multiple responsibilities. As a conscientious provider, you know that you must do this every day in order to care for your patients, to perform the things you need to do to live and work successfully, and to be open to new opportunities.

If you establish a list of goals, you may want to have a small "check off" section in your journal that you can, on a daily basis, use to quantify the work you are doing toward your goal. Having a goal list and process also makes global goals more manageable and less intimidating at a time when we may feel stressed and overwhelmed.

NOTES ON SETTING GOALS

Make sure your goals are realistic. If you struggle with tests, it may not be feasible to have scoring 100% on the exam as your goal. A more modest, but still impressive, goal for you may be to score 90% or above (we are familiar with many practitioners and students who simply desire to pass, and that is an entirely reasonable goal).

Allow enough time for your plan. For example, it probably is not a good idea to study 12 hours a day for 5 days prior to the examination. You have probably heard several times throughout your academic career about the futility of cramming. That said, students always have, and probably always will, cram. Interestingly enough, research indicates that those who do not cram usually score better.

Strive for a sense of peace. Any test is just that, a test. It is a reflection of how well you took an exam on a given day and time. It does not define you as a human being or even qualify your skills as a PA. The problem is, with a job, perhaps a family, and some semblance of a social life, giving peace a chance is not always feasible. Perhaps you might go for a balance and accept that you will do the best you can do—period.

Allow for changes in your plan. A job, a family, and a social life all can interfere with your study plan. You must reassess what your particular life responsibilities are and put together a reasonable block of time for study.

Set up a system of rewards for yourself when you do well. For example, going to a movie after you complete a certain amount of study or having a meal during a study group session presents a change of routine and revitalizes everyone. We suspect that the well-balanced clinician who may not be working most of the time to pay off school loans and the like already has many skills in this regard and, we hope, already is well skilled in how to use them.

PREPARATION

You must allow sufficient time for the execution of your goal plan. We suggest you begin your study at least 6 months prior to actually taking the examination. Unfortunately, the consequences of failure are significant (e.g., loss of certification, job, exam fees). Fortunately, those taking the PANRE may sit for the exam two or three more times, depending on when you initially take the PANRE. Those who are practicing PAs have the option of taking the PANRE in the fifth year to relieve some of the pressure.

You must allot enough time to prepare adequately for the exam(s). You need to know what type of learner you are and what study methods work best for you. If you are disciplined and unlikely to stray from your study schedule, you may do better studying on your own. If you are easily distracted or get overwhelmed, you may benefit from studying in a group. Modern technology can even allow you to study with friends/classmates who are hundreds of miles away via email, instant messaging, or a conference call. The adage "Nothing succeeds like success" is especially true when selecting study group members. Try to find others who are motivated, organized, and share your purpose. You need to identify the sources you will use to study. Notes from your PA school classes can be a good starting point (although we caution you to seek more recent materials if you graduated more than 5 or 10 years ago), as well as standardized textbooks, test preparation books, and multimedia learning modules.

STRESS MANAGEMENT

We would like to point out that wellness and stress management are essential to success in almost any endeavor. However, we recognize that not every one of us follows the tenets of stress management. Certainly, we recognize that stress management can be difficult following 3 days on call. Our hope is that you will use the tips presented that may be helpful to you.

During the exam preparation process, it is very important to maintain your physical and emotional well-being. Most people tend to perform well when they are calm and focused. Even a minor illness can get in the way of your success. Therefore, your goal-setting should include attention to proper nutrition, exercise, and health maintenance. You should plan your food intake around your study times so that you are not trying to study just after a heavy meal, when you feel sluggish. During study time, light snacks such as fruits or vegetables are a good choice.

If you are a "caffeine freak" (and what medical practitioner could do without this necessary fuel?), this is probably not the time to attempt to quit your habit—being irritable and edgy will not enhance your success. Likewise, if you are a smoker (and obviously you should quit), it is probably best to put off quitting until after the testing process. It usually does not help to consume alcohol during study periods, because it will affect your attention and may distract you from your goal for that session. If you are taking medication that affects your study skills, see your health care provider and determine if there are other options. Regular exercise will do much to protect your health during this study period. You can even make a walk or quick run part of your study routine. You may feel calmer and more focused upon your return. This could allow you to better utilize your time.

However you structure your nutrition and exercise during the exam preparation period, the most important thing is to be consistent. If you can stick with your plan until test time, your likelihood of success is better than those who do not have a plan.

If you find that you tend to become very anxious in a testing scenario, the more you can familiarize yourself with the process, the better you will feel during the "real" test. Taking practice examinations with a time limit can help you to feel more comfortable during the examinations. This review book is equipped with a 300-question practice test that we hope will assist you in this process. If you have severe symptoms of test anxiety, such as persistent tachycardia, diaphoresis, gastrointestinal upset, or profound negative feelings, you may wish to consult your health care provider. There are many options for treating such anxiety, including cognitive therapy, behavior modification, and medication. If you are lucky enough to be very good friends with a psychologist, we suggest you stay in touch.

PREPARING FOR THE DAY

Be sure to schedule your PANCE or PANRE realistically. For example, many times, PANCE test-takers are in a whirlwind of activity following graduation. They may need to move, close their affairs at their school, or even get married. Try to schedule your exam for a time that will be convenient and when you will not have multiple demands on your attention. In other words, make the exam the priority for that period.

Once you have scheduled your exam, it would be helpful to do a little research in order to make sure you understand the content of the examination. The areas of interest in the PANCE/PANRE (as set forth by the National Commission on the Certification of Physician Assistants [NCCPA]; www.nccpa.net) are:

- History and Physical Examination Findings
- Laboratory/Diagnostic Studies
- Differential Diagnoses
- Preventive Medicine
- Clinical Therapeutics
- Pharmacology
- Basic Sciences

You should determine the site(s) where you may take your examination. If possible, go there and become familiar with the facility. You will need your testing confirmation from NCCPA and identification. You should not take anything else with you into the test center. Testing centers provide lockers for test-takers to secure valuables. Be sure you know two routes to the facility for the test day in case of bad traffic, roadwork, etc. It is a good idea to find out where the restroom facilities are. Remember that you can only take an erasable sheet (dry-erase boards) and grease pencil into the testing room with you. You will need to notify the proctor if you need to leave the testing room for any reason during the exam.

Once you know where your test facility is, we suggest you perform visualization exercises centering on your success. Picture yourself driving to the exam site, meeting the proctor, and beginning your exam. In short, picture yourself succeeding on test day. Positive images such as this will help offset doubts and anxiety that may occur on or around test day. Just as a marathon runner decreases training before a race, you will also want to cut back somewhat on your study time in the days before the exam (probably 5 days before). "Cramming" will not help you at this point; it might even make you perform poorly because it may confuse you and create more anxiety. A good rule of thumb is to study approximately one-half of your "usual" study time in the 3 to 5 days leading up to the exam. Be sure to get plenty of sleep and make an effort to get some exercise to offset the natural feelings of anxiety you may encounter.

Once the exam is over, you should be able to say honestly that you have done the best you could on that test that day. Once you do that, GO HOME! Plan a special activity for later that day to reward yourself for your efforts. Usually, it is not helpful to call classmates to discuss the exam; this could confuse you and may cause you to doubt your performance. Years of PA education have shown us that you should reward those in your life who have helped you to prepare for this examination. Remember, your family probably "studies" with you as you prepare.

TECHNICAL ASPECTS OF THE EXAMINATION

It is important to remember that few, if any, test-takers know everything about every item on an examination. If someone scores 75 out of 100 questions correctly, they answered 25 questions incorrectly. However, they did answer the *majority* of the questions correctly.

The PANCE and PANRE consist entirely of multiple-choice questions. Some of the questions involve images of physical findings, electrocardiograms, and radiographs. That is, they are all multiple choice with four (and sometimes five) responses. The examinee should read each stem (*question part*) and identify key words. If you cannot determine the truth of the statement, just assume that it is true and look for any factors that would make it false. Answer the question before reading the possible responses. Eliminate obvious distracters. Look for extreme modifiers (e.g., *all*, *none*, *best*, *absolutely*, *worse*, *only*, *invariably*, *no one*, *everyone*, *certainly not*); these usually indicate the answer is false.

Try to avoid frustration with a question that may have more than one possible answer. Remember, you are looking for the *most* appropriate, the *most* likely, or the *best* choice. For example, if someone presents with chest pain radiating down her left arm and the question is "Which of the following is the most likely diagnosis?" your answer choices may be:

A. Myocardial infarction
B. Congestive heart failure
C. Costochondritis
D. Gastroesophageal reflux disease (GERD)

The problem with this question is that you do not receive a complete set of information (this sometimes happens). We learn, as clinicians, to eliminate the most deadly of diagnoses in the care and treatment of patients. Therefore, you should clinically eliminate myocardial infarction, followed by congestive heart failure. Still, a major problem exists. We know that the "typical" patient presenting to the emergency room with this problem likely has or is having a myocardial infarction. He may be having any of the other choices. In this case, pick the myocardial infarction choice until or unless you receive more information.

You should also watch for such words such as *never*, *always*, and *only*. This usually points in one direction. Additionally, when eliminating choices, watch for the item that stands out. For example, going back to our example, what would you do if the choices were:

A. Myocardial infarction
B. Congestive heart failure
C. Costochondritis
D. Gout

Obviously, gout has nothing to do with the set of circumstances presented. Thus, it is probably not the answer. This narrows down the possible answer to one of three choices.

Textbooks, review books, and instructors throughout time have admonished students not to guess on any question. We feel this does not reflect reality. Therefore, we will bite our collective literary tongues and offer tips in what we shall call "educated surmising." You can call it guessing if that helps. So, if you must, make your best educated guess (or surmise). Remember that, statistically, incorrect answers are in the B and C positions. However, do not change your answer because it is the third B in a row. The test questions are usually in random order. In addition, in several studies of large medical schools, students who answered according to their first impulse generally answered correctly, because the brain's subconscious typically brings up the correct answer. In general, the odds are statistically against you changing an answer to the correct one. Unless you are *absolutely* sure about a different answer, you should generally go with your first instinct.

FOR EACH QUESTION

Read each question carefully and identify the subject area. Identify what the question asks. Perhaps try the "cover" technique (try to answer without looking at the answers provided). You can also try the "True/False" technique (try to complete the stem or question using each response and discard those that do not work); that is, is this statement *true* or is it *false*? If two answers appear correct, eliminate the one that seems to have the least relevance to the question. If in doubt, there is no penalty in guessing, or "educational surmising," and remember you have a statistical chance of selecting the correct answer.

SAMPLE QUESTIONS

Consider the following sample questions. Key words in the question are in italics. We provided information regarding each answer option in parentheses.

1. Which of the following is the *most common* cause of nongonococcal urethritis in men younger than age 35?
   A. *Pseudomonas aeruginosa* (Very rare, not usually in urinary tract, and not in young men.)
   B. *Escherichia coli* (Not common in men, especially young men.)
   C. *Chlamydia trachomatis* (Common in young men, causes symptoms.)
   D. *Trichomonas vaginalis* (Common, but does not cause symptoms in men.)

Answer: C

2. A *45-year-old man* presents to the emergency department with a *fracture* of the femur following an automobile accident. He is pale, has a blood pressure of 100/60 mmHg, and a pulse of 110 beats per minute. Which of the following would be the *most important* initial step in the management of this patient?
   A. Insert a large-bore IV cannula, obtain blood, and begin fluid therapy. (Gaining access is most important.)
   B. Apply a splint and order a radiograph of the femur. (The patient is going into shock, and splinting takes awhile.)
   C. Obtain a radiograph of the abdomen and chest. (The patient is going into shock, and, again, this takes awhile.)
   D. Perform a careful physical exam with particular reference to the affected extremity. (This is not a bad thing, but it is not the most important considering the patient's condition.)

Answer: A

3. Which of the following agents is the treatment of choice to *reverse propoxyphene* overdose?
   A. Methadone (An opioid, not used for an overdose.)
   B. Naloxone (This is good for an overdose.)
   C. Phenytoin (This is an antiseizure medication, but it can be used for digoxin overdose.)
   D. Thiamine (Used for EtOH overdose.)

Answer: B

4. A 30-year-old patient presents with a *sudden onset* of vertigo, nausea, and vomiting that began 2 days ago. He states that he is unable to sit up or get out of bed without precipitating the symptoms (*postural element*). He denies any other associated neurologic symptoms or hearing changes. His past medical history is unremarkable except for an upper respiratory infection that resolved spontaneously. Which of the following is the *most likely* diagnosis?
   A. Acute labyrinthitis (Generally follows a recent upper respiratory tract infection.)
   B. Benign positional vertigo (Does not have an acute onset.)
   C. Menière's syndrome (Involves hearing loss and tinnitus, which patient denies.)
   D. Transient ischemic attack (The patient is only 30, so this is unlikely.)

Answer: A

5. The *triad* of symptoms that constitutes *Menière's* syndrome includes tinnitus and chronic deafness. Which of the following is the third component?

A. Ataxia (This is a consequence of the disease.)
B. Diplopia (If so, get a CAT scan.)
C. Dysphagia (Worry about recurrent laryngeal nerve paralysis.)
D. Vertigo (This is a symptom.)

Answer: D

CONCLUSION

Finally, we suggest that you reflect in a global sense regarding these examinations. The vast majority of those who take these examinations pass them—usually on the first try. Overwhelmingly, past statistics favor your success. One only has to examine the Web sites of PA programs around the country to see this. The recertification examination has similar pass rates—if not better. The NCCPA publishes the numbers as to how many pass the boards yearly, and they are very good. We believe this is so, for the most part, because most practicing PAs are competent practitioners. This knowledge, coupled with some good study (perhaps a good review book or two) should, and usually does, result in success. We wish you success in your test-taking and in your careers.

Contributors

EDITORS

David Paulk, EdD, PA-C
Academic Coordinator and Associate Professor
Department of Medical Science and Community Health
Arcadia University
Glenside, Pennsylvania

Donna M. Agnew, MT (ASCP), MSPAS, PA-C
Associate Director and Assistant Professor
Department of Medical Science and Community Health
Arcadia University
Glenside, Pennsylvania

CONTRIBUTING AUTHORS

Renee E. Amori, MD
Attending Physician, Division of Endocrinology
Cooper University Hospital
University of Medicine and Dentistry of New Jersey
Camden, New Jersey

Gwenn Amos, OD
Assistant Professor
Salus University
Elkins Park, Pennsylvania

Jennifer L. Arnold, MHS, PA-C
Main Line Cardiothoracic Surgery
Lankenau Hospital
Wynnewood, Pennsylvania

John A. Batsis, MD
Instructor in Medicine
Fellow, Geriatric Medicine
Division of Primary Care Internal Medicine
Mayo Clinic College of Medicine
Rochester, Minnesota

Robert Bettiker, MD
Assistant Professor of Medicine
Section of Infectious Diseases
Temple University
Philadelphia, Pennsylvania

Contributors

Charles D. Bortle, MEd, RRTNPS, NREMT-P
Director of Logistics and Field Operations
Department of Emergency Medicine
Albert Einstein Medical Center
Philadelphia, Pennsylvania

Dale Bryansmith, MD
Greater Philadelphia Cancer and Hematology Specialists
Philadelphia, Pennsylvania

Richard L. Commaille, PA-C
Program Director
Physician Assistant Post-Graduate Residency in Surgery
The Hospital of Central Connecticut
New Britain, Connecticut

Jill M. Cowen, MSPAS, PA-C
Instructor of Pediatrics
Penn State Hershey Children's Heart Group
Hershey, Pennsylvania

Eleanor Davis, PA-C
Department of Urology
Thomas Jefferson University
Philadelphia, Pennsylvania

Rachel Catanzaro Ditoro, MSPAS, PA-C
Assistant Professor and Clinical Coordinator
Department of Medical Science and Community Health
Arcadia University
Glenside, Pennsylvania
Honorary Faculty
University of Birmingham
Birmingham, England

Wendy Eaton, MSPAS, PA-C
Central Bucks Specialists Cardiology
Doylestown, Pennsylvania

Keith Herzog, MD
Assistant Professor of Pediatrics
College of Medicine
Drexel University
Philadelphia, Pennsylvania
Attending Physician
St. Christopher's Hospital for Children
Philadelphia, Pennsylvania

Irvin H. Hirsch, MD
Department of Urology
Clinical Professor of Urology
Thomas Jefferson University
Philadelphia, Pennsylvania

Jonathan T. Hirsch, PA-C
M-C-B Orthopedics and Sports Medicine
Doylestown, Pennsylvania
DFES Emergency Medicine
Christiana Hospital
Newark, Delaware
Adjunct Faculty Physician Assistant Program
Arcadia University
Glenside, Pennsylvania

Robert Howard, PT, MD
Assistant Director of Emergency Medicine
Chestnut Hill Hospital
Philadelphia, Pennsylvania

Melissa Kohler Justice, PA-C, MHS
Department of Medical Imaging
Chestnut Hill Hospital
Philadelphia, Pennsylvania

Tep Kang, PharmD, BCPS
Pharmacy Specialist, Critical Care
Christiana Care Health System
Newark, Delaware

Barry Korn, DO, DPM, DAAPM
Medical Director
Center for Pain Management
Cherry Hill, New Jersey
Adjunct Professor
Department of Medical Science and Community Health
Arcadia University
Glenside, Pennsylvania

Michael Lucca, MD, FACEP, FAAEM
Adjunct Assistant Professor
Department of Emergency Medicine
Drexel University College of Medicine
Philadelphia, Pennsylvania
Associate Director, Emergency Medicine
Holy Redeemer Hospital
Meadowbrook, Pennsylvania
Clinical Adjunctive Professor
Department of Medical Science and Community Health
Arcadia University
Glenside, Pennsylvania

Pamela L. Meyer, DO
Dermatological Associates
Hellertown, Pennsylvania
Clinical Adjunctive Professor
Department of Medical Science and Community Health
Arcadia University
Glenside, Pennsylvania

Contributors

Douglas Nadel, MD
ENT Associates of Bucks and Montgomery Counties
Doylestown, Pennsylvania

Nicole M. Orzechowski, DO
Instructor in Medicine
Mayo Clinic College of Medicine
Fellow, Division of Rheumatology
Rochester, Minnesota

Mark L. Pe, MD
Clinical Professor of Urology
Department of Urology
Thomas Jefferson University
Philadelphia, Pennsylvania

Mary Puckett, PhD, PA-C
21st Century Oncology
Clyde, North Carolina

Tabassum Salam, MD, FACP
Associate Residency Program Director
Department of Medicine
Christiana Care Health System
Newark, Delaware
Associate Medical Director
Department of Medical Science and Community Health
Arcadia University
Christiana, Delaware

Jon Shapiro, MD
Adjunct Professor
Department of Medical Science and Community Health
Arcadia University
Philadelphia Health Associates—Gastroenterology
Philadelphia, Pennsylvania

Richard D. Siegel, MD
Assistant Professor of Medicine
Division of Endocrinology, Diabetes, and Metabolism
Department of Medicine
Tufts Medical Center
Tufts University School of Medicine
Boston, Massachusetts

Christopher R. A. Sim, MPAS, PA-C
Associate Director and Assistant Professor
Physician Assistant Program
Department of Medical Science and Community Health
Arcadia University
Newark, Delaware

Les A. Szekely, MD, FCCP, DABSM
Bucks County Medical Associates
Doylestown, Pennsylvania

Paul Y. Takahashi, MD, FACP, AGSF
Assistant Professor of Medicine
Consultant, Division of Primary Care Internal Medicine
Mayo Clinic College of Medicine
Rochester, Minnesota

Henry D. Unger, MD, FACEP
Chair, Department of Emergency Medicine
Holy Redeemer Hospital
Clinical Assistant Professor of Emergency Medicine
Drexel University
Adjunct Professor of Medical Science
Department of Medical Science and Community Health
Arcadia University
Glenside, Pennsylvania

Irwin Wolfert, MD
Medical Director
Department of Medical Science and Community Health
Arcadia University
Glenside, Pennsylvania
General Medical Practice
Abington, Pennsylvania

Dermatology

Pamela L. Meyer, DO

1. A 45-year-old man presents with an asymptomatic rash of both elbows, which he has experienced for several years. It is annular and papular with central clearing and has not changed over time. No over-the-counter treatment has been helpful. Which of the following is the most appropriate action to take regarding this patient's condition?

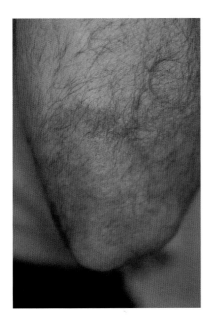

   A. Ketoconazole 350 mg orally for 14 days
   B. Thyroid and fasting-glucose studies
   C. Intramuscular injection of triamcinolone
   D. Permethrin topical application nightly for 7 days

2. A 17-year-old male presents with the following painful skin eruption. Which of the following is the most likely diagnosis?

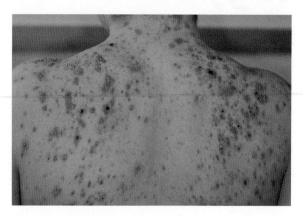

   A. Papular acne
   B. Pustular acne
   C. Cystic acne
   D. Scarring acne

3. A 67-year-old male presents with the following nonhealing, scaly scalp lesions, which have been present for several years. However, the number of lesions is increasing, and over-the-counter moisturizers have not been helpful. Which of the following statements is true regarding this condition?

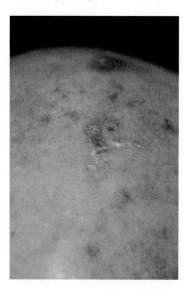

   A. Wide excisions with flaps or grafts would be appropriate treatment.
   B. 82% of the lesions will become squamous cell carcinoma within a year.
   C. Cryotherapy with liquid nitrogen would be appropriate treatment.
   D. 25% of the lesions will become basal cell carcinoma within a year.

4. The following skin infection is most likely caused by which of the following?

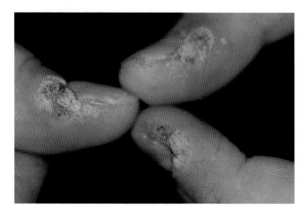

    A. Human papilloma virus #16 or #18
    B. A pox virus
    C. Human papilloma virus #2
    D. Herpes simplex virus

5. Which of the following tests would most likely support the diagnosis of the following skin condition?

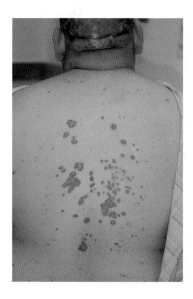

    A. Wood's lamp
    B. Bacterial culture
    C. Auspitz sign
    D. Swab for viral culture

6. A 30-year-old male presents with a 3-month-old pruritic rash of his buttocks. He has tried over-the-counter moisturizers, which help with the itching, but he notes that the rash is progressing. He admits having something similar last year that cleared spontaneously. He denies any other pertinent medical history. Which of the following would be the most appropriate first-line therapy for this patient's condition?

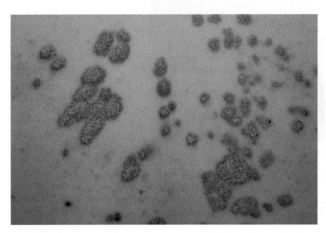

   A. Topical application of a class I steroid daily for 4 weeks with calcipotriene cream at the opposite time of day
   B. Intramuscular injection of prednisolone at 40 mg/ml with oatmeal baths daily at home
   C. A course of a clindamycin oral antibiotic for 10 days with a topical antibiotic such as mupirocin
   D. Topical application of ketoconazole cream twice daily for 4 weeks with a 10-day course of oral terbinafine

7. A 40-year-old female presents with an enlarging growth on the scalp. She states she was born with the growth, however it recently started changing in size. You correctly diagnose her with a nevus sebaceous lesion. Which of the following statements is true regarding this lesion?

   A. Nevus sebaceous tumors require complete excision.
   B. Nevus sebaceous is a hair-follicle tumor associated with amelanotic melanoma in 72% of cases.
   C. Nevus sebaceous is a type of kerion and requires oral antifungal therapy.
   D. Nevus sebaceous is a tumor of the eccrine sweat glands and resolves when perspiration stops.

8. A 60-year-old female presents with an intensely pruritic, diffuse rash that began a week after a family reunion. She has already been to the emergency room, where she received a steroid injection. She is taking 50 mg of diphenhydramine to sleep at night. However, the rash continues to progress and now covers most of her body. She admits waking from sleep because of the itch. She actively scratches the rash during your examination. Which of the following statements is true regarding this patient's condition?

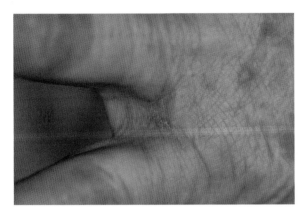

- **A.** Her home needs fumigation.
- **B.** Ivermectin is a first-line therapy.
- **C.** The infection primarily involves the hair follicles.
- **D.** The causative agent is *Sarcoptes scabeii var. hominis*.

9. A 26-year-old female presents with a rash for the past 4 months. She denies any associated symptoms. The rash continues to progress despite treatment with over-the-counter topical acne medications and hydrocortisone. She denies any new oral medications or other pertinent medical history; however, she admits to trying a new toothpaste and shampoo within the last 6 months. Which of the following is this patient's most likely diagnosis?

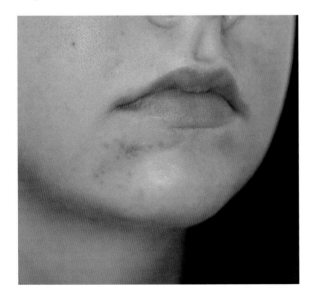

- **A.** Perioral dermatitis
- **B.** Acne vulgaris
- **C.** Acne rosacea
- **D.** Impetigo

10. A 55-year-old male presents with a nonhealing, painful lesion. Which of the following is the most likely diagnosis?

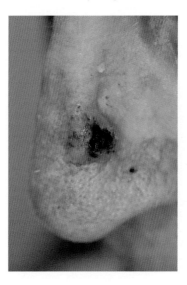

   A. Amelanotic melanoma
   B. Squamous cell carcinoma
   C. Basal cell carcinoma
   D. Keratoacanthomaten

11. A 49-year-old female presents with a history of recent travel to China on business. She developed an itchy and weeping rash upon her return to the United States. She has not tried any treatment and needs a "cure" before she goes back to China in 2 weeks for an extended visit. She admits to a history of high blood pressure, well controlled with a calcium-channel blocker, and exercise-induced asthma along with occasional seasonal allergies, which she controls with over-the-counter diphenhydramine, as needed. She denies any pertinent dermatologic history. Which of the following would be the most appropriate first-line therapy for this patient?

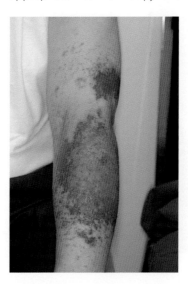

   A. Topical and/or oral steroids, with education about the need for moisturizers and proper bathing habits.
   B. Oral immunosuppressive and topical antikeratolytic therapy
   C. Penicillin G benzathine
   D. Topical antifungal therapy

12. A 53-year-old male presents with a year-long change to his fingernails. He is concerned that he may have a fungal infection. Which of the following is the most likely diagnosis?

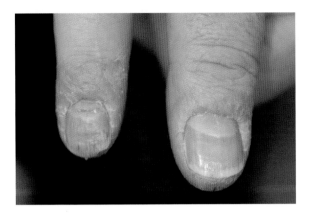

    A. Onychomycosis
    B. Eczema of the nail
    C. Lichen planus
    D. Paronychia

13. A 76-year-old female presents with a scaly rash of her nose for the past 18 months. She denies any associated symptoms. She states it gets worse in the summer and better in the winter, but never completely clears. She also admits picking at the site, which occasionally bleeds. Which of the following is true regarding this patient's condition?

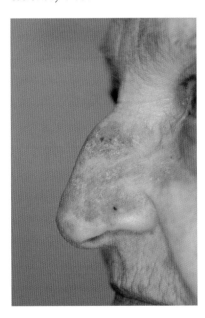

    A. Treatment of this condition could include cryotherapy, imiquimod cream, or curettage and electrodesiccation.
    B. Treatment options are limited, but she can use either a low-potency topical steroid or petrolatum.
    C. This condition worsens with exposure to sunlight, therefore necessitating daily sunscreen and referral to a rheumatologist.
    D. Treatment of this condition could include frequent hair-washing with a ketoconazole shampoo.

14. A 74-year-old male presents with a very tender lesion on the antehelix of the right ear that he first noticed approximately 9 months ago. He states that he can no longer sleep on that side because of the discomfort. Which of the following would be the most appropriate treatment?

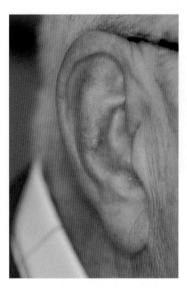

   A. Surgical removal of the lesion with skin grafting, because it may extend into the ear cartilage.
   B. Relieve pressure on that side and perform an intralesional injection of triamcinolone.
   C. Recommend close monitoring of serum uric acid levels and dietary purine restrictions.
   D. This lesion is common in patients who have had excessive sun exposure, therefore no treatment is necessary.

15. A 16-year-old female presents with a history of hair loss initially noticed by her hairstylist 3 months ago (see below). She has been using over-the-counter minoxidil twice daily and has already noticed the hair growing back. Which of the following is the most likely diagnosis?

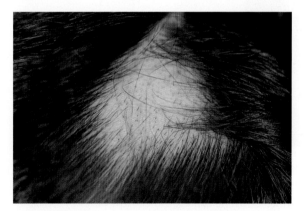

   A. Tinea capitis
   B. Telogen effluvium
   C. Alopecia areata
   D. Discoid lupus

16. A 27-year-old male complains of an enlarging growth on his neck below his beard area. He admits shaving over it occasionally, causing it to bleed. Which of the following would be the most appropriate treatment for this patient?

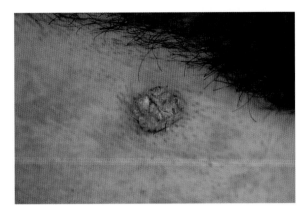

   A. Imiquimod cream at bedtime and covering the growth with duct tape
   B. Shave removal with electrodesiccation
   C. Cryotherapy, although several treatments might be required
   D. Mohs surgery

17. A 29-year-old female presents with a diffuse rash that has worsened over the past few weeks. She admits to itching and burning, especially at night, but does not awaken from sleep. She also states that the symptoms are worse after a shower or after she gets out of the hot tub. Which of the following would be the most appropriate management of this patient?

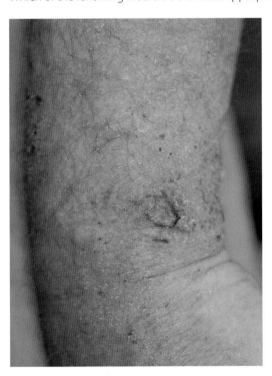

   A. Treat with an oral cephalosporin antibiotic and drain the hot tub for a thorough cleaning.
   B. Prescribe oral trimethoprim/sulfamethoxazole and apply topical mupirocin in the nares at night.
   C. Use moisturizers, stay out of the hot tub, and apply a moderately potent topical steroid twice daily for 2 weeks.
   D. Apply clotrimazole cream twice daily for 4 weeks.

18. A 21-year-old female presents with a new growth. She is concerned it might be cancerous, because of its rapid growth. She denies any tenderness, bleeding, or drainage from the site. Which of the following would *not* be part of an appropriate differential diagnosis?

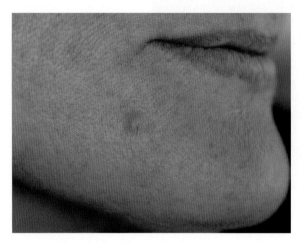

  A. Dermal nevus
  B. Junctional nevus
  C. Compound nevus
  D. Pilar nevus

19. A 26-year-old male presents to your clinic with his wife with a history of a changing mole. His wife states that it has become larger and darkened in color. The patient admits to significant sun exposure in the past, but has been diligent with sunscreen in the last 2 years since his marriage. He denies any symptoms. He denies any family history of skin cancer. He and his wife are well versed in Internet knowledge of skin lesions, specifically melanomas. They ask you for information regarding this lesion and the "ABCDs" of melanoma. Which of the following statements is true?

  A. The ABCDs of melanoma indicate that this is probably a Clark's Level II lesion with superficial spreading.
  B. The ABCDs of melanoma do not apply to this lesion, because it is not a melanoma, but rather a nonsuspicious nevus.
  C. The ABCDs of melanoma require a lesion to display at least three of the four suspicious features.
  D. The ABCDs of melanoma are **A**symmetry, **B**order irregularity, **C**olor variation, and **D**iameter greater than 6 mm.

20. A 47-year-old female presents with a large growth. She recently noticed that it was becoming "itchy." She remembers seeing these same lesions on her mother as she aged and worries that this is an "age spot." Upon physical examination, you notice a raised, almost "stuck-on" lesion with distinct color variation. Which of the following is the most likely diagnosis?

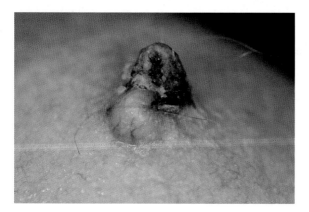

A. Seborrheic keratosis
B. Actinic keratosis
C. Malignant melanoma
D. Dermal nevus

21. An 86-year-old man presents for evaluation of an arm rash that resolved before the appointment. However, upon examination you notice a growth on the chest. He has no history regarding the lesion. Which of the following would be the most appropriate treatment of this lesion?

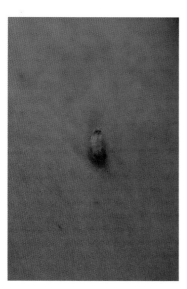

A. Cryotherapy alone or in combination with radiation.
B. No treatment is necessary, because the lesion will fall off in due time.
C. Shave and curettage, sending the specimen for biopsy.
D. Treat the lesion by electrodesiccation.

22. A 19-year-old male presents with a "weird," mildly pruritic rash. He describes the appearance of a single, larger spot on the chest that developed several weeks ago and many smaller spots erupting more recently. He currently takes no medication and denies any changes in his soaps, detergents, or moisturizers. Which of the following statements would be *false* regarding this patient?

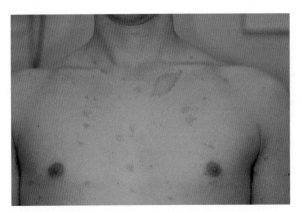

   A. Herald patch occurs in 80% of cases.
   B. The rash is self-limited, lasting an average of 3 months.
   C. The rash indicates a genetic predisposition to psoriasis.
   D. Treatment can include topical steroids.

23. A 36-year-old female presents with a complaint of "red spots" on her skin. She admits seeing these on her body in the past, but has recently seen them on her face. Which of the following statements is *incorrect* regarding this patient's lesions?

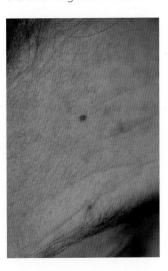

   A. The diagnosis is cherry angioma or hemangioma.
   B. These are a cutaneous manifestation of intestinal polyps.
   C. Treatment with electrodesiccation is appropriate.
   D. Recurrence after treatment is very common.

24. A 37-year-old male presents with a pruritic rash of the buttock and groin areas. He has tried over-the-counter antifungal creams and hydrocortisone, but the rash keeps recurring. Your patient is concerned that the rash is so persistent. Which of the following most likely explains the recurrence?

  A. He has chronic tinea pedis and keeps reinfecting himself from the untreated source.
  B. He has made the infection worse by using topical steroids with antifungal creams.
  C. This is a chronic rash that requires almost constant oral therapy.
  D. This is a cutaneous T-cell lymphoma, which resembles tinea, and requires chemotherapy.

25. A 62-year-old male presents with a history of hair loss that started in patches around the neck and parietal regions of the scalp. The hair loss is progressive. Furthermore, this will probably result in complete loss of scalp hair. Which of the following best explains this man's disease progression?

  A. Alopecia androgenica, alopecia areata, alopecia totalis
  B. Alopecia areata, alopecia effluvium, alopecia universalis
  C. Alopecia areata, alopecia totalis, alopecia universalis
  D. Alopecia androgenica, alopecia effluvium, alopecia totalis

26. A 44-year-old female complains of a newly discovered skin change on the side of her nose. Which of the following is the most likely diagnosis?

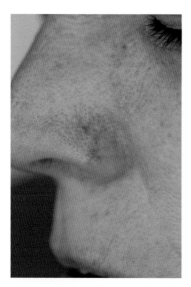

  A. Telangiectasia
  B. Spider hemangioma
  C. Rosacea
  D. Hemangioma narum

27. A 33-year-old male presents with a changing "mole." He denies any other medical history. He admits that the lesion has been intensely pruritic of late. He states that it was noticed by a family member, so he is not sure when the change first occurred. Which of the following would be the most appropriate management of this patient?

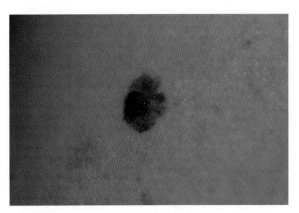

   A. Monitor with photos and measurements every 3 months to determine if change is actually occurring.
   B. Reassure the patient that this is a benign "barnacle" and that he should expect to see more of them.
   C. Perform a fungal culture to confirm a fungal infection and treat with a topical antifungal.
   D. Perform a punch biopsy or complete excision with a referral to a surgical oncologist as soon as possible.

28. A 51-year-old male presents with a recent thumbnail change. He states that the nail can be extremely tender. The patient worries this could be an infection that would destroy the nail. He admits to being an excessive hand washer and is always clipping the nails short. He denies any trauma specifically to that nail. Which of the following statements would be *false* concerning this patient?

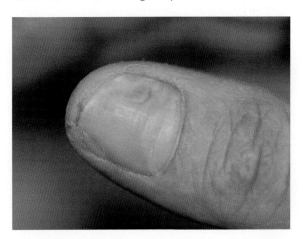

   A. The microtraumas of constant nail clipping probably caused a combination of infections.
   B. Diagnostic tests should include a bacterial, a fungal, and a viral culture.
   C. Prophylactic treatment should be with oral terbinafine, topical class I steroid, and oral acyclovir.
   D. This condition is common in individuals who have obsessive-compulsive disorder (OCD).

29. Which of the following are prognostic indicators for the skin cancer shown below?

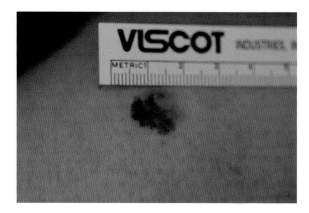

   A. Breslow thickness and Clark's level
   B. Civatte's thickness and Burrow's evaluation
   C. Koebner phenomenon and Von Zumbusch depth
   D. The five Ps and sentinel lymph node

30. A 77-year-old male presents with a nonhealing growth of the scalp. He recounts a history of trauma to the area with the comb approximately 6 months ago. He has tried a topical triple-antibiotic ointment without success. Which of the following statements regarding this lesion is correct?

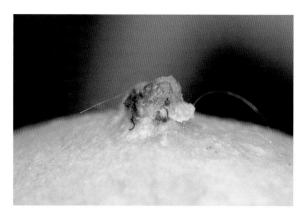

   A. This basal cell carcinoma is a sun-induced lesion and has a metastatic rate of 33%.
   B. This squamous cell carcinoma is a genetically oriented lesion best removed by Mohs surgery.
   C. This cutaneous horn is often associated with squamous cell carcinoma best removed by shave and curettage.
   D. This keratoacanthoma is more often associated with alcoholics best removed by cryotherapy.

31. The lesion shown below is located on the back of an elderly female at the location of the clasp of her bra line. She admits scratching it against the door jam (for relief) whenever possible. It has been present for more than 2 years. Which of the following is the most likely diagnosis?

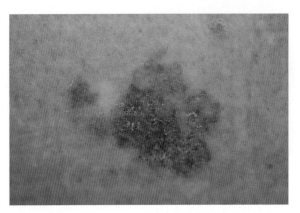

- **A.** Chronic contact dermatitis
- **B.** Bowen disease
- **C.** Psoriasis
- **D.** Chronic cutaneous lupus erythematosus.

32. A 34-year-old male presents to the office with a complaint of an enlarging shoulder mass. He states it has a foul odor and occasionally drains. He denies medication usage except for a daily aspirin for cardioprotective reasons. Which of the following would be an *inappropriate* treatment for this patient's lesion?

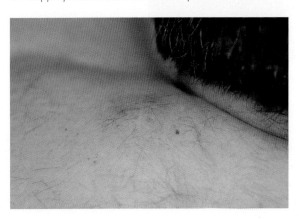

- **A.** Incision and drainage with or without packing
- **B.** Incision and drainage with or without oral antibiotics
- **C.** Intralesional injection with triamcinolone
- **D.** Wide excision after cessation of aspirin therapy

33. A 61-year-old Hispanic female presents with a long, but intermittent, history of a rash on the palms and soles. She states that the rash begins as small pustules or blisters and coalesces to form plaques. She is concerned, because her condition seems to be worsening and she finds it painful to walk. Her past medical history includes frequent canker sores, migraines, and well-controlled hyperlipidemia. Which of the following is the most likely diagnosis?

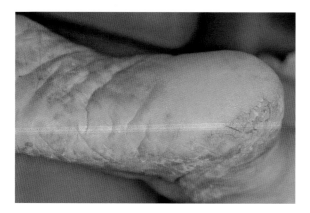

   A. Pustular tinea pedis
   B. Erythema multiforme minor
   C. Palmoplantar pustular psoriasis
   D. Secondary syphilis

34. A 24-year-old female presents with a complaint of "bumps" around the eye area. She thought that they were pimples, and tried over-the-counter acne medication without any improvement. She admits to squeezing them; however, she is unable to express drainage from the lesions. She denies additional symptoms and has no significant past medical history except for an appendectomy at 8 years of age. Which of the following best describes this patient's condition?

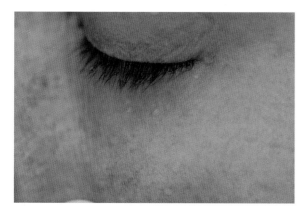

   A. Syringoma
   B. Milia
   C. Sebaceous hyperplasia
   D. Neurofibroma

35. An elderly woman has had an ulcerated basal cell lesion on her nose for almost 2 years. Which of the following is a *false* statement concerning basal cell carcinoma?

   A. The five types of basal cell carcinoma are nodular, cystic, sclerosing, morpheaform, and pigmented.
   B. Basal cell carcinoma is primarily sun induced, particularly in those with fair skin.
   C. Gorlin's syndrome is a genetic defect that causes multiple basal cell carcinoma lesions.
   D. Basal cell carcinoma progresses by soft tissue extension and lymph node metastasis approaches 43%.

36. A 65-year-old grandmother developed an intensely pruritic, generalized rash on her body. She has tried using over-the-counter antihistamines, hydrocortisone, and soaking in oatmeal baths. Her medical history is significant for diabetes controlled with oral hypo-glycemic agents and insomnia treated with alprazolam. You suspect that the rash might be infectious, but she denies any of her relatives or friends having similar symptoms. She states that the rash burns while in the shower and that nothing calms the intensity of the itch, especially in her "private parts." Which of the following statements is true?

   A. In a male patient, this same skin condition would not affect the genitals.
   B. This is not a sexually transmitted condition in young adults.
   C. The symptoms are often cyclical, depending on the hatching of eggs.
   D. Preventative therapy includes high doses of vitamin A.

37. A 22-year-old obese female presents with a complaint of "dry skin" on her buttocks. She claims to have used "every moisturizer over the counter" without success. Physical exami-nation reveals a serpiginous and scaly eruption with excoriation overlying the buttock and posterior thigh area. Which of the following is the most appropriate management of this patient's condition?

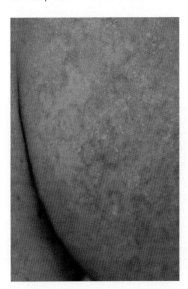

   A. Treatment with an oral antihistamine until the rash resolves
   B. Topical treatment with mupirocin ointment for 2 weeks
   C. Topical treatment with a fluorinated glucocorticoid cream daily for 1 week
   D. Topical treatment with an antifungal for 4 weeks

38. A diabetic patient complains of an axillary rash. On inspection, you note satellite lesions around the periphery. Which of the following best describes these lesions?

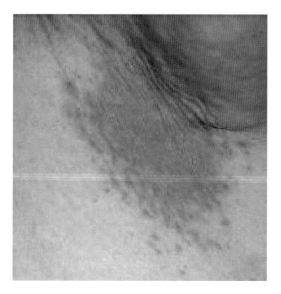

A. Cherry angiomas
B. Cutaneous candidiasis
C. Psoriasis
D. Tinea corporis

39. A patient presents with the following lesions. He denies any constitutional symptoms or sexual activity. Which of the following is the most likely diagnosis?

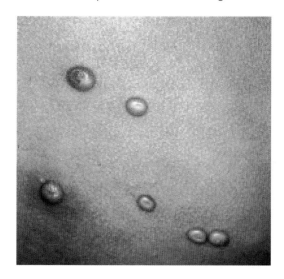

A. Acne vulgaris
B. Herpes simplex type I
C. Molluscum contagiosum
D. Varicella zoster (shingles)

40. A male patient presents with lesions. He states he thought it was a pimple, and that he "popped" it to make it go away. However, the area became inflamed and then very pruritic. Which of the following is the most likely diagnosis?

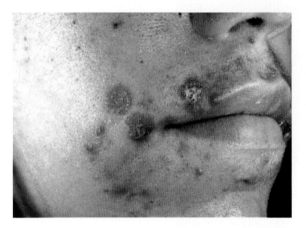

    A. Cystic acne
    B. Impetigo
    C. Tinea versicolor
    D. Herpes simplex type I

41. A male patient presents for a routine examination because he is seeking a primary care practitioner. He notes he has had spots over much of his body for much of his life. Your examination reveals a depigmentation of the epidermis over much of his trunk in an irregular pattern that does not fluoresce with a Wood's lamp. The lesions are not pruritic or painful. Which of the following is the most likely diagnosis?

    A. Tinea versicolor
    B. Spider nevi
    C. Verruca vulgaris
    D. Vitiligo

42. A male patient from Colombia presents with the following lesions on his back. He states that frequently a "dusty scale" covers the lesions and that they tend to stay white during the summer when the rest of his skin darkens. Which of the following diagnostic modalities would confirm your diagnosis?

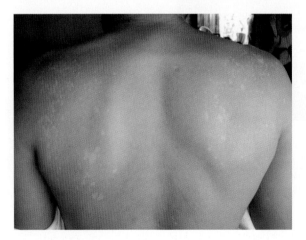

    A. KOH examination
    B. Blood culture
    C. Wood's lamp examination
    D. Viral culture

ANSWERS

1. **The correct answer is B.** This patient has granuloma annulare (GA), a common dermatologic condition of unknown cause. It appears most often over the dorsa of the hands, elbows, knees, and feet and in places that are subject to frequent, mild injury. It is most often seen in older children and young adults. The lesion often is symmetrical and formed by skin-colored, firm papules that can expand to form rings. GA usually has no symptoms, although there may be mild pain. In most cases, treatment is unnecessary, because the lesions resolve in nearly 75% of cases. Topical or injectable cortisone may prove useful in symptomatic cases. A more severe form of this disease is generalized granuloma annulare, in which lesions are found diffusely over the body, often with moderate to severe pruritus. GA occasionally is associated with diabetes, thyroid disease, and HIV infection, but most people with GA are otherwise healthy. Therefore, it is prudent to screen for thyroid or glycemic problems. Because this patient is asymptomatic, intramuscular injections of triamcinolone would not be useful. However, if this patient has psoriasis, kenalog injections would be appropriate. Ketoconazole is useful for tinea, and permethrin is appropriate for patients with scabies.

2. **The correct answer is C.** The pathophysiology of acne includes four factors: follicular hyperkeratination, sebum overproduction stimulated by androgens with subsequent plugging of the follicle, *Propionibacterium acnes*, and inflammation. Acne demonstrates a spectrum of progression and symptom severity, from comedomes to papulopustules to nodules and cysts. Treatment modalities are based on the severity and grade of acne and may include topical retinoids, topical or oral antibiotics, benzoyl peroxide, hormone therapy, or isotretinoin. This patient has cystic acne. Cystic acne (nodulocystic acne) appears with large pus-filled or nodular comedones. An acne cyst is typically 5 mm or more in diameter. The cysts are usually painful, and scarring is common. Scarring acne is usually the aftermath of the acne condition itself, most likely of the nodulocystic type. Patients who squeeze an acne cyst may cause a deeper infection resulting in a more painful inflammation that lasts longer than if the cyst had been left alone. Cystic acne is common across the larger surfaces of the body, such as in this case. Acne patients need referral to a dermatologist for probable treatment with isotretinoin, a systemic retinoid. Isotretinoin is a teratogen and requires two negative pregnancy tests prior to initiation of treatment and mandatory contraception counseling. The clinician should obtain CBC, lipid panels, and liver enzymes at baseline and repeat monthly in addition to a pregnancy test.

3. **The correct answer is C.** This patient probably has actinic keratosis. Many consider actinic keratosis to be an early form of squamous cell carcinoma, although disagreement still exists in the dermatologic community. Cryotherapy is an effective and well-accepted therapy for actinic keratosis, even for uncomplicated squamous cell carcinoma. However, actinic keratosis may be diffuse, with unapparent lesions in adjacent skin. Regional therapy with 5-fluorouracil or imiquimod is highly successful in the treatment of early lesions. The thought that most become squamous cell carcinoma within a year is irrelevant, because many in the dermatologic community believe them to be one and the same. Wide excisions with flaps or grafts would be inappropriate for this condition and should be reserved for extensive skin carcinoma, such as melanoma. Actinic keratosis does not convert to basal cell carcinoma, so this choice is also incorrect.

4. **The correct answer is C.** This patient has verruca vulgaris, or the common skin wart. Human papilloma virus #2 causes this lesion. Human papilloma virus strains #16 and #18 typically cause infections of the genital tract and are implicated in cervical dysplasia and carcinoma. Poxvirus is the etiologic agent of molluscum contagiosum, characterized by skin-colored papules with a central umbilication. Herpes simplex virus produces grouped, confluent vesicles on an erythematous base that are often painful.

5. **The correct answer is C.** This patient has psoriasis. Auspitz sign, named after the Austrian dermatologist Heinrich Auspitz, is the appearance of punctate bleeding spots after the removal of psoriatic scales. It results from the capillaries being so close to the surface of the skin directly beneath the plaques. The clinician may see this in other conditions that present with scaling lesions, such as actinic keratosis and Darier's disease. Wood's lamp is a useful tool to make the diagnosis of tinea corporis, whereas a bacterial culture would reveal conditions such as impetigo or meningococcemia. A viral swab would be useful to determine the presence or absence of viruses such as herpes zoster.

6. **The correct answer is A.** This patient has psoriasis. No cure is available; however, treatment can be highly useful in alleviating symptoms. The appropriate treatment depends on the extent of the disease. For this patient (mild–moderate psoriasis), the most appropriate treatment is application of a topical steroid cream. Phototherapy is useful for patients with moderate to severe psoriasis, and oral or parenteral therapy is appropriate for patients with systemic psoriasis.

7. **The correct answer is A.** Researchers first described nevus sebaceous in 1895. It is a circumscribed hamartomatous lesion composed predominantly of sebaceous glands. The risk of malignancy is difficult to establish with precision, and malignant change may occur at any age. Because of this risk, many authorities recommend complete surgical excision, preferably before puberty, because the lesion thickens and the risk of malignancy increases with age. Full-thickness skin excision is usually required. Current recommendations do not include topical destruction, because it may mask malignant changes underneath the surface. Primary reconstruction is usually possible. It is not usually associated with amelanotic melanoma, and oral antifungal therapy would be useless. Although true that sebaceous or oil glands are the primary cells associated with this tumor, the mere absence of sweating will not reduce the tumor.

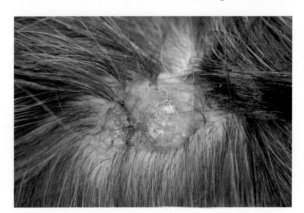

8. **The correct answer is D.** This patient has scabies, and the causative agent is *Sarcoptes scabeii var. hominis*. Infestation is common, occurs worldwide, and affects people of all races and social classes. Scabies spreads rapidly in crowded conditions where there is frequent skin-to-skin contact between people, such as in hospitals, institutions, child-care facilities, and nursing homes. Patients usually present with excoriated papules and ridged burrows, primarily in areas of few or no hair follicles, such as seen in the webbing between the fingers; the skin folds on the wrist, elbow, and knee; the penis; the breast; and the shoulder blades. Patients complain of intense pruritus, especially at night and over most of the body. Secondary bacterial infections are common. Once away from the human body, the mite only lives for 2 to 3 days, so fumigation of the household is unnecessary. Permethrin or lindane serves as an appropriate first-line treatment.

9. **The correct answer is A.** This patient has perioral dermatitis, characterized by small papulopustular lesions that become confluent and demonstrate a rim around the ver-

milion border of the lips void of any lesions. Females are predominantly affected and, although the etiology remains unknown, the condition worsens with administration of potent topical fluorinated steroids. Unlike acne vulgaris, comedomes are not associated with perioral dermatitis. Rosacea is a chronic acneiform condition that presents with erythema, telangiectasias, and papulopustular lesions without comedomes. Rhinophyma can also occur; however, this occurs more commonly in men with rosacea. Impetigo, typically a lesion of younger children, represents a superficial infection of the epidermis usually caused by *Staphylococcus aureus*, Group A *Streptococcus*, or both. The lesions are generally more widespread and present clinically as weepy, erythematous, honey-crusted erosions. Untreated impetigo can develop into ecthyma.

10. **The correct answer is C.** This patient has basal cell carcinoma. A shave and curettage with electrodessication would be the most appropriate treatment. Basal cell carcinoma is the most common form of skin cancer, as well as the most benign, especially if detected early. These lesions are known to invade deeper tissue and bone when left untreated, however. The typical basal cell lesion is a pearly nodule with telengectasias that forms central erosions with rolled borders leading to a rodent ulcer. Squamous cell carcinomas (some think of it as actinic keratosis) are brownish, flaky lesions, unlike what is pictured here. Regional therapy with 5-fluorouracil or imiquimod is highly successful in the treatment of early apparent lesions. Excision is appropriate for significant carcinomas. Amelanotic melanoma implies a melanoma without the characteristic darkening of the lesion. It has an irregular shape and usually a faintly pigmented border. These lesions are especially dangerous, due to delays in diagnosis, and thus the melanoma may have spread by the time of diagnosis. Patients with amelanotic melanoma require referral to a surgical oncologist as soon as possible. A keratoacanthomaten typically occurs on sun-exposed, hair-bearing areas of the body as a fast-growing nodule that has a central depression of keratinized material. Some authors have referred to it as a form of squamous cell carcinoma, although the literature is mixed. Many of these lesions will spontaneously regress in months to years, leaving a scar, whereas others will become more destructive and metastasize like squamous cell carcinoma. Because of this uncertainty, many practitioners opt for wide excision of the lesion in lieu of close monitoring.

11. **The correct answer is A.** This patient has atopic dermatitis. Atopic dermatitis, also known as atopic eczema, is a noncontagious skin disease characterized by xerosis and chronic skin inflammation. There is often an associated family history for atopy, such as allergies and asthma. The most appropriate first-line treatment for this condition would be topical and/or oral steroids (depending on the severity), along with education regarding effective use of moisturizers and proper bathing habits. Oral immunosuppressive therapy such as methotrexate along with an antikeratolytic agent would be appropriate therapy for patients with psoriasis. Treatment with penicillin G benzathine, referral to an infectious disease specialist, along with reporting to the state health department, would be appropriate treatments for syphilis. Topical antifungal therapy would be first-line treatment for patients with tinea infections.

12. **The correct answer is D.** This patient has a paronychia. A fungal culture will likely show no growth. Paronychia is typically a painful, bacterial soft-tissue infection that occurs when there is a breakdown between the nail and the nail fold. Fungal infections do cause paronychias; however, they are less common than bacterial infections. In acute paronychia, patients often present with a history of nail manipulation (intentional or not), or minor trauma to the fingertip, with a presenting complaint of pain, tenderness, and swelling in one of the lateral folds of the nail. Patients with chronic paronychia complain of symptoms lasting 6 weeks or longer, with episodic inflammation, pain, and swelling occurring most often after an exposure to water or a moist environment. Onychomycosis (tinea unguium) refers to a fungal infection that affects the toenails or the fingernails. It may involve any component of the nail unit, including the nail bed,

matrix, or nail plate. The nail may become discolored, hyperkeratotic, and brittle. It can cause pain, discomfort, and disfigurement and may produce serious physical and occupational limitations. However, many patients with this condition remain asymptomatic. KOH preparations typically show multinucleated hyphae. Treatment typically involves topical or oral antifungals. Eczema of the nails represents an inflammatory process that generally coincides with an atopic history. Nails may be pitted or demonstrate transverse grooves. Lichen planus dermatitis presents as shiny, flat-topped papules that often have an angular shape. These lesions often have a reddish-purplish color with a shiny cast due to a very fine scale. The disease can occur anywhere on the skin, but often favors the inside of the wrists and ankles, the lower legs, the back, and the neck. It affects the mouth, genital region, hair, and nails in some individuals. In approximately 10% of cases, the nails are affected. The nail plate appears thin, with grooved ridges. In some cases, the nail may darken and lift up off the nail bed distally, also known as onycholysis. The nails may stop growing and eventually shed.

13. **The correct answer is A.** This patient has actinic keratosis. The correct treatment of this condition includes cryotherapy, imiquinod or curettage, and electrodesiccation. A low-potency topical steroid or petrolatum would not prove useful. Excessive exposure to sunlight may cause her condition, but it is not *worsened* by sun exposure. However, almost any patient could benefit from application of a sunscreen with an SPF factor of at least 30. Referral to a rheumatologist would imply she has the discoid rash associated with systemic lupus erythematosus (SLE), for which there is no clinical evidence. Frequent hair washing with a ketoconazole shampoo is an appropriate treatment option for a patient with seborrheic dermatitis.

14. **The correct answer is B.** This patient has chondrodermatitis nodularis chronica helicis (CNH). This is a common, benign, painful condition of the helix or antehelix of the ear, which often affects middle-aged or older men. The exact cause of CNH is unknown, although most authorities believe the cause to be prolonged and excessive pressure on the ear. Nodules are firm, tender, well demarcated, and round to oval, with a raised, rolled edge and central ulcer or crust. The primary treatment goal should be to relieve or eliminate pressure at the site of the lesion. This is often difficult because of the patient's preference or necessity to sleep on the side of the lesion. A pressure-relieving prosthesis can be fashioned by cutting a hole from the center of a bath sponge. Topical antibiotics may relieve pain caused by secondary infections. Topical and intralesional steroids also may be effective in relieving discomfort. Collagen injections may bring relief by providing cushioning between the skin and cartilage. One treatment modality has been cryotherapy, although with mixed results. Historically, clinicians utilized surgical removal (localized to the affective area) as a treatment modality with these patients. The surgical removal treatment along with skin grafting would most likely occur in cases of squamous cell carcinoma or melanoma in which extensive resection and grafting would be appropriate. The clinician should monitor uric acid levels and restrict dietary purines in patients with gouty tophi. Tophi are nodules composed of uric acid crystals that deposit in the soft tissue areas of the body. A keratoacanthoma results from excessive sun exposure, but would manifest as a rapidly growing nodular lesion. True keratacanthomas will frequently self-regress, yet some are more aggressive and can even metastasize, supporting the belief that it may be a subtype of squamous cell carcinoma and warrant excision.

15. **The correct answer is C.** This patient has alopecia areata, which is a self-limited, non-scarring hair loss usually involving the scalp. Exclamation-point hairs (i.e., hairs that are tapered at the proximal base of the shaft), if present, support the diagnosis. Treatment with minoxidil typically provides spotty results. Intralesional steroid injections have been fairly successful in the treatment of this condition. Current research indicates this condition to be an autoimmune disorder that causes suppression of or complete ces-

sation of hair growth. Some of the literature shows evidence that T cell lymphocytes cluster around the affected follicles, causing inflammation and subsequent hair loss. Emotional stress may contribute to the condition. This condition is also associated with an increased risk of developing other autoimmune diseases, such as systemic lupus erythematosus (SLE). Tinea capitis (also called ringworm of the scalp) is a skin disorder that usually affects only children. It can be persistent and contagious; however, it often disappears spontaneously at puberty. Treatment with an oral and/or a topical antifungal agent would effectively treat this condition. Telogen effluvium is a form of nonscarring alopecia characterized by diffuse hair shedding, often with an acute onset. Telogen effluvium is a reactive process caused by metabolic or hormonal stress or by medications. Generally, recovery is spontaneous and occurs within 6 months. Physiologic stress is, however, the most common cause of telogen effluvium. Because this condition is self-limited, reassurance is often all that is necessary. Discoid lupus erythematosus (DLE) is a chronic skin condition of sores with inflammation and scarring favoring the face, ears, and scalp and, at times, other body areas. These lesions develop as red, inflamed patches with a scaling and crusty appearance. When lesions occur in hairy areas, such as the beard or scalp, permanent scarring and hair loss can occur. The exact cause is unknown, but current research shows the cause to be autoimmune, with the immune system attacking normal skin. Cortisone ointment applied to the skin in the involved areas will often improve the lesions and slow their progression. Cortisone injections into the lesions will also treat discoid lupus and usually are more effective than cortisone ointment. Alternatively, calcineurin inhibitors, pimecrolimus cream, or tacrolimus ointment may be used. Imiquimod reports to be helpful in a few patients. These patients require referral to a rheumatologist.

16. **The correct answer is C.** The patient has verruca vulgaris, or the common wart. Cryotherapy would be most appropriate in this patient. Due to the extensive nature of the lesion, the clinician may need to provide several treatments. Imiquimod cream at bedtime would be more useful for patients with squamous cell carcinoma. Shave removal with electrodessication would not be appropriate due to the likelihood of recurrence. This treatment would be more useful in patients with seborrheic keratosis. The clinician should reserve Mohs surgery for surgical removal of skin cancers, particularly when preservation of normal tissue is desired.

17. **The correct answer is C.** This patient has eczema. Proper treatment would include avoidance of the hot tub, increased moisturization, and the use of a moderately potent topical steroid twice a day for 2 weeks. Clotrimazole cream would be useful in candidal infections, which this woman does not have. Oral trimethoprim/sulfamethoxazole therapy, along with topical mupriocin to the nares to reduce nasal carriage, would be appropriate if this was a methicillin-resistant *Staphylococcus aureus* (MRSA) infection. Finally, an oral cephalosporin would be appropriate if this was a hot-tub folliculitis. As an added precaution, the astute clinician might advise the patient to routinely drain and clean her hot tub as an appropriate additional preventative measure.

18. **The correct answer is D.** A pilar nevus is a harmatamatous lesion that typically presents with rubbery nodules and darkened hair within or surrounding it. All of the other nevi tend also to be brown or black, frequently lightening in color as they progress. Another term for this is the common mole. The rubbery nodules and darkened hair tend to differentiate this nevus from the common mole.

19. **The correct answer is D.** The ABCD acronym for melanoma screening was first devised in 1985 by Friedman, Rigel, and Kopf in the *Journal of Clinical Cancer* for the purpose of providing primary care practitioners and the lay public a useful mnemonic. It was hoped that this mnemonic would aid in the early recognition of potentially curable cutaneous malignant melanoma. Now, the well-known parameters of **A**symmetry, **B**order irregularity, **C**olor variation, and **D**iameter greater than 6 mm are used universally in all forms of

medical education along with the lay media in order to provide simple parameters for appraisal of pigmented cutaneous lesions that may need further evaluation. In 2004, in the *Journal of the American Medical Association* (*JAMA*), Naheed, Shaw, and Rigel, et al. suggested adding a fifth letter, "E" to signify a lesion **E**volving over time. The authors describe "evolving lesions" as lesions that have changed with respect to size, shape, symptoms (e.g., tender or pruritic), surface (e.g., bleeding), or varying in shades of color. Other researchers support this as cited in the article, although some authors term the "E" as enlargement. The *JAMA* authors believe this falls short as enlargement refers only to the size of the lesion alone and ignores the other changes melanoma may undergo. We advise the clinician to research the article(s) as listed in the end matter for further understanding.

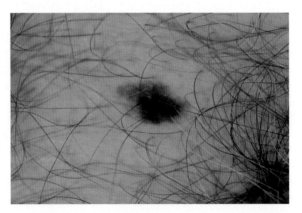

20. **The correct answer is A.** This is a seborrheic keratosis. In the past, patients and clinicians alike called this an "age spot," because it is the most common benign tumor in older individuals. Although the specific etiology is unknown, they are more common in sun-exposed areas. It can be treated by either cryotherapy or shave removal. Actinic keratosis is a crusty, hyperkeratotic scale that sometimes has a flaky appearance. In some literature, it is another name for pre-squamous cell carcinoma. It is also known as solar keratosis. Melanoma is a typically darkened, irregularly shaped lesion that is highly malignant. It requires wide excision and referral to a surgical oncologist. A dermal nevus, also known as a common mole, may be brown or black, frequently lightening in color as it progresses. Treatment is typically unsuccessful, because they have a high recurrence rate.

21. **The correct answer is C.** This patient has a cutaneous horn. The appropriate treatment would be to shave and curettage and send the specimen for routine laboratory analysis, because these can predispose to squamous cell carcinoma. Cryotherapy alone or in combination with radiation is reserved for someone with the actual diagnosis of carcinoma, such as squamous cell carcinoma or melanoma. There is no evidence that this lesion will "fall off" in due time. Electrodessication would be appropriate for a pedunculated seborrheic keratosis.

22. **The correct answer is C.** This is the classic clinical presentation of pityriasis rosea. Prodromal symptoms of malaise, fever, headache, and arthralgias may precede the eruption of the salmon-colored, scaly herald patch. A generalized rash follows the herald patch 1 to 2 weeks later, which typically lasts up to 3 months, with an average duration of 2 to 6 weeks. The rash generally localizes to the trunk and proximal extremities. Lesions tend to follow skin lines, accounting for the typical "Christmas tree distribution." Usually, no treatment is necessary, although the literature reports some success in children older than 2 years of age with erythromycin. There are reports that antihistamines and topical steroids may provide symptomatic relief. UVB phototherapy or sunlight exposure may also provide improvement in this condition. There is no evidence that this genetically

predisposes patients to psoriasis. The practitioner may consider serologic testing, because secondary syphilis is in the differential diagnosis for this exanthem.

23. **The correct answer is B.** These are cherry hemangiomas, which are the most common vascular proliferation noted in dermatology. They often appear as small cherry red macules, as noted. They are a result of dilated venules and are benign. Clinicians should treat these lesions only in situations of irritation or hemorrhage or when the patient finds them to be cosmetically undesirable. Treatment can consist of shave excision, electrodesiccation, curettage, pulsed-dye laser, or cryotherapy. Recurrence after treatment is common in many cases. There is no evidence that these are cutaneous indicators of intestinal polyps. Hyperpigmented macules around the lips and mucocutaneous membranes are suggestive of intestinal polyps, as seen in the inherited disorder known as Peutz-Jeghers syndrome.

24. **The correct answer is A.** This patient has tinea cruris. His condition is probably due to reinfection from a chronic tinea pedis condition. Topical steroids may decrease the inflammation when used in conjunction with antifungals. There is no indication in this patient that oral therapy would be of any benefit. Furthermore, the lack of other complaints, including lymphadenopathy, makes it unlikely that this patient has chronic T cell lymphoma (CTCL) even though the skin manifestations can resemble some of this patient's signs/symptoms. For example, mycosis fungoides, first described in 1806, is the most common form of CTCL. Patients with this condition would present with other systemic complaints as described.

25. **The correct answer is C.** Alopecia areata is a self-limited condition thought to be an autoimmune disorder that causes suppression of or complete cessation of hair growth. Some of the literature shows evidence that T cell lymphocytes cluster around the affected follicles, causing inflammation and subsequent hair loss. Alopecia totalis is the loss of all scalp hair. Current thinking believes it to be an autoimmune disorder exacerbated by stress. Alopecia universalis is also an autoimmune disorder that involves the loss of all body hair, including eyebrows and eyelashes. If a person were to lose hair in this autoimmune-sequential fashion, it would be as noted. Alopecia androgenica is male-pattern baldness, which presents as thinning or hair loss on the crown and in the frontotemporal regions. Alopecia effluvium, or telogen effluvium, is the transient, diffuse loss of hair due to a shift of the hair follicles into a telogen, or resting phase, usually noticed as the person grooms daily. The following picture shows an early point in the progression of this condition.

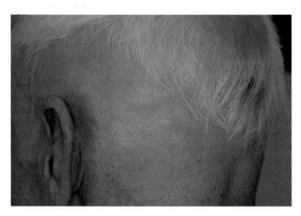

26. **The correct answer is B.** This patient has a spider hemangioma, or spider nevus. It frequently presents in pregnant females. These acquired lesions are most common on the face, neck, upper part of the trunk, and arms. Rapid development of numerous prominent spider angiomas may occur in patients with hepatic cirrhosis, malignant liver

disease, and other hepatic dysfunctions. A common characteristic is an elevated blood estrogen level (as in pregnancy). Electrodesiccation and laser treatment both can be effective for facial spider angiomas. Telangectasias are very similar to varicose veins and are the small visible superficial veins often called spider veins. These frequently appear on the legs. Rosacea is a skin disease that affects the middle third of the face, causing persistent redness over the areas of the face and nose. It is prominent in areas that normally blush, which include the forehead, the chin, and the lower half of the nose. The tiny blood vessels in these areas dilate and become more visible through the skin, appearing like tiny red lines (called telangiectasias). Papulopustular lesions can occur in rosacea, resembling acne. Hemangioma narum is the most common tumor of infancy, and thus would not be likely with this patient.

27. **The correct answer is D.** This patient has malignant melanoma and requires referral to a surgical oncologist as soon as possible for a punch biopsy and probable complete wide excision and other treatment modalities. A fungal culture and treatment with a topical antifungal would be appropriate if this patient had a tinea condition, such as tinea nigra. Benign "barnacles," also known as seborrheic or solar keratosis, could warrant observation and/or treatment if they progress or prove bothersome. Monitoring the lesion with photographs and measurements every 3 months to watch for change would be appropriate with dysplastic nevi.

28. **The correct answer is C.** This patient probably has onychomycosis or tinea unguium of his nail. Prophylactic treatment with the listed drugs would be inappropriate, especially antiherpetic acyclovir without a confirmed diagnosis. Microtrauma of constant nail clipping could very well contribute to this patient's condition. This condition frequently occurs in patients with obsessive-compulsive disorder. It is entirely appropriate to obtain bacterial and viral swabs along with a fungal culture to confirm the diagnosis.

29. **The correct answer is A.** This patient has malignant melanoma. Breslow thickness refers to the tumor thickness in millimeters following removal, whereas Clark's level refers to the thickness in relation to skin structures. Civatte's thickness refers to skin damage from a variety of skin conditions, including syphilis. Burrowing is typically defined by most dictionaries as "to construct by tunneling." Burrow's evaluation refers to the tunnels or burrows located in the skin. This can be contrasted with Burrow's solution, which is an astringent containing aluminum acetate. The Koebner phenomenon is the development of isomorphic lesions in the traumatized, uninvolved skin of patients seen in patients with a variety of skin conditions, such as psoriasis and lichen planus. Von Zumbusch refers to the condition of pustular psoriasis. The sentinel node refers to the first node that receives cancerous cells when they metastasize. The five (or six in some texts) Ps refer to the morphologic characteristics of lichen planus: pruritic, polygonal, planar (flat-topped), purple, papules and plaques.

30. **The correct answer is C.** This patient has a cutaneous horn of obviously some depth and extent. These can be associated with squamous cell carcinoma, and therefore require removal by shave and curettage. This lesion is not necessarily sun induced, and metastatic rates are nebulous, so A is incorrect. It is not genetically oriented, and Mohs surgery would be inappropriate for this patient unless the diagnosis of squamous cell is confirmed, then it can be considered. This lesion is not generally associated with alcoholics, as would a keratoacanthoma; therefore, there is no indication for cryotherapy.

31. **The correct answer is B.** This is Bowen disease, first described in 1912. Bowen disease is a squamous cell carcinoma (SCC) in situ with the potential for significant lateral spread. Larger lesions can reach several centimeters in diameter. The most appropriate treatment is by curettage. Auspitz sign is pinpoint capillary bleeding that occurs after psoriasis scales have been removed due to the superficial location of the blood vessels. It was named after Heinrich Auspitz, the Austrian dermatologist. Currently, there is no cure for psoriasis;

however, treatment can be useful in alleviating symptoms. The appropriate treatment depends on the extent of the disease. For mild–moderate psoriasis, the most appropriate treatment is application of a topical steroid cream. Phototherapy would be useful for patients with moderate to severe psoriasis, and oral or parenteral therapy would be appropriate for patients with systemic psoriasis. Patients with chronic cutaneous lupus erythematosus require referral to a rheumatologist for definitive treatment.

32. **The correct answer is C.** This patient has an epidermoid inclusion cyst. Epidermal inclusion cysts are the result of the implantation of epidermal elements in the dermis. Asymptomatic epidermoid cysts do not need to be treated. Uninfected inflamed cysts may respond to an intralesional injection of triamcinolone; however, this patient's lesion is obviously infected and inflamed, so this would not be an appropriate treatment. Incision and drainage followed by treatment with antistaphylococcal oral antibiotics is the most appropriate management for this condition. Incision and drainage is a fast and simple method of dealing with epidermoid cysts. However, recurrence is frequent, because the keratin-producing lining of the cyst is not removed, which may necessitate wide excision.

33. **The correct answer is C.** This patient has palmoplantar pustular psoriasis (Von Zumbusch disease). The palms and soles can become very dry and thickened, often with deep painful cracks (fissures) that can significantly interfere with activities. Palmoplantar psoriasis tends to be a chronic recurrent condition. Tobacco smokers commonly present with the pustular form; however, unfortunately, giving up smoking does not always result in clearance of the psoriasis. Treatment depends on the extent of the disease. Topical treatments of mild psoriasis of the palms and soles are appropriate, whereas more severe psoriasis usually requires PUVA or systemic agents, such as retinoids. Tinea pedis may be associated with recurrent cellulitis, because fungal pathogens provide a portal for bacterial invasion of subcutaneous tissues. Patients with refractory disease may require an evaluation for underlying immunosuppression or diabetes. These patients may present with painful "bumps" or pustules; however, this is not the case in this patient. Erythema multiforme minor presents acrally as symmetrically distributed, erythematous, expanding macules or papules that evolve into classic iris or target lesions with bright red borders and central petechiae, vesicles, or purpura. The clinician is advised to monitor the patient carefully, as the lesions may coalesce and become generalized. The lesions may be macular, papular, or wheals. Furthermore, the rash favors palms and soles, dorsum of the hands, and extensor surfaces of the extremities and face. This patient's presentation does not fit the clinical picture of erythema multiforme minor. Secondary syphilis occurs approximately 1 to 6 months (commonly 6 to 8 weeks) after the primary infection. A symmetrical reddish-pink nonpruritic rash may appear on the trunk and extremities. The rash can involve the palms of the hands and the soles of the feet. In moist areas of the body, the rash becomes flat, broad, whitish lesions known as condylomata lata.

34. **The correct answer is A.** This patient has a syringoma, which is a ductal tumor of a benign nature with a genetic disposition. Typical treatment involves electrodesiccation. Milia are keratin deposits usually caused by oil-based products. These also have a genetic disposition and are best treated with extraction. Milia are more whitish in appearance and frequently seen in newborns. Hypertrophy of the sebaceous glands, also known as sebaceous hyperplasia, has a genetic disposition. The most appropriate treatment of this condition is electrodessication. Neurofibromatosis is a condition of disfiguring nerve cell tumors ("elephant-man" disease); patients with this condition need referral for genetic counseling. Treatment is typically surgical and generally palliative, because these tumors frequently reoccur.

35. **The correct answer is D.** Basal cell carcinoma is the most common skin carcinoma. It progresses slowly over time and rarely metastasizes via lymph nodes. Typically, basal cell

carcinoma presents with localized destruction. All of the other choices are true regarding the characteristics of basal cell carcinoma.

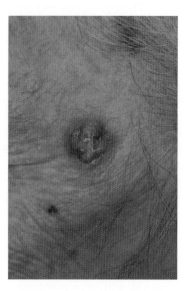

36. **The correct answer is C.** This patient has scabies, and the causative agent is *Sarcoptes scabeii var. hominis*. Infestation is common, found worldwide, and affects people of all races and social classes. Scabies spreads rapidly under crowded conditions where there is frequent skin-to-skin contact between people, such as in hospitals, institutions, childcare facilities, and nursing homes. Patients usually present with pimple-like irritations, burrows, or rash of the skin, especially in the webbing between the fingers; the skin folds on the wrist, elbow, and knee; and the penis, the breast, and the shoulder blades. Patients complain of intense itching, especially at night and over most of the body. The scratching frequently causes patients to excoriate their skin and create secondary bacterial infections. Permethrin or lindane is an appropriate first-line treatment. The patient may contract scabies from skin-to-skin contact. However, scabies is not a sexually transmitted infection. High doses of vitamin A would not prove preventative.

37. **The correct answer is D.** This patient's most likely diagnosis is tinea corporis (ringworm), and treatment with a topical antifungal for 4 weeks will most likely resolve her symptoms. The lesions of tinea corporis typically present as well-demarcated plaques that demonstrate peripheral enlargement with an area of central clearing.

38. **The correct answer is B.** Candidiasis is an infection most commonly caused by the yeast *Candida albicans*. Superficial infections of skin and mucous membranes are the most common types of candidial infections of the skin. Common types of candidal skin infections include diaper dermatitis, intertrigo, interdigitous infection, perianal dermatitis, and candidal balanitis. In certain subpopulations, candidal infection of the skin has increased in prevalence in recent years, principally because of the increased number of immunocompromised patients. KOH preparation is the easiest and most cost-effective method for diagnosing cutaneous candidiasis, but its use is not acceptable as a confirmatory diagnosis without supporting clinical evidence. A culture from an intact pustule, skin biopsy tissue, or desquamated skin can help to support the diagnosis. Microscopic examination of skin scrapings prepared with calcofluor white stain is a simple way of detecting the yeasts and pseudohyphae of *C. albicans*. *Candida albicans* produces a distinct bright color in a pattern characteristic of the organism when viewed under a fluorescence microscope. Treatment includes the use of antifungal creams and, if severe enough, oral antifungals. This patient does not have psoriasis. Currently, there is no cure for psoriasis; however, treatment may be highly useful in alleviating symptoms. The appropriate treat-

ment depends on the extent of the disease. For patients with mild–moderate psoriasis, the most appropriate treatment is application of a topical steroid cream. Phototherapy is useful for patients with moderate to severe psoriasis, and oral or parenteral therapy is appropriate for patients with systemic psoriasis. Wood's lamp is highly useful to make the diagnosis of tinea corporis. Additionally, KOH preparations would show septate hyphae of dermatophytes. The characteristic beefy-red appearance and satellite lesions of this rash and its location lend one to suspect candidiasis over tinea corporis.

39. **The correct answer is C.** Molluscum contagiosum is a viral skin infection that causes pearl-like raised papules or nodules on the skin. The virus originates in the pox family. It typically spreads through contact with contaminated objects, such as toys, clothing, or towels; however, sexual spread can occur. These lesions may be confused with herpes, but unlike herpes (also a viral infection that spreads sexually), the lesions are painless. Immunocompromised individuals tend to have the worse cases of this condition. It is common in children. Typically, the condition is self-limited, and therefore not treated. However, in those with more severe conditions, scraping, freezing, or other surgical removal may be appropriate. These modalities frequently lead to scarring. The lesions ultimately disappear within months to a few years. Acne vulgaris typically presents with the comedome of acne (closed "whiteheads" or open "blackheads"). These lesions typically appear as a whitehead of pus surrounded by an erythematous base. Topical antibiotics can be useful in the treatment of these lesions. Papular acne, another subtype of acne vulgaris, is a swelling without the whitehead but still with the erythematous base. Benzoyl peroxide washes are useful for this condition. Varicella zoster is a skin eruption usually along dermatome lines that occurs in individuals who were previously infected with the herpes virus. These lesions are painful and frequently require antivirals and narcotic analgesics.

40. **The correct answer is B.** This patient has impetigo. Impetigo is a bacterial skin condition characterized by pruritic, crusting skin lesions. It is more common in children who live in unhealthy conditions; however, it may be seen in adults following other skin disorders—in this patient's case, a probable minor skin ulcer or acne eruption. It typically begins as a pruritic and painful blister that eventually oozes and forms a honey-colored crust. These lesions usually spread through direct transmission as the patient scratches the primary lesions. Treatment of mild infections typically includes topical antimicrobial creams, such as mupirocin; however, more severe lesions require oral therapy. Although this patient may have had acne vulgaris with an attendant whitehead, this is no longer the case, and bacterial overgrowth probably led to the current condition. Tinea versicolor is a benign fungal disease that causes scaly macules or papules on the skin. As the name implies (*versi* means several), the condition can lead to discoloration of the skin, with colors ranging from white to red to brown; however, the skin can be hypo- or hyperpigmented. Frequently, a fine dustlike scale covers the lesion. There may be mild pruritus, although this is the exception rather than the rule. The condition is not contagious, because the causative fungal pathogen (*Malassezia furfur*) is a normal inhabitant of the skin. Most patients complain of cosmetic disfigurement. The most common locations for lesions are the trunk, chest, abdomen, neck, and sometimes the proximal extremities. Patients generally notice the condition during the summer months, because tanning highlights the skin color discrepancy. Herpes is an infection caused by a herpes simplex virus (HSV). Oral herpes causes lesions around the mouth or face. Genital herpes affects the genitals, buttocks, or anal area. Genital herpes is a sexually transmitted infection (STI). Typically, the lesions present as vesicular groupings of painful lesions. These lesions may become pruritic, but the hallmark is their proclivity to become painful.

41. **The correct answer is D.** This patient has the characteristic lesions of vitiligo. Vitiligo is a specific type of leukoderma characterized by depigmentation of the epidermis, which can range from partial to extensive in nature. Vitiligo is an acquired progressive

disorder in which some or all of the melanocytes in the interfollicular epidermis, and occasionally those in the hair follicles, selectively are destroyed. Clinically, it appears as sharply circumscribed, cosmetically disturbing white spots that stand out. The condition is sharply noticeable if the patient is tan, because there is a clear difference between the tanned skin and the lesions of vitiligo. The most common sites of involvement are the face, neck, and scalp, as well as areas subjected to repeated trauma, including bony prominences and the forearm or the distal phalanges. There is no single therapy for vitiligo, because the response is highly variable. Treatment options include systemic phototherapy, PUVA treatment, and/or narrowband UV-B phototherapy. Verruca vulgaris, or the common wart, is a viral infection that causes raised growths, which may be located almost anywhere. Treatment ranges from excision to freezing of the lesions. Spider nevi or common moles most frequently appear in pregnant females. These acquired lesions are found most commonly on the face, neck, upper part of the trunk, and arms. Rapid development of numerous prominent spider angiomas may occur in patients with hepatic cirrhosis, malignant liver disease, and other hepatic dysfunctions. Tinea versicolor is a benign fungal disease that causes scaly macules or papules on the skin. As the name implies (*versi* means several), the condition can lead to discoloration of the skin, with colors ranging from white to red to brown; however, the skin can be hypo- or hyperpigmented. Frequently, a fine dustlike scale covers the lesion. There may be mild pruritus, although this is the exception rather than the rule. The condition is not considered contagious, because the causative fungal pathogen is a normal inhabitant of the skin. Most patients complain of cosmetic disfigurement. The most common location for lesions is the trunk, chest, abdomen, neck, and sometimes the proximal extremities. Patients generally notice the condition during the summer months, because tanning highlights the skin-color discrepancy. Confirmation of the diagnosis is by KOH examination, which demonstrates the characteristic short, cigar-butt hyphae that are present in the diseased state. The KOH finding of spores with short mycelium is also known as the "spaghetti and meatballs" sign of tinea versicolor. For better visualization, ink blue stain, Parker ink, methylene blue stain, or Swartz-Medrik stain can enhance the KOH preparation. The ultraviolet black (Wood's) lamp can be used to demonstrate the coppery-orange fluorescence of tinea versicolor. However, in some cases, the lesions appear darker than the unaffected skin under the Wood lamp, but they do not fluoresce, therefore this is not usually diagnostic.

42. **The correct answer is A.** This patient has tinea versicolor. Tinea versicolor is a benign fungal disease that causes scaly macules or papules on the skin. As the name implies (*versi* means several), the condition can lead to discoloration of the skin, with colors ranging from white to red to brown; however, the skin can be hypo- or hyperpigmented. Frequently a fine dustlike scale covers the lesion. There may be mild pruritus, although this is the exception rather than the rule. The condition is not considered contagious, because the causative fungal pathogen is a normal inhabitant of the skin. Most patients complain of cosmetic disfigurement. The most common locations for lesions are the trunk, chest, abdomen, neck, and sometimes the proximal extremities. Patients generally notice the condition during the summer months, because tanning highlights the skin-color discrepancy. The diagnosis confirms with KOH examination, which demonstrates the characteristic short, cigar-butt hyphae that are present in the diseased state. The KOH finding of spores with short mycelium is also known as the "spaghetti and meatballs" sign of tinea versicolor. For better visualization, ink blue stain, Parker ink, methylene blue stain, or Swartz-Medrik stain enhances the KOH preparation. The ultraviolet black (Wood's) lamp can be used to demonstrate the coppery-orange fluorescence of tinea versicolor. However, in some cases, the lesions appear darker than the unaffected skin under the Wood lamp, but they do not fluoresce, therefore this is not usually diagnostic. Special media are required for culture. Because the diagnosis is made clinically and can be confirmed with a KOH preparation, cultures are rarely obtained. With blood examination,

no definitive deficiencies of normal antibodies or complement are present in patients with tinea versicolor; however, research is ongoing in this area.

REFERENCES

Bolognia, J., Jorizzo, J., and Rapini, R. P. (2008). *Dermatology*, Mosby Medical Publishers, Elsevier, Philadelphia, PA.

Callen, J. P., Greer, K. E., Paller, A. S., and Swinyer, L. J. (2000). *Color Atlas of Dermatology*, 2nd ed. Saunders Publishing, Philadelpha, PA.

du Vivier, A. (2002). *Atlas of Clinical Dermatology*, 3rd ed. Churchill-Livingstone Publishers, Elsevier, Philadelphia, PA.

Friedman R. J., Rigel D. S., Kopf A. W. (1985). "Early detection of malignant melanoma: The role of physician examination and self-examination of the skin." *A Cancer Journal for Clinicians* 35: 130–151.

Naheed R. A., Shaw, H. M., Rigel, D. S., Friedman, R. J., McCarthy, W. H., Osman, I., Kopf, A. W., and Polsky, D. (2004). "Early diagnosis of cutaneous melanoma: revisiting the ABCD criteria." *Journal of the American Medical Association* 292: 2771–2776.

Ophthalmology

Gwenn Amos, OD

1. A patient presents to your office with a blowout fracture. Which of the following clinical signs would increase your suspicion for entrapment of the inferior rectus muscle?

   A. Diplopia in upgaze
   B. Exophthalmos
   C. Negative forced-duction test
   D. Pain on attempted upgaze

2. A patient with a history of chronic sinusitis and frontal headaches presents with a complaint of recent onset of eye pain. Which of the following bones of the orbit is a likely proximal route of invasion of a mucocele from the sinuses?

   A. Zygomatic (malar) bone
   B. Greater wing of the sphenoid bone
   C. Lesser wing of the sphenoid bone
   D. Ethmoid bone

3. An object at infinity located "behind" the retina best describes which of the following?

   A. Emmetropic eye
   B. Hyperopic eye
   C. Myopic eye
   D. Astigmatic eye

4. The concept of astigmatism is best described by which of the following?

   A. Unequal refracting powers in the principal meridians of the cornea.
   B. One eye is hyperopic, the fellow eye is myopic.
   C. Unequal refracting powers in the principal meridians of the crystalline lens.
   D. The eye cannot be corrected to 20/20, but the reason is not attributed to structural changes in the eye or visual pathway.

5. Which of the following statements is the most accurate definition of *strabismus*?

   A. Disconjugate binocular eye movements.
   B. A deviation present only after binocular vision has been interrupted, such as by occlusion of one eye.
   C. Reduced visual acuity in the absence of detectable organic disease.
   D. Deviation from perfect ocular alignment under binocular viewing conditions.

6. While examining the corneal reflex using a penlight, you notice that the corneal reflex in the OD is approximately 1.5 mm nasal to the center of the pupil. The corneal reflex in the OS centers over the pupil. Which of the following best estimates this deviation?

   A. Right exotropia
   B. Right esotropia
   C. Indeterminable, because you are not stimulating accommodation
   D. Indeterminable without performing a cover–uncover test

7. Which of the following is the best description of presbyopia?

    A. An anomaly of accommodation due to changes in the crystalline lens

    B. A markedly lowered amplitude of accommodation for a particular age

    C. A common refractive error or ametropia

    D. Fatigue of accommodation due to accommodative exertion to overcome exophoria at near

8. Which of the following is the most accurate statement regarding the components of the crystalline lens of the eye?

    A. The lens has the highest protein content of any tissue of the body.

    B. The lens does not have pain fibers.

    C. The lens does not have blood vessels.

    D. The lens does not have nerves.

9. Which of the following statements about the abducens nerve (VI) and the extraocular muscle it innervates is true?

    A. The extraocular muscle innervated by the abducens nerve is the medial rectus muscle.

    B. A palsy of the abducens nerve results in significant proptosis.

    C. A palsy of the abducens nerve results in horizontal diplopia.

    D. The action of the muscle innervated by the abducens nerve is adduction.

10. Which of the following statements about the trochlear nerve (IV) and the extraocular muscle it innervates is true?

    A. The muscle innervated by the trochlear nerve is the inferior oblique muscle.

    B. The action of the muscle innervated by the trochlear nerve is to intort the eye.

    C. The trochlear nerve is least subject to injury because of its anatomy and intracranial course.

    D. A palsy of the trochlear nerve results in horizontal diplopia.

11. Which of the following statements about the oculomotor nerve (III) and the extraocular muscles it innervates is true?

    A. The muscles innervated by the oculomotor nerve include the medial rectus and the inferior rectus muscles

    B. A complete palsy of the oculomotor nerve results in limitation of ocular movement in all fields of gaze.

    C. Pupil-involved, third-nerve palsies are less ominous than pupil-sparing, third-nerve palsies.

    D. Ptosis does not commonly accompany third-nerve palsy.

12. Which of the following is not typically a function of the ciliary body?

    A. Accommodation

    B. Control of the amount of light entering the eye

    C. Uveoscleral outflow of aqueous humour

    D. Aqueous humour formation

13. Which of the following actions best explains how the ciliary muscle variably focuses the lens?

    A. Slight constriction of the pupil

    B. Decreasing convexity of the anterior surface of the lens

    C. Decreasing convexity of the posterior surface of the lens

    D. Releasing tension on the zonular fibers

14. Which statement about the innervation to the ciliary muscle of the eye is most often true?

   A. All three portions of the ciliary muscle are innervated by cranial nerve III.
   B. Innervation of the ciliary muscle is via sympathetic nerves.
   C. Faulty innervation to the ciliary muscle results in the common condition known as presbyopia.
   D. Topical instillation of miotics has no effect on the ciliary muscle.

15. Which of the following is the most common cause of diplopia?

   A. Uncorrected refractive error
   B. Keratoconus
   C. Binocular vision abnormalities
   D. Nerve palsies

16. Lesions in the visual pathway anterior to the chiasm (i.e., lesions of the retina or optic nerve), typically result in which type of visual field defects?

   A. Congruous homonymous hemianopias
   B. Incongruous homonymous hemianopias
   C. Bitemporal defects
   D. Unilateral defects

17. Which of the following visual field defects typically occur as a result of chiasmal lesions in the visual pathway?

   A. Congruous homonymous hemianopias
   B. Incongruous homonymous hemianopias
   C. Bitemporal defects
   D. Unilateral defects

18. Which of the following visual field defects typically occur as a result of lesions in the optic tract of the visual pathway?

   A. Congruous homonymous hemianopias
   B. Incongruous homonymous hemianopias
   C. Bitemporal defects
   D. Unilateral defects

19. Which of the following visual field defects typically occur as a result of lesions in the occipital lobe of the visual pathway?

   A. Congruous homonymous hemianopias
   B. Incongruous homonymous hemianopias
   C. Bitemporal defects
   D. Unilateral defects

20. Which of the following is the most common cause of acquired cataract in children?

   A. Metabolic disease
   B. Trauma
   C. Drug toxicity
   D. Acquired ocular infections

21. Under which of the following conditions should surgical intervention for congenital lens opacities be urgently undertaken?

   A. If detected after the first 2 months of life
   B. If detected as leukocoria by the parents
   C. Symmetric bilateral opacities
   D. Unilateral, dense, central opacities

22. A 24-year-old construction worker presents with a history of a foreign body in the left eye from 3 days ago. Although the foreign-body sensation is decreasing, his vision is worsening, and he notes a more general discomfort of the eye globe. Which of the following diagnostic techniques will *not* assist in localizing the foreign body?

A. Orbital soft-tissue CT scan
B. Ultrasonography
C. MRI of the globe
D. Orbital soft-tissue x-ray

23. Which of the following agents are contraindicated for the treatment of corneal abrasions that result from foreign-body removal?

A. Topical antibiotic drops
B. Antibiotic ointment
C. Topical anesthetic drops
D. Topical cycloplegic drops

24. Which of the following is the major mechanism for vision loss in primary open-angle glaucoma?

A. Intraocular pressure elevation
B. Retinal ganglion cell atrophy
C. Retinal nerve fiber layer thinning
D. Optic nerve head ischemia

25. A patient presents complaining of pain in the eye accompanied by a frontal headache and nausea. In addition to visual blur, the patient notes halos when looking at lights. Which of the following is usually the most likely cause of this condition?

A. Glaucomatocyclitic crisis
B. Inflammatory open-angle glaucoma
C. Pigmentary glaucoma following exercise
D. Acute angle-closure glaucoma

26. Which of the following patients is most at risk for primary open-angle glaucoma?

A. A 32-year-old myopic white male with hypertension and diabetes
B. A 32-year-old emmetropic Hispanic male with a family history of blindness (maternal uncle) of unknown etiology
C. A 48-year-old hyperopic white female with a history of diabetes and large optic cups
D. A 48-year-old myopic African American female with a younger sister who has a visual field defect from glaucoma

27. Which of the following is *not* typically a common cause of sudden, painless vision loss?

A. Retinal artery occlusion
B. Ischemic optic neuropathy
C. Optic neuritis
D. Retinal detachment

28. Which of the following distinguishes a hordeolum from a chalazion of the eyelid?

A. A hordeolum involves the meibomian glands.
B. A hordeolum is characterized by localized swelling.
C. Treatment of a hordeolum consists of warm compresses.
D. A hordeolum is caused by *Staphylococcal* infections.

29. Which of the following best describes the condition of misdirected eyelashes impinging on the cornea?

A. Distichiasis
B. Trichiasis
C. Entropion
D. Epicanthus

30. Which of the following is *not* usually considered a critical sign of dacryocystitis?

A. Secondary conjunctivitis
B. Mucoid discharge can be expressed from the lacrimal sac through the lacrimal punctum
C. Tearing
D. Localized periorbital swelling

31. Which of the following populations most commonly present with acute infectious dacryoadenitis?

A. Young adults, in association with infectious mononucleosis
B. Adults, in association with gonorrhea
C. Children, as a complication of mumps, measles, or influenza
D. Patients with sarcoidosis

32. Which of the following is the most appropriate critical sign distinguishing a diagnosis of orbital cellulitis from preseptal cellulitis?

A. Eyelid edema
B. Warmth of affected eyelid
C. Mild fever
D. Pain with eye movement

33. Which of the following conditions would *not* typically trigger an evaluation for retinoblastoma in children?

A. Strabismus
B. Retinal hemorrhages
C. Leukocoria
D. Ocular inflammation

34. Which of the following signs and symptoms is inconsistent with central retinal artery occlusion (CRAO)?

A. Marked afferent pupillary defect
B. Scattered retinal hemorrhages
C. Attenuated retinal arterioles
D. Foveolar cherry-red spot

35. A 66-year-old African American female with hypertension and diabetes presents for routine monitoring of her systemic conditions. She mentions an annoying blind spot in the visual field of one eye. Upon examination with direct ophthalmoscopy, you notice superficial retinal hemorrhages in a sector of the retina that do not cross the horizontal raphe. Which of the following conditions most likely explains this problem?

A. Hypertensive retinopathy
B. Hemiretinal vein occlusion
C. Branch retinal artery occlusion
D. Branch retinal vein occlusion

36. A 25-year-old African American female presents with complaint of bilateral red eyes. She has no discharge from either eye and notes only mild irritation. Vision is within normal limits. Her boyfriend accompanies her into the exam room and answers questions for her whenever she hesitates for even a brief moment. She has taken two aspirin this morning for a headache. Her history and exam are otherwise unremarkable. Which of the following is the most likely diagnosis for this patient's red eyes?

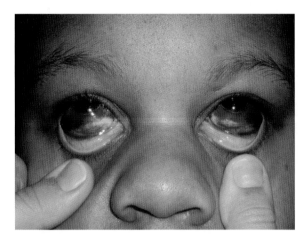

A. Acute hemorrhagic conjunctivitis, OU
B. Bacterial conjunctivitis, OU
C. Subconjunctival hemorrhage, OU
D. Scleritis, OU

37. A full-time spectacle-wearing patient presents with a unilateral red eye, pain, photo-phobia, lacrimation, and slightly decreased vision. The corneal lesions, shown below, are located in the epithelium. The patient has a mild inflammatory reaction in the anterior chamber. The patient reports having seen a dermatologist earlier that same day for a skin rash. Which of the following is the most likely diagnosis?

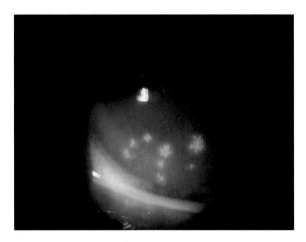

A. Acanthamoeba keratitis
B. Varicella-zoster viral keratitis
C. Recurrent corneal erosion
D. Herpes simplex keratitis

38. A 58-year-old African American male presents with a tender, red eyelid that is warm to the touch. He is unable to open the eye because of eyelid edema. He has no restriction or pain upon testing of ocular motilities. There is chemosis of the conjunctiva. The patient reports no drug or environmental allergies. Which of the following is the most appropriate course of treatment for this patient?

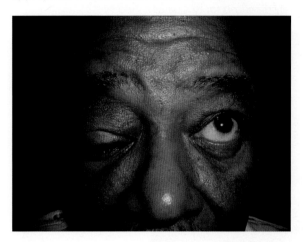

   A. Hospitalization with IV antibiotics and appropriate palliative care
   B. Hospitalization with oral antibiotics and appropriate palliative care
   C. Oral antibiotics and appropriate palliative care
   D. Antibiotic ointment to the affected lid area and appropriate palliative care

39. Which of the following signs usually accompanies bacterial conjunctivitis?

   A. Purulent discharge
   B. Mucous discharge
   C. Serous discharge
   D. Tearing

40. A 62-year-old male presents with sudden, painless vision loss; an afferent pupillary defect; and the clinical appearance shown below. Which of the following is *not* typically an associated systemic condition?

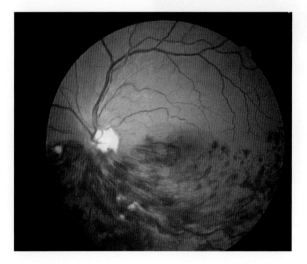

   A. Diabetes
   B. Cardiovascular disease
   C. Hypertension
   D. Giant cell arteritis

41. A patient presents with a moderate headache that occurred upon wakening this morning. The headache is located in the occipital region. On examination, you find severe acute hypertension and the clinical ophthalmoscopic findings shown below. Which of the following is the most critical aspect of management to preserve this patient's vision?

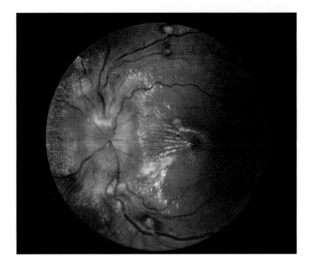

    A. Panretinal photocoagulation
    B. Lumbar puncture
    C. NSAIDs
    D. Judicious lowering of blood pressure

42. A typical clinical picture of hypertensive retinopathy is shown below. Which of the following differential diagnoses most closely resembles the ophthalmoscopic findings seen with this condition?

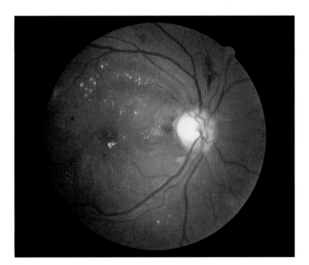

    A. Collagen vascular disease
    B. Radiation retinopathy
    C. Diabetic retinopathy
    D. Anemia

43. A patient presents with a complaint of pruritic, watery eyes with a purulent discharge that he is unable to resolve with warm compresses or an antibiotic cream prescribed by his optometrist. Which of the following is the most likely diagnosis?

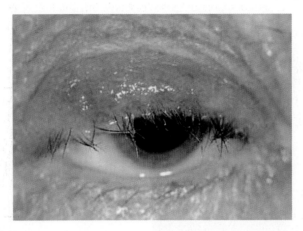

    A. Viral conjunctivitis
    B. Bacterial conjunctivitis
    C. Blepharitis
    D. Chalazion

44. A 69-year-old male presents with a history of visual changes consisting of severe vision loss in one eye. It initially presented with an inability to read street signs and newsprint, progressing to the current situation. He complains of loss of central vision, but not peripheral visual loss. He is unable to drive, read, or recognize people's faces. Which of the following is the most likely diagnosis?

    A. Macular degeneration
    B. Acute-angle closure glaucoma
    C. Cataract
    D. Open-angle glaucoma

45. Which of the following terms best describes bleeding in the anterior chamber of the eye?

    A. Conjunctivitis
    B. Blepharitis
    C. Hyphema
    D. Corneal abrasion

46. Which of the following results in a triangular, yellowish patch or bump on the white of the eye, most often on the side closest to the nose? It does not usually grow on the cornea.

    A. Pterygium
    B. Pinguecula
    C. Hordeolum
    D. Chalazion

ANSWERS

1. The correct answer is A. Diplopia and pain can occur in a blowout fracture, even without entrapment. A forced-duction test will be positive, so a negative forced-duction test helps in the elimination of the diagnosis. Diplopia can occur with a variety of situations, ranging from excessive alcohol consumption to a blowout fracture. However, in patients with a blowout fracture with entrapment of the inferior rectus muscle, diplopia especially in upgaze is a common cause. Pain is a nebulous symptom to make the diagnosis, as most (if not all) patients report pain with this injury, regardless of muscle entrapment. You would expect pain on upgaze regardless of the presence or absence of muscle entrapment. Most patients with blowout fracture present with enophthalmos, not exophthalmos.

2. **The correct answer is D.** The frontal sinus situates above the orbit, the maxillary sinus below the orbit, and the ethmoid and sphenoid sinuses medially to the orbit. Both the maxillary bone and the ethmoid bone are susceptible to erosion from sinus infection. However, the "paper thin" ethmoid bone is the thinner of the two bones, therefore more susceptible to problems. The zygomatic (malar) bone, the greater wing of the sphenoid bone, and the lesser wing of the sphenoid bone are located laterally and posteriorly in the orbital cavity and are less subject to sinus infection.

3. **The correct answer is B.** In an emmetropic eye, an object at infinity focuses on the retina. In a myopic eye, an object at infinity focuses in front of the retina. In an astigmatic eye, an object at infinity focuses at two separate points, neither of which focuses on the retina. In a hyperopic eye, an object at infinity focuses behind the retina.

4. **The correct answer is A.** By definition, an astigmatic eye has differing refracting powers in different meridians of the cornea. The cornea is responsible for approximately 70% of the refractive power of the eye. One hyperopic eye and one myopic eye is an exaggerated definition of anisometropia. The lens, a biconvex structure of the eye, contributes significantly to the refractive power of the eye, but to a lesser extent than the cornea. Although either lens surface could contribute an astigmatic component to the overall refractive error of the eye, it is typically minor in comparison to the amount contributed by the cornea. Amblyopia refers to an eye that is not correctable to 20/20 for reasons that are not attributable to structural changes in the eye or the visual pathway.

5. **The correct answer is D.** Vergences are disconjugate binocular eye movements. This is movement of the eyes in opposite directions, such as in convergence or divergence. Latent strabismus or phoria is deviation present after the interruption of binocular vision. Amblyopia refers to reduced visual acuity in the absence of detectable organic disease. Strabismus, misalignment of the eyes under binocular viewing conditions, can occur in any direction.

6. **The correct answer is A.** The right eye is deviated in an outward direction, thus the light displaces in a nasal direction. Although accommodation is not sufficiently stimulated to make the Hirschburg method an accurate measure of the deviation, it does provide information about the direction of the deviation. With practice, the clinician can make estimates of the magnitude of the deviation. Neutralization of the deviation with the use of prisms in conjunction with the unilateral cover test using an accommodative target provides an accurate measure of the magnitude of the deviation.

7. **The correct answer is A.** Although often discussed as a common refractive disorder, presbyopia is an anomaly of the accommodative system that results with increasing loss of elasticity to the crystalline lens. Individuals who show markedly low amplitude of accommodation for their particular age have an insufficiency of accommodation. An individual who suffers from fatigue of accommodation is best managed with convergence training in conjunction with therapy to better maintain accommodation.

8. **The correct answer is A.** The lens is composed of approximately 65% water and 35% protein. It also has trace minerals, potassium, and both oxidized and reduced forms of ascorbic acid and glutathione.

9. **The correct answer is C.** The abducens nerve innervates the lateral rectus muscle, which is responsible for abduction of the eye. The horizontal diplopia resulting from sixth-nerve palsy worsens at distance.

10. **The correct answer is B.** The trochlear nerve innervates the superior oblique muscle, which is responsible for intorsion of the eye. Because the trochlear nerve is the most slender of the cranial nerves and has the longest course, it is most subject to injury. A palsy of the trochlear nerve can result in vertical or oblique diplopia.

11. **The correct answer is A.** Complete palsies of the third nerve result in restriction of ocular muscles in all directions of gaze with the exception of temporal (abduction) gaze. Pupil-involved third-nerve palsies require hospitalization due to a common etiology of aneurysm. Pupil-spared third-nerve palsies most often result from microvascular disease. Ptosis commonly accompanies third-nerve palsies. Pain may or may not accompany third-nerve palsies.

12. **The correct answer is B.** The ciliary body, like the iris and choroid, is part of the uveal tract. The iris, not the ciliary body, controls the amount of light entering the eye by the adjustment of the pupil's size.

13. **The correct answer is D.** The ciliary muscle exerts action on the lens primarily by means of the zonular fibers of the lens. When the lens is flat and not accommodating, the zonular fibers are taut; the ciliary muscle is not contracting. When the ciliary muscle does contract, the result is release of the tension on the zonular fibers, which allows the lens to assume its natural (more spherical) shape. Accommodation describes the increase in curvature of both the anterior and posterior surfaces of the lens. The pupil constricts slightly during the process of accommodation. Pupillary constriction alone, however, does not alter the shape of the lens to the extent that a change in focus occurs.

14. **The correct answer is A.** The outer longitudinal, middle radial and inner circular portions of the ciliary muscle receive their innervation from the parasympathetic fibers of cranial nerve III. Loss of elasticity in the crystalline lens is responsible for presbyopia. Pilocarpine, a common topical miotic, causes contraction of the longitudinal muscles of the ciliary body. In turn, this produces tension on the scleral spur and trabecular meshwork lamellae, which results in increased aqueous outflow and decreased intraocular pressure. Because the sphincter muscles of the iris receive their innervation from cranial nerve III, instillation of pilocarpine results in pupillary constriction, also known as miosis.

15. **The correct answer is C.** Although uncorrected refractive error, monocular diplopia from keratoconus, and nerve palsies can all cause diplopia, binocular vision abnormalities are the most common cause.

16. **The correct answer is D.** Lesions of the retina or optic nerve, anterior to the chiasm, result in unilateral visual field defects. Lesions of the chiasm typically result in bitemporal visual field defects. Contralateral homonymous visual defects result from lesions in the visual pathway posterior to the chiasm. A lesion of the optic tract results in incongruous homonymous visual field defects. A lesion in the occipital lobe results in congruous homonymous visual field defects. The more posteriorly the lesion is located, the more congruous the visual field defect.

17–19. Lesions of the retina or optic nerve, anterior to the chiasm, result in unilateral visual field defects. Lesions of the chiasm typically result in bitemporal visual field defects. Contralateral homonymous visual defects result from lesions in the visual pathway posterior to the chiasm. A lesion of the optic tract results in incongruous homonymous visual field defects. A lesion in the occipital lobe results in congruous homonymous visual field defects. The more posteriorly the lesion is located, the more congruous the visual field defect. **17. The correct answer is C. 18. The correct answer is B. 19. The correct answer is A.**

20. **The correct answer is B.** Blunt or penetrating trauma is the most common cause of acquired cataract in children. Drug toxicity, metabolic diseases, acquired ocular infections, and ocular inflammation are other causes of acquired cataract in children.

21. **The correct answer is D.** Deprivation amblyopia is permanent if not treated within the first 2 months of life. The size, density, and location of congenital opacities, if detected within the first 2 months of life, determine the necessity for urgent surgical intervention. Many dense cataracts may go undetected by parents. Cataracts may be symmetric; however, they may not be large or dense enough to warrant urgent surgical intervention. Bilateral congenital cataracts that do warrant urgent surgical intervention demand as short a time interval as possible before cataract surgery is undertaken on the fellow eye in order to prevent deprivation amblyopia. Cases of dense, unilateral opacities appearing centrally in the lens, typically greater than 2 mm in size, require urgent surgical intervention to prevent deprivation amblyopia of the affected eye.

22. **The correct answer is C.** An orbital soft-tissue CT scan or radiograph can be helpful in localizing an intraocular foreign body. These scans are also important for medicolegal purposes. Ultrasonography is helpful to rule out the presence of an intraocular foreign body. Slit lamp biomicroscopy, direct ophthalmoscopy, and binocular indirect ophthalmoscopy are also indicated when patients present with a history of foreign-body trauma or foreign-body sensation. Magnetic resonance imaging (MRI) is strictly contraindicated in these cases, because a metallic foreign body under the influence of a magnetic field can become a high-velocity projectile that threatens the health of the eye or vision.

23. **The correct answer is C.** Topical antibiotic drops or ointment are proper medications for the treatment of corneal or conjunctival abrasions induced iatrogenically during foreign-body removal. Whether to deliver via drops or ointment depends on a number of factors, including if the clinician intends to patch the eye, the patient's visual requirements, and the severity of the abrasion. The severity of the abrasion may indicate prophylactic treatment for a secondary inflammation using cycloplegic drops. Use of even mild cycloplegic drops can make the eye more comfortable and is often overlooked as adjunctive therapy. Topical anesthetics should not be considered as part of the therapeutic regimen for corneal abrasions because of the propensity for delayed healing, masking of complications, and corneal scarring.

24. **The correct answer is B.** Retinal ganglion cell atrophy leads to thinning of the nerve fiber layer and the inner nuclear layer of the retina. In turn, axons are lost in the optic nerve, leading to atrophy and enlargement of the optic cup. Increased intraocular elevation generally influences ganglion cell atrophy slowly over many years in cases of primary open-angle glaucoma. Ganglion cell atrophy in cases of normal-tension glaucoma may be associated with ischemia of the optic nerve as well as damage from intraocular pressures in a normal range.

25. **The correct answer is D.** Glaucomatocyclitic crisis (Posner-Schlossman syndrome), inflammatory open-angle glaucoma, and pigmentary glaucoma can all present with elevated intra-ocular pressure (IOP). In all of these conditions, however, the angle is open. Pain and photophobia may accompany both glaucomatocyclitic crisis and inflammatory open-angle glaucoma. If vision is affected, vision loss is minimal. A patient with pigmentary glaucoma may experience visual blur and halos, especially after exercise or pupillary dilation, which causes the release of excessive pigment into the anterior chamber and subsequent corneal edema from the IOP spike. However, the patient does not experience dramatic pain, headache, or nausea. Only acute angle-closure glaucoma results in the combination of symptoms described.

26. **The correct answer is D.** Risk factors for glaucoma include age (over 45), black race, myopia, systemic vascular disease (including hypertension and/or diabetes), glaucoma in the contralateral eye, a family history of blindness, and vision loss secondary to glaucoma.

27. **The correct answer is C.** Patients experiencing optic neuritis have pain with eye movements. Neither retinal artery or vein occlusions, ischemic optic neuropathy, vitreous hemorrhage, nor retinal detachment has accompanying pain, although all can lead to sudden vision loss.

28. **The correct answer is D.** Both hordeolum and chalazion may involve the meibomian glands. Hordeolum may also involve glands of Zeiss or glands of Moll. Both are characterized by localized swelling, which may be painful or tender, although this is more characteristic of hordeolum. Initial treatment involves warm compresses. Without resolution of a hordeolum within 48 hours, incision and drainage is indicated for the infected lump. Chalazion is a sterile granulomatous inflammation.

29. **The correct answer is B.** Distichiasis is a condition of accessory eyelash growth. Entropion is inward turning of the eyelid margin. Folds of skin over the medial canthi distinguish epicanthus.

30. **The correct answer is A.** Tearing accompanies both acute and chronic dacryocystitis. Applying pressure over the tear sac usually expresses mucoid material through the punctum. Pain, redness, and swelling radiate from the nasal aspect of the lower eyelid. Despite constant discharge of mucoid material into the conjunctival cul de sac, conjunctivitis rarely accompanies dacryocystitis.

31. **The correct answer is C.** Dacryocystitis can arise from a bacterial etiology or a viral etiology in children, young adults, or older adults. When presenting in patients with sarcoidosis, it occasionally presents bilaterally. However, it is most common in children.

32. **The correct answer is D.** Along with pain on attempted eye movement, ocular motilities may be restricted in cases of orbital cellulitis. Fever is likely to be more severe in cases of orbital cellulitis than in preseptal cellulitis. In addition, in cases of orbital cellulitis the conjunctiva(e) is/are chemotic and injected.

33. **The correct answer is B.** Until a retinoblastoma grows large enough to produce leukocoria, it typically remains unnoticed. Retinoblastoma can also produce strabismus or ocular inflammation. Because this is a life-threatening tumor, presentation of any of these conditions in childhood warrants evaluation for this primary malignant tumor.

34. **The correct answer is B.** Ophthalmoscopically, the retina appears as opaque white following a CRAO, with a cherry-red spot in the foveolar region. The retinal arterioles attenuate and may show boxcarring, and there is typically an afferent pupillary defect. Scattered retinal hemorrhages and cotton-wool spots may be visualized in the retina following a central retinal vein occlusion (CRVO).

35. **The correct answer is D.** Hypertensive retinopathy and diabetic retinopathy present in both eyes and do not respect the horizontal raphe. A hemiretinal vein occlusion would affect more than a sector of the retina. The patient would complain of loss of either the upper or the lower half of her vision, rather than a blind spot. Branch retinal artery occlusion has characteristic fundoscopic signs, including retinal edema in the area supplied by the occluded vessel. Superficial hemorrhages occurring with a branch retinal vein occlusion occur alongside the occluded retinal vein and only rarely cross the midline.

36. **The correct answer is C.** Bilateral subconjunctival hemorrhages are less common than sectoral monocular subconjunctival hemorrhages. They are more likely to occur in cases of trauma or if the patient has a bleeding disorder. Acute hemorrhagic conjunctivitis has

a viral etiology. Patients are symptomatic for pain, photophobia, irritation, lid swelling, and tearing, in addition to the subconjunctival hemorrhages. Note the marked absence of inferior palpebral injection, a hallmark sign for bacterial conjunctivitis. The absence of eye pain and decreased vision help to rule out scleritis as the diagnosis for this case.

37. **The correct answer is D.** The corneal lesion in herpes simplex keratitis occurs in the epithelium. Corneal lesions in varicella-zoster viral keratitis occur in the stroma. Initial symptoms for acanthamoeba keratitis are more significant than the clinical findings, including epithelial and subepithelial infiltrates. Patients often have a history of soft contact lens wear. Healing corneal erosions often appear as pseudodendrites. Patients will have a history of eye pain upon awakening from sleep.

38. **The correct answer is C.** This is a case of preseptal cellulitis. The patient is not experiencing pain or restriction of eye movements, thereby differentiating the condition from orbital cellulitis. Hospitalization is not required unless the patient is noncompliant with treatment recommendations, including follow-up care, or does not improve after several days of administration of oral antibiotics. The clinician should hospitalize children younger than 5 years of age with preseptal cellulitis. Palliative care includes warm compresses and antibiotic ointment if a secondary conjunctivitis is present.

39. **The correct answer is A.** Allergic conjunctivitis produces a mucous discharge. Viral conjunctivitis produces a serous discharge. Red eyes from acute uveitis, acute glaucoma, and corneal abrasions result in tearing.

40. **The correct answer is D.** All of the conditions listed occur with central retinal artery occlusion. Giant cell arteritis does not occur in patients with retinal vein occlusions.

41. **The correct answer is D.** If blood pressure lowers too quickly in cases of malignant hypertension, the patient can go blind.

42. **The correct answer is B.** The clinical picture of radiation retinopathy appears ophthalmoscopically most similar to hypertensive retinopathy. Radiation retinopathy typically develops within a few years of irradiation of the eye or adnexa. Collagen vascular disease shares only cotton-wool spots with the signs of hypertensive retinopathy. The hemorrhages seen in diabetic retinopathy are dot-and-blot type rather than the flame-shape hemorrhages typically seen in hypertensive retinopathy. Arteriolar attenuation is not common in diabetic retinopathy. Retinal changes from anemia appear predominantly with hemorrhages.

43. **The correct answer is C.** This patient has blepharitis. It usually affects the skin of the eyelids, more specifically, the lid margins where the hair follicles are located. Blepharitis typically occurs when there is bacterial overgrowth of the oil follicles at the lid margin. Although it is tenacious and difficult to treat, the patient is not usually at risk for loss of vision. Treatment involves good hygiene and sometimes repetitive antibiotics. If there is an underlying condition, such as psoriasis, the clinician should treat the underlying condition as well. Oral steroids may also be useful. Conjunctivitis, or "pink eye," commonly originates from a viral or bacterial infection of the lining of the conjunctiva(e). Interestingly, the literature supports different treatments. If there is *confirmed* bacterial conjunctivitis, then intraoptic antibiotics should be administered for 2 to 3 days; viral conjunctivitis usually is treated empirically. Contrary to popular belief, vision loss is not a typical outcome, and even without treatment, most cases of bacterial conjunctivitis improve. Warm compresses and good hygiene are also important in these cases. A chalazion is a swelling of an eye gland from a blockage—either viral or bacterial—and, interestingly, may be the result of blepharitis.

44. **The correct answer is A.** This is a chronic age-related condition that occurs when the macula deteriorates as a result of age. The macula is the area responsible for central vision, hence the symptoms. The condition can progress rapidly or slowly, and it may

affect both eyes. Although it is currently irreversible, early identification and treatment are necessary to reduce symptoms. Photocoagulation or photodynamic therapy have been utilized with some success with this condition. Open-angle glaucoma is caused by an increase in intraocular pressure that affects the optic nerve, thus causing blindness. This loss of vision is usually painful and sudden. It is a true medical emergency. Open-angle glaucoma typically occurs more gradually and causes a loss of peripheral vision. The clinician should realize that the nomenclature changes over time. The acute angle-closure literature suffered through the years by the lack of a standard definition as well as specific diagnostic criteria. Recently, there has been a significant movement to standardize the definitions of the various forms of angle-closure disease. Primary angle-closure glaucoma, primary angle closure, acute angle closure, and acute angle-closure glaucoma have been interchangeable. Currently, acute angle closure is defined as at least two of the following symptoms: a history of intermittent blurring of vision associated with halos, sudden ocular pain, and nausea/vomiting. Furthermore, upon examination, the patient should present with at least three of the following signs: conjunctival injection, corneal epithelial edema, a mid-dilated nonreactive pupil, IOP >21 mm Hg, and a shallow chamber in the presence of occlusion. Cataracts are typically cloudiness that develops over the lens of the eye and does not usually present with acute vision loss.

45. **The correct answer is C.** Hyphema refers to a bleed in the anterior chamber of the eye (the space between the cornea and the iris). Conjunctivitis and blepharitis are viral or bacterial infections of the conjunctiva or lid margins, respectively. A corneal abrasion does not usually result in bleeding.

46. **The correct answer is B.** A pinguecula does not grow onto the cornea, although it frequently appears on the nasal aspect of the eye. If it appears to grow onto the cornea, then it is termed a *pterygium* (meaning "winglike" from the Greek *ptreygion*). A hordeolum, the common sty, and a chalazion are meibomian gland lipogranulomas. Chalazions represent chronic, nontender, hard granulomatous inflammation of the meibomian glands. Hordeolums are tender and more characteristic of an acute, focal, infectious process. They can involve the gland of Zeis (more common with external styes) or the meibomian gland (internal styes).

REFERENCES

Cullum, R. D., and Chang, B. (1994). *The Wills Eye Manual; Office and Emergency Room Diagnosis and Treatment of Eye Disease.* Lippincott–Raven Publishers, Philadelphia, PA.

Grosvenor, T. P. (1989). *Primary Care Optometry.* Professional Press Books, Fairchild Publications, New York.

Paton, D., Hyman, B. N., and Justice, J. (1976). *Introduction to Ophthalmoscopy.* The Upjohn Company, Michigan.

Riordan-Eva, P., and Whitcher, J. (2004) *Vaughan & Ashbury's General Ophthalmology.* Lange Medical Books/McGraw-Hill Medical Publishing Division, New York.

Varma, R. (1997) *Essentials of Eyecare; The Johns Hopkins Wilmer Handbook.* Lippincott–Raven Publishers, Philadelphia, PA.

CHAPTER

3

Ear, Nose, and Throat

Douglas Nadel, MD
Donna M. Agnew, MT (ASCP), MSPAS, PA-C

1. Which of the following conditions causes sensorineural hearing loss?

    A. Cerumen impaction
    B. Presbycusis
    C. Serous otitis media
    D. Tympanic membrane perforation

2. A patient presents complaining of intermittent drainage from his left ear, which he describes as a thin, yellow discharge. On otoscopic examination, you note a retracted tympanic membrane and adherent to the incus with a perforation. Which of the following is the most appropriate diagnosis?

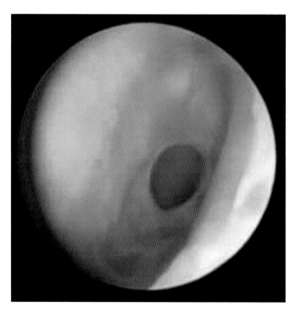

    A. Chronic otitis media
    B. Menière's disease
    C. Ossicular discontinuity
    D. Otosclerosis

3. Which of the following is *not* a known complication of acute otitis media?

    A. Facial nerve paralysis
    B. Meningitis
    C. Otosclerosis
    D. Tympanic membrane perforation

49

4. A 39-year-old male presents complaining of severe vertigo associated with persistent nausea and episodic vomiting for 2 days that is slowly resolving since waking this morning. He denies any fever, hearing loss, tinnitus, recent travel, constipation, diarrhea, vigorous weight training, or diving. Which of the following is the most likely diagnosis?

   A. Inner ear barotraumas
   B. Labyrinthitis
   C. Menière's disease
   D. Vestibular neuritis

5. A 5-year-old boy presents to the emergency department complaining of a severe sore throat. On physical examination, he is drooling, has stridorous inspirations, and is febrile, with a temperature of 102°F. A lateral neck radiograph demonstrates the prevertebral soft tissues. You also ordered an MRI, the results of which are below. Which of the following is the most likely diagnosis?

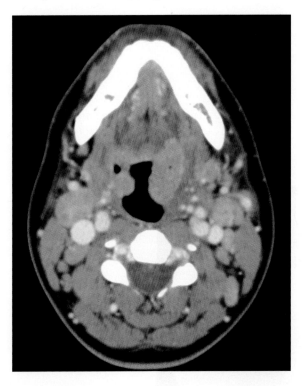

   A. Cervical adenitis
   B. Epiglottitis
   C. Peritonsillar abscess
   D. Retropharyngeal abscess

6. Which of the following types of tinnitus is of most concern?

   A. An intermittent high-pitched ring
   B. A chirping sound resembling crickets
   C. A low-pitched buzzing sound
   D. A pulsatile sound similar to a heartbeat

7. Koplik's spots appear as white grains of sand on the buccal mucosa and are seen in the early stages of which of the following viral diseases?

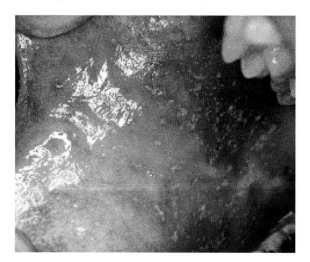

A. Parvovirus B19
B. Rubeola
C. Rubella
D. Varicella

8. Which of the following best describes an acoustic neuroma?

A. A viral infection of the vestibular nerve that causes severe vertigo
B. Progressive demylination of the acoustic nerve that leads to sensorineural hearing loss
C. A schwannoma arising in the eighth cranial nerve that causes gradual, unilateral hearing loss
D. The involution of squamous epithelium through the tympanic membrane

9. A 62-year-old female notes swelling under her right jaw after eating. It lasts about half an hour, then spontaneously resolves. Which of the following is the most likely cause of this problem?

A. Cervical tuberculosis
B. Lymphoma
C. A stone in the submandibular gland or Wharton's duct
D. Parotitis

10. Which of the following would be the *least* appropriate treatment for the condition shown below?

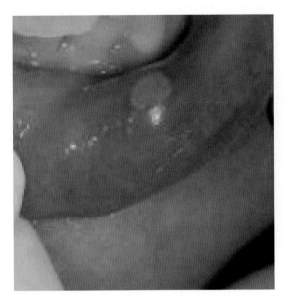

    A. Analgesics
    B. Antibiotics
    C. Oral rinses
    D. Surgical excision

11. A 17-year-old male presents complaining of sore throat and malaise. On physical examination, you note that his palantine tonsils are enlarged and erythematous. You also note white exudates. The patient's uvula symmetrically rises. On palpation, the patient has some discrete, slightly tender nodes along the posterior cervical chain. Which of the following is the most likely clinical diagnosis?

    A. Leukoplakia
    B. Mononucleosis
    C. Peritonsillar abscess
    D. Vincent's angina

12. A 71-year-old female presents complaining of progressive pain and swelling in her neck over the past week. She had a molar extracted 10 days ago. On examination, the floor of the mouth and the anterior neck is firm, hard, and erythematous. Which of the following diagnoses is most consistent with this patient's history and physical findings?

    A. Ludwig's angina
    B. Sublingual sialolithiasis
    C. Submandibular sialadenitis
    D. Vincent's angina

13. A patient complains of recurrent episodes of vertigo, hearing loss, and tinnitus lasting several hours at a time. Which of the following is the most likely diagnosis?

    A. Benign paroxysmal positional vertigo
    B. Labyrinthitis
    C. Menière's disease
    D. Serous otitis media

14. A 22-year-old male presents to the emergency department after sustaining a traumatic contusion to the left side of his face during an altercation earlier in the evening. On examination, there is some edema and ecchymosis surrounding the left eye. The patient is unable to look up with the left eye, as this results in diplopia. Radiologic findings are below. Which of the following injuries did he most likely suffer?

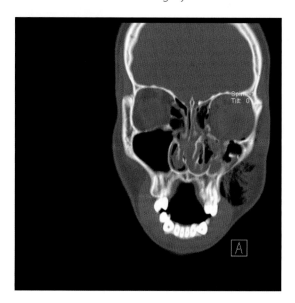

  A. Frontal sinus fracture
  B. LeFort fracture
  C. Orbital floor (blowout) fracture
  D. Zygomatic (tripod) fracture

15. A 33-year-old female with a medical history of asthma (adequately controlled with an inhaled steroid) complains of odynophagia and tender white patches on the roof of her mouth. The physical examination reveals creamy white patches overlying an erythematous base on the posterior palate and anterior pillars. These exudates remove easily upon gentle pressure with a depressor. She denies any fever, chills, otalgia, nasal congestion, or postnasal drip. Which of the following is the most likely diagnosis?

  A. Leukoplakia
  B. Lichen planus
  C. Oral candidiasis
  D. Strep pharyngitis

16. Which of the following are the typical findings associated with acute mastoiditis?

  A. Ipsilateral facial weakness and postauricular ecchymosis
  B. Ptosis, miosis, and anhidrosis
  C. Protrusion of the pinna, postauricular erythema, and tenderness
  D. Tinnitus, vertigo, and sensorineural hearing loss

17. Which of the following anatomical sites is usually responsible for anterior epistaxis?

  A. Kiesselbach's plexus
  B. The sphenopalantine foramen
  C. The hiatus semilunaris
  D. Woodruff's plexus

18. Which of the following systemic diseases is directly associated with oral manifestations?
    A. Rheumatoid arthritis
    B. Sjögren's syndrome
    C. Tuberculosis
    D. Wegener's granulomatosis

19. Which of the following is the most common initial presenting symptom of laryngeal carcinoma?
    A. Hemoptysis
    B. Hoarseness
    C. Stridor
    D. Weight loss

20. In which of the following circumstances is an emergency tracheostomy *least* indicated?
    A. Status asthmaticus
    B. An airway-obstructing foreign body
    C. Blunt trauma to the head and neck
    D. Stridor secondary to subglottic carcinoma

21. Routine examination of a patient's ear reveals a few white, chalky patches on the tympanic membrane. The eardrum is mobile on pneumatic otoscopy. Which of the following is the most likely diagnosis?
    A. Acute otitis media
    B. Cholesteatoma
    C. Serous otitis media
    D. Tympanosclerosis

22. A 40-year-old male presents complaining of nasal congestion that has progressively worsened over the past 6 months. On inspection, the left nasal cavity appears obstructed by a pale, flesh-colored, pedunculated, round mass, as seen on nasal endoscopy. Which of the following is the correct diagnosis?

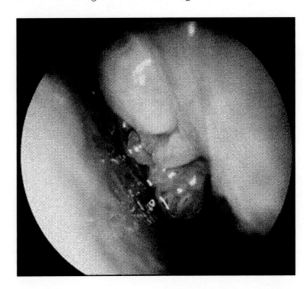

    A. Nasal polyposis
    B. Osler-Weber-Rendu syndrome
    C. Septal hematoma
    D. Vasomotor rhinitis

23. Sampter's triad includes nasal polyps, aspirin sensitivity, and which of the following?

    A. Allergic rhinitis
    B. Asthma
    C. Bronchiectasis
    D. Eczema

24. A patient fell down a flight of stairs and landed directly on his face. Which of the following findings is most suggestive of a septal hematoma?

    A. Bilateral bulging of the septum into the nasal cavities
    B. Dried blood in the nares and friable mucosa
    C. Periorbital ecchymosis
    D. Septal deviation

25. Which of the following tests best evaluates for acoustic neuroma?

    A. Audiogram
    B. Caloric stimulation
    C. Head CT with contrast
    D. Gadolinium-enhanced MRI

ANSWERS

1. **The correct answer is B.** Presbycusis commonly presents as sensorineural loss, which typically occurs in adults with advancing age. It usually presents gradually, is progressive, and involves high-frequency sounds. Patients may note diminished hearing in the presence of increased background noise. Conductive hearing loss results from dysfunction or pathology of the middle or inner ear. Causes include otitis media, perforation of the tympanic membrane, or impacted cerumen in the ear canal. Sensory hearing loss usually results from deterioration of the cochlea, and neural hearing loss usually occurs with pathology of the eighth cranial nerve.

2. **The correct answer is A.** Chronic otitis media usually presents because of recurrent acute otitis media. It can also occur in conjunction with other diseases and/or secondary to trauma. The tympanic membrane is usually perforated. Frequently, the aural mucosa shows changes, such as polypoid degeneration, which replaces granulation tissue. Osteitis and sclerosis of the tympanic membrane may also occur. Otosclerosis may appear on the tympanic membrane, as mentioned in the question. Otosclerosis is a progressive disease affecting the bone surrounding the inner ear that tends to run in families. Ossicular discontinuity or disruption frequently occurs due to a choleasteatoma. Ménière's disease is a syndrome that frequently results in vertigo, tinnitus, and hearing loss. Ménière's disease is a condition of the inner ear and does not usually present with damage.

3. **The correct answer is C.** Facial nerve paralysis, meningitis, and tympanic membrane perforation can all result from unresolved or untreated otitis media due, in part, to bacterial proliferation. Otosclerosis is a progressive disease affecting the bone surrounding the inner ear that tends to run in families. It usually originates in the stapes and can be corrected through a surgical replacement (stapedectomy).

4. **The correct answer is D.** Vestibular neuritis, or neuronitis, is a paroxysmal attack of vertigo that may persist for days or weeks. It usually is a one-time occurrence. Auditory function usually is not impaired. The physical examination will reveal nystagmus and absent response to caloric stimulation unilaterally or bilaterally. The treatment is usually

supportive, although diazepam or meclizine has proven useful during the acute vertigo attack. All of the other conditions are usually longer-lived and chronic in nature.

5. **The correct answer is D.** Pharyngeal abscesses (especially peritonsillar) typically present with marked pain and a toxic-appearing, febrile patient. Patients may present with odynophagia, trismus, and some deviation of the palatine tonsil with contralateral deviation of the uvula. Patients frequently demonstrate a "hot potato" voice and drool due to difficulty swallowing secretions secondary to pain. Epiglottitis (actually just above the glottis) also presents as this patient did. Patients with epiglottitis may progress to airway compromise and, as such, are a medical emergency. The oropharyngeal findings are out of proportion to the patient's complaints of pain, but any manipulation of the pharyngeal structures may cause airway compromise. The MRI differentiates the two conditions. Epiglottitis presents with the so-called "thumbprint" sign caused by enlargement of the epiglottitis. The radiograph in this situation shows widening of structures consistent with space-occupying swelling of the pharyngeal structures—in this case, a retropharyngeal abscess. Treatment of peritonsillar abscesses includes drainage, antibiotic coverage of group A strep and oropharyngeal anaerobes, and steroids to reduce inflammation.

6. **The correct answer is D.** Tinnitus is the perception of abnormal ear or head noises in the absence of external stimuli. Normally, patients have intermittent periods of mild, high-pitched tinnitus without any sequelae or other problems. Aspirin, NSAIDs, and loop diuretics commonly cause tinnitus. Pulsatile or unilateral tinnitus may be indicative of conditions that are more serious. Patients with pulsatile tinnitus should have a thorough workup in order to identify the sites of turbulent flow or vaso-occlusive abnormalities. Muscle spasms frequently cause the clicking or chirping noises and are not as much of a concern.

7. **The correct answer is B.** Koplik's spots are pathognomonic of measles or rubeola. They usually appear 2 days before the generalized rash of measles occurs and may last 1 to 4 days as tiny, crystal-appearing lesions (resembling table salt) on the buccal or labial mucosa. They usually appear opposite the second molars and frequently appear on the vaginal mucosa. Parvovirus B19, also called erythema infectiosum and fifth disease, has a "slapped-cheek" appearance to the face and a generalized reticular rash. The exanthema associated with rubella begins on the face and progresses caudally, with desquamation in areas of rash clearing. The rash associated with varicella appears as a pearl or a dewdrop on a rose petal and occurs in crops. Lesions typically occur in various stages, from macular progressing to papular, vesicular, and pustular, and finally crusting over with eschar.

8. **The correct answer is C.** An acoustic neuroma, also known as a vestibular schwannoma, is one of the most common intracranial tumors. It is located along the eighth cranial nerve and is usually unilateral. These tumors are usually benign and arise within the internal auditory canal, growing to encompass the cerebellopontine angle, which eventually compresses the pons and results in hydrocephalus. Patients typically present with unilateral, gradual hearing loss.

9. **The correct answer is C.** Patients with sialolithiasis typically present with postprandial pain and swelling. They often have a history of acute sialadenitis. Because of their location, the stones may move, with spontaneous resolution of the associated pain. Repeated episodes of sialadenitis are frequently associated with stricture and chronic infection. Lymphoma, tuberculosis, and parotitis would likely be associated with other constitutional symptoms, such as fever and malaise. Lymphoma presents in the lymph nodes. Parotitis (mumps) is a paramyxoviral disease spread by respiratory droplets that produces inflammation of the salivary glands. Although parotid enlargement is frequently exacerbated by the ingestion of acidic foods, it generally persists for approximately 1 week before

resolving. Cervical tuberculosis occurs frequently in childhood and causes destruction of the cervical vertebrae; it may also present with a retropharyngeal abscess.

10. **The correct answer is D.** This patient has stomatitis, also known as aphthous ulcers or canker sores. The cause remains uncertain, although research shows an association with the herpes virus. The literature also notes an association with increased stress, although the findings are more nebulous in this regard. Treatment is nonspecific and consists of topical corticosteroids and analgesics, which serve to provide symptomatic relief. Other treatment options include tetracycline or minocycline rinses, lysine, vitamin C, and vitamin B complex and are of variable efficacy. Some patient may benefit from "magic mouthwash," a 1:1:1 mixture of viscous lidocaine, diphenhydramine hydrochloride, and magnesium hydroxide antacid. There should be further investigation as to the etiology when aphthous ulcers occur with symptoms of arthritis, genital ulcers (Behçet's), urethritis (Reiter's), diarrhea (Crohn's), conjunctivitis, or uveitis.

11. **The correct answer is B.** Mononucleosis is a viral illness typically caused by the Epstein-Barr virus. Physical examination reveals lymphadenopathy, fever, malaise, and splenomegaly (up to 50% of patients). The lymphadenopathy is typically along the posterior cervical chain and is usually painful. Leukoplakia is a white patch or plaque that represents a premalignant oral lesion. It typically does not remove upon rubbing the mucosal surface. Heavy tobacco and/or alcohol consumption is a risk factor for the development of leukoplakia. Patients with peritonsillar abscess typically present with a more toxic picture and an asymmetrical rise of the uvula on physical examination. Vincent's angina, or necrotizing ulcerative gingivitis, typically occurs in young adults under stress. An acute gingival inflammation and necrosis often present with bleeding, fever, halitosis, and cervical lymphadenopathy.

12. **The correct answer is A.** Ludwig's angina one of the most common deep neck infections. It is actually a cellulitis of the sublingual and submaxillary spaces and is often the result of a mandibular infection. The patient typically presents with edema and erythema of the upper neck and mouth. The tongue may displace superiorly and posteriorly if the cellulitis spreads. This typically follows significant dental procedures, such as an extraction. Sublingual and submandibular sialadenitis most commonly effect the parotid or submandibular gland. Sialadenitis presents as an acute swelling of the gland, along with increased pain and edema, especially when eating meals. There is marked tenderness of the duct opening. Sialadenitis usually follows dehydration or a chronic illness. Vincent's angina, or necrotizing ulcerative gingivitis, typically occurs in young adults under stress. It is an acute gingival inflammation and necrosis, often presenting with bleeding, fever, halitosis, and cervical lymphadenopathy.

13. **The correct answer is C.** Menière's disease frequently results in vertigo and all its attendant symptoms, as described in the question. Menière's disease is a condition of the inner ear of unknown etiology. Caloric testing typically reveals loss of impairment of thermally induced nystagmus on the involved side. With labryinthitis, patients suffer from continuous, severe vertigo (worse with head movement), lasting several days to weeks, accompanied by nausea, vomiting, and nystagmus. Patients often have a history of a viral infection a few weeks prior to the onset of symptoms. Patients will experience gradual improvement and eventual recovery. There is associated hearing loss and tinnitus. Benign paroxysmal positional vertigo is the most common type of vertigo experienced by patients. Symptoms are transient, lasting less than 1 minute, and are directly associated with changes in head position. It can occur spontaneously in elderly patients or result from trauma, infection of the inner ear, or debris accumulation in the semicircular canals. Serous otitis media results from a blocked Eustachian tube, with resultant transudation of trapped fluid. Serous otitis may be due to an anatomical blockage, as seen in children with enlarged adenoids or cleft palates or those with allergies or ENT infections. It may

manifest as hearing impairment or speech delay. This is especially common in children because of the narrow, horizontally placed Eustachian tubes.

14. **The correct answer is B.** This radiograph clearly shows a blowout fracture with subsequent displacement of the orbital globe. Fracture of the bony orbit can result in entrapment of the extraocular muscles and subsequent diplopia. Additional complications that may occur include retinal detachment and hyphema. Frontal sinus fractures are not usually apparent on standard radiographs and, as such, a CT scan is the diagnostic procedure of choice for such injuries. LeFort fractures are a classification system used to describe maxillary fractures. Maxillary and zygomatic fractures present with significant malar depression and paresthesias of the infraorbital nerves.

15. **The correct answer is C.** Oral candidiasis, or thrush, is a painful, white curdlike patch overlying erythematous mucosa. The patches remove easily when scraped with a tongue blade. In patients with lichen planus or leukoplakia, there is usually no underlying erythema. Lichen planus presents with pruritic, violet-colored papules with flattened tops that also present with fine white streaks and "lacy" appearances along the mucosa. Patients with hepatitis C may present with these lesions. These lesions are sometimes seen in strep pharyngitis, but typically they lie more posteriorly and are easily removed by rubbing the mucosa. Leukoplakia is a white patch not easily removed upon rubbing the mucosal surface; it is considered a precancerous lesion.

16. **The correct answer is C.** Acute suppurative mastoiditis usually follows several weeks of inadequately treated otitis media. It typically presents with postauricular pain, erythema, and a spiking fever. Protrusion of the pinna may occur due to the space-occupying swelling. The other symptoms are not usually present in this situation. Ptosis, miosis, and anhidrosis constitute the triad of Horner's syndrome, which is secondary to a defect in the sympathetic innervation to the face. Tinnitus, vertigo, and sensorineuronal hearing loss are encountered in Menière's disease.

17. **The correct answer is A.** Anterior epistaxis is the most common form of epistaxis and is usually more manageable than posterior epistaxis due to easy access. Anatomically, Kiesselbach's plexus is located over the anterior septum and is responsible for anterior bleeds, whereas Woodruff's plexus situates over the posterior middle turbinate and is a common source of posterior bleeds.

18. **The correct answer is B.** Sjögren's syndrome is an autoimmune disorder that manifests with sicca (dryness of the eyes, mouth, and other mucus membranes). It results from lymphocytic infiltration and destruction of exocrine glands, primarily the salivary and lacrimal glands. Treatment includes cholinergic agents to stimulate secretions. The clinician should suspect tuberculosis in a patient with persistent cough, night sweats, fatigue, and weight loss. Oral manifestations are not generally associated with tuberculosis. Wegener's granulomatosis is a chronic vasculitis that typically presents with rhinorrhea, chronic sinus inflammation, and nasal cartilage collapse, leading to a saddle nose deformity. Patients may also demonstrate subglottal stenosis, pulmonary infiltrates, and glomerulonephritis, leading to renal failure.

19. **The correct answer is B.** The most common initial presenting symptom of laryngeal carcinoma is hoarseness. Less common symptoms include odynophagia, dysphagia, persistent cough, halitosis, referred otalgia, hemoptysis, and stridor. Weight loss would likely be a late manifestation of disease progression.

20. **The correct answer is A.** The management of status asthmaticus includes aggressive pharmacologic treatment. Because of its many risks, endotracheal intubation and mechanical ventilation should be considered only in refractory cases. Tracheostomy plays no role in the treatment of status asthmaticus. It usually proves useful in the treatment

of upper-airway foreign-body obstruction, head and neck blunt trauma, and obstruction due to laryngeal carcinoma.

21. **The correct answer is D.** Tympanosclerosis is the deposition of hyaline and calcifications on the tympanic membrane and subepithelium resulting from recurrent infections of the middle ear or trauma (perforation or myringotomy tubes). Acute otitis media is noted with a hypomobile, erythematous eardrum. Cholesteatoma may be congenital or acquired and is a slow-growing lesion of stratified squamous epithelium that erodes surrounding bony structures, leading to a conductive hearing loss. It presents with a malodorous otorrhea, dizziness, vertigo, and, in some cases, facial nerve paralysis. Serous otitis secondary to Eustachian tube dysfunction may be noted by a retracted tympanic membrane and tiny bubble formation on otoscopic examination.

22. **The correct answer is A.** Nasal polyps are pale, mucosal, edematous masses commonly seen in patients with allergic rhinitis. They may result in chronic obstruction and a diminished sense of smell. Osler-Weber-Rendu syndrome is an inherited disorder of the blood vessels that can cause excessive bleeding. The syndrome is also called hereditary hemorrhagic telangiectasia, or HHT. Septal hematoma is a blood-filled tumor resulting from trauma. Vasomotor rhinitis presents with increased clear nasal discharge and edematous turbinates, but not to the extent shown here.

23. **The correct answer is B.** Sampter's triad includes nasal polyps, aspirin sensitivity, and asthma.

24. **The correct answer is A.** Septal hematomas, which typically result from trauma, are space-occupying lesions that may present as described in the question. Dried blood in the nares along with friable mucosa may be the result of trauma (secondary to self-manipulation) or perhaps epistaxis. Septal deviation typically causes breathing difficulties, especially when sleeping but does not usually cause a visible bulge.

25. **The correct answer is D.** Acoustic neuroma, also called vestibular schwannoma, is a benign slow-growing tumor involving the eighth cranial nerve. It accounts for nearly 80% of tumors found within the internal auditory canal or cerebellopontine angle. This tumor is best visualized on MRI with gadolinium and appears as a "light-bulb" shaped lesion. With progressive tumor growth, patients experience headache, unilateral hearing loss, facial paresthesias and weakness, rotational vertigo, and disequilibrium.

REFERENCES

Alho, O. P., Teppo, H., Mäntyselkä, P., and Kantola, S. (2006). "Head and neck cancer in primary care: Presenting symptoms and the effect of delayed diagnosis of cancer cases." *Canadian Medical Association Journal* 174(6): 779–784.

Crummer, R. W., and Hassan G. A. (2004). "Diagnostic approach to tinnitus." *American Family Physician* 69(1): 120–126.

Fauci, A. S., Braunwald, E., Kasper, D. L., Hauser, S. L., Longo, D. L., Jameson, J. L., and Loscalzo, J. (2008). *Harrison's Textbook of Internal Medicine*, 17th ed. McGraw-Hill Medical Publishing, New York.

Galioto, N. J. (2008). "Peritonsillar abscess." *American Family Physician* 77(2): 199–202.

Goldman, L., and Ausiello, D. (2008). *Cecil Medicine*, 23rd ed. Saunders Elsevier, Philadelphia, PA.

Gonsalves, W. C., Chi, A. C., and Neville, B. W. (2007). "Common oral lesions: Part II masses and neoplasia." *American Family Physician* 75:509–512.

Kancherla, V. S., and Hanson, I. C. (2006). "Mumps resurgence in the United States." *Journal of Allergy and Clinical Immunology* 118(6): 1393–1412.

Lockwood, A. H. (2005). "Tinnitus." *Neurologic Clinics* 23(3): 893–900.

McBride, D. R. (2000). "Management of aphthous ulcers." *American Family Physician* 62:149–154, 160.

Mavragani, C. P., and Moutsopoulos H. M. (2007). "Conventional therapy of Sjögren's syndrome." *Clinical Reviews in Allergy and Immunology* 32(3): 284–291.

National Institute on Deafness and Other Communication Disorders. (1997). "Presbycusis." (Online). Available at www.nidcd.nih.gov/health/hearing/presbycusis.asp. Accessed: April 27, 2008.

Polensek, S. H. (2008). "Labyrinthitis." In *Ferri's Clinical Advisor Instant Diagnosis and Treatment.* Mosby Elsevier, Philadelphia, PA.

Porter, G. T. (2008). "Epistaxis." (Online). Available at www.utmb.edu/otoref/grnds/Epistaxis-2002-04/Epistaxis-2002-04.htm. Accessed: April 27, 2008.

St. Martin, M. B., and Hirsch, B. E. (2008). "Imaging of hearing loss." *Otolaryngologic Clinics of North America* 41(1): 157–178, vi–vii.

Tierney, Jr., L. M., McPhee, S. J., and Papadakis, M. A. (2008). *Current Medical Diagnosis and Treatment.* McGraw-Hill Companies, Inc., New York.

Weisberg, S. S. (2007). "Measles." *Disease-a-Month* 53(10): 467–528.

Pulmonology

Les A. Szekely, MD, FCCP, DABSM
Donna M. Agnew, MT (ASCP), MSPAS, PA-C

1. Which of the following best characterizes the pathologic changes in asthmatic patients?
   A. Airway inflammation with mucous plugging of the small airways
   B. Alveolar collapse with shunting of deoxygenated blood
   C. Repeated patterns of eosinophilic pulmonary infiltrates
   D. Parenchymal scarring, glandular dilation, and impaired ciliary function

2. A 26-year-old female with a medical history of reactive airway disease presents complaining of chest tightness and persistent, non-productive cough. She is generally well-maintained on a combined steroid and long-acting beta-agonist inhaler. She notes that her tightness and cough have worsened to the point that she more frequently uses her albuterol inhaler. Which of the following would *not* be part of the appropriate management of this patient?
   A. A leukotriene inhibitor
   B. A prednisone taper or a prednisone burst
   C. A mast cell stabilizer
   D. An antimicrobial for atypical organisms

3. A 13-year-old male presents with a history of an intermittent cough productive of thick, purulent sputum that is worse at night and upon awakening in the morning. His mother notes that the cough is associated with wheezing on occasion. She is concerned her son may have developed asthma. She notes that the coughing is more frequent and persistent. The patient does not have a significant past medical history of respiratory difficulties. You perform a full workup consisting of pulmonary function tests (PFTs), chest x-ray, and sputum culture. The culture showed 4+ *Pseudomonas aeruginosa*. The chest radiograph shows bronchiectasis, and the PFTs indicates nonspecific airflow obstruction. Which of the following should be the next diagnostic study in the evaluation of this patient?
   A. CT scan of the chest
   B. Sweat chloride test
   C. V/Q scan
   D. Bronchoscopy

4. Which of the following tests is the most noninvasive diagnostic test for patients with pulmonary embolism?
   A. D-dimer
   B. Helical CT scan
   C. Pulmonary angiography
   D. V/Q scan

5. A 19-year-old college student presents to student health services with a hacking, dry, nonproductive cough of 2 days duration. She has a fever of 101°F, malaise, and head-ache. She denies chills. Which of the following organisms is most likely causing her symptoms?

   A. *Streptococcus pneumoniae*
   B. *Haemophilus influenzae*
   C. *Mycoplasma pneumoniae*
   D. *Chlamydia pneumoniae*

6. A 21-year-old college basketball player presents to the emergency department with a sudden onset of shortness of breath and left-sided pleuritic chest pain that occurred 2 hours after practice. He denies a significant past medical history. He is not on any medications and denies allergies. The chest radiograph is below. Which of the following is the most appropriate treatment?

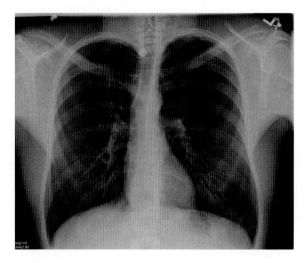

   A. Needle decompression and chest tube placement
   B. Admission to the hospital for anticoagulation therapy
   C. Parenteral antimicrobials
   D. Percutaneous drainage of effusion

7. Which of the following etiologic agents of pneumonia typically does not transmit via person-to-person contact?

   A. *Mycoplasma pneumoniae*
   B. *Klebsiella pneumoniae*
   C. *Legionella pneumophila*
   D. *Streptococcus pneumoniae*

8. A 43-year-old female Russian immigrant presents with an initially dry cough that is now productive of blood-tinged sputum, fever, and drenching night sweats. She also notes a 20-pound unintentional weight loss. Her chest radiograph is below. Which of the following is the most likely diagnosis?

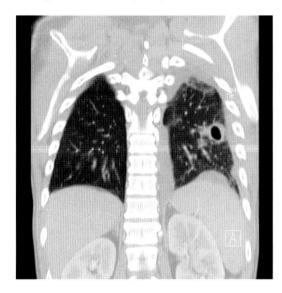

    A. Sarcoidosis
    B. Pulmonary fibrosis
    C. Aspergillosis
    D. Tuberculosis

9. A high-resolution CT is ordered to further evaluate a 2-cm, solitary pulmonary nodule identified on the chest radiograph of a 62-year-old female complaining of a chronic cough. Which of the following radiographic findings would be most suggestive of a benign lesion?

    A. Dense calcifications in a central pattern
    B. Peripheral halos
    C. Spiculated margins
    D. Thick walled (>16 mm) cavitary lesions

10. A 57-year-old patient with a longstanding history of snoring and daytime somnolence submits to polysomnography testing. The results identify approximately seven to eight apneic episodes per hour accompanied by significant arterial oxygen desaturations. Which of the following treatment modalities is both curative for obstructive sleep apnea and has been proven to reduce hypoxia?

    A. Nasal continuous positive airway pressure (CPAP)
    B. Oral prosthesis
    C. Supplemental oxygen via nasal cannula
    D. Uvulopalatopharyngoplasty (UPPP)

11. Which of the following respiratory diseases resulting from occupational exposures demonstrates a "ground glass" or "honeycomb" appearance of the lung parenchyma on radiograph?

    A. Asbestosis
    B. Berylliosis
    C. Coal worker's pneumoconiosis
    D. Silicosis

12. Which of the following is the most common presenting symptom of a patient with pulmonary embolism?

    A. Cough
    B. Dyspnea
    C. Hemoptysis
    D. Wheeze

13. Deficiencies or dysfunction in which of the following anticoagulant proteins is the most common inherited cause of a hypercoagulable state leading to deep vein thrombosis (DVT) and pulmonary embolism?

    A. Antithrombin III
    B. Factor V Leiden
    C. Lupus anticoagulant
    D. Protein C

14. Which of the following treatments for chronic obstructive pulmonary disease (COPD) has proven efficacy in altering the course of the disease?

    A. Inhaled bronchodilators
    B. Inhaled steroids
    C. Smoking cessation
    D. Surgical lung reduction

15. A 36-year-old African American female presents with generalized malaise and dyspnea. The chest radiograph reveals bilateral hilar and mediastinal adenopathy. Subsequent tissue biopsy via flexible bronchoscopy reveals a noncaseating granuloma containing multinucleated giant cells. Sputum for acid-fast stain was negative, with cultures still pending. Labs were unremarkable, with the exception of a moderate elevation in angiotensinogen-converting enzyme. What of the following is the most likely diagnosis?

    A. Adenocarcinoma
    B. Lymphoma
    C. Sarcoidosis
    D. Tuberculosis

16. Because of their significant bactericidal activity and low toxicity profile, which of the following medications, when used in the treatment of tuberculosis, are included as part of any four-drug regimen?

    A. Ethambutol and rifampin
    B. Isoniazid and ethambutol
    C. Isoniazid and pyrazinamide
    D. Isoniazid and rifampin

17. Which of the following antihypertensive medications is inappropriate for a 53-year-old female with asthma?

    A. ACE inhibitor
    B. Beta blocker
    C. Calcium-channel blocker
    D. Thiazide diuretic

18. A 61-year-old female with a history of emphysema secondary to an alpha$_1$-antitrypsin deficiency is now 9 months status-post a single lung transplant. Her postoperative history includes two episodes of acute rejection that were successfully treated with intravenous high-dose corticosteroids. She admits to malaise and progressive exertional breathlessness. Pulmonary function tests (PFTs) reveal an obstructive airflow pattern. She denies fever, dyspnea, or cough. Which of the following is the most likely diagnosis?

A. Atelectasis
B. Bronchiolitis obliterans
C. Posttransplant rejection
D. Secondary infection

19. Which of the following is the single most common respiratory complaint for which patients seek medical treatment?

A. Cough
B. Dyspnea
C. Hemoptysis
D. Wheezing

20. Which of the following antihypertensive medications has a nonproductive cough as a commonly encountered adverse side effect?

A. Alpha blockers
B. Angiotensin-converting enzyme inhibitors
C. Beta blockers
D. Calcium-channel blockers

21. A 31-year-old female presents complaining of a persistent cough for the past 3 to 4 weeks. She recounts an onset of a low-grade fever and coryza about a month ago, which has since resolved. She describes bouts of "coughing fits" over the past week, with associated shortness of breath and two episodes of posttussive vomiting. The cough appears to be worse at night. Which of the following is the most appropriate next step in the management of this patient?

A. Obtain a sputum culture and prescribe a fluoroquinolone antibiotic.
B. Prescribe a narcotic cough suppressant for symptomatic relief.
C. Recommend a mucolytic and beta-agonist inhaler to reduce airway hyperresponsiveness.
D. Submit a nasopharyngeal swab culture and prescribe a macrolide antibiotic.

22. Which of the following best describes the pathophysiology of emphysema?

A. Destruction of alveolar septa
B. Hyperirritability of the tracheobronchial tree
C. Hypertrophy of mucus-producing glands in the large airways
D. Mucus plugging of the small airways

23. Which of the following patients is most at risk for developing active tuberculosis?

A. A 57-year-old patient with acute myelogenous leukemia
B. A 61-year-old patient on hemodialysis for end-stage renal disease
C. A 33-year-old patient with HIV infection
D. A 72-year-old patient with silicosis

24. A 71-year-old male with a past medical history of hypertension, coronary artery disease, and COPD presents to the emergency department complaining of pleuritic chest pain and shortness of breath. Initial assessment finds him to be afebrile, normotensive, and mildly tachypneic, with a respiratory rate of 24. Stat arterial blood gases on room air are as follows:

pH 7.34; $PaCO_2$ 62 mmHg; PaO_2 60 mmHg; HCO_3 32 mEq/L.

Which of the following best describes this patient's acid-base disorder?

A. Compensated metabolic acidosis
B. Compensated respiratory acidosis
C. Metabolic acidosis
D. Respiratory acidosis

25. You are the hospitalist paged to evaluate a ventilated patient who is described by the ICU charge nurse as becoming acutely agitated, dyspneic, and cyanotic. On exam, a cursory inspection reveals decreased oxygen saturations, asymmetric chest expansion, and left tracheal deviation. The patient had a Swan-Ganz catheter placed via a right subclavian approach just prior to his change in status. Which of the following is the most likely diagnosis?

A. Acute myocardial infarction
B. Left-side pneumothorax
C. Pulmonary air embolus
D. Right-side pneumothorax

26. Which of the following viruses causes croup?

A. Adenovirus
B. Influenza
C. Parainfluenza
D. Respiratory syncytial virus

27. On postoperative morning rounds, you note a temperature of 38.4°C on a patient who is 1-day status-post bowel resection, secondary to a small bowel obstruction. Which of the following is the most likely cause of the patient's fever?

A. Atelectasis
B. Intra-abdominal abscess
C. Peritonitis
D. Pneumonia

28. Which of the following patients is most likely to produce a false high reading on pulse oximetry?

A. A patient who is hypovolemic
B. A patient suffering from smoke inhalation
C. A patient who is in septic shock
D. A patient who is a hypothermic drowning accident survivor

29. Which of the following bacteria is the most common pathogen isolated in cases of community-acquired pneumonia?

A. *Chlamydia pneumoniae*
B. *Klebsiella pneumoniae*
C. *Mycoplasma pneumoniae*
D. *Streptococcus pneumoniae*

30. Which of the following spirometry parameters best assesses obstructive lung disease?

A. ERV (expiratory reserve volume)
B. FEV1% (forced expiratory volume)
C. RV (residual volume)
D. FVC (forced vital capacity)

31. Which of the following is most likely to produce a transudative pleural effusion?

   A. Congestive heart failure
   B. Empyema
   C. Malignancy
   D. Pancreatitis

32. A 41-year-old male presents complaining of a hacking nonproductive cough for the past 2 to 3 months that is now associated with fever, chills, fatigue, and a 10-pound weight loss. With his 20-pack-year history of smoking, you obtain a chest x-ray, which reveals interstitial infiltrates extending from the perihilar areas in a "butterfly" pattern, sparing the apices. You perform a bronchioalveolar lavage, which confirms your suspicion of infection with *Pneumocystis jirovecii*. Which of the following is the treatment of choice for this patient?

   A. Clindamycin
   B. Dapsone
   C. Pentamidine
   D. Trimethoprim-sulfamethoxazole (TMP-SMX)

33. A preoperative chest radiograph on a 56-year-old male with a 60-pack-year history of tobacco abuse reveals bilateral peripheral lung masses. Of which of the following histologic types of bronchogenic lung cancer is this finding most suggestive?

   A. Adenocarcinoma
   B. Large cell carcinoma
   C. Small cell carcinoma
   D. Squamous cell carcinoma

34. A 63-year-old retired plumber presents complaining of shortness of breath and right-sided chest pain for the past several weeks. The initial chest x-ray reveals a right middle lobe pleural effusion. A thoracentesis demonstrates a hemorrhagic exudate. A biopsy confirms your diagnosis of malignant pleural mesothelioma. Which of the following is the greatest risk factor for the development of this type of lung cancer?

   A. Asbestos exposure
   B. Cigarette smoking
   C. Oncogenic predisposition
   D. Radiation exposure

35. A 22-month-old toddler presents to the emergency department via EMS in acute respiratory distress. On exam, you note nasal flaring, intercostal retractions, a faint inspiratory stridor, and wheezing. He is afebrile and tachypneic, with an SaO_2 on room air of 91%. A stat chest radiograph reveals hyperinflation of the right lung with a left mediastinal shift. Which of the following is the most likely diagnosis?

   A. Acute epiglottitis
   B. Asthma exacerbation
   C. Atelectasis
   D. Foreign-body aspiration

36. An elderly man presents to the emergency department with acute onset of fever, altered mental status, right pleuritic chest pain, and a cough that is productive of maroon-colored gel-like sputum. EMS states the patient was picked up downtown lying over a steam vent. You detect a strong odor of alcohol as you approach the patient. A physical examination reveals rales, dullness to percussion, and increased tactile fremitus over the right upper lobe. Which of the following organisms is the most likely cause of pneumonia in this patient?

   A. *Chlamydia pneumoniae*
   B. *Klebsiella pneumoniae*
   C. *Mycoplasma pneumoniae*
   D. *Streptococcus pneumoniae*

37. Which of the following scenarios represents the most common cause of acute respiratory distress syndrome?

A. A 73-year-old patient with aspiration of gastric contents
B. A 41-year-old patient with a salicylate overdose
C. A 68-year-old patient with urosepsis
D. A 39-year-old patient with aortic aneurysm who has received multiple transfusions

38. Which of the following is the most common cause of respiratory distress in a preterm infant?

A. Apnea
B. Birth asphyxia
C. Hyaline membrane disease
D. RSV pneumonia

39. A 33-year-old female presents complaining of acute onset of a sharp, stabbing left anterior chest pain and shortness of breath once a day. She states that she has "trouble taking in a full breath" secondary to the pain. She denies fever, hemoptysis, or relief with change in position. She received treatment for pneumonia with a fluoroquinolone antibiotic approximately 2 weeks ago. On completion of the antibiotic, her cough became less productive, but it remains persistent. Physical examination reveals rales in the left lung base with an associated friction rub. Which of the following is the most likely diagnosis and recommended treatment for this patient?

A. Pneumothorax, chest tube placement
B. Pleurisy, anti-inflammatory and analgesic medications
C. Pulmonary embolism, anticoagulation therapy
D. Pericarditis, anti-inflammatory medications

40. In which of the following conditions would Cheyne-Stokes breathing be *least* likely?

A. End-stage left ventricular failure
B. Metabolic acidosis
C. Neurologic disease
D. Sleeping at high altitudes

41. A 51-year-old male presents to the emergency department via EMS after being found unconscious on the floor of his apartment by a neighbor. The history obtained from the neighbor reveals that he has been out of work for over a year on disability for a back injury, for which he became increasingly depressed. He underwent a period of physical therapy, but when that proved to be unsuccessful he had spinal disk surgery 3 months ago. He complained of postoperative pain treated with narcotic pain medications, with only minimal relief. His initial lab screening reveals normal glucose, BUN, creatinine, and electrolytes; a drug screen positive for opioids; and the following arterial blood gas profile: pH 7.34, pCO_2 55, and HCO_3 29. Assuming that there is only one physiologic abnormality, which of the following best describes this acid-base disturbance?

A. Metabolic acidemia
B. Metabolic alkalemia
C. Respiratory acidemia
D. Respiratory alkalemia

42. Which of the following is the most identifiable predisposing factor for the development of asthma?

A. Atopy
B. Exercise
C. Gastroesophageal reflux
D. Stress

43. A 73-year-old male presents with an acute exacerbation of a chronic condition. His chest radiograph is shown below. Which of the following should *not* be included in the pharmacologic treatment of this patient?

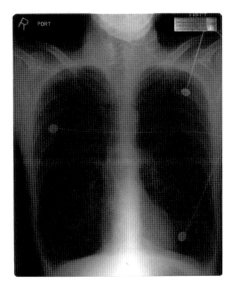

- **A.** Broad-spectrum antibiotic
- **B.** Inhaled ipratropium chloride and beta agonist
- **C.** Systemic corticosteroids
- **D.** Theophylline

44. Which of the following is *not* a recognized benefit of lung-reduction surgery for the treatment of severe emphysema?

- **A.** Increased exercise tolerance
- **B.** Improvement in pulmonary function spirometry
- **C.** Improved mortality
- **D.** Symptomatic relief of dyspnea

45. A 37-year-old male presents to the emergency department in acute renal failure. He admits to symptoms of a "cold"—fever, chills, arthralgias, and myalgias—over the past week. He became alarmed this morning when he had an episode of hemoptysis of 2 tablespoons of bright red blood. Which of the following tests would *not* support a diagnosis of Goodpasture's syndrome in this patient?

- **A.** ANCA (antibodies to neutrophil cytoplasmic antigens)
- **B.** Anti-GBM (antibodies to the glomerular basement membrane)
- **C.** ASO titer (antistreptolysin O titer)
- **D.** Renal biopsy

ANSWERS

1. The correct answer is A. Asthma is a syndrome of unknown etiology characterized by airway obstruction and airway hyperresponsiveness. It is usually secondary to environmental or allergic stimuli leading to bronchoconstriction and airway inflammation. The inflammation is due to infiltration with mast cells and eosinophils. Mucous production is increased, leading to small-airway plugging, which, in effect, acts as a valve, letting air in but not out with the same efficiency. Alveolar collapse typically occurs in atelectasis. Eosinophilic infiltrates occur with acute eosinophilic syndrome. Parenchymal scarring, glandular dilation, and impaired ciliary function occur with cystic fibrosis.

2. **The correct answer is D.** Although the use of antimicrobials for atypical organisms, such as *Mycoplasma*, is an area of ongoing research, current recommendations do not suggest their use. All of the choices remaining are appropriate to consider in a patient with moderate-to-persistent asthma.

3. **The correct answer is B.** Cystic fibrosis is an autosomal-recessive gene-mutation defect that inhibits the function of chloride channels. It manifests with the symptoms as described in the question. Patients typically are younger than age 18, although because of treatment advances more adults are presenting with the disease (40% of cases). A sweat chloride test confirms the diagnosis. A CT scan would be useful when looking for masses and other lesions. V/Q scans typically identify perfusion defects. A bronchoscopy is a highly invasive procedure that would not yield high diagnostic results, and thus would not be warranted in this patient.

4. **The correct answer is B.** In patients with pulmonary embolism, the gold-standard test is pulmonary angiography. However, this test is invasive and could lead to complications such as renal compromise, allergic reactions to contrast media, or arrhythmia. If the practitioner is considering a noninvasive test with a high diagnostic yield, then the helical CT scan is the test of choice. D-dimer is nonspecific for pulmonary embolism. The V/Q scan often is equivocal in patients, thus necessitating further testing.

5. **The correct answer is C.** This patient presents with the typical presentation of *Mycoplasma*. *Streptococcus pneumoniae* patients are usually elderly and frequently present with shaking chills. Patients in college age groups are probably immunized against *Haemophilus influenzae*. *Chlamydia pneumoniae* often is associated with symptoms of sore throat and hoarseness.

6. **The correct answer is A.** This patient has an obvious pneumothorax, probably spontaneous. He requires immediate needle decompression and chest tube placement. A delay in treatment could result in further shifting of respiratory structures, leading to a tension pneumothorax. The chest radiograph shows no evidence of effusion, so drainage is not necessary. Admission to the hospital is warranted; however, no evidence of pulmonary embolism exists, thus anticoagulation is not appropriate. Because there is no evidence of an infectious process, antimicrobials are unnecessary.

7. **The correct answer is C.** *Legionella pneumophila* spreads via contaminated water sources. The first occurrence and identification of this disease occurred during an American Legion conference in Philadelphia in 1976. Ultimately, investigators isolated a contaminated air-conditioning system as the culprit harboring the bacterium. It does not transmit via person-to-person contact, as do the other agents listed.

8. **The correct answer is D.** This patient has pulmonary tuberculosis. It is common in patients from Russia, the Pacific Rim, Sub-Saharan Africa, Latin America, and the Indian subcontinent. Frequently, these patients do not have access to adequate care or treatment of their disease. The typical presentation is as noted in the question. Patients usually have pulmonary infiltrates and cavitation on chest radiograph. Patients with sarcoidosis typically have bilateral hilar and right peritracheal lymphadenopathy. The chest film rarely shows cavitation, as is normally seen in tuberculosis. Patients with aspergillosis frequently present with a patchy infiltration that can lead to a necrotizing pneumonia frequently seen in immunocompromised patients and patients with asthma. Pulmonary fibrosis usually is found in patients older than age 65 who have idiopathic disease and a typical pleural-based "honeycomb" pattern of fibrosis on CT. Patients with tuberculosis who receive delayed treatment or no treatment may show a miliary pattern, as shown below.

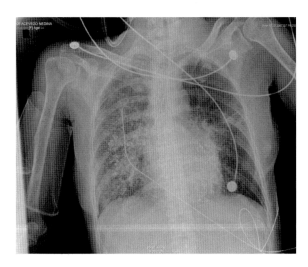

9. **The correct answer is A.** Calcifications seen with malignant pulmonary lesions tend to be stippled, few in number, and located eccentrically. Peripheral halos, speculated margins, and thick walls usually occur with malignant lesions.

10. **The correct answer is A.** Treatment of obstructive sleep apnea includes weight reduction and avoidance of alcohol and sedatives. Mechanical oral appliances that protrude the mandible and tongue forward are modestly effective in mild-to-moderate cases.

11. **The correct answer is A.** Asbestosis typically demonstrates linear opacities that initiate in the lung bases and progress superiorly with disease progression (see below). Beryllium causes the formation of granuloma. Inhaled coal dust particles are surrounded by alveolar macrophages and appear as discrete opacities on x-ray, usually in the upper lobes. "Eggshell" calcifications along the periphery of the hilar lymph nodes exemplify the radiographic findings of silicosis. The patient in this radiograph also has a right basilar lung mass.

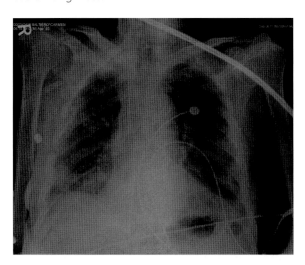

12. **The correct answer is B.** Dyspnea occurs in approximately 75% of patients with pulmonary embolism, and tachypnea is the most frequent sign. Dyspnea, syncope, and cyanosis occur in significant pulmonary embolisms, whereas a small embolism might present with cough, hemoptysis, or pleuritic chest pain, especially on inspiration.

13. **The correct answer is B.** Factor V Leiden deficiency is more common than all the other hypercoagulable states combined. It also accounts for a much higher rate of recurrent thrombosis in a patient who has completed and discontinued a standard course of anticoagulation therapy.

14. **The correct answer is C.** Smoking cessation is the only treatment for COPD proven to change the progression of the disease. Inhaled bronchodilators and steroids provide symptomatic relief but do not halt the long-term decline in lung function. Lung-volume reduction surgery improves exercise tolerance in severe cases but does not alter disease course.

15. **The correct answer is C.** Although sarcoidosis can affect any organ tissue, nearly 90% of cases present with granulomatous inflammation of the lung. It has a higher incidence in women, especially African American, and the onset of presentation usually occurs in the third or fourth decades. Patients may be asymptomatic and diagnosed as the result of abnormal findings on a chest radiograph. Symptoms can be nonspecific, such as fever, malaise, or dyspnea. Associated findings such as hepatosplenomegaly, parotid gland enlargement, or erythema nodosum should raise suspicion for the disease. Angiotensin-converting enzymes (ACE) levels are generally elevated in patients with active disease and decline with treatment and clinical improvement. The mainstay of treatment is corticosteroid therapy when end-organ effects are documented.

16. **The correct answer is D.** The goal of tuberculosis treatment is twofold: to eliminate tubercle bacilli while preventing the emergence of resistant strains. It is for this reason that current recommendations advocate a four-drug regimen. Isoniazid and rifampin are included in the four-drug regimen because they are bactericidal to both intracellular and extracellular organisms. Isoniazid can cause hepatotoxicity and peripheral neuropathy. Rifampin causes orange discoloration of body secretions. The addition of pyrazinamide may reduce bacterial load early in the course of treatment and can result in uricemia. Ethambutol and streptomycin may serve to protect against the development of drug resistance. Optic neuritis can be a side effect of ethambutol use. Ototoxicity and nephrotoxicity may occur with streptomycin.

17. **The correct answer is B.** Blockade of B2 receptors in bronchial smooth muscle may lead to increased airway resistance in patients with asthma.

18. **The correct answer is B.** Bronchiolitis obliterans is a chronic rejection complication seen in lung transplant patients. Early lesions of inflammation occur in the small-airway epithelium, which leads to granulation tissue deposition in the airway lumen, leading to partial or complete obstruction. Previous acute rejections and a history of symptomatic Cytomegalovirus infections are risk factors for the development of this condition.

19. **The correct answer is A.** Acute cough, defined as lasting fewer than 3 weeks, usually follows upper respiratory infections. Chronic cough, defined as lasting longer than 8 weeks, in immunocompetent patients may be due to a variety of conditions, including postnasal drip, asthma, chronic bronchitis, gastroesophageal reflux disease (GERD), bronchiectasis, or ACE inhibitor use.

20. **The correct answer is B.** Angiotensin-converting enzymes (ACE) inhibitors exert their vasodilator effect by inhibiting the conversion of angiotensin I to angiotensin II (a potent vasoconstrictor) and by blocking the inactivation of bradykinin. The cough is secondary to the accumulation of bradykinin. The cough can develop at any time during the course of treatment and is not dose related. The cough often is associated with a tickling or scratchy sensation in the throat. Resolution often occurs approximately 3 to 5 weeks following discontinuation of the medication.

21. **The correct answer is D.** A prolonged, paroxysmal cough lasting longer than 2 to 3 weeks associated with shortness of breath and posttussive vomiting is highly suspicious for *Bordetella pertussis* infection. This paroxysmal stage generally lasts 2 to 4 weeks and follows the catarrhal stage, during which patients experience low-grade fever, coryza, lacrimation, malaise, and mild cough. Lymphocytosis sometimes occurs in pediatric patients with whooping cough. A nasopharyngeal swab culture makes the diagnosis and is positive in about 75% of children and 50% of adults when specimens are submitted within 2 weeks of onset of symptoms. The treatment of choice is erythromycin, but macrolide antibiotics have demonstrated excellent activity against *B. pertussis*.

22. **The correct answer is A.** The pathophysiology of emphysema involves the distention of the air spaces distal to the terminal bronchiole with destruction of the alveolar walls, without evidence of fibrosis. Hyperirritability and mucus plugging are seen in asthma, whereas mucous gland hypertrophy is indicative of chronic bronchitis.

23. **The correct answer is C.** Although all of these patients are at increased risk, the single most potent risk factor for the development of active tuberculosis is HIV coinfection. The risk is directly proportional to the degree of cellular immunity depression, ultimately the CD4 count.

24. **The correct answer is B.** With a decreased pH, increased $PaCO_2$, and increased HCO_3, the patient demonstrates compensated respiratory acidosis. He essentially retains CO_2 because of impaired ventilation, and his kidneys attempt to compensate by reabsorbing more bicarbonate to maintain a more homeostatic pH. In chronic compensated respiratory acidosis, for every 10 point rise in pCO_2 above 40 mmHg, there is a 0.03 decrease in pH from 7.40.

25. **The correct answer is D.** Iatrogenic pneumothorax is a complication of invasive procedures such as cannulation of the subclavian vein, thoracentesis, intercostal nerve blocks, bronchoscopy, and percutaneous lung biopsy. It occurs more often with apical procedures, because airflow is greater in the apices than in the lung bases. An increased angle of the needle or too deep a placement can nick the parietal pleura, promoting air accumulation in the pleural cavity. Mechanical ventilation serves to exacerbate this condition, leading to a tension pneumothorax.

26. **The correct answer is C.** Parainfluenza viruses (particularly serotype 1) cause croup, or laryngotracheobronchitis, in children. Symptoms include coryza, sore throat, hoarseness, and cough. In severe cases, the cough may progress to a barklike cough associated with stridor, leading to hypoxia and airway obstruction.

27. **The correct answer is A.** Atelectasis is responsible for nearly 90% of febrile episodes in the first 48 hours postoperatively. It affects one-quarter of patients who undergo abdominal surgeries. Causes include obstruction secondary to intubation or anesthetic agents. In most cases, the cause is due to the closure of small bronchioles. Shallow breathing and difficulty in hyperinflation of the lungs secondary to pain also contribute to the risk for atelectasis. You would not expect infectious causes of fever to present so acutely after a surgical procedure.

28. **The correct answer is B.** On pulse oximetry, carboxyhemoglobin would be falsely counted as oxyhemoglobin, which would show an inaccurately high percent oxygen saturation. Hypovolemia, shock, and hypothermia would result in decreased perfusion, leading to false low readings.

29. **The correct answer is D.** Approximately two-thirds of bacterial isolates in cases of community-acquired pneumonia are *Streptococcus pneumoniae*. On sputum gram stain, the organism appears as gram-positive diplococci aligned end to end, often seen intracellularly in neutrophils. On a blood agar plate, the organism is an alpha-hemolytic mucoid

colony due to its capsule, which serves as a virulence factor. A polyvalent pneumococcal vaccine provides capsular antigenic exposure to 23 common strains of *S. pneumoniae*. The vaccine prevents or reduces the severity of infection in immunocompromised patients, those older than age 65, and those suffering with a chronic disease.

30. **The correct answer is B.** COPD presents with hyperinflation of the lungs and airway narrowing, which lead to an increase in airway resistance and the loss of elastic lung recoil. This results in diminished maximal expiratory flow rates and air trapping within the lungs, increasing the expiratory reserve volume, residual volume, and functional residual capacity in patients with COPD. FEV1% is of clinical value because it not only reflects the pathophysiology of COPD, but remains insensitive to patient effort beyond a threshold minimum in spirometry testing.

31. **The correct answer is A.** Pleural effusions classify as transudates or exudates based on the sample determination of total protein, glucose, lactate dehydrogenase (LDH), and white blood count and differential. Transudates represent normal capillary integrity and the absence of pleural disease. They occur due to increased hydrostatic pressure (congestive heart failure being the cause of 90% of cases), decreased oncotic pressure (hypoalbuminemia and cirrhosis with ascites), and a negative pleural pressure gradient (atelectasis). Pleural disease, impaired capillary permeability, or decreased lymphatic drainage may cause exudates. Infections and cancer are the two most common causes of exudative effusions.

32. **The correct answer is D.** Trimethoprim-sulfamethoxazole (TMP-SMX) is the drug of choice because of its low cost and exceptional bioavailability. It is most frequently administered in its oral form, but may be given via IV in patients who are experiencing nausea, vomiting, or intractable diarrhea. Other standard therapies include parenteral pentamidine, trimetrexate plus leucovorin, dapsone, clindamycin, primaquine, and atovaquone. Supplemental oxygen and adjunctive corticosteroids help maintain oxygen saturation. *Pneumocystis carinii* reclassified from a protozoan to a fungus and renamed *Pneumocystis jirovecii* in 2001. Pneumocystis pneumonia remains the most common life-threatening opportunistic infection in AIDS patients, and often occurs in patients with CD4 counts less than 200 cells/mm^3. Infection presents with fever, exertional dyspnea, cough, and retrosternal chest tightness. Atypical presentation may be with spontaneous pneumothorax, especially in patients on aerosolized pentamidine prophylaxis. Chest radiographs generally demonstrate diffuse infiltrates in a classic "butterfly" pattern extending from the perihilar region, but may be normal in about 10 to 15% of patients.

33. **The correct answer is A.** Bronchogenic carcinoma accounts for nearly 90% of primary lung cancers, with cigarette smoking being the leading cause. The four histologic types of bronchogenic carcinoma, in order of occurrence, are adenocarcinoma, squamous cell carcinoma, large cell carcinoma, and small cell carcinoma. Adenocarcinoma develops from the mucous glands and most commonly presents as peripheral masses. Squamous cell carcinoma forms as sessile or polypoid masses from bronchial epithelium, which accounts for their central location. Initial metastasis is local. The presence of metastasis may be discovered through the presence of hilar adenopathy or mediastinal widening on chest radiograph. Large cell carcinoma represents a diverse group of tumors that may present either centrally or peripherally and progress rapidly in mass effect. Small cell carcinoma is bronchial in origin and extends locally in the mediastinum. Depending on the location of the lesion, sputum cytology, bronchial washing and brushing, bronchioalveolar lavage, or needle or open biopsy may make the diagnosis.

34. **The correct answer is A.** Studies confirm a strong association between past asbestos exposure and the development of malignant mesothelioma. Other risk factors include radiation and SV40 virus. Although cigarette smoking exacerbates asbestosis and increases

the risk of bronchogenic carcinoma in asbestos workers, no direct correlation exists between smoking and the development of mesothelioma.

35. The correct answer is D. Foreign-body aspiration should always be included in the differential diagnosis of a child younger than 4 years old who presents in acute respiratory distress.

36. The correct answer is B. *Klebsiella pneumoniae* is a common etiologic agent of community-acquired lobar pneumonia in alcoholic men older than age 40. These patients typically have comorbidities such as diabetes mellitus or COPD. Complications include cavitary lesions, abscess formation, and empyema.

37. The correct answer is C. The most common cause of acute respiratory distress syndrome (ARDS) is sepsis (in approximately 50% of cases) followed by trauma. As the patient in choice C has urosepsis, he is most likely to present this condition. Acute respiratory distress syndrome is characterized by an acute onset of hypoxia secondary to alveolar damage and diffuse, noncardiogenic pulmonary infiltrates. Predisposing factors include infection, aspiration, shock, trauma, massive transfusions, and drug ingestion.

38. The correct answer is C. Hyaline membrane disease is caused by a decrease in surfactant. Surfactant is responsible for reducing the surface tension in the alveolus during expiration. The alveoli remain partially open, thus maintaining a residual functional capacity. Diminished levels of surfactant, poor lung compliance, and atelectasis may progress to respiratory failure. Treatments include supplemental oxygen, nasal CPAP, administration of exogenous surfactant, and intubation, if necessary. Prenatal corticosteroids, such as betamethasone, given to the mother may accelerate lung maturity in the infant.

39. The correct answer is B. A sharp, knifelike pain that worsens with inspiration, coughing, and sneezing typically describes pleuritic chest pain. It is caused by inflammation and fluid accumulation in the pleural space, leading to an abrasive friction rub auscultated on physical exam. It generally resolves within a few weeks and should be conservatively managed with anti-inflammatory and pain medication. Pericarditis may also present as a sharp, usually substernal, chest pain and a noted friction rub; however, the pain usually worsens by lying flat and is relieved by sitting up and leaning forward.

40. The correct answer is B. In Cheyne-Stokes respiration there is oscillating periods of hyperpnea and apnea (alternating changes in rate and tidal volume) resulting in hypoxia. It may present in patients with congestive heart failure, stroke, or traumatic brain injury or during sleep at high altitudes. Biot's respiration is the rhythmic cluster of quick, shallow breaths followed by periods of apnea, generally due to medulla damage. Kussmaul breathing is characterized by deep, large-volume breathing, which is a respiratory compensation (blowing off CO_2) to compensate for a metabolic acidosis.

41. The correct answer is C. Using the classic normal arterial blood gas values of pH 7.4, pCO_2 40, and HCO_3 24, this is classified as an acidemia with a pH of less than 7.4. Next you must decide if this is metabolic or respiratory acidemia. Notice that both CO_2 and HCO_3 are abnormal. Now ask yourself: "Which of these has changed in the same physiologic direction as the pH?" Specifically, "Which one has changed in the direction that would create more acid?" The answer is that the change in pCO_2 to 55 is in the same physiologic direction as the change in pH, because more CO_2 creates more H^+ ions.

$CO_2 + H_2O \rightarrow$ carbonic anhydrase $\rightarrow H_2CO_3 \rightarrow$ carbonic anhydrase $\rightarrow H^+ + HCO_3$

The patient therefore has respiratory acidemia. Notice that the increase in HCO_3 is *not* in the same physiologic direction as the pH change, because if the increase in HCO_3 were the *primary change* causing the change in pH, the pH would be higher (alkaline), because more HCO_3 increases pH. The increase in pCO_2 is the primary change, the low pH is the effect, and the high HCO_3 is the kidney's *compensation* in attempt to keep the pH from becoming too acidic. The likely cause of this patient's increase in CO_2 is his respiratory depression from opioid overdose.

42. **The correct answer is A.** Allergen exposure is one of the most precipitating triggers for asthma exacerbations. Symptoms may occur immediately upon exposure or 4 to 6 hours later, as seen in delayed asthma attacks. Common inhaled allergens such as dust mites, cat dander, tobacco smoke, and seasonal pollen lead to airway hyperresponsiveness and inflammation.

43. **The correct answer is D.** As the radiograph shows, this patient clearly has COPD. There is no indication for theophylline therapy in a patient with an acute exacerbation of chronic COPD. However, if the patient currently takes theophylline on a regular basis, the theophylline should be continued with maintenance of serum levels in the therapeutic range.

44. **The correct answer is C.** Improvement in mortality rates secondary to lung-reduction surgery is uncertain, with no recognized reduction in mortality when compared to medical management.

45. **The correct answer is C.** Goodpasture's syndrome consists of the triad of diffuse alveolar hemorrhage, glomerulonephritis, and the production of antibodies to the glomerular basement membrane. Antiglomerular basement membrane serologic assays help to confirm the diagnosis and monitor efficacy of treatment. Both cytoplasmic and perinuclear ANCA antibodies are present in approximately one-third of patients during the syndrome's clinical course. Renal biopsy makes the definitive diagnosis. Streptolysin-O is an enzyme produced by *Streptococcus pyogenes* (group A *Streptococcus*). Antibody to streptolysin-O is of diagnostic value in confirming a past group A strep infection in a patient with the sequelae of scarlet fever, rheumatic fever, or glomerulonephritis. Infection with *S. pyogenes* is not associated with pulmonary hemorrhage or hemoptysis.

REFERENCES

Fauci, A. S., Braunwald, E., Kasper, D. L., Hauser, S. L., Longo, D. L., Jameson, J. L., and Loscalzo, J. (2008). *Harrison's Textbook of Internal Medicine*, 17th ed. McGraw-Hill Medical Publishing, New York.

Goldman, L., and Ausiello, D. (2008). *Cecil Medicine*, 23rd ed. Saunders Elsevier, Philadelphia, PA.

Gordon, B. R. (2008). "Asthma history and presentation." *Otolaryngologic Clinics of North America* 41(2): 375–385.

Stein, P., Woodard, P., Weg, J., Wakefield, T., Tapson, V., Sostman, H., Sos, T., Quinn, D., Leeper, Jr, K., and Hull, R. (2007). "Diagnostic pathways in acute pulmonary embolism: Recommendations of the PIOPED II investigators." *American Journal of Medicine* 119(12): 1048–1055.

Tierney, Jr., L. M., McPhee, S. J., and Papadakis, M. A. (2008). *Current Medical Diagnosis and Treatment*. The McGraw-Hill Companies, New York.

Wilmott, R. W. (2007). "Cystic Fibrosis Foundation guidelines for diagnostic sweat testing." *Journal of Pediatrics* 151(1): A2.

Cardiology

Jennifer L. Arnold, MHS, PA-C
Jill M. Cowen, MSPAS, PA-C
Wendy Eaton, MSPAS, PA-C

1. A 16-year-old female has been experiencing dizziness with positional changes and oc-casional palpitations for 6 months. She denies any overt syncopal spells, but states that she feels as if she has almost passed out on occasion. Witnesses state that she often looks pale and "clammy" when she complains of dizziness. No symptoms have occurred during physical activity. Her beverage consumption consists of an iced latte every morning, diet soda at lunch, a glass of water with dinner, and two hypercaffeinated drinks while doing her homework. The family history is benign, and her past medical history is otherwise unremarkable. Her orthostatic vital signs are as follows:

    - Supine, blood pressure (BP) 106/78 mmHg, pulse 68 bpm
    - Standing after 1 minute, BP 104/64 mmHg, pulse 78 bpm
    - Standing after 5 minutes, BP 102/62 mmHg, pulse 98 bpm (patient felt dizzy)

    A mid-systolic click is appreciated at the apex when the patient is moved from the supine to standing position. There is no murmur. The remainder of the physical exam is normal. Her electrocardiogram (ECG) shows normal sinus rhythm, normal P wave height and morphology, normal PR interval, normal QT interval, and normal ventricular forces. Which of the following is the most likely cause of her symptoms?

    A. Intermittent paroxysmal supraventricular tachycardia
    B. Intermittent nonsustained ventricular tachycardia
    C. Hypertrophic cardiomyopathy
    D. Neurocardiogenic presyncope

2. Which of the following is the most likely cardiac pathology based on the clinical exam findings in question 1?

    A. Tricuspid valve prolapse
    B. Mitral valve prolapse
    C. Hypertrophic cardiomyopathy
    D. Ventricular septal defect

3. Which of the following is the most appropriate first-line treatment for the patient in question 1?

    A. Eliminate caffeinated beverages and increase water intake.
    B. Prescribe fludrocortisone 0.1 mg by mouth twice daily.
    C. Prescribe midodrine 5 mg by mouth three times daily.
    D. Refer the patient to an electrophysiologist for radiofrequency ablation.

4. If the patient from question 1 had the ECG shown below, which of the following would be the most likely cause of her symptoms?

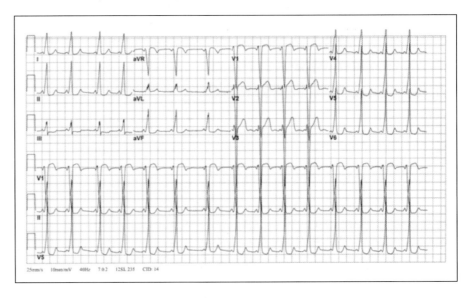

A. Intermittent supraventricular tachycardia in the setting of Wolff-Parkinson-White (WPW) syndrome
B. Intermittent ventricular tachycardia in the setting of long QTc syndrome
C. First-degree atrioventricular block
D. Complete heart block

5. A 65-year-old African American male enters the emergency department with complaints of chest discomfort. He appears uncomfortable and diaphoretic and is breathing irregularly. The ECG showed ST segment elevation in three leads. He has received morphine, oxygen, three doses of nitroglycerin, and aspirin without relief of his symptoms. Which of the following is the most appropriate next line of treatment?

A. Call the cardiothoracic surgery team for immediate coronary artery bypass grafting (CABG).
B. Observe the patient on telemetry for 24 hours.
C. Rush the patient to the catheterization laboratory for a cardiac catheterization and possible percutaneous transannular coronary angioplasty (PTCA).
D. Schedule the patient for a nuclear stress test to assess coronary artery patency with exercise.

6. The electrocardiogram for the patient in question 5 demonstrates ST segment elevation in leads V1, V2, and V3. Which of the following areas of the heart is affected?

A. Anterior wall
B. Posterior wall
C. Lateral wall
D. Inferior wall

7. A 35-year-old male comes into your office with a history of mild exertional chest pain that has been occurring for 3 months. He shares with you that his father had a heart attack at age 45. The patient appears to be well, is breathing comfortably, is not diaphoretic, and is not pale or cyanotic. His blood pressure in your office is 136/90 mmHg; his pulse is 75 bpm. The physical exam is otherwise normal. His resting ECG in your office is also unremarkable. Which of the following would be the most appropriate recommendation for this patient?

   A. Tell him that this is most likely musculoskeletal pain and that he should use a non-steroidal anti-inflammatory (NSAID) when needed.
   B. Because of the patient's family history, schedule him for a cardiac catheterization to image his coronary arteries.
   C. Schedule him for a graded exercise test to look for exercise-induced myocardial ischemia.
   D. Tell this patient that his symptoms are most likely related to exercise-induced asthma and schedule pre- and postexercise spirometry.

8. The patient in question 7 had the following fasting lipid profile: total cholesterol (TC) of 270 mg/dl, low-density lipoprotein (LDL) of 204 mg/dl, high-density lipoprotein (HDL) of 35 mg/dl, triglycerides of 160 mg/dl, and total-to-HDL ratio of 7:72. Which of the following would be the best treatment option based on the lipid panel and his positive family history of myocardial infarction?

   A. A low-fat, low-cholesterol diet and increased aerobic exercise
   B. An HMG coreductase inhibitor (statin); a low-fat, low-cholesterol diet; and exercise
   C. Gemfibrozil in conjunction with diet and exercise modifications
   D. A bile-acid sequestrant, such as cholestyramine, to block excessive cholesterol intake at the bowel level

9. The results of the graded-exercise test for the patient in question 7 are shown below. Which of the following would be the next step in treating this patient?

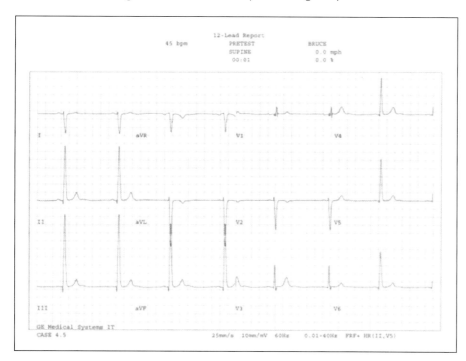

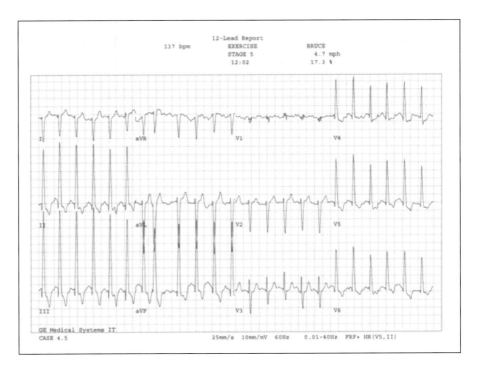

A. Send the patient home with instructions to avoid strenuous exercise.
B. Send the patient to the cardiac catheterization laboratory to evaluate coronary artery anatomy and the degree of blockage.
C. Send the patient to the operating room for immediate coronary artery bypass graft.
D. Tell the patient that these are nonspecific findings.

10. Which of the following is the most common pathogen responsible for subacute bacterial endocarditis following dental or nonsterile surgical procedures?

A. *Haemophilus influenzae*
B. *Moxarella catarrhalis*
C. *Streptococcus viridans*
D. *Streptococcus pneumoniae*

11. A 25-year-old IV drug user presents with a fever that has lasted for several days. A II/VI systolic ejection murmur along the left lower sternal border is found on physical examination. Additional findings include tender red nodules at the end of the fingers and toes; small, painless hemorrhagic lesions on the palms and soles; and linear hemorrhagic streaks under the nails. Which of the following is the most likely diagnosis?

A. Rheumatic fever
B. Kawasaki disease
C. Pulmonary stenosis
D. Subacute bacterial endocarditis

12. A tall, thin, 16-year-old male comes into your office for the first time. Physical exam findings are as follows: height greater than 95% for age; weight 50% for age; pectus carinatum; scoliosis; hyperflexibility of joints (particularly the elbows); arm-span-to-height ratio greater than 1.05; and arachnodactyly, demonstrated by a positive wrist and thumb sign. Which of the following should be your main cardiac concern for this patient?

A. Aortic stenosis
B. Aortic root dilatation
C. Bicuspid aortic valve
D. Mitral valve stenosis

13. A 65-year-old female presents with intermittent complaints of palpitations. She cannot remember the exact onset of her symptoms. She is otherwise healthy. Her physical exam demonstrates an irregular heart rhythm at 75 bpm and blood pressure of 110/70 mmHg. She appears well, with no diaphoresis, pallor, or cyanosis. Respirations are unlabored. Lung fields are clear to auscultation bilaterally. There are no murmurs, rubs, or gallops, and no jugular venous distention (JVD). Pulses are 2+ and equal throughout, with no edema, clubbing, or cyanosis. The remainder of her physical exam is within normal limits. Her ECG is shown below. Which of the following is the most appropriate treatment option?

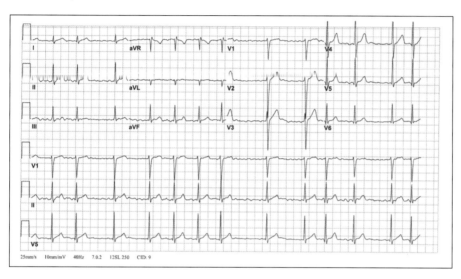

A. Attempt DC cardioversion in the office.
B. Schedule the patient for a transesophageal echocardiogram to exclude the presence of an atrial thrombus prior to attempting cardioversion.
C. Administer adenosine to convert the patient to normal sinus rhythm.
D. Administer lidocaine to convert the patient to normal sinus rhythm.

14. A 3-year-old boy presents to the emergency room with a 7-day history of fever, with a maximum temperature of 104°F. He appears very uncomfortable. Physical exam findings include bilateral nonexudative conjunctivitis; erythemic tongue, with red, dry, cracked lips; diffuse scarlatina-form rash; erythema of the palms and soles with desquamation; and bilateral cervical lymphadenopathy. His heart exam demonstrated normal heart rate and rhythm. You note a vibratory, II/VI systolic ejection murmur at the left sternal border. His pulses were 2+ and equal throughout. The remainder of the physical exam was unremarkable. He has no known allergies, is not taking any medications, and his immunizations are up-to-date. Which of the following is the most likely diagnosis?

A. Juvenile rheumatoid arthritis
B. Kawasaki disease
C. Rocky Mountain Spotted Fever
D. Stevens-Johnson syndrome

15. Which of the following is the main cardiac concern for the patient in question 14?

A. Coronary artery aneurysm formation
B. Aortic stenosis
C. Aortic insufficiency
D. Mitral valve insufficiency

16. A 13-year-old male presents to your office with complaints of bilateral knee pain and low-grade fever for 4 days. While talking with the patient, you note that he has a tremor. Physical exam findings include a new II/VI blowing systolic murmur heard at the apex. There is no click. You treated this patient for strep pharyngitis 3 weeks ago. Which of the following is the most likely diagnosis?

   A. Juvenile rheumatoid arthritis
   B. Mitral valve prolapse with mitral insufficiency
   C. Rheumatic fever
   D. Lyme disease

17. Rheumatic fever most commonly affects which of the following two heart valves?

   A. Tricuspid and pulmonary
   B. Aortic and mitral
   C. Aortic and pulmonary
   D. No heart valves are affected.

18. A 16-year-old male comes to your office for a sports physical. He notes intermittent leg pain, but has otherwise been asymptomatic. His blood pressure in the right arm is 150/86 mmHg. Other physical findings include a I-II/VI systolic murmur heard in the left interscapular region of the back. His pulses are 2+ to 3+ in the upper extremities and 1+ in the lower extremities. There appears to be a 1- to 2-second delay between the brachial and femoral pulse with palpation. Which of the following is the most likely cause of his symptoms?

   A. Peripheral vascular disease
   B. Essential hypertension
   C. Renal insufficiency
   D. Coarctation of the aorta

19. Which of the following is the treatment of choice for the ECG shown below?

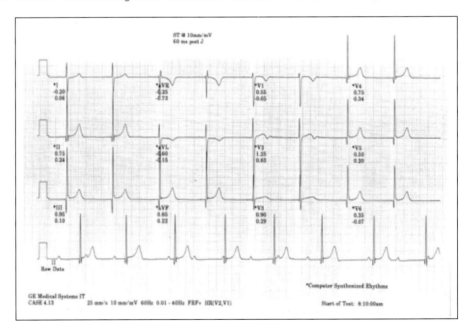

   A. digoxin
   B. Pacemaker implantation
   C. atropine
   D. epinephrine

20. A 75-year-old woman enters the emergency department with complaints of a moderate headache and trouble walking. She has a facial droop, slurred speech, and difficulty raising her left arm. She currently undergoes treatment for hypertension. Which of the following is the next most appropriate action?

    A. Obtain a CT scan (without contrast) of the head to rule out intracerebral hemorrhage prior to consideration of thrombolytic therapy.

    B. Obtain a CT scan (with contrast) of the head to rule out intracerebral hemorrhage prior to consideration of thrombolytic therapy.

    C. Obtain an MRI to rule out intracerebral hemorrhage prior to consideration of thrombolytic therapy.

    D. Perform no diagnostic studies prior to beginning thrombolytic therapy.

21. A 25-year-old female presents to the emergency department with complaints of chest pain for the last 3 to 4 days. She states that the pain is relatively constant, but admits that sitting up and leaning forward relieves her symptoms somewhat. She has a past medical history significant for lupus. She states that she had an upper respiratory infection with fever 1 to 2 weeks ago. Her ECG demonstrates global ST segment elevation. Which of the following is the most likely diagnosis?

    A. Acute myocardial infarction

    B. Pulmonary embolus

    C. Pericarditis

    D. Costochondritis

22. A 35-year-old female presents to the emergency department complaining of palpitations. Her vital signs are as follows: heart rate 180 bpm, respirations 14 per minute and regular, blood pressure 120/80 mmHg. Her lungs are clear. No other symptoms are reported. Her ECG is shown below. Which of the following is the appropriate treatment?

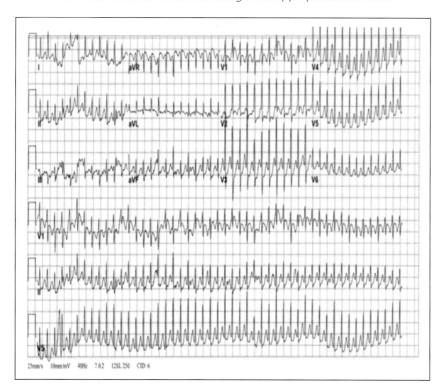

    A. Atropine

    B. Lidocaine

    C. Adenosine

    D. Diltiazem

23. A 40-year-old African American male has had elevated blood pressure during three separate visits. His blood pressure in your office today is 140/85 mmHg. Basic metabolic profile, urinalysis, and renal ultrasound are all normal. Which of the following is the most appropriate treatment for this patient?

A. atenolol
B. enalapril
C. lisinopril
D. losartan

24. A 65-year-old male complains of chest discomfort, fatigue, and shortness of breath for 2 to 3 days. He states that he had "real bad heartburn" 3 days ago. His blood pressure is 98/62 mmHg; his pulse is 65 bpm and regular. Respirations are unlabored. ECG shows Q waves in leads II, III, and aVF. Blood work demonstrates a normal CK-MB and normal troponin I. Which of the following is the most likely diagnosis?

A. Acute lateral-wall myocardial infarction
B. Old lateral-wall myocardial infarction
C. Acute inferior-wall myocardial infarction
D. Old inferior-wall myocardial infarction

25. A 45-year-old female involved in a restrained motor vehicle accident has developed tachycardia and tachypnea. A friction rub is auscultated over the left sternal border. She has a narrow pulse pressure, and pulsus paradoxus is noted. Which of the following is the most appropriate treatment?

A. Pericardiocentesis
B. Diuretic therapy with furosemide
C. Digoxin to improve ventricular function
D. Atenolol to correct the tachycardia

26. A 54-year-old male presents to the emergency department with a 20-minute history of crushing, substernal chest pain. His vital signs include a BP of 147/82 mmHg, heart rate of 73 bpm, and pulse ox of 96% on room air. He has an initial ECG that reveals 3-mm ST elevations in leads II, III, and aVF. Which of the following best describes his ECG findings?

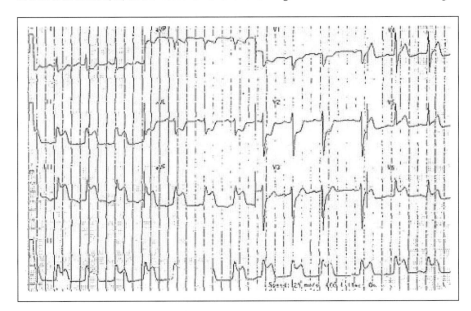

A. Pericarditis
B. Acute inferior-wall myocardial infarction
C. Acute lateral-wall myocardial infarction
D. Pulmonary embolus

27. Which of the following is the hallmark sign of Wolff-Parkinson-White syndrome on an ECG?

    A. Hyperacute T waves

    B. S1, Q3, T3

    C. Delta waves

    D. Diffuse ST elevation

28. Which of the following laboratory diagnostic tests should be included in the initial workup for atrial fibrillation?

    A. TSH

    B. C-reactive protein

    C. Homocysteine level

    D. Leukocyte count

29. Patients with known coronary artery disease should strive for which of the following LDL cholesterol goals?

    A. 200 to 300 mg/dl

    B. Less than 200 mg/dl

    C. 100 to 150 mg/dl

    D. Less than 100 mg/dl

30. Which of the following is *not* a typical sign of cardiac failure?

    A. Ascites

    B. Hepatojugular reflux

    C. Jugular venous distention

    D. Discordant blood pressures

31. A 23-year-old male presents with a 2-week history of waxing and waning chest pain that is worse in the supine position. On physical exam, you auscultate a cardiac rub. Which of the following would his ECG most likely reveal?

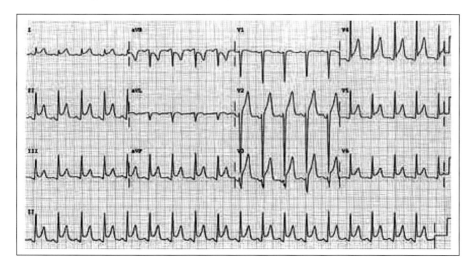

    A. Hyperacute T waves

    B. Delta waves

    C. Diffuse ST elevation

    D. Sinus tachycardia

32. A 23-year-old male presents with a 2-week history of waxing and waning chest pain that is worse in the supine position. You auscultate a cardiac friction rub on physical exam. He also describes a 5-day history of fever, cough, and malaise. Which of the following clinical scenarios best describes this patient?

A. Acute pericarditis
B. Acute myocardial infarction
C. Pericardial effusion
D. Pulmonary embolus

33. A 78-year-old female presents to the emergency department with a 1-week history of increased shortness of breath. On physical exam, she is noted to have a III/VI systolic murmur that is best heard at the right second interspace. Which of the following murmurs best describes this situation?

A. Aortic stenosis
B. Mitral stenosis
C. Aortic regurgitation
D. Mitral regurgitation

34. Which of the following pathological changes is typically associated with acute cardiac or ischemic events?

A. Acute vasospasm and associated hypertension
B. Heavily calcified atherosclerotic plaque with significant vessel occlusion
C. Thrombosis formation at the site of a ruptured atherosclerotic plaque
D. Vessel occlusion/obstruction by atherosclerotic plaque

35. A 49-year-old male is status-post lateral-wall myocardial infarction 1 day ago. He is currently awaiting coronary artery bypass graft (CABG) surgery. He is on heparin and a nitroglycerin drip. Suddenly, he develops stabbing chest pain and shortness of breath. On auscultation of the heart, you hear a new harsh holosystolic murmur along the left sternal border, and you palpate a thrill in the same area. The patient's cardiac index has dropped and his pulmonary artery (PA) pressures have increased. Which of the following is the most likely cause of the patient's chest pain?

A. Mitral stenosis
B. Postinfarction atrial septal defect
C. Left ventricular aneurysm
D. Postinfarction ventricular septal defect

36. Which of the following is the most common cause of mitral stenosis?

A. Rheumatic fever secondary to group A streptococcal pharyngitis
B. Rheumatic fever secondary to *Haemophilus influenzae* infection
C. Idiopathic calcification of the valve
D. Atrial myxomas

37. A 70-year-old woman presents complaining of increasing dyspnea. She states that the dyspnea used to be on exertion, but now occurs at rest and at night and is accompanied by orthopnea. On physical exam, there is 2+ pedal edema, rales in the bilateral lung bases, and a low-pitched diastolic rumble auscultated at the apex with the bell of the stethoscope. The patient's chest x-ray is shown below. Which of the following is the most likely diagnosis?

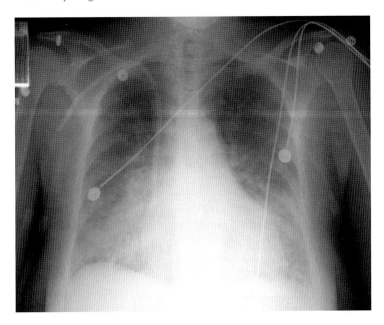

- **A.** Tricuspid regurgitation
- **B.** Aortic regurgitation
- **C.** Aortic stenosis
- **D.** Mitral stenosis

38. With regard to the patient in question 37, which of the following is the next most appropriate diagnostic study?

- **A.** Arteriogram
- **B.** Transesophageal echocardiogram (TEE)
- **C.** Chest CT
- **D.** Electrocardiogram (ECG)

39. Which of the following valves is the most likely to become infected in a patient with infective endocarditis?

- **A.** Tricuspid (native)
- **B.** Pulmonic (prosthetic)
- **C.** Aortic (native)
- **D.** Mitral (prosthetic)

40. Which of the following physiologic changes can occur in mitral regurgitation, but typically does not occur in mitral stenosis?

- **A.** Chronic volume overload in left ventricle
- **B.** Symptoms of dyspnea and pulmonary edema
- **C.** Right ventricular failure
- **D.** Pulmonary arterial hypertension

41. A 70-year-old male presents complaining of increasing shortness of breath while climbing the steps in his home. Two weeks prior to this event, he was able to climb eight steps without feeling short of breath, now he can only climb four steps before stopping to "catch his breath." He denies chest pain, orthopnea, paroxysmal nocturnal dyspnea (PND), and cough. On physical examination, you note jugular vein distension, 1+ pedal edema, and slight bibasilar rales. Which of the following New York Heart Association classes would best describe this patient's heart failure?

A. Class IV
B. Class III
C. Class II
D. Class I

42. Which of the following is a congenital heart disease characterized by downward displacement of the septal and posterior leaflets of the tricuspid valve into the right ventricle?

A. Ebstein anomaly
B. Marfan syndrome
C. Coarctation of the aorta
D. Ventricular septal defect

43. A 68-year-old female postop patient is in the ICU on maximum doses of norepinephrine and dobutamine. Her hemoglobin is 10 mg/dL. The nurse is unable to keep her blood pressure above 90/50 mmHg with volume (D5-1/2normal saline), and she has a positive Kussmaul sign along with pulsus paradoxus. Her emergent CT is shown below. Which of the following is the most appropriate treatment?

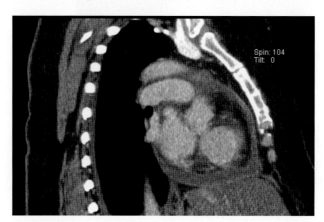

A. Thoracentesis
B. Tube thoracostomy
C. Pericardiocentesis
D. Blood transfusion

44. Which of the following correctly describes the chest radiograph shown below?

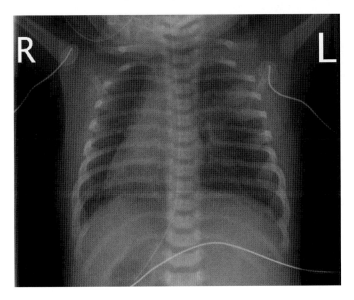

A. Mesocardia
B. Dextrocardia with situs inversus
C. Levocardia
D. Dextrocardia with situs solitus

45. Which of the following heart sounds is due to the flow of blood from the atria to the ventricles as the mitral and tricuspid valves open during early diastole? (In older adults, this sound is indicative of congestive heart failure.)

A. S_3
B. S_1
C. S_4
D. S_2 split

46. Which of the following symptoms, as described by patients, is most consistent with right-side heart failure?

A. "I have difficulty breathing while climbing stairs."
B. "I have a gnawing pain just under my lower right rib."
C. "I need to sleep upright in a recliner to breathe."
D. "I sometimes wake up at night gasping for air."

47. A 69-year-old male who is 5 weeks status-post anterior-wall myocardial infarction presents to your office complaining of a persistent low-grade fever and pleuritic chest pain that worsens with deep inspiration for the past 2 to 3 days. The patient is mildly tachycardic, and the ECG shows no acute changes. On auscultation, you note a transient pericardial friction rub at the left sternal border. Spiral CT of the chest is negative, and an echocardiogram reveals a small pericardial effusion. Which of the following is the most likely diagnosis?

A. Community-acquired pneumonia
B. Costochondritis
C. Dressler's syndrome
D. Pulmonary embolism

48. Which of the following is *not* an anatomical finding in the congenital heart defect known as tetralogy of Fallot?

    A. Atrial septal defect
    B. Overriding aorta
    C. Pulmonic stenosis
    D. Right ventricular hypertrophy

ANSWERS

1. **The correct answer is D.** Neurocardiogenic presyncope, also known as vasovagal presyncope, is an inappropriate increase in vagal efferent activity, often resulting from a precedent increase in sympathetic cardiac stimulation. The patient's dizziness with positional changes, palpitations, and history of pallor and diaphoresis reflect this disorder; however, these symptoms are also associated with cardiac dysrhythmia. As such, the diagnosis of neurocardiogenic presyncope is often a diagnosis of exclusion. Positive orthostatic vital signs (eliciting symptoms with position change, increase in heart rate by 30 bpm, or drop in systolic blood pressure greater than 20 mmHg) are consistent with neurocardiogenic presyncope. Additionally, this patient is most likely dehydrated, because most of her fluid consumption contains caffeine (a diuretic), which would predispose her to neurocardiogenic symptoms. Lack of symptoms with exercise is reassuring; symptoms with exercise should receive further evaluation for a cardiac dysrhythmia or structural heart defect. Additionally, there is no family history of cardiomyopathy, cardiac dysrhythmia, or sudden death. Intermittent supraventricular tachycardia is less likely, because her PR interval is normal (no pre-excitation/delta wave), suggesting Wolff-Parkinson-White syndrome. Ventricular tachycardia is unlikely, because her QTc interval is normal. If her QTc interval prolongs, she would be at risk for development of torsades de pointe, a form of ventricular tachycardia that will quickly decompensate to ventricular fibrillation. In addition, the patient's heart size is normal, because there is no indication of ventricular enlargement on the ECG. Increased ventricular mass is associated with an increased risk for development of ventricular ectopy. Because her heart size is normal, hypertrophic cardiomyopathy would be incorrect.

2. **The correct answer is B.** A mid-systolic click heard at the apex is diagnostic for mitral valve prolapse. This click often accentuates when the patient is moved from supine to standing, as well as from standing to squatting. Tricuspid valve prolapse produces a mid-systolic click along the left sternal border and is often located higher on the chest compared to the click of mitral valve prolapse. Occasionally, patients with hypertrophic cardiomyopathy may have a harsh systolic ejection murmur heard at the left sternal border. A harsh holosystolic murmur is associated with a ventricular septal defect.

3. **The correct answer is A.** Once the diagnosis of neurocardiogenic presyncope is established, the first line of therapy is lifestyle modifications. Eliminating caffeinated beverages, increasing noncaffeinated fluid intake, and increasing salt intake (to improve intravascular volume) will resolve symptoms in 90 to 95% of patients. Fludrocortisone (a glucocorticoid) once daily is the next line of therapy if lifestyle modifications alone are not enough. Midodrine hydrochloride (a vasopressor) may be used if lifestyle modifications are ineffective and fludrocortisone is contraindicated. If electrocardiogram changes predispose the patient to a cardiac dysrhythmia, then the patient should be referred to an electrophysiologist. This patient's electrocardiogram was "normal."

4. **The correct answer is A.** The presence of a delta wave (short PR interval with slurred R wave) is diagnostic for Wolff-Parkinson-White (WPW) syndrome. This would predispose the patient to development of supraventricular tachycardia. The patient's QTc interval is normal, thus eliminating long QTc syndrome as an answer. First-degree AV block is

defined as a PR interval greater than 0.2 seconds, or "one big box." Complete heart block is present when there is complete disassociation of the P wave (atrial contraction) from the QRS complex (ventricular contraction). This is not present in this electrocardiogram.

5. **The correct answer is C.** This patient is having a myocardial infarction. His electrocardiogram shows isolated ST segment elevation, indicating myocardial injury (evolving heart attack). After receiving the appropriate medications in the emergency department, admission to the cardiac catheterization laboratory for a coronary angiography and possible percutaneous transluminal coronary angioplasty (PTCA) is most appropriate. Sending the patient to the operating room prior to obtaining the angiogram would be incorrect, because revascularization of the patient without surgery may be possible. Observing this patient for 24 hours would not be appropriate, due to the fact that this patient did not respond to initial medical therapy and requires immediate intervention to minimize myocardial injury/death. The patient will require further testing at some point, most likely a nuclear stress test. However, revascularization of the heart muscle must be accomplished first in this case.

6. **The correct answer is A.** V1, V2, and V3 are associated with the anterior wall of the heart. Posterior-wall injury would be associated with ST segment depression in V1 and V2. ST segment elevation in V5 and V6 would be associated with lateral-wall injury. ST segment elevation in leads II, III, and aVF indicate inferior-wall injury.

7. **The correct answer is C.** The patient is clinically stable with a mildly elevated blood pressure. The family history of early coronary artery disease is of concern; however, more testing is required before scheduling an invasive study, such as a catheterization. If the patient had a positive stress test, then cardiac catheterization is indicated. Angina, asthma, and musculoskeletal pain are all included in the differential diagnosis of chest pain. Exercise-related asthma is often associated with a postexercise cough, which the patient did not report. Additionally, because of the patient's family history of coronary disease, and only after a coronary cause of symptoms has been ruled out should the clinician consider asthma studies. Musculoskeletal pain is a common cause of chest pain in young people; however, because of the patient's family history the differential of musculoskeletal pain is not a consideration as a cause of the patient's pain until angina is ruled out.

8. **The correct answer is B.** According to the Adult Treatment Panel III (ATP III), this patient has a moderate to high risk of developing coronary artery disease. Therefore, statin treatment for treatment of LDL cholesterol would be indicated. The patient's risk factors include a positive family history for coronary disease, hypertension, and an LDL cholesterol greater than 200 mg/dl. With multiple risk factors, the treatment goal is to lower the patient's LDL cholesterol to less than 130 mg/dl. Diet and exercise alone would be inadequate given the patient's overall risk of coronary disease. If the patient's triglycerides were elevated, then gemfibrozil is indicated. A bile-acid sequestrant may lower the LDL cholesterol to a minor degree (approximately 15%), but would be ineffective as a monotherapy to reach the patient's treatment goal.

9. **The correct answer is B.** A horizontal ST segment depression of 2.0 mm is seen in multiple leads at peak. The criterion for a positive stress electrocardiogram is greater than 1.0 mm of horizontal or downsloping ST segment depression measured 80 msec from the J point. The false positive rate is 10 to 30% when using this criterion; however, this significantly decreases when 2.0 mm of ST segment depression occurs. With a positive stress test, the patient requires cardiac catheterization. The patient does not require coronary artery bypass graft (CABG) surgery until after he has undergone a cardiac catheterization and it has been determined that percutaneous transannular coronary angioplasty or stent placement would not be possible. With a positive stress test, this patient requires further evaluation (cardiac catheterization) prior to discharge.

10. **The correct answer is C.** *Streptococcus viridans* is associated with approximately 90% of cases of subacute bacterial endocarditis contracted following dental procedures. *Haemophilus influenzae*, *Moxarella catarrhalis*, and *Streptococcus pneumoniae* are common causes of community-acquired pneumonia and acute otitis media.

11. **The correct answer is D.** Endocarditis should always be suspected in patients with a fever and history of IV drug use. Clinical findings for endocarditis include Osler nodes, Janeway lesions, and splinter hemorrhages. Clinical findings for Kawasaki disease include non-exudative bilateral conjunctivitis, mucosal erythema, strawberry tongue, erythema of palms and soles with desquamation, and cervical lymphadenopathy. Rheumatic fever typically follows a *β-hemolytic Streptococcal* infection of the pharynx. Clinical findings of rheumatic fever include polyarthritis, carditis, chorea, erythema marginatum (rash), and subcutaneous nodules. A systolic ejection murmur at the left upper sternal border would be consistent with pulmonary stenosis.

12. **The correct answer is B.** The patient has the clinical symptoms of Marfan syndrome, a genetic, systemic connective tissue disease. Patients with Marfan syndrome are at risk of aortic root dilatation and aortic dissection. Aortic stenosis, bicuspid aortic valve stenosis, and mitral valve stenosis are not associated with Marfan syndrome.

13. **The correct answer is B.** The ECG shows atrial fibrillation. There is no distinct P wave, and the ventricular response is irregular. The patient is stable with an appropriate blood pressure and stable heart rate; however, it unknown how long the patient has been in atrial fibrillation. With complaints of palpitations over an extended period, the clinician must assume that the onset of atrial fibrillation is greater than 24 to 48 hours. As such, a transesophogeal echocardiogram is appropriate to rule out clot formation in the atrial appendage. Furthermore, the patient should receive anticoagulation for 3 weeks prior to undertaking DC cardioversion. There is no indication to use adenosine, currently used for medical conversion of supraventricular tachycardia. Lidocaine is an appropriate medication for conversion of ventricular tachycardia or ventricular fibrillation to sinus rhythm.

14. **The correct answer is B.** Clinical findings of Kawasaki disease include nonexudative bilateral conjunctivitis, mucosal erythema, strawberry tongue, erythema of the palms and soles with desquamation, scarlatiniform rash, and cervical lymphadenopathy. The murmur is consistent with a functional murmur, which is audible because of increased blood flow through the heart in the setting of fever. Fever, joint pain, and a salmon-pink macular rash are associated with juvenile rheumatoid arthritis. Patients with Rocky Mountain Spotted Fever have onset of high fever, myalgias, severe and persistent headache, and a maculopapular rash on the soles, palms, and extremities. This rash eventually spreads centrally; however, there is usually no desquamation. Erythema multiforme presents with papules that develop target lesions. It is typically associated with Stevens-Johnson syndrome.

15. **The correct answer is A.** The risk of coronary artery aneurysm formation in patients with Kawasaki disease is 25% among those who do not receive treatment. Treatment with intravenous immunoglobulin (IVIG) within 14 days of the onset of fever currently decreases the risk of coronary artery aneurysm formation to less than 2%. Valve disease is not associated with Kawasaki disease. Aortic insufficiency and mitral valve insufficiency are associated with rheumatic fever.

16. **The correct answer is C.** This patient has clinical findings suspicious for rheumatic fever. Rheumatic fever is a clinical diagnosis based on Jones criteria and documentation of a strep infection of the pharynx. According to the Jones criteria, patients must exhibit either two major criteria or one major and at least two minor criteria. Major criteria include polyarthritis, carditis (aortic insufficiency and mitral valve insufficiency), Sydenham chorea, erythema marginatum (rash), and subcutaneous nodules. The patient meets one

major and two minor criteria: a new, blowing systolic murmur at the apex suggestive of new onset mitral insufficiency (indicative of carditis, major criterion); multijoint pain (arthralgias, minor criterion); and fever (minor criterion). Although joint pain is consistent with juvenile rheumatoid arthritis, these patients do not usually present with carditis. Patients with Lyme disease can also develop joint pain, but these patients present with conduction abnormalities (first-degree AV block), not valve disease. Auscultation revealed no physical findings, thus mitral valve prolapse is unlikely.

17. **The correct answer is B.** The aortic valve and mitral valve are the two valves most commonly affected by rheumatic fever. The most common cause of noncongenital tricuspid stenosis is rheumatic fever; however, the incidence of rheumatic tricuspid stenosis is still less than rheumatic aortic and mitral valve disease. The pulmonary valve is not affected by rheumatic fever.

18. **The correct answer is D.** Systemic hypertension in conjunction with weak pulses in the lower extremities and a palpable brachial/femoral delay are diagnostic for coarctation of the aorta. Additionally, a murmur at the left interscapular region of the back can often be heard. Patients with mild coarctation are often asymptomatic in infancy but develop upper extremity hypertension during adolescence. The patient's complaint of leg pain (claudication) is due to decreased arterial blood flow to the lower extremities as a result of coarctation. Claudication is also commonly associated with peripheral vascular disease (narrowing/occlusion of the peripheral arteries) caused by atherosclerosis. Atherosclerosis to the degree needed to cause claudication is unlikely in a 16-year-old patient. Patients with renal insufficiency may present with systolic hypertension; however, these patients would have normal four-extremity pulses. Patients with essential hypertension would also have normal four-extremity pulses.

19. **The correct answer is B.** The patient is in complete (third-degree) heart block. There is no association between the atrial complexes (P waves) and the ventricular complexes (QRS complex). As such, the patient requires pacemaker placement to reestablish atrial/ventricular synchrony. Digoxin is inappropriate in this case as it may be a cause of complex heart block in patients with digitalis toxicity. Atropine will increase the atrial rate, but will have no effect on the ventricular rate. Epinephrine is an antiarrhythmic used in asystole and ventricular tachycardia/fibrillation and would not be indicated for this patient.

20. **The correct answer is A.** In patients displaying symptoms of a stroke, the clinician should rule out intracerebral hemorrhage. Therefore, a CT scan without contrast should be performed prior to considering thrombolytic therapy. A CT scan is preferred over an MRI in an acute stroke patient, due to the fact that a CT scan is performed faster, and an MRI does not detect intracerebral hemorrhage well within the first 48 hours of a bleeding episode. Administering thrombolytic therapy to a patient with stroke symptoms resulting from an intracerebral hemorrhage would be detrimental.

21. **The correct answer is C.** This patient has pericarditis, as indicated by pleuritic chest pain and global ST segment elevation seen on ECG. Pericarditis often occurs following a febrile illness. Patients with autoimmune syndromes commonly present in this fashion. A pulmonary embolus would not have the finding of global ST segment elevation on ECG. Acute myocardial infarction would not have global ST segment elevation, rather ST segment elevation isolated to a specific region of the heart. Costochondritis, or chest wall pain, usually has a normal ECG.

22. **The correct answer is C.** Provided the patient does not have serious underlying heart disease, paroxysmal supraventricular tachycardia usually does not have serious side effects and most attacks will resolve spontaneously. Mechanical measures consisting of various Valsalva maneuvers have proven successful in interrupting attacks. Adenosine is the best choice from among the pharmacologic selections due to its brief duration

of action and negative inotropic activity should this type of therapy be employed. Because the half-life is less than 10 seconds, it must be given rapidly. Atropine is more appropriate for patients in severe bradycardia. Lidocaine blocks aberrant foci in the heart and therefore is typically administered in more serious situations. Diltiazem could be given intravenously; however, it has a longer half-life and therefore is not generally the first-line drug.

23. **The correct answer is D.** First-line pharmacotherapy for systemic hypertension is considered to be diuretics and angiotensin-converting enzyme (ACE) inhibitors. African Americans typically respond poorly to ACE inhibitors. Angiotensin receptor blockers (ARBs) are more efficacious in this specific population. β-blockers would also be efficacious; however, they are typically not used as a first-line therapy.

24. **The correct answer is D.** The patient has had an old inferior-wall myocardial infarction. Presence of a Q wave is diagnostic for myocardial infarction; however, the patient's CK-MB is no longer elevated. Serum CK-MB normalizes within 48 hours of myocardial cell death. Troponin I may be elevated for 5 to 7 days. Leads II, III, and aVF are associated with the inferior wall. Leads V5 and V6 are associated with the lateral wall.

25. **The correct answer is A.** The patient has cardiac tamponade most likely resulting from trauma. Pericardiocentesis is required to drain the excess fluid in the pericardium causing restriction of ventricular filling and decreased cardiac output. Diuretic therapy may be useful in mild, stable cases of pericardial effusion, but is inappropriate for this patient due to the severity of her symptoms. Ventricular filling and function are impaired due to the excess fluid in the pericardial sac. Until removal of the fluid is accomplished, medical therapy to improve ventricular function would be ineffective. The patient is tachycardic as a compensatory measure in an attempt to maintain cardiac output in the setting of decreased stroke volume. The tachycardia usually corrects once the excess pericardial fluid is removed.

26. **The correct answer is B.** ECG changes consistent with acute inferior-wall myocardial infarctions are as described in the question. Reciprocal ECG changes occasionally are observed during the initial period of the acute infarction, presenting with ST segment depressions in leads V1 to V3, 1, or aVL. Typical ECG findings in patients with pericarditis include diffuse concave-upward ST-segment elevation and, occasionally, PR-segment depression. Lateral wall AMI changes are usually confined to leads 1 and aVL. Reciprocal ECG changes occasionally are observed during the initial period of the acute infarction, presenting as ST-segment depressions in the inferior leads (2, 3, and aVF) or leads V1 and V2. ECG findings in pulmonary embolus are neither sensitive nor specific.

27. **The correct answer is C.** Wolff-Parkinson-White (WPW) syndrome presents with three characteristic findings on ECG (shown below): QRS widening, a delta wave(s), and a shortened PR interval. Segers, Lequime, and Denolin actually named the delta wave, even though it has been erroneously attributed to Wolff, Parkinson, and White. It occurs due to pre-excitation of the ventricles via a congenital bypass tract. It refers to the shape of the wave and not to any other cause. Ischemic/infarction episodes or pericarditis typically present with hyperacute T waves and diffuse ST elevations.

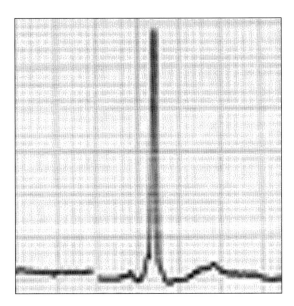

28. The correct answer is A. Atrial fibrillation is the most common cardiac complication of patients with hyperthyroidism and may present in 10 to 15% of these patients. This is usually due to the influence of the thyroid hormone on atrial muscle cells. Patients with poor cardiac fitness and unstable angina present with elevated C-reactive protein levels. Characteristic ECG findings of angina usually involve ST-T changes, and typically not atrial fibrillation. Elevated homocysteine levels are associated with a greater risk of myocardial injury due to ischemia in acute coronary syndromes. ECG findings in patients with leukocytosis are normal or indeterminate.

29. The correct answer is D. The literature shows that patients with known coronary artery disease benefit from increased high-density lipoprotein (HDL) and lowered total cholesterol and low-density lipoprotein (LDL) levels. An LDL count less than 100 mg/dl is ideal for all patients; 100 to 150 mg/dl is considered to be near or above ideal; whereas a count over 200 mg/dl is now considered excessively high.

30. The correct answer is D. Typical signs of cardiac failure include pulmonary congestion, peripheral edema, ascites, a distant apical beat on auscultation, hepatojugular reflux, and jugular venous distention. Patients with such conditions as abdominal aortic aneurysms typically present with discordant blood pressures.

31. The correct answer is C. This patient has acute pericarditis. Typical ECG findings of this condition are diffuse ST elevations. Wolff-Parkinson-White (WPW) delta waves and hyperacute T waves may present in ischemic or infarction episodes. Sinus tachycardia is nonspecific and can apply to a variety of conditions.

32. The correct answer is A. This patient presents with acute pericarditis, which is characterized by waxing and waning pain aggravated with supine positions. Pericardial friction rubs are frequently diagnostic of this condition. The patient's 5-day history of fever, cough, and malaise points strongly to a viral origin. Acute myocardial infarction pain syndromes are not positional, nor do they tend to wax and wane or typically follow a viral episode. Pulmonary embolism is also not waxing and waning or positional. Pericardial effusion tends to present with a constricting chest pain that is progressive and not intermittent.

33. The correct answer is A. The simplest way of understanding this murmur is by the location where the clinician best hears the abnormal sound. The aortic valve sounds transmit to the right second interspace, and the pulmonic sounds to the left second interspace. The mitral and tricuspid valvular sounds transmit best in the lower-left sternal border areas. Therefore, the practitioner now must determine whether the systolic murmur is one of aortic stenosis or regurgitation. The practitioner can classify systolic murmurs as aortic and tricuspid stenosis and/or mitral and pulmonic regurgitation. Typically, diastolic murmurs are mitral and pulmonic stenosis and aortic and tricuspid regurgitation. Furthermore, the murmur of aortic stenosis frequently presents in the elderly population.

34. **The correct answer is C.** The initial injury that occurs in atherosclerosis is damage to the endothelial cells lining the blood vessels. Factors that could lead to this injury include increased levels of oxidized low density lipoproteins (LDL-C), infectious agents, free radicals formed by cigarette smoking, or perhaps the shearing stress placed on endothelial cells due to hypertension. Endothelial cell wall injury triggers a cascade of events, which include the secretion of mediators that modulates the inflammatory response. They phagocytose the increased amount of lipoproteins from the LDLs and transform into foam cells. The arterial wall thickens as more LDLs uptake by macrophages and an atheroma is formed. An atheroma is a core of lipids and necrotic cellular debris resulting from dying foam cells. The smooth muscle cells produce collagen, which forms a fibrous cap over the atheroma. As compensation for the growth of the atheroma, the vessel dilates and allows for continuous blood flow. Eventually, the size of the atherosclerotic plaque encroaches on the lumen of the blood vessel causing a reduction in blood flow. Plaque develops most commonly in areas of increased turbulence, such as when the direction of blood flow changes at branches or bifurcations. The continuous elaboration of proteolytic enzymes by the macrophages under the fibrous cap initiates a breakdown of the collagen. As a result, the cap weakens and eventually ruptures. The atheroma and its thrombotic material are exposed and lead to the formation of a thrombus and ensuing emboli. This precipitating event could (and frequently does) lead to a myocardial infarction.

35. **The correct answer is D.** Extensive myocardial damage subsequent to occlusion of a major coronary vessel can result in septal necrosis and rupture. This usually occurs within the first week of an infarction. The presence of a ventricular septal defect is suggested by the loud holosystolic murmur, which reflects the left-to-right shunting across the ruptured septum. Such patients usually develop acute pulmonary edema and cardiogenic shock. A left ventricular aneurysm results from occlusion of a major vessel, which produces an extensive transmural infarction. The two most common presentations are ischemic syndromes and congestive heart failure (no murmur). Mitral stenosis may occur as a result of rheumatic fever; thickened valve leaflets and shortened chordae tendinae causing decreased forward output and increased pulmonary venous pressures, thus causing congestive heart failure. The murmur is a low-pitched diastolic rumble with an opening snap heard best with the bell at the apex. Atrial septal defects (ASDs) do not usually occur following a myocardial infarction.

36. **The correct answer is A.** The most common cause of mitral stenosis is rheumatic fever secondary to group A strep pharyngitis. The etiologic agent for acute rheumatic fever is group A beta-hemolytic strep, not *Haemophilus influenzae*. Idiopathic calcification can occur, but is an uncommon cause. Atrial myxomas do not cause mitral stenosis.

37. **The correct answer is D.** Mitral stenosis occurs in later decades. The most common presentation is dyspnea, fatigue, and decreased exercise tolerance. The classic MS murmur is a low-pitched diastolic rumble with opening snap, heard best by placing the bell at the apex. The stenotic valve causes back up of blood in the left atrium, then to the pulmonary circulation, causing pulmonary hypertension, congestive heart failure, and Kerley B lines on chest x-ray. The AR classic murmur is decrescendo diastolic, and dyspnea usually does not occur until later in the disease. The AS murmur is a crescendo-decrescendo systolic ejection murmur, loudest at the right second interspace radiating to the neck.

38. The correct answer is B. Transesophageal echocardiogram (TEE) is the best diagnostic tool to assess heart function and valvular disease.

39. The correct answer is D. Infective endocarditis attacks prosthetic valves first, most commonly on the left side of the heart. As the mitral valve is anatomically on the left side of the heart (which, as most practitioners know, is the largest section of the heart), then reason dictates this would be the valve most often affected. It is postulated that prosthetic valves become infected first due to the foreign-body nature of the devices. Porcine valves have been used in past years in an attempt to reduce this; however the literature has not shown statistically significant differences between the two. As is well known, the pulmonic valve is on the right side of the heart and is less likely to become infected.

40. The correct answer is A. Mitral regurgitation (MR) and mitral stenosis (MS) can cause symptoms of dyspnea and pulmonary edema, right ventricular failure, and pulmonary hypertension. However, only in MR is the left ventricle subjected to chronic volume overload due to the leaky mitral valve and some volume flowing backward. This in turn causes less forward progress, which results in more blood volume left in the ventricle.

41. The correct answer is B. Class III demonstrates marked limitation of physical activity, which causes fatigue, palpitations, dyspnea, or angina. Class IV is the inability to carry out any physical activity without discomfort, with symptoms present at rest. Class II has a slight limitation of physical activity. Ordinary activity results in fatigue, palpitations, dyspnea, or angina pain. Class I has no limitation of physical activity.

42. The correct answer is A. Ebstein anomaly is a congenital heart disease characterized by downward displacement of the septal and posterior leaflets of the tricuspid valve into the right ventricle below the AV junction. Marfan syndrome is an inherited disorder of connective tissue related to a defect in fibrillin-1 protein and lesions of the eyes, lungs, skeletal system, and cardiovascular system. Coarctation of the aorta is the narrowing of the thoracic aorta just distal to the origin of the left subclavian artery. Ventricular septal defect (VSD) is a defect in the interventricular septum.

43. The correct answer is C. Pericardiocentesis is the best choice to relieve cardiac tamponade. If a surgical team is available, it is best to take a postoperative patient back to the operating room to explore where the blood is coming from. There is no need for a blood transfusion, because the patient's hemoglobin is 10.

44. The correct answer is B. No explanation necessary; however, for additional information, the clinician is advised to study the CT scan shown below.

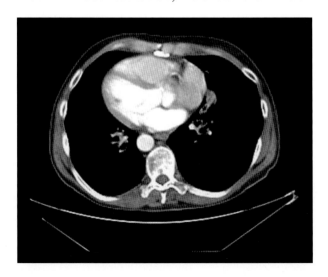

45. The correct answer is A. Although S3 may be physiologic in children and young adults, in older adults it is suggestive of ventricular volume overload often due to congestive heart failure. Auscultation of this is best during ventricular filling after S2. S1 is heard when the mitral valve closes and marks the beginning of systole. S4 is an atrial gallop representing atrial contraction, therefore auscultation of this occurs just prior to S1. An S2 split represents closure of the aortic and pulmonic valves; there is a loud component then a softer component.

46. The correct answer is B. Right-sided heart failure usually results from left-sided heart failure. The chief presenting symptoms of congestive heart failure include exertional dyspnea, eventually leading to dyspnea at rest; orthopnea; paroxysmal nocturnal dyspnea (PND); nonproductive cough; and nocturia. Right-sided heart failure manifests with dependent edema, elevated jugular venous pressure, hepatomegaly, and liver congestion. These symptoms may be perceived as right upper abdominal discomfort due to hepatic congestion and liver capsular distention, so the clinician is advised to be vigilant in this regard.

47. The correct answer is C. Dressler's syndrome is an inflammatory response characterized by low-grade fever, chest pain, and pericardial effusion, which can occur approximately 1 to 6 weeks following pericardiotomy or myocardial infarction. Complications can include constrictive pericarditis or cardiac tamponade.

48. The correct answer is A. Tetralogy of Fallot involves the following anatomic malformations: overriding aorta, pulmonic stenosis, ventricular septal defect, and right ventricular hypertrophy. It results in low oxygenation saturations, and treatment is with corrective surgery.

REFERENCES

American Heart Association. (2007). *Advanced Cardiovascular Life Support Provider Manual*. American Heart Association, Dallas, TX.

Bojar, R. (2004). *Manual of Perioperative Care in Adult Cardiac Surgery*, 4th ed. Blackwell Publishing, Malden, MA.

Cohn, L. (2008). *Cardiac Surgery in the Adult*, 3rd ed. McGraw-Hill Publishers, New York.

D'Amore, P. J., (2005). "Evolution of C-reactive protein as a cardiac risk factor." *Laboratory Medicine* 36(4): 234–238.

Dudek, R. (2005). *High-Yield Heart*. Lippincott, Williams and Wilkins, Philadelphia, PA.

Hay, W. W. J., and Hayward, M. J. (2001). *Current Pediatric Diagnosis and Treatment*, 15th ed. McGraw-Hill Publishers, New York.

Lilly, L. S. (ed.). (1998). *Pathophysiology of Heart Disease*, 2nd ed. Lippincott, Williams and Wilkins, Philadelphia, PA.

McPhee, S. J., Papadakis, M. A., and Tierney, L. M. (2008). *Current Medical Diagnosis and Treatment*, 47th ed. McGraw-Hill Publishers, New York.

National Institutes of Health. (2004). "Update on cholesterol guidelines: More-intensive treatment options for higher risk patients." (Online). Available at www.nih.gov/news/pr/jul2004/nhlbi-12.htm. Accessed July 19, 2007.

Park, M. K. (2002). *Pediatric Cardiology for Practitioners*, 4th ed. Mosby Publishers, St. Louis, MO.

Prasad, R., and Kahan, S. (2006). *In a Page Cardiology*. Lippincott, Williams and Wilkins Publishers, Philadelphia, PA.

Way, L., and Doherty, G. (2006). *Current Surgical Diagnosis and Treatment*, 12th ed. McGraw-Hill Publishers, New York.

Electrocardiography

Charles Bortle, MEd, RRTNPS, NREMT-P

1. Leads I, II, and III encircle the heart in one plane and together define which of the following?

    A. Einthoven's triangle
    B. The unipolar leads
    C. The R-wave progression
    D. The anterior wall

2. Which of the following is the inherent firing rate of the junctional pacemaker?

    A. 100 to 120 bpm
    B. 80 to 100 bpm
    C. 40 to 60 bpm
    D. 20 to 40 bpm

3. When applying a typical three-lead cardiac monitor, the red lead is typically placed on which of the following?

    A. Right leg or lower abdomen
    B. Left arm or upper thorax
    C. Right arm or upper thorax
    D. Left leg or lower abdomen

4. The PR interval is measured from which of the following?

    A. The beginning of the P wave to the beginning of the QRS complex
    B. The end of the P wave to the end of the QRS complex
    C. The beginning of the P wave to the end of the P wave
    D. The end of the P wave to the end of the QRS complex

5. The rhythm shown below is an example of which of the following?

    A. Second-degree heart block, type I
    B. Third-degree heart block
    C. Second-degree heart block, type II
    D. Idioventricular rhythm

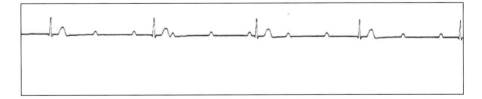

6. This 12-lead ECG demonstrates which of the following?

    A. Anterior-wall injury pattern

    B. Inferior-wall injury pattern

    C. Lateral-wall ischemia pattern

    D. Inferior-wall reciprocal change

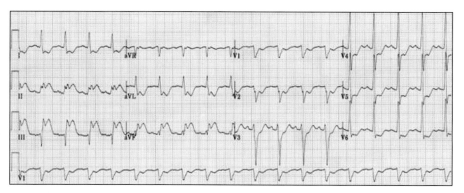

7. This 12-lead ECG demonstrates which axis?

    A. Normal axis

    B. Left axis shift

    C. Right axis shift

    D. Extreme left axis shift

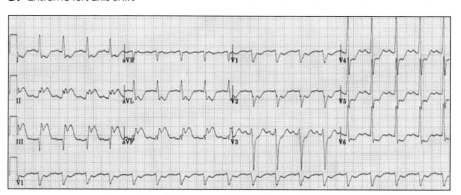

8. The rhythm shown below is an example of which of the following?

    A. Second-degree A/V block, type I

    B. Second-degree A/V block, type II

    C. Complete heart block

    D. Bundle branch block

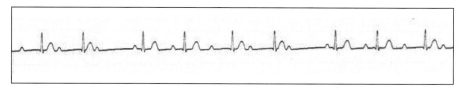

9. What does the following ECG illustrate?

    A. Multifocal premature atrial contractions
    B. Back-to-back premature ventricular contractions
    C. Frequent unifocal premature junctional contractions
    D. Multifocal premature ventricular contractions

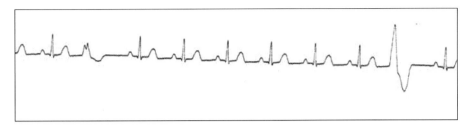

10. What does the following rhythm strip illustrate?

    A. Atrial tachycardia
    B. Supraventricular tachycardia
    C. Ventricular tachycardia
    D. Accelerated idioventricular rhythm

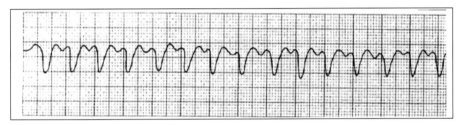

11. In the following illustration, which of the following is the R wave?

    A. The first negative deflection of the QRS complex
    B. The first positive deflection of the QRS complex
    C. The second negative deflection of the QRS complex
    D. The predominant component of all QRS complexes

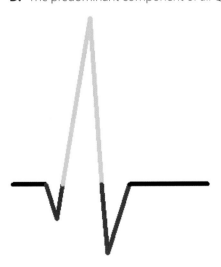

12. The rhythm shown below best illustrates which of the following?

    A. Ventricular tachycardia

    B. Sinus tachycardia

    C. Wolff-Parkinson-White syndrome

    D. Supraventricular tachycardia

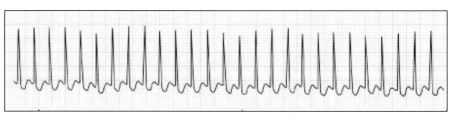

13. A patient appears to be in a sinus rhythm except that his rate rhythmically increases and decreases with respirations. This phenomenon is known as which of the following?

    A. Ashberger's phenomenon

    B. Sick sinus syndrome

    C. Lown-Ganong-Levine syndrome

    D. Sinus arrhythmia

14. Which of the following rhythms is the hallmark of atrial fibrillation?

    A. Irregularly irregular

    B. Regularly irregular

    C. Irregularly regular

    D. Paradoxically irregular

15. A consistent QRS complex that demonstrates a "swooping upstroke" is consistent with which of the following?

    A. Wenckebach's phenomenon

    B. Digitalis toxicity

    C. Wolff-Parkinson-White syndrome

    D. Bundle branch block

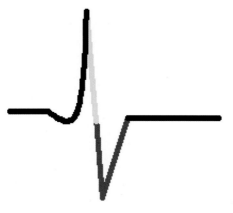

16. The complex shown below demonstrates a downward-sloping ST segment that resembles a soup ladle. This morphology is consistent with which of the following?

    A. Wolff-Parkinson-White syndrome
    B. Hyperkalemia
    C. Posterior-wall infarction
    D. The digitalis effect

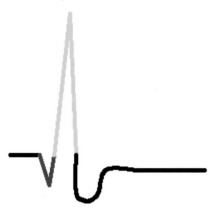

17. A patient who consistently has an ectopic complex every third beat, as shown below, is best described as being in which of the following?

    A. Bigeminy
    B. Trigeminy
    C. Back-to-backs
    D. Trifascicular block

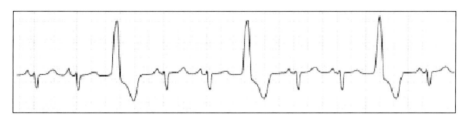

18. Which of the following best describes the rhythm shown below?

    A. Ventricular tachycardia
    B. Atrial tachycardia with aberrancy
    C. Ventricular pacemaker
    D. Idioventricular rhythm

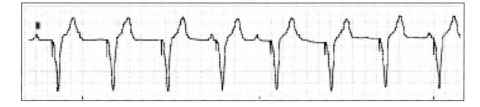

19. A patient with the rhythm shown below would be described as having had which of the following?

    A. A run of ventricular tachycardia

    B. A sudden-death episode

    C. A trimodal ectopic event

    D. A demand pacemaker activation

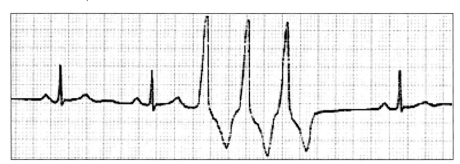

20. Which of the following best describes this ECG finding of a patient with hyperkalemia in the 6.0 to 7.0 mEq/L range?

    A. Shortened PR interval

    B. Left bundle branch block

    C. Tachycardia

    D. Peaked T waves

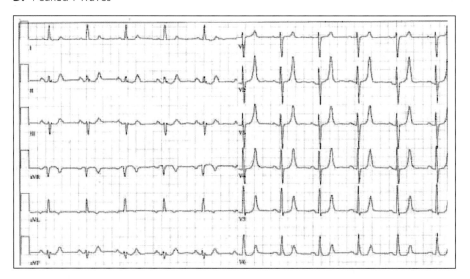

21. This 12-lead ECG best demonstrates which of the following shifts?

    A. Right axis shift

    B. Left axis shift

    C. Normal axis

    D. Extreme left axis shift

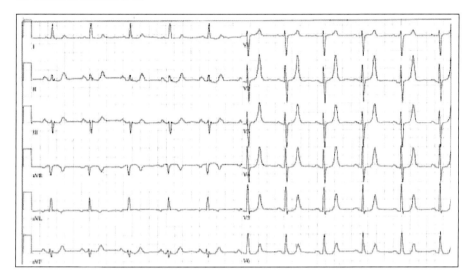

22. Which wall of the myocardium predominantly receives its blood supply from the left anterior descending coronary artery?

    A. Inferior wall

    B. Lateral wall

    C. Anterior wall

    D. Posterior wall

23. Which leads in a 12-lead ECG are typically associated with the inferior wall?

    A. Leads II, III, and aVF

    B. Leads I and aVL

    C. Leads V1 through V4

    D. Lead aVR

24. Of patients having an inferior-wall infarction, 10 to 50% may be "preload dependent" because they are also experiencing which of the following?

    A. Pulmonary embolus

    B. Bundle branch block

    C. Right ventricular myocardial event

    D. Pericardial effusion

25. How many ECG electrodes does it take to perform a 12-lead ECG?

    A. 14

    B. 12

    C. 10

    D. 8

26. What is the function of the electrode on the right leg when performing a 12-lead ECG?

    A. It allows you to view the inferior wall.

    B. It is the ground.

    C. It allows you to view the MCL1 lead.

    D. It allows you to view the right ventricle.

27. In an unremarkable12-lead ECG, the aVR is typically which of the following?

  A. An inverted lead
  B. An upright lead
  C. A diagnostic lead
  D. A triphasic lead

28. Which of the following best describes this adult ECG tracing?

  A. Hyperkalemia
  B. Hypothermia
  C. Bundle branch block
  D. Cardiac ischemia

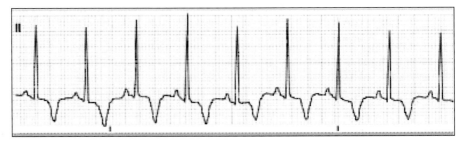

29. Which of the following is the most obvious pathology demonstrated on this 12-lead ECG tracing?

  A. Anterior-wall injury
  B. Inferior-wall ischemia
  D. Lateral-wall reciprocal change
  E. Posterior-wall infarction

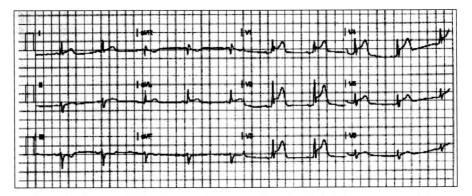

Questions 30–33 refer to the following electrocardiogram:

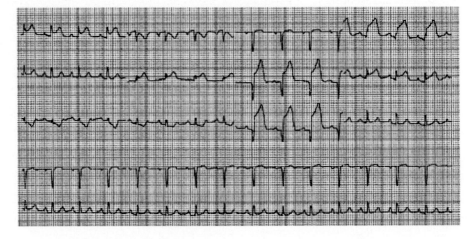

30. Which of the following is consistent with myocardial injury in the anterior wall?

    A. Peaked T waves
    B. Inverted T waves
    C. Tombstone Ts
    D. Widened QRS complex

31. To a lesser degree, the same pattern of injury is typically seen in which of the following?

    A. Lateral wall
    B. Inferior wall
    C. Reciprocal wall
    D. Right ventricle

32. Leads III and aVF demonstrate which of the following?

    A. Hyperkalemia
    B. Left ventricular hypertrophy
    C. A reciprocal change
    D. A right-axis shift

33. Which of the following would you see if you were to observe only lead II in this patient?

    A. Significant ischemic changes
    B. Signs of electrolyte imbalance
    C. Impending sudden death
    D. Nothing impressive

34. Why does this 12-lead ECG demonstrate a bundle branch block?

    A. The T waves are inverted in V5 and V6.
    B. The QRS complexes are all wider than 0.12 seconds.
    C. The rate is slow and irregular.
    D. The QT interval is prolonged.

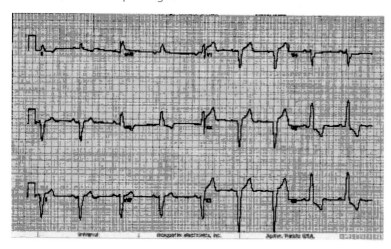

35. The axis on this 12-lead ECG demonstrates which of the following?

    A. Right shift

    B. Extreme left shift

    C. Left shift

    D. Normal axis

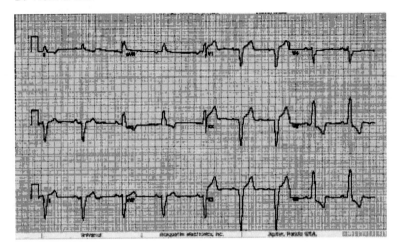

36. Which of the following best describes the rhythm shown below?

    A. Sinus rhythm with artifact

    B. Junctional tachycardia

    C. Atrial fibrillation

    D. Ventricular fibrillation

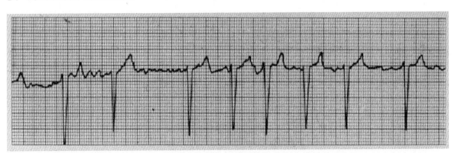

37. Which of the following best demonstrates the rhythm shown below?

    A. Ventricular fibrillation

    B. Atrial fibrillation

    C. Ventricular tachycardia

    D. Torsades de pointe

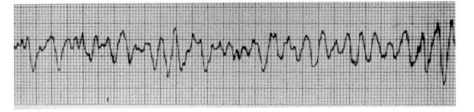

38. What portion of the normal ECG complex typically represents repolarization of the ventricles?

    A. The P wave
    B. The QRS complex
    C. The PR interval
    D. The T wave

39. Which of the following heart blocks demonstrates a progressively lengthening PR interval until a QRS complex is "dropped"?

    A. Second-degree, type II
    B. Second-degree, type I
    C. Third-degree
    D. Second-degree, type III

40. Which of the following is the normal width of a QRS complex?

    A. Less than 0.20 seconds (five small blocks on typical ECG paper)
    B. Less than one-half the R-to-R interval
    C. Less than 2 millivolts
    D. Less than 0.12 seconds (three small blocks on typical ECG paper)

41. Which of the following is true of a typical premature ventricular contraction (PVC)?

    A. It comes early in the cardiac cycle and has a noncompensatory pause.
    B. It comes late in the cardiac cycle interpolated between two normal beats.
    C. It comes early in the cardiac cycle and has a compensatory pause.
    D. It comes late in the cardiac cycle and blocks the next QRS.

42. Your patient is attached to a standard three-lead cardiac monitor, allowing you to see leads I, II, and III. You suddenly lose the signal in leads II and III, but can still see lead I. Which electrode came off?

    A. Left leg
    B. Right leg
    C. Left arm
    D. Right arm

43. Which of the following identifies a left ventricular hypertrophy on a 12-lead ECG?

    A. QT segment lengthening
    B. Notched R waves, or "rabbit ears," in the anterior leads
    C. Increased amplitude in the QRS complexes in the V leads
    D. A right axis shift

44. This rhythm strip best demonstrates which of the following?

    A. An idioventricular rhythm
    B. A sinus bradycardia
    C. A bundle branch block
    D. A junctional rhythm

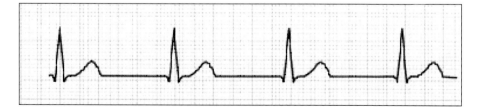

45. What does this rhythm best demonstrate?

    A. An artifact
    B. A ventricular flutter
    C. Sinus arrest
    D. Torsades de pointe

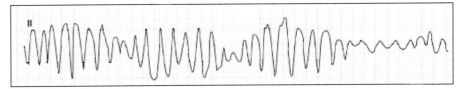

46. A patient has not survived his cardiac event and has received a pronouncement of death. Ten minutes later, a "code" is paged to the same room, and you are shown the rhythm strip below. The patient is apneic and pulseless. Which of the following best describes this cardiac activity?

    A. An interpolated beat
    B. An agonal beat
    C. A premature ventricular contraction
    D. An external electrical stimulus

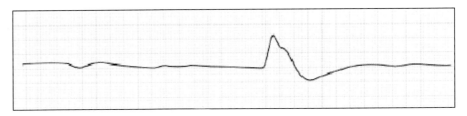

47. A patient demonstrates the rhythm shown below, yet he is apneic and pulseless. Which of the following best describes this situation?

    A. Pulseless electrical activity (PEA)
    B. Electro/mechanical dissociation (EMD)
    C. Pulsus paradoxus (PP)
    D. A/V dissociation (CHB)

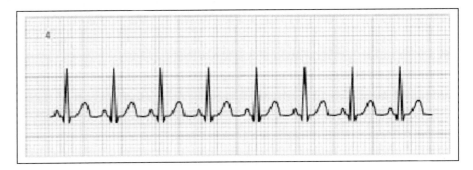

48. Which of the following ECG abnormalities best describes a group of syndromes probably caused by congenital issues with ion channels?

    A. Short sinus syndromes
    B. Long QT syndromes
    C. Poor R wave progression
    D. Early repolarization

ANSWERS

1. **The correct answer is A.**

2. **The correct answer is C.**

3. **The correct answer is D.**

4. **The correct answer is A.**

5. **The correct answer is B.**

6. **The correct answer is B.** Although there are many malignant changes on this graph, the most obvious is the ST elevation in II, III, and aVF (inferior-wall injury). There is a reciprocal change in the lateral wall (I and aVL), as well as ST depression in the anterior leads.

7. **The correct answer is A.** The axis is normal because the QRS is predominantly upright in leads I and aVF.

8. **The correct answer is A.**

9. **The correct answer is D.**

10. **The correct answer is C.**

11. **The correct answer is B.**

12. **The correct answer is D.** The QRS is narrow, making a supraventricular origin much more likely than a ventricular origin.

13. **The correct answer is D.**

14. **The correct answer is A.**

15. **The correct answer is C.**

16. **The correct answer is D.**

17. **The correct answer is B.**

18. **The correct answer is C.**

19. **The correct answer is A.** Three premature ventricular contractions (PVCs) in a row constitute a run of V-tach. Some might also call it a "triplet."

20. **The correct answer is D.** Hyperkalemia typically causes the following ECG changes: Peaked T waves at approximately 6.5. The QRS begins to widen, and the P wave shrinks as the PR interval elongates at approximately 7.5. Then the P wave is absent, and the QRS continues to widen, becoming almost sinusoidal at 8.5.

21. **The correct answer is B.** The graph demonstrates a left axis shift, because the QRS is upright in lead 1 and predominantly negative in aVF

22. **The correct answer is C.**

23. **The correct answer is A.**

24. **The correct answer is C.**

25. **The correct answer is C.**

26. **The correct answer is B.** The right-leg lead is the ground and can actually be placed anywhere on the patient.

27. **The correct answer is A.** aVR is typically "upside down." A common error in acquiring an ECG is to accidentally reverse the arm leads, or switch the arm and leg leads. In either of these cases, aVR will appear upright (positive deflection). Many practitioners look at aVR first to help confirm that the technician or person obtaining the ECG properly performed the test.

28. **The correct answer is D.** Symmetrically flipped T waves are the classic sign of ischemia. ST elevation indicates injury, and significant Q waves represent infarction.

29. **The correct answer is A.** The most obvious change on this graph is the profound ST elevation in V1 through V4, which is indicative of anterior-wall injury.

30. **The correct answer is C.**

31. **The correct answer is A.** Because both the left anterior descending coronary artery (anterior wall) and the circumflex artery (lateral wall) both arise from the right coronary artery, it is not uncommon to see both falls suffering similar ischemic changes when the lesion is high.

32. **The correct answer is C.** The clear ST depression in leads III and aVF reflects an inverted mirror image of the lateral-wall (I and aVL) changes. It is a reciprocal change.

33. **The correct answer is D.** Because lead II is the only unremarkable lead on this ECG, it would be possible to miss the event on this patient if only lead II was monitored and no 12-lead ECG was obtained.

34. **The correct answer is B.** The critical indicator of bundle branch block is a QRS width greater than 0.12 seconds, *not* "rabbit ears."

35. **The correct answer is C.** Lead I is upright, and lead aVF is negative. The axis shift lends support to this being a left bundle branch block.

36. **The correct answer is C.**

37. **The correct answer is A.** V-fib is chaotic and irregular. Torsades follows a repeating pattern.

38. **The correct answer is D.**

39. **The correct answer is B.**

40. **The correct answer is D.**

41. **The correct answer is C.**

42. **The correct answer is A.** Leads I, II, and III are bipolar, meaning that it takes two electrodes to produce the lead. Leads II and III share the left-leg electrode; in lead I the left-leg electrode serves only as the ground.

43. **The correct answer is C.**

44. **The correct answer is D.** No P waves and a rate in the 40 to 60 bpm range.

45. **The correct answer is D.** Note the repeating pattern that switches from predominantly positive to predominantly negative and then back again.

46. **The correct answer is B.**

47. The correct answer is A. PEA is any organized cardiac rhythm without a pulse. It is a more inclusive term than EMD.

48. The correct answer is B.

REFERENCES

American Heart Association. (2003). *ACLS Principles and Practice*. American Heart Association, Dallas, TX.

Dubin, D. (2000). *Rapid Interpretation of EKGs*, 6th ed. Cover Publishing, Tampa, FL.

Grauer, K. (1998). *A Practical Guide to ECG Interpretation*, 2nd ed. Mosby Publishers, St. Louis, MO.

Liu, R. (2006). "Right ventricular infarction." (Online). Available at www.emedicine.com/med/topic2039.htm. Accessed March 15, 2008.

Gastroenterology

Jon Shapiro, MD

1. Which of the following patients requires the most urgent visualization of the esophagus?
   A. 26-year-old male with intermittent dyspepsia
   B. 50-year-old male with dysphagia
   C. 23-year-old pregnant female with heartburn
   D. 45-year-old female with two episodes of self-limited hiccoughs

2. Which of the following conditions is associated with adenocarcinoma of the esophagus?
   A. Colon cancer
   B. Gallstones
   C. Barrett's metaplasia
   D. Duodenal ulcers

3. Which of the following events typically precedes bleeding from a Mallory-Weiss tear?
   A. Third trimester of pregnancy
   B. Violent coughing
   C. Prolonged diarrhea
   D. Gingivitis

4. Which of the following is usually associated with squamous cell carcinoma of the esophagus?
   A. Cigarette smoking and alcohol intake
   B. Barrett's esophageal lesions
   C. High content of gliadin in wheat bread
   D. Vitamin B_{12} deficiency

5. A 35-year-old banker has suffered mild reflux for years. After his reflux failed to respond to initial therapy, he received the diagnosis of moderate esophagitis without metaplasia following endoscopy. Which of the following recommendations for lifestyle modification is *not* appropriate in this patient?
   A. Elevation of the head of the bed
   B. Avoidance of fatty foods
   C. Elimination of fiber from the diet
   D. Avoidance of excessive intake of chocolate and caffeine

6. Following a stroke, a 76-year-old woman has begun choking when she drinks her iced tea. Which technique is most likely to provide useful information about her swallowing?
   A. Routine upper GI series
   B. Obstruction series
   C. Endoscopy
   D. Videofluoroscopy of swallowing

7. Why do esophageal varices tend to occur in the distal esophagus?
   A. There is no serosal lining.
   B. This is where the mucosa transitions toward the gastric type.
   C. This is the location of potential portosystemic anastomoses.
   D. Smooth muscle cells predominate in the muscularis layer.

8. A 42-year-old man undergoes an esophagogastroduodenoscopy (EGD) and is discovered to have a benign gastric ulcer on biopsy. Which of the following bacteria is associated with his ulcer?
   A. *Salmonella typhi*
   B. *Escherichia coli*
   C. *Staphylococcus aureus*
   D. *Helicobacter pylori*

9. Which of the following reasons explains why duodenal ulcers seen on upper GI radiographs do not undergo routine biopsy?
   A. The incidence of duodenal cancer is low.
   B. *Helicobacter pylori* only *infects* the stomach.
   C. Duodenal ulcers do not bleed.
   D. The small bowel cannot be biopsied without causing a perforation.

10. A 30-year-old woman undergoes workup for iron deficiency anemia and abdominal pain. Biopsy of the duodenum on endoscopy reveals flattened villi and lymphocytic infiltrates below the mucosa. Which of the following food components would this patient be most sensitive to?
    A. Complex carbohydrates
    B. Lactose
    C. Animal protein
    D. Gluten

11. Which of the following typically found in the small bowel by contrast radiography or technetium scan most likely explains gastrointestinal tract bleeding in a teenager?
    A. Meckel's diverticulum
    B. Lymphoma
    C. Adenocarcinoma
    D. Lipoma

12. Several years after a complete gastric resection for cancer, an 80-year-old man develops an abnormal gait and macrocytic anemia. Malabsorption of which of the following best explains this presentation?
    A. Calcium
    B. Iron
    C. Magnesium
    D. Vitamin B_{12}

13. Following a gunshot wound to the abdomen, a 27-year-old male has his ileum and ascending colon resected. Despite reanastomosis of the remaining bowel, he suffers persistent watery diarrhea. There is no nocturnal diarrhea. He has had no travel and no recent antibiotics. Which of the following is the most specific and effective therapy for his diarrhea?
    A. Oral narcotics
    B. Anticholinergics
    C. Cholestyramine
    D. Fiber supplementation

14. Which of the following can improve the effectiveness of oral replacement of pancreatic enzymes?

    A. Proton-pump inhibitors
    B. Loperamide
    C. Lactose
    D. Calcium

15. Which of the following does not travel through the hepatic circulation but rather is absorbed through the lymphatic system?

    A. Disaccharides
    B. Iron
    C. Polypeptides
    D. Chylomicrons

16. Which of the following is not a major causative factor in the genesis of peptic ulcer disease?

    A. Hypocalcemia
    B. Acid hypersecretion
    C. Nonsteroidal anti-inflammatory (NSAID) medications
    D. Infection with *Helicobacter pylori*

17. Which of the following flours is *least* likely to cause symptoms in a person with celiac disease?

    A. Wheat
    B. Oat
    C. Rice
    D. Bleached white

18. Which of the following does *not* contribute to the diagnosis of acute cholecystitis?

    A. Pericholecystic fluid
    B. Thickened gallbladder wall
    C. Dilated common bile duct
    D. Gallstones within the gallbladder

19. A 32-year-old woman originally diagnosed with ulcerative colitis (UC) develops a series of chronic draining fistulae on her perineum. Which of the following explains why her UC diagnosis is incorrect?

    A. The correct diagnosis is lymphocytic colitis.
    B. As a disease restricted to the mucosal layer, ulcerative colitis does not cause fistulization.
    C. The lack of hemorrhage rules out Crohn's disease.
    D. Granulomatous disease more often affects the jejunum or ileum.

20. Which of the following physical findings is most suggestive of acute cholecystitis?

    A. Rebound tenderness
    B. Epigastric tenderness
    C. Fluid wave
    D. Murphy's sign

21. An 18-year-old unrestrained driver develops left-sided shoulder pain following a motor vehicle accident. Chest, rib, and shoulder radiographs reveal no abnormalities. The patient develops hypotension. A CT scan of the abdomen is below. Which of the following is the most likely diagnosis?

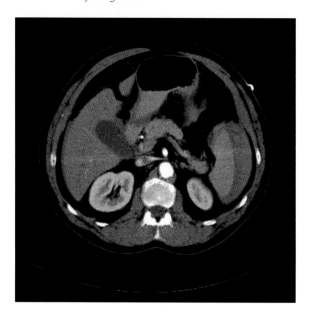

- **A.** Splenic rupture
- **B.** Ruptured aorta
- **C.** Gallbladder torsion
- **D.** Mallory-Weiss tear

22. An 18-year-old female college student has a history of chronic diarrhea and previous hematemesis from a Mallory-Weiss tear. On examination, she is thin and pale. She has erosions in the enamel of her teeth. She does not have enlarged lymph nodes. Her chest is clear, and the abdominal exam is benign. Laboratory evaluation reveals alkalosis. Which of the following therapies is the best treatment for this patient?

- **A.** Metoclopramide to enhance gastric emptying
- **B.** Loperamide to slow colonic transport
- **C.** Psychological consultation for a possible eating disorder
- **D.** Ursodeoxycholic acid to prevent gallstone formation

23. A 34-year-old man has long-standing complicated Crohn's disease with diarrhea. He has fistulas from his jejunum to his colon. Which mechanism is *least* likely contributing to his diarrhea?

- **A.** Small-bowel mucosal inflammation
- **B.** Stasis in the bowel with bacterial overgrowth
- **C.** Fat malabsorption from bile acid depletion
- **D.** Hypermotility of the colon

24. Which nutrient class empties most slowly from the stomach?

- **A.** Protein
- **B.** Complex carbohydrates
- **C.** Fat
- **D.** Simple sugars

25. A 64-year-old patient with diabetes has gradually developed postprandial fullness. She has nausea after dinner and occasionally regurgitates partially digested food long after the completion of a meal. Which of the following medications will be most useful in relieving her symptoms?

  A. Histamine type-2 receptor blockers, such as ranitidine
  B. Proton-pump inhibitors, such as omeprazole
  C. Calcium-containing antacids
  D. Metoclopramide

26. Which of the following best describes the mucosal changes of Barrett's esophagitis?

  A. Metaplasia
  B. Hyperplasia
  C. Hypertrophy
  D. Dysplasia

27. After weight loss, a 54-year-old man presents complaining of chest pain and regurgitation. You make the diagnosis of achalasia. Which manometric abnormality is *not* typical of this esophageal disorder?

  A. Hypertensive lower esophageal sphincter (LES)
  B. Incomplete relaxation of the LES
  C. Lack of peristalsis in the distal one-third of the esophagus
  D. Esophageal hyperperistalsis

28. Which of the following is best absorbed in the proximal small bowel as opposed to other segments of the intestine?

  A. Free water
  B. Iron
  C. Vitamin B_{12}
  D. Bile acids

29. Which of the following is *not* a risk factor for development of gallstones?

  A. Rapid weight loss
  B. Hemolysis
  C. Systolic hypertension
  D. Pregnancy

30. Which of the following is *not* an indication for surgery for peptic ulcer disease?

  A. Gastric outlet obstruction from an antral ulcer
  B. Gastric perforation
  C. Persistent bleeding
  D. Proximal location

31. Hypersecretion of what substance causes the hyperacidity associated with the Zollinger-Ellison syndrome?

  A. Gastrin
  B. Calcium
  C. Somatostatin
  D. Vasoactive intestinal peptide

32. You admit an 80-year-old woman for chemotherapy-induced neutropenia and fever. She receives empirical treatment with broad-spectrum antibiotics. Seven days later, she develops watery diarrhea. Which of the following antibiotic regimens should you start for her diarrhea after placing her in contact isolation?

  A. Metronidazole for *Clostridium difficile*
  B. Cephalexin for *Staphylococcus aureus*
  C. Vancomycin for methicillin-resistant *Staphylococcus aureus* (MRSA)
  D. Biaxin for *Salmonella typhi*

33. Which of the following is *not* helpful in the prevention and treatment of traveler's diarrhea?

    A. Avoidance of raw fruit and vegetables

    B. Bismuth

    C. Avoiding all tap water except ice

    D. Ciprofloxacin twice a day at the start of the diarrhea

34. Which extraintestinal manifestation of inflammatory bowel disease is more common in ulcerative colitis than in Crohn's disease?

    A. Arthritis

    B. Rashes

    C. Perianal abscesses

    D. Primary sclerosing cholangitis

35. An otherwise-healthy 45-year-old business executive tries to donate blood. The clinician advises her to consult her primary care office to discuss a possible chronic hepatic infection. Which of the following *cannot* be the cause?

    A. Hepatitis A

    B. Hepatitis B

    C. Hepatitis C

    D. Hepatitis D (delta)

36. Analyze the following serologic pattern and pick the clinical scenario that is the best fit. The patient feels well. He has no fever, icterus, or signs of cirrhosis on physical examination.

Hepatitis B: HBsAg–, anti-Hbs+

Hepatitis A: Hepatitis A IgG+ and IgM–

    A. Acute hepatitis A infection; immune to hepatitis B

    B. Chronic hepatitis A infection; immune to hepatitis B

    C. Immune to hepatitis A; chronic hepatitis B infection

    D. Immune to hepatitis A and B

Questions 37–39 refer to the same patient.

37. A 65-year-old male alcoholic presents with melena. He is not experiencing pain, nausea, or emesis. Which of the following sources of gastrointestinal bleeding is *least* likely?

    A. Gastritis

    B. Duodenal ulcer

    C. Colonic diverticulosis

    D. Gastric ulcer

38. Two months later, this same patient presents with shortness of breath and increasing abdominal girth. Paracentesis yields cloudy fluid with 600 WBCs per ml; 80% of these are polymorphonucleocytes. Which of the following is the next best step in evaluation and treatment?

    A. Culture the fluid and await sensitivities

    B. Call for immediate surgical intervention

    C. Perform a liver biopsy

    D. Start empiric antibiotics

39. The following year, the patient presents with worsening ascites. At this time, his serum albumin is 3.0. The ascitic fluid level albumin is 2.3. Which of the following is the most likely reason for this laboratory profile?

    A. This is a typical presentation of alcoholic cirrhosis.

    B. This is not consistent with portal hypertension.

    C. This is not consistent with malignant ascites.

    D. The paracentesis was probably contaminated.

40. Which of the following abnormalities is seen in both Crohn's disease and ulcerative colitis?

    A. Mucosal inflammation
    B. Fistulization
    C. Granulomas
    D. Transmural involvement

41. Which of the following does *not* correlate with the severity of acute pancreatitis?

    A. The appearance of the pancreas on the abdominal CT scan
    B. Serum amylase level
    C. Hypoxemia
    D. Hypocalcemia

42. Which of the following is the best method to diagnose perforation of a hollow intra-abdominal organ?

    A. Upright x-ray of the abdomen
    B. CT of the abdomen
    C. Ultrasound of the abdomen
    D. Physical examination

43. Which of following patients has the highest risk of developing carcinoma of the colon? The patient's colonoscopy is shown below.

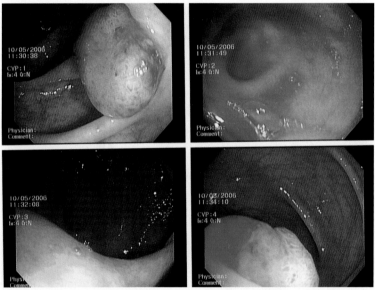

Courtesy of Christina Czyrko, MD

    A. A patient with familial adenomatous polyposis
    B. A patient with a previously cured rectal carcinoma
    C. A patient with 20 years of active ulcerative colitis
    D. A patient with three prior adenomatous polyps

44. Which of the following is the most common indication for hepatic transplantation in the United States?

    A. Nonalcoholic steatohepatitis
    B. Autoimmune hepatitis
    C. Hepatitis B
    D. Hepatitis C

45. Which of the following type of kidney stones is particularly associated with Crohn's disease?

A. Cholesterol
B. Hemosiderin pigment
C. Oxalate
D. Calcium pyrophosphate

46. A 12-year-old girl refers to you because of abnormal liver function tests. Her ALT and AST are normal. Her alkaline phosphatase level is twice the upper limit of normal. She denies abdominal pain or jaundice. She further denies nausea or weight loss. The physical examination is noncontributory. Which of the following is the next best step?

A. Order ultrasound of the liver, gallbladder, and bile ducts to evaluate the anatomy.
B. Order a CT of the abdomen to evaluate the anatomy.
C. Obtain a serum aldolase to see if the enzyme elevation is muscle based.
D. Obtain a serum GGT to see if the enzyme elevation is hepatobiliary based.

47. Charcot's triad represents the typical presentation of cholangitis. Which of the following is *not* part of the triad?

A. Pain
B. Ascites
C. Fever
D. Jaundice

48. Hypersecretion of which hormone is *not* associated with diarrhea?

A. Vasoactive intestinal peptide (VIP)
B. Somatostatin
C. Gastrin
D. Insulin

49. A 72-year-old male presents following a routine physical with his primary care practitioner due to the presence of heme-positive stools. His only complaint is an unintentional weight loss of 20 pounds over the past month and some vague abdominal pain. You obtain a barium enema, shown below. Which of the following is the most likely diagnosis?

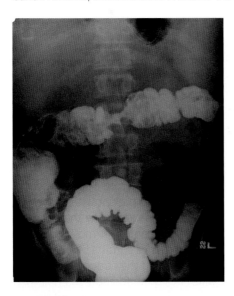

A. Sigmoid carcinoma
B. Transverse colon carcinoma
C. Crohn's disease
D. Ulcerative colitis

ANSWERS

1. **The correct answer is B.** Several symptoms—bleeding, early satiety, weight loss, and dysphagia—represent a high degree of diagnostic urgency, because they may indicate a malignant disease. Dyspepsia is a vague and common symptom for which empiric treatment is appropriate. Reflux symptoms during pregnancy are relatively frequent and rarely represent serious pathology. Prolonged hiccoughs may represent lesions in the upper gastrointestinal tract or in the thorax, and therefore warrant complete imaging. Occasional hiccoughs, however, are not a cause for concern.

2. **The correct answer is C.** Barrett's metaplasia is a change of the normal squamous cell mucosa to a glandular tissue that resembles the epithelial layer of the intestines. Barrett's metaplasia is a premalignant condition that warrants endoscopic surveillance. Adeno-carcinoma of the colon, duodenal ulcers, and cholelithiasis bear no direct relationship to esophageal cancer.

3. **The correct answer is B.** Pregnancy causes many gastrointestinal manifestations and complications, including fatty liver, increased incidence of gallstones, reflux esophagitis, and protracted vomiting. Nausea and vomiting are more common in the first trimester and could lead to a Mallory-Weiss tear. There is a more direct connection to answer B. Violent retching or coughing can lead to upward prolapse of esophageal mucosa. The torsion can result in bleeding. The symptoms are usually that of self-limited upper gastrointestinal bleeding with hematemesis of gross blood or coffee ground type emesis. Gingivitis can lead to dental problems and possibly other systemic effects due to the presence of high bacterial titers. It is not a cause of Mallory-Weiss lesions.

4. **The correct answer is A.** Tobacco consumption and alcohol intake are synergistically involved in the development of squamous cell carcinoma of the esophagus. The risk is dose related, with an extremely high relative risk associated with heavy use of both products. Barrett's esophagus is associated with adenocarcinoma of the esophagus. Gliadin is the antigen involved in celiac disease. Vitamin B_{12} deficiency causes hematologic and neurologic problems. Severe iron deficiency correlates with an unusually high incidence of esophageal carcinoma.

5. **The correct answer is C.** The literature and lay media alike report many lifestyle recommendations to reduce acid reflux. Although they are frequently rational, there is less than perfect evidence to support them. It is thought that avoidance of fatty foods, chocolate, caffeine, and nicotine reduces reflux via several mechanisms: reduced acid production, improved gastric emptying, and better bicarbonate secretion. Elevating the head of the bed and not eating close (within 3 hours) to bedtime may also improve symptoms. These latter two measures are probably the most effective. Dietary fiber does not affect the volume of gastroesophageal reflux or its symptoms.

6. **The correct answer is D.** Videofluoroscopy best delineates the static and dynamic details of the complex process of swallowing. Assistance from a speech/swallowing therapist can help with diagnosis and education of the patient with dysphagia. The routine upper gastrointestinal series involves still exposures while the patient is observed swallowing barium on a fluoroscopy screen. Dynamic wall motion and mucosal details are not generally seen well. The obstruction series consists of an upright chest radiograph and abdominal films. It is good at surveying the abdomen, particularly at zeroing in on possible obstruction of the intestines or perforation of a hollow viscus. However, it is not a good test for diagnosing dysphagia. Endoscopy performs well in visualizing masses, mucosal abnormalities, and large strictures. However, it can miss subtle strictures and peristalsis.

7. **The correct answer is C.** The connection between the portal and systemic venous systems occurs through preexisting connections at the microscopic level. As portal pressure rises, these connections enlarge and decompress the portal system by returning blood directly to the vena cava, bypassing the liver. The anatomy of the esophagus leads to early spread of cancer because of the lack of serosal lining. Striated muscle (voluntary) is prevalent in the proximal esophagus. Smooth muscle predominates in the distal esophagus, but this is not relevant to the location of varices.

8. **The correct answer is D.** *Helicobacter pylori* is the causative agent in the majority of peptic ulcers involving the stomach or the duodenum. The formation of ulcers depends on factors of bacterial aggressiveness as well as host response. *Helicobacter pylori* contributes to a spectrum of illness, from minimal inflammation (gastritis) to carcinoma. *Salmonella* infection of the gastrointestinal tract can cause diarrhea. Low gastric acid decreases the amount of bacteria needed to infect an individual. *Escherichia coli* is a prevalent gram-negative colonizer of the colon. Varieties of *E. coli* can cause invasion of the bowel wall and secretory and inflammatory diarrhea. *Staphylococcus aureus* is an inhabitant of the skin and is responsible for a large portion of soft-tissue infections.

9. **The correct answer is A.** Ulcers of the stomach may hide an underlying carcinoma. It is necessary to biopsy all gastric ulcers and follow them until complete healing. Carcinoma of the small bowel is sufficiently uncommon to allow empiric treatment of duodenal ulcers without biopsy. The other statements are false. *Helicobacter pylori* can infect the stomach and duodenum. Duodenal ulcers may bleed when they erode into the underlying tissue. When larger vessels are involved, the bleed tends to be more profuse. It is possible to obtain endoscopic biopsies of the small bowel safely. This rarely causes perforation.

10. **The correct answer is D.** Gluten sensitivity underlies the increasingly recognized disorder of celiac disease. A cell-mediated response to a component of many grains causes damage to the epithelial and subepithelial layers of the proximal small bowel. Malabsorption then ensues with subsequent abdominal symptoms. Mild cases may remain asymptomatic for many years. When symptoms occur, they commonly include abdominal cramping, diarrhea, and anemia. Deficiency of lactase leads to malabsorption of dairy products in many people, particularly adults. The symptoms overlap with those of irritable bowel syndrome and celiac disease. Animal protein and complex carbohydrates are not relevant to this case.

11. **The correct answer is A.** Meckel's diverticulum is an embryonic remnant formed in some individuals by the failure of a normal developmental structure to regress. It can present with bleeding or obstruction. The bleeding typically occurs as a result of acid production from the ectopic gastric-type mucosa. Lymphoma and adenocarcinoma are cancerous tissues that occur rarely and are unusual causes of small intestinal bleeding. Lipomas are common submucosal lesions throughout the gastrointestinal tract. They usually cause no symptoms.

12. **The correct answer is D.** Vitamin B_{12} absorption is a complex process requiring gastric secretion of acid and intrinsic factor. Surgical resection and chronic gastritis are two common causes of vitamin B_{12} malabsorption. It manifests as megaloblastic anemia and neurologic damage characterized by lower-extremity sensory deficits, spasticity, and gait disturbance. Cognitive dysfunction can occur as well. Gastric resection could affect absorption of other vitamins, nutrients, and trace elements, but such malabsorption does not lead to the same clinical presentation.

13. **The correct answer is C.** This clinical scenario suggests bile-acid malabsorption. With this likely diagnosis, it is reasonable to try a resin, such as cholestyramine, that can bind

the excess bile acid and prevent the subsequent secretory diarrhea. Narcotics, anticholinergics, and fiber supplements all have clinical utility in other situations.

14. **The correct answer is A.** Digestive enzymes are very sensitive to denaturation by acid. The bicarbonate-rich environment of the small-bowel lumen typically protects these enzymes. Proton-pump inhibitors can thus improve the efficacy of these oral replacements. Loperamide is a brand of antidiarrheal medication. Lactose is a disaccharide in milk. Many adults poorly absorb this disaccharide. Some individuals do need calcium supplementation, but this will not enhance digestion.

15. **The correct answer is D.** Triglyceride-rich chylomicrons are absorbed across the small intestinal mucosa directly into the lymphatic system. They travel to the venous system through the thoracic duct. The majority of nutrients are absorbed into the intestinal venous system, which feeds the liver via the portal vein.

16. **The correct answer is A.** Hypocalcemia does not cause excess acid production and does not contribute to ulcerogenesis; however, there is literature supporting an implication in peptic ulcer formation. Hyperparathyroidism would also predispose one to peptic ulcer formation due to excessive calcium production. *Helicobacter pylori* infection and use of NSAIDs are the cause of the vast majority of peptic ulcers. Acid hypersecretion occasionally contributes to ulcer production. The cause may also be idiopathic or caused by the Zollinger-Ellison syndrome.

17. **The correct answer is C.** Any form of wheat flour is pathogenic for patients with gluten sensitivity. There is variable blame for oats as a cause of inflammation in celiac patients. Some authors consider oats to be safe for most diets, but it is best to eliminate all gluten from the diet. This is due to the fact that even small quantities may worsen the disease and increase the risk of eventual cancer. Rice flour is well tolerated and safe.

18. **The correct answer is C.** Ultrasound does not provide a single diagnostic clue to acute cholecystitis. A dilated common bile duct indicates a pathology that is obstructing the ampulla of Vater or the common duct itself. This is not a sign of acute cholectystitis. Cholecystitis, or acute inflammation of the gallbladder, likely occurs due to obstruction of the cystic duct by a stone. Some of the diagnostic clues for acute cholecystitis include fluid around the gallbladder (pericholecystic); a thickened gallbladder wall; stones in the gallbladder or cystic duct; and tenderness when the ultrasound probe is pushed down over the gallbladder (ultrasonic Murphy's sign).

19. **The correct answer is B.** With ulcerative colitis, inflammation limits to the mucosal surface (see photo A). This patient probably has Crohn's disease. Because of the transmural inflammation in Crohn's disease, penetration and tunneling can lead to fistulas and abscesses. Lymphocytic colitis relates to collagenous colitis. Patients present with watery diarrhea and a normal mucosal appearance on colonoscopy. Mucosal biopsies reveal the characteristic collagen deposits in the colonic wall. Although hemorrhage is more common with ulcerative colitis, it certainly can occur in Crohn's disease. Granulomatous disease is difficult to see, particularly in the limited tissue sample provided by an endoscopic biopsy. Therefore, the absence of granulomata is not a criteria to exclude Crohn's disease. Ulcerative colitis is typically associated surface inflammation and is limited to the colon. Crohn's disease can occur anywhere from the mouth to the anus and oftentimes has skip lesions (areas of disease interspersed with normal intestine, as noted in photo B).

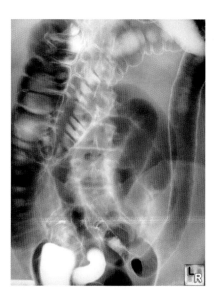

A. Ulcerative colitis

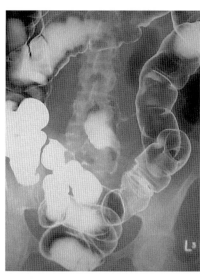

B. Skip lesions and cobblestoning

20. **The correct answer is D.** Murphy's sign is tenderness on palpation of the right upper quadrant of the abdomen. It results when there is pressure on the underlying inflamed gallbladder in acute cholecystitis. Rebound tenderness is one of the signs of peritoneal irritation. It is not specific for gallbladder disease. Epigastric tenderness can occur in pancreatitis, gastritis, and esophagitis, among other diseases, as well as cholecystitis. A fluid wave is one of the physical examination maneuvers used to diagnose the presence of ascites.

21. **The correct answer is A.** This history is suggestive of splenic rupture. The patient's abdominal CT scan confirms the diagnosis. This injury can occur in contact sports and motor vehicle accidents from trauma to the abdomen. Bleeding into the peritoneum causes pain, which may radiate to the shoulder and scapula following the phrenic nerve distribution. Rupture of the aorta can also happen in the same clinical setting. It may show up with a different pain presentation and without the radiation to the shoulder. Torsion of the gallbladder is rare and not trauma related. The patient would complain of right-sided pain. Mallory-Weiss tears result from coughing or retching and has the dramatic presentation of an upper gastrointestinal bleed.

22. The correct answer is C. With the scenario as described, one must be suspicious of an eating disorder. Laxative abuse is common among people with eating disorders. Mallory-Weiss tears and dental erosions can result from repeated self-induced emesis. This patient shows no clear clinical picture for gastroparesis. Decreased appetite, abdominal pain, and postprandial vomiting are some of the difficulties typically seen in this disorder. An empiric trial of loperamide is sometimes appropriate in the treatment of diarrhea. However, the clinician should investigate chronic diarrhea for a specific etiology to guide the treatment. Ursodeoxycholic acid is effective therapy in some hepatic ailments. It can be prophylaxis against the formation of gallstones during rapid weight loss.

23. The correct answer is D. When colonic contents contaminate the small bowel, the bacterial level rises. The subsequent overgrowth can cause steatorrhea and diarrhea. Small-bowel inflammation is present in this patient and contributes to the chronic symptoms. As the bacteria deconjugate bile acids, the bile pool depletes, further lowering the pool of bile acids available to digest fats. Colonic hypermotility is not a major contributor to diarrhea in this clinical scenario.

24. The correct answer is C. If there are osmotically active particles in the duodenum, such as peptides and fatty acids, this can cause neurohumeral signaling to slow gastric emptying. Fat decelerates gastric emptying the most. This makes sense physiologically because this nutrient class is the most difficult to digest.

25. The correct answer is D. When patients present with gastroparesis, diabetes is commonly the cause. The failure of the stomach to empty properly leads to fullness, abdominal pain, nausea, and vomiting. This contributes to the larger picture of autonomic disturbance that occurs in long-standing diabetes. Metoclopramide will assist in gastric emptying.

26. The correct answer is A. Barrett's esophageal changes are metaplastic. The tissue type changes from the normal squamous cell lining to an intestinal-type lining. *Hyperplasia* refers to an increase in cell number, whereas *hypertrophy* refers to an increase in cell size. *Dysplasia* is a spectrum of tissue changes, from normal to cancerous. With dysplasia, the cells appear more unusual in terms of morphology and misalignment in the epithelial layer. There is a direct relationship to dysplasia and risk of future cancer development. If there is much dysplasia, then there is a greater risk.

27. The correct answer is D. Achalasia is a motility disorder affecting the lower esophagus. It causes swallowed contents to remain in the esophagus because of the failure of the lower esophageal sphincter to relax. The baseline pressure of the sphincter is very high. The lack of peristalsis in the distal portion of the esophagus also contributes to the stasis.

28. The correct answer is B. The proximal small bowel excels at iron absorption. Water is absorbed well throughout the gastrointestinal tract. The colonic mucosa absorbs water from the fecal stream without much nutrient absorption or secretion. Vitamin B_{12} and bile acids are specifically absorbed in the distal ileum. Loss of the terminal ileum, even a short segment, may contribute more to steatorrhea than the comparable loss of intestine elsewhere.

29. The correct answer is C. Systolic hypertension does not cause cholelithiasis. Hemolysis causes bilirubin-based bile stones. Weight loss and pregnancy are both associated with stasis and poor gallbladder contraction.

30. The correct answer is D. Proximal location of a peptic ulcer is not particularly relevant to its management. The initial approach to gastric outlet obstruction from ulcer should be conservative. Close observation of the patient with the use of nasogastric suction to empty the stomach along with proton-pump inhibitors to reduce the gastric acid output may be helpful. If this does not reduce the local edema and open the pylorus, then surgery may be called for. Perforation by an ulcer can cause peritonitis and sometimes pancreatitis. Should this occur, surgical intervention is necessary to oversew the ulcer. The inability to control bleeding by medications and/or endoscopic intervention could require surgical intervention or treatment by an interventional radiologist.

31. **The correct answer is A.** Each of the listed substances can be caused by hormonal hypersecretion by various tumors. Zollinger-Ellison syndrome typically results due to a gastrin-secreting tumor that is usually located in the pancreatic or duodenal region. Its manifestations include aggressive peptic ulcer disease and diarrhea. Hypercalcemia can cause increased secretion of gastric acid in a gastrin-independent pathway. Somatostatin oversecretion leads to diabetes, gallstones, and steatorrhea. Vasoactive intestinal peptide oversecretion causes secretory diarrhea.

32. **The correct answer is A.** Antibiotic-associated diarrhea (pseudomembranous colitis) usually occurs 5 to 10 days after the start of antibiotic treatment. It occurs due to the presence of toxin-producing strains of *Clostridium difficile*, and it is routinely treated with metronidazole. This infection has become increasingly common and now appears in the community, as well as its more common presence in the hospital. Cephalexin, as a member of the cephalosporin family, is a common cause of pseudomembranous colitis. *Staphylococcus aureus* has not been implicated to date in antibiotic-associated diarrhea. Vancomycin may prove useful in the treatment of stubborn *C. difficile* infections. Because the intravenous route does not provide sufficient antibiotic levels in the colonic lumen, it is usually administered by mouth or via a gastric route. Although *Salmonella* species can cause gastroenteritis, they have no relationship with antibiotic-associated diarrhea.

33. **The correct answer is C.** Consumption of untreated water can lead to infection with pathologic enteric bacteria. Freezing the water into ice cubes does not reliably prevent transmission of these diarrhea-causing organisms. Bismuth and quinolone can prevent or lessen the severity of the diarrhea. Only well-washed peeled fruit is safe for consumption.

34. **The correct answer is D.** Primary sclerosing cholangitis is an immune process seen more often in patients with ulcerative colitis than in those with Crohn's disease. Various forms of arthritis can occur with either form of inflammatory bowel disease. Perianal abscesses, such as fistulas, occur more often in Crohn's disease.

35. **The correct answer is A.** Hepatitis A causes a spectrum of disease severity in its presentation as acute infection. Of the viruses listed, it is the only one *incapable* of establishing chronic infection.

36. **The correct answer is D.** The presence of antibodies to each virus suggests immunity to both viruses. IgM antibody would suggest acute infection. Hepatitis B surface antigen presence would indicate viremia, with either acute or chronic infection. Hepatitis A does not cause a chronic infection, as is seen with hepatitis B and C.

37. **The correct answer is C.** Melena is digested blood that has a characteristic appearance and odor. It represents bleeding from the upper gastrointestinal tract, usually from a site proximal to the jejunum. Colonic diverticular bleeding is likely to present with bright red blood from the rectum. Each of the other lesions is a gastroduodenal lesion that usually presents with melena.

38. **The correct answer is D.** This is a chronologic sequence. A man has abused alcohol for many years and presumably has developed cirrhosis and portal hypertension. This presents with abdominal swelling, increasing girth, and dyspnea. Evaluation of the abnormal intra-abdominal fluid requires investigation of the possibility of spontaneous bacterial peritonitis. This occurs without the perforation of an organ, such as an ulcer or

colonic diverticulum, thus the "spontaneous" nature of the peritonitis. It happens in the setting of preexisting ascites. The presence of more than 250 polymorphonucleocytes per milliliter suggests this diagnosis. It is neither safe nor necessary to await the culture results. The clinician should begin immediate antibiotics to cover *Pneumococcus* and intestinal gram-negative rods. Neither a liver biopsy nor a surgical consult is required at this time.

39. **The correct answer is B.** In order to characterize the ascites and determine its cause, the serum and ascitic fluid concentrations of albumin should be measured. The difference (gradient) helps to classify the ascites as being caused by portal hypertension or another pathophysiologic event. A serum-ascitic fluid albumin difference greater than 1.1 helps confirm that portal hypertension is the culprit. The practitioner should consider other possible etiologies such as carcinoma or tuberculosis when the gradient is less than 1.1. In this case, the gradient is 0.7, thus B is the correct answer.

40. **The correct answer is A.** Fistulization, formation of granulomas, and involvement of all layers of the bowel wall characterize Crohn's disease. Both Crohn's disease and ulcerative colitis manifest with mucosal inflammation.

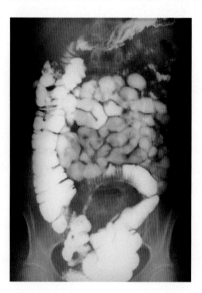

41. **The correct answer is B.** During the course of inflammation of the pancreas, digestive enzymes release into the circulation in very high concentrations. This leads to the utility of the serum amylase and lipase in diagnosing acute pancreatitis. The level of their rise, however, does not correlate with the course or severity of the disease. The appearance of the pancreas on a contrast CT of the abdomen is useful for prognostication. The pancreas may appear normal in mild pancreatitis. Severe pancreatitis presents with apparent bleeding, inflammation, abnormal collections of fluid, and erasure of normal anatomic boundaries. Hypoxemia and hypocalcemia represent metabolic changes that could secondarily occur due to the systemic effects of the pancreatitis. Both of these diagnostic criteria are useful in grading the severity of acute pancreatitis.

42. **The correct answer is A.** To diagnose free air under the diaphragm, clinicians have traditionally used the the simple, quick, and inexpensive obstruction series. Free air under the diaphragm is a sign of perforation of an intra-abdominal organ. A simple abdominal radiograph will tell you what you need to know. This test is elegant in its simplicity in our age of advanced imaging modalities. CT scan of the abdomen frequently demonstrates air outside of the intestinal lumen, but it involves more time, expense, and radiation, and therefore is not the best choice. Neither ultrasound nor physical examination is sensitive to the presence of air free in the peritoneum.

43. The correct answer is A. Each group represents individuals with a higher-than-average risk for the development of colorectal carcinoma (CRC). Patients with familial adenomatous polyposis inherit the propensity for multiple colonic polyps, as well as some extra-colonic neoplasms. The risk of developing colorectal cancer is almost 100% by the time the patient reaches his or her mid-40s. A history of previous colonic polyps or cancer significantly increases the risk of future cancer. The risk of CRC estimates to be between 10 and 20% after 20 years of ulcerative colitis. As shown in the photograph accompanying this question, the patient has a colonic polyp, and thus the clinician should follow this patient closely. An additional photograph of colonic polyps, shown below, will help to increase the reader's understanding of this common problem.

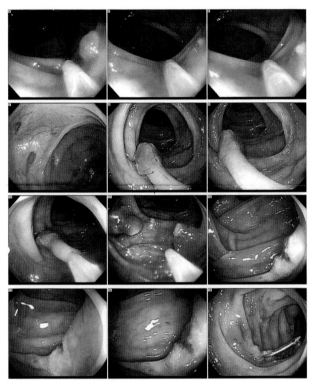

Courtesy of Christina Czyrko, MD

44. The correct answer is D. Approximately 35,000 new cases of hepatitis C are diagnosed each year, and close to 4 million people are currently infected in the United States. In the absence of an effective vaccine, such as exists for hepatitis B, hepatitis C remains a prevalent ailment and a frequent cause of cirrhosis and end-stage liver disease. It is currently the most frequent illness necessitating liver transplantation.

45. The correct answer is C. Urinary oxalate can be unusually high in patients with malabsorption. Current thought is that calcium in the intestine binds to malabsorbed fats and then is carried out in the fecal stream. This means that the calcium ions are no longer available to complex with oxalic acid. The acid is therefore absorbed more than normal. The urine then excretes this acid, where its concentration is further increased by the dehydration that can accompany inflammatory bowel disease.

46. The correct answer is D. The normal levels of some laboratory tests should adjust depending on a patient's age. Alkaline phosphatase originates in the bone and in the hepatobiliary system. The "upper limit of normal" from most labs will not adjust for the high bone growth and turnover that accompany the adolescent growth spurt. Because this is expected, imaging of the liver and bile ducts will not be necessary in this young woman without symptoms. If the clinician requires further proof, the GGT should demonstrate the hepatic origin of the enzyme elevation. Confusion can sometimes occur in the interpretation of liver tests because the transaminases ALT and AST produce in the muscle tissue as well as in the liver. Aldolase and other muscle-based enzymes can be helpful in clearing up any confusion. This, however, is not relevant to alkaline phosphatase.

47. **The correct answer is B.** Fever, pain, and jaundice represent the triad of symptoms suggestive of bile duct obstruction and cholangitis. Ascites is the collection of an abnormal amount of intraperitoneal fluid, which occurs as a result of many pathophysiologic events. It is unrelated to cholangitis or cholelithiasis.

48. **The correct answer is D.** Insulin hypersecretion is associated with hypoglycemia. Secretion of each of the other hormones is a potential cause of diarrhea. Vasoactive peptide causes chloride-dependent secretion of fluid and electrolytes. Overproduction of somatostatin likewise causes steatorrhea and frequent loose stools. Excessive gastrin release causes secretion of fluid and, more important, malabsorption through inactivation of digestive enzymes.

49. **The correct answer is B.** The results of the barium enema clearly show the typical apple-core lesion of colon carcinoma. It is located in the transverse colon. The patient's vague abdominal pain and weight loss coupled with heme-positive stools seals the diagnosis. Crohn's disease and ulcerative colitis are typically associated with more abdominal pain, along with bloody diarrhea.

REFERENCES

Abeloff, M. D., Armitage, J. O., Neiderhuber, J. E., Kastan, M. B., and McKenna, W. G. (2004). *Clinical Oncology*, 3rd ed. Churchill-Livingstone, Philadelphia, PA.

Behrman, R. E., Kliegman, R. M., and Jenson, H. B. (2004). *Nelson Textbook of Pediatrics*, 17th ed. Saunders Publishing, Philadelphia, PA.

Brunicardi, F. C., Andersen, D. K., Billiar, T. R., Dunn, D. L., Hunter, J. G., Matthews, J. B., Pollock, R. E., and Schwartz, S. I. (2006). *Schwartz's Principles of Surgery*, 8th ed. McGraw-Hill Publishers, New York.

Cohen, J., and Powderly, W. G. (2004). *Infectious Diseases*, 2nd ed. Mosby–Elsevier, Philadelphia, PA.

Davila, R. E., Rajan, E., Adler, D. G., Egan, J., Hirota, W. K., Leighton, J. A., Qureshi, W., Zuckerman, M. J., Fanelli, R., Wheeler-Harbaugh, J., Baron, T. H., and Faigel, D. O. (2005). ASGE guideline: the role of endoscopy in the patient with lower-GI bleeding. *Gastrointestinal Endoscopy* 62(5): 656–660.

Feldman, M., Freidman, L. S., and Brandt, L. J. (2006). *Sleisenger and Fortran's Gastrointestinal and Liver Diseases*, 8th ed. Saunders Publishing, Philadelphia, PA.

Friedman, S. (2006). Cancer in Crohn's disease. *Gastroenterology Clinics of North America*. 35(3): 621–639.

Goldman, L., and Ausiello, D. (2004). *Cecil Textbook of Medicine*, 22nd ed. Saunders, Philadelphia, PA.

Harrell, L. E., and Hanauer, S. (2004). Mesalamine derivatives in the treatment of Crohn's disease. *Gastroenterology Clinics of North America* 33(2): 303–317.

Kasper, D. L., Braunwald, E., Fauci, A. S., Hauser, S. L., Longo, D. L., Jameson, J. L., and Isselbacher, K. J. (eds.). (2005). *Harrison's Principles of Internal Medicine*, 16th ed. The McGraw-Hill Companies, Inc., New York.

Mettler, Jr., F. A. (2005). *Essentials of Radiology*, 2nd ed. Elsevier–Saunders, Philadelphia, PA.

Tintinalli, J. E., Kelen, G. D., Stapczynski, J. S., Ma, O. J., and Cline, D. M. (2004). *Tintinalli's Emergency Medicine*. McGraw-Hill Publishers, New York.

Townsend, C. M., and Mattox, K. L. (2004). *Sabiston Textbook of Surgery*, 17th ed. Saunders–Elsevier, Philadelphia, PA.

Orthopedics

Jonathan T. Hirsch, PA-C
Robert Howard, PT, MD
David Paulk, EdD, PA-C

1. A 19-year-old boy falls onto his outstretched hand while playing basketball. He has pain in the anatomical snuffbox upon palpation. His initial x-rays are noncontributory. Which of the following is *not* appropriate management of this patient?

   A. Immediate immobilization by thumb spica splint or casting.
   B. Repeat radiographs or perform an MRI in 10 to 14 days if the clinical exam is still suggestive of a fracture.
   C. Radiographs should include scaphoid or navicular views initially.
   D. If initial wrist x-rays are negative, the patient may return to sports in 48 hours.

2. A 20-year-old wrestler presents to the emergency department after injuring his shoulder. He fell backward during practice and put his right hand behind him to break his fall. He has injured this same shoulder several times in the past. He is in severe pain. He cannot move the shoulder and is holding his right arm slightly abducted. He is reluctant to let you passively move the shoulder and seems to have numbness over the lateral aspect of the right shoulder region as well. The radiograph is shown below. Which of the following is the most likely diagnosis?

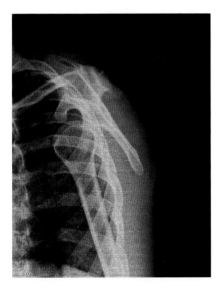

   A. Fracture of the distal clavicle
   B. Calcific tendonitis
   C. Biceps tendon rupture
   D. Anterior shoulder dislocation

3. A 30-year-old male with a known seizure disorder presents to the emergency department with confusion in an obvious postictal state along with significant left shoulder pain. He is unable to move his left shoulder. The radiograph is shown below. Which of the following is the most likely diagnosis?

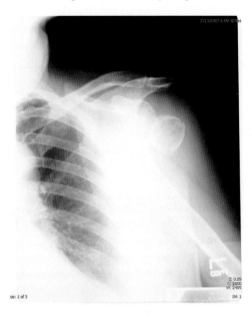

A. Anterior shoulder dislocation
B. Posterior shoulder dislocation
C. Humeral shaft fracture
D. Scapular or clavicular fracture

4. A 10-year-old boy was tackled by his brother while playing football. He immediately felt pain near his left shoulder. He is having trouble moving his shoulder as well. On physical exam, he has palpable tenderness medial to his shoulder about halfway over toward his neck. His shoulder is not swollen, and he can use his elbow without difficulty. However, he does have what looks like a swollen lump halfway between his shoulder and his neck anteriorly. His radiograph is shown below. Which of the following is the most likely diagnosis?

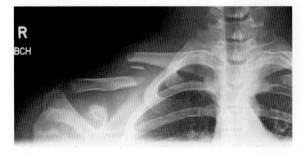

A. Rotator-cuff tear
B. Posterior shoulder dislocation
C. Humeral fracture
D. Clavicle fracture

5. An 80-year-old man presents with a complaint of pain in his upper arm. He states that he heard a "pop" in his upper arm while bowling last night and immediately afterward felt pain and was unable to use the arm to lift a bowling ball. On physical exam, he has ecchymosis of the upper arm and a visible bulge about halfway down his upper arm. Which of the following is the most likely diagnosis?

A. Anterior shoulder dislocation
B. Biceps tendon tear
C. Elbow fracture
D. Acromioclavicular joint sprain

6. A 20-year-old man presents complaining of right-hand pain after punching a wall in anger the day before. He complains of pain on the ulnar aspect side of his hand. On physical exam, he has marked swelling and ecchymosis of the ulnar side of his hand. The radiograph is below. Which of the following is *not* true regarding this injury?

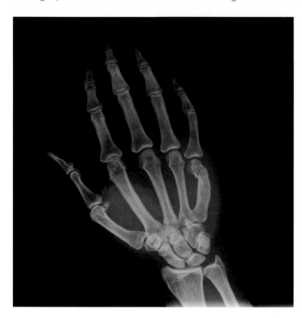

A. The patient probably has a boxer's fracture, or fracture of the neck of the fifth metacarpal.
B. The greater mobility of the fourth and fifth metacarpals makes them more likely to be fractured than the other metacarpals.
C. Emergent management includes immobilization in an ulnar gutter splint in the position of function.
D. Avascular necrosis usually occurs with this injury.

7. A 25-year-old woman falls on an icy sidewalk and lands on her right hand. She immediately feels pain in her elbow but denies other injuries. On physical exam, she has swelling around the elbow joint and cannot extend or supinate her elbow. The radiographs are shown below. Which of the following is the most likely diagnosis?

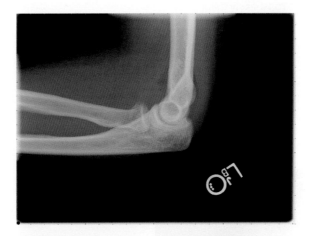

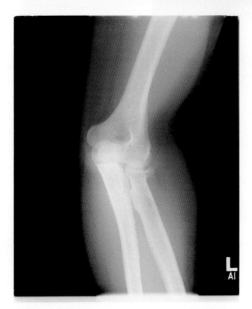

   A. Olecranon bursitis
   B. Anterior shoulder dislocation
   C. Radial head fracture
   D. Distal radial fracture

8. Which of the following is *false* regarding the innervation of the hand?

   A. The median nerve innervates the thenar eminence for both sensory and motor functions.
   B. The patient should abduct and adduct fingers against resistance to check the function of the radial nerve.
   C. The radial nerve innervates much of the skin on the dorsum of the hand.
   D. The ulnar nerve innervates muscles on the small-finger side of the hand, which is responsible for the majority of the strength utilized when an object is grabbed.

9. In nontraumatic back pain, "red flags" in a patient's history or physical might lead the clinician to believe that the back pain is something more than just a musculoskeletal problem. Which of the following patients with low back pain is *least* likely to raise a red flag?

   A. A 25-year-old female IV drug abuser with back pain and a fever
   B. An 11-year-old with back pain and no apparent injury
   C. A 40-year-old woman with a history of ovarian cancer
   D. A 35-year-old construction worker with a complaint of back pain when lifting at work

10. An 80-year-old man presents to your office with low back pain. Which of the following is the *least* likely etiology?

    A. Prostatitis
    B. Abdominal aortic aneurysm
    C. Osteoarthritis
    D. Osteopenia

11. Which of the following is the *least* important part of the neurologic examination in patients with low back pain?

    A. Evaluate strength in ankle plantar flexors to test motor function at the S1/S2 level.
    B. Evaluate the popliteal reflex to test L5.
    C. Evaluate the Achilles reflex to test S1.
    D. Evaluate the extensor hallucis longus or (great toe dorsiflexor) to test L5.

12. Which of the following is not a key part of the diagnosis of a patient with cauda equina syndrome?

    A. Bladder dysfunction (usually overflow incontinence)
    B. Perineal numbness or numbness in the inner thighs (saddle paresthesias)
    C. Bilateral radiating leg pain below the knees
    D. Hip pain

13. An 82-year-old woman falls on the ice. Emergency medical services (EMS) transports her to the emergency department. On physical exam, she has a shortened, externally rotated left leg and has increased pain in the same hip. She is somewhat more comfortable when lying quietly, but screams in pain with any movement. She is very tender to palpation over her proximal thigh and has swelling in that area. The radiograph is shown below. Which of the following is the most likely diagnosis?

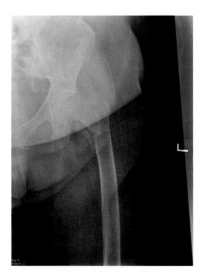

    A. Hip dislocation
    B. Distal femoral fracture
    C. Hip fracture
    D. Pelvic fracture

14. A 45-year-old male presents limping into your office. He tells you that he was playing basketball with his kids yesterday and felt a "pop" near his knee when he jumped up to get a rebound. He immediately felt pain and had a hard time with ambulation afterward. On physical exam, he is unable to extend the knee fully, has swelling at his proximal knee, and has a palpable defect at his suprapatellar region. Which of the following is the most likely diagnosis?

A. Quadriceps tendon rupture
B. Knee dislocation
C. Achilles tendon rupture
D. Chondromalacia patella

15. A 35-year-old skier is referred to your office. She has pain in her knee after twisting it while skiing. She thinks that she heard a "pop" and then felt pain and swelling. On physical exam, she has a knee effusion and laxity on Lachman's test as well as laxity on the anterior drawer test. Which of the following is the most likely diagnosis?

A. Lateral collateral ligament injury
B. Patellar tendon rupture
C. Chondromalacia patella
D. Anterior cruciate ligament injury

16. A 20-year-old football player presents with a complaint of knee pain after "being hit on the outside of his knee when carrying the football." On physical exam, he has localized tenderness over the medial joint line along with laxity and pain on valgus stress of the knee. Which of the following is the most likely diagnosis?

A. Lateral collateral ligament tear
B. Patellar dislocation
C. Chondromalacia patella
D. Medial collateral ligament injury

17. A 13-year-old soccer player presents complaining of bilateral knee pain that worsens when he plays soccer. He notes that the pain seems to feel better after resting for a day or two. On physical exam, he has tenderness and swelling over both knees at the level of the tibial tuberosities. Which of the following is the most likely etiology of his knee pain?

A. Chondromalacia patella
B. Bilateral tibial stress fractures
C. Cruciate ligament injuries
D. Osgood-Schlatter disease

18. A 40-year-old accountant enters your office with an obvious limp. He complains of pain near the back of his ankle. He notes that he was running the bases yesterday during a softball game and heard a "pop" in the back of his ankle and felt pain in the same area. He could not run after the injury. On physical exam, he has ecchymosis from his heel up to his calf, a palpable defect above his calcaneus posteriorly, and is unable to plantar flex the foot against resistance. Which of the following is the most likely diagnosis?

A. Achilles tendon rupture
B. Ankle sprain
C. Calcaneal bursitis
D. Peroneal tendonitis

19. A 21-year-old volleyball player comes to the emergency department after twisting her ankle while playing volleyball. She complains of pain over the outside of her ankle and swelling. She can walk, but only with pain. On physical exam, she has pain on inversion of the ankle and palpable tenderness just inferior to the lateral malleolus. On ligament testing with inversion, she has slight joint laxity with pain. Which of the following is the most likely diagnosis?

    A. Moderate or grade II lateral ankle sprain
    B. Deltoid ligament tear
    C. Distal tibial fracture
    D. Retrocalcaneal bursitis

20. A 3-year-old girl presents to the pediatric office where her parents brought her. She was playing with her older brother today, and he was swinging her around by her arms. Immediately afterward, she began to cry and stopped using her right arm. On physical exam, she sits quietly and holds her right arm with the elbow extended and the forearm pronated. She has no swelling or ecchymoses, but refuses to move her right elbow. You obtain a radiograph of the right elbow and it is negative for fracture. Which of the following is the most likely diagnosis?

    A. Radial head fracture
    B. Distal humeral fracture
    C. Subluxation of the radial head (nursemaid's elbow)
    D. Ulnar shaft fracture

21. A 32-year-old male playing tennis lunged for a ball going down the sideline. Upon doing so, he felt a sudden pain in the back of his leg. Which of the following positive physical examination findings would be consistent with his injury?

    A. Thomas' test
    B. Homans' test
    C. Tailor's test
    D. Thompson's test

22. A 61-year-old female with a long-standing history of cervical neck arthritis presents to your office with complaints of paresthesias in the second and third fingers of her left hand. She admits this has been present for 6 to 8 months. Which test would clinically confirm a diagnosis of carpal tunnel syndrome versus a cervical radiculopathy?

    A. Phalen's test
    B. Finkelstein's test
    C. Froment's test
    D. Grip strength

23. A 28-year-old male involved in a motor vehicle accident has a direct impact injury to the dashboard of his car, striking his knee. His radiograph is shown below. Which of the following is the most pressing concern for this patient?

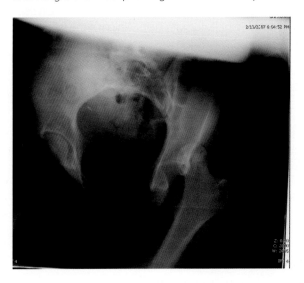

A. Avascular necrosis of the femoral head
B. Chronic greater trochanteric bursitis
C. Eventual fatigue fracture with a return to sporting activities
D. Fibromyositis

24. A 31-year-old male is playing volleyball. He strikes the tip of his second finger of his right hand on the ball when trying to block an opponent's shot. He has pain at the distal interphalangeal joint and decreased motion. Radiographs show a small avulsion fracture of the proximal aspect of the distal phalanx. This is also associated with the patient being unable to extend his finger. The radiograph is shown below. Which of the following best describes this patient's injury?

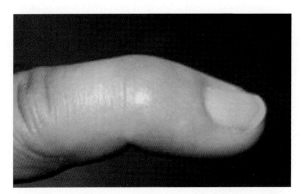

A. Boutonnière deformity
B. Mallet finger
C. Dupuytren's contracture
D. Trigger finger

25. A 73-year-old woman was watering her lawn when she tripped over the hose, landing on the ground with most of the impact on her right hyperflexed hand. Her radiograph is shown below. Which of the following statements most appropriately applies to this fracture?

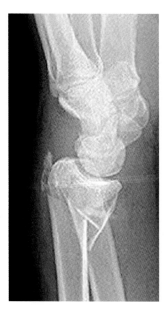

A. If the fracture is stable, it can be casted without trying to reduce the displaced fracture.
B. The complications of such a fracture will be associated with median nerve or radial artery damage.
C. The common name for this fracture is Colles' fracture.
D. The most appropriate treatment for this fracture is to wrap a bulky dressing around the injured area until the swelling subsides and then casting the patient in a long arm cast for 6 weeks.

26. A 62-year-old white male, whose father is from Norway, presents to your office with a chief complaint of hand pain and some functional deficit (difficulty extending his finger). Exam reveals a palpable thickening which resembles a callus in a cordlike presentation. A picture of his problem is shown below. Which of the following best describes what this patient is developing?

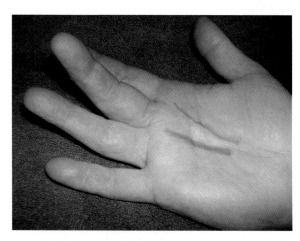

A. Dupuytren's contracture
B. Carpal tunnel syndrome
C. Trigger finger
D. De Quervain's tenosynovitis

27. Which of the following best describes the fracture shown in the radiograph below?

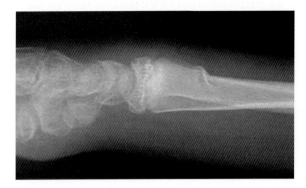

   A. Fatigue
   B. Impacted
   C. Torus
   D. Epiphyseal

28. A 19-year-old sophomore on the local university football team sustained an impact injury from an opponent's helmet to his anterior lower leg. He continued playing and finished the game. He has since developed increasing pain and now presents at the emergency department. The radiographs are normal. On physical examination, passive plantar flexion of the ankle provokes extreme pain that is disproportionate to the injury. He also has some sensory hypoesthesia. Which of the following should be your most pressing concern?

   A. Occult tibia fracture
   B. Achilles tendon rupture
   C. Compartment syndrome
   D. Deep vein thrombosis

29. A 27-year-old woman fell onto her outstretched hand while playing tennis. She demonstrates exquisite tenderness with palpation of the anatomical snuffbox. Her radiograph is shown below. Which of the following is *false* regarding this patient?

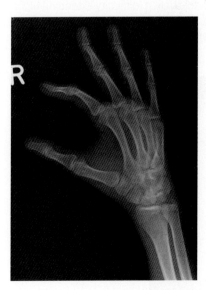

   A. Nonunion and osteonecrosis are common complications of scaphoid fractures.
   B. The bone scan shows decreased uptake in the area of the scaphoid.
   C. Radiographs should be taken again 10 to 12 days post injury.
   D. If anatomical snuffbox tenderness is present, treat it as a scaphoid fracture until proven otherwise.

30. A 32-year-old golfer stepped out of the golf cart on the eighth hole, twisting his ankle. He has pain in his foot, and radiographs confirm a fracture toward the proximal portion of the fifth metatarsal. Which of the following best describes this fracture?

    A. Jones fracture
    B. Torus fracture
    C. Bennett's fracture
    D. Smith's fracture

31. Which of the following terms best describe an acutely painful, erythematous great toe that is warm to the touch accompanied by a recently elevated uric acid level?

    A. Pogoniasis
    B. Podobromidrosis
    C. Tophyperidrosis
    D. Podagra

32. A healthy, athletic 21-year-old female falls while skiing. She sustained a compound fracture of her fifth metacarpal. You evaluate her in the emergency department, and the fracture is reducible. She states she has minimal pain. Which of the following would be most appropriate as her initial treatment?

    A. Ulnar gutter splint with referral to orthopedic office
    B. Short arm cast with follow-up for x-ray in 1 week to confirm fracture position
    C. Emergent open irrigation of wound site and antibiotics
    D. Short arm cast with immediate referral to orthopedic office

33. A 14-year-old boy fell skateboarding. He has pain in his elbow. His radiograph is shown below. How would you describe this injury?

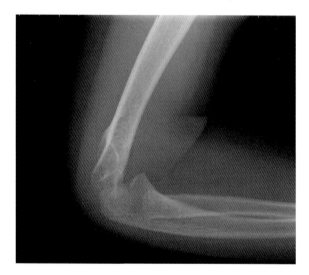

    A. Greenstick fracture
    B. Occult fracture
    C. Fatigue fracture
    D. Pathologic fracture

34. Which of the following statements is *false* regarding Lyme disease?

    A. Cranial nerve palsy can present.
    B. Common rash is erythema multiforme.
    C. The knee is the most commonly affected joint should arthritis develop in an untreated patient.
    D. The disease is named after a town in Connecticut.

35. A 7-year-old girl has fallen off the monkey bars. She sustained a fracture of her distal radius that involves the growth plate (epiphysis). On radiograph, the fracture runs through the epiphyseal line. Which Salter classification would this represent?

   A. I
   B. II
   C. III
   D. IV

36. A 39-year-old patient has a past history of a shoulder dislocation. He experiences discomfort in his shoulder with external rotation maneuvers of his right arm (e.g., taking off his glasses at night and putting them on the nightstand while lying in bed). You are concerned about his shoulder stability. Which of the following clinical tests best describes placing the patient's arm at 90° abduction and then externally rotating his shoulder?

   A. Sulcus sign
   B. Jerk test
   C. Apprehension sign
   D. Impingement sign

37. Which of the following is *false* regarding fractures of the fifth metacarpal neck?

   A. It is caused by direct impact on the metacarpal head in a clenched-fist.
   B. It is commonly referred to as a Salter fracture.
   C. Palmar displacement is common.
   D. It is commonly referred to as a boxer's fracture.

38. An 18-year-old field hockey player stopped to reverse her direction as the play transitioned from offense to defense. She felt a "pop" as her knee buckled and developed swelling. Aspiration of her knee yielded a hemarthrosis. An anterior cruciate ligament (ACL) tear is suspected. Which of the following exam maneuvers would be positive for an ACL tear?

   A. Straight-leg raise
   B. Lachman's test
   C. McMurray's test
   D. Posterior drawer test

39. A 62-year-old male field hockey coach stopped to reverse his direction as his team's play transitioned from offense to defense. He felt a "pop" as his knee buckled and developed swelling. Aspiration of his knee yielded a hemarthrosis. You suspect a quadriceps tendon rupture. Which of the following exam maneuvers would be positive for a quadriceps tendon rupture?

   A. Straight-leg raise
   B. Lachman's test
   C. Valgus stress test
   D. McMurray's test

40. A 51-year-old female presents with foot pain that improves when she removes her shoes. The physical exam reveals pain between the third and fourth toes. Her pain increases when squeezing the metatarsal heads together with medial/lateral compression. Which of the following is the most likely clinical diagnosis?

   A. Plantar callus
   B. Plantar fasciitis
   C. Hammer toe
   D. Morton neuroma

41. An 8-year-old boy who plays multiple sports complains of posterior heel pain in his right foot. Which of the following is the most likely diagnosis?

    A. Sever's disease
    B. Kohler's disease
    C. Freiberg's infraction
    D. Charcot-Marie-Tooth disease

42. A 13-year-old boy just finished his soccer season and is now playing basketball in school. He has pain in the front of his knees (right greater than left) that worsens with activities and improves with rest and ice. Which of the following is the most likely diagnosis?

    A. Gaucher disease
    B. Osgood-Schlatter disease
    C. Legg-Calvé-Perthes disease
    D. Reiter syndrome

43. An 82-year-old female presents to discuss progressive motion deficits and pain in her "arthritic hands." She has osteoarthritis, and visually you notice deformity and swelling of the distal interphalangeal joints of her fingers, as shown below. Which of the following best describes these nodules?

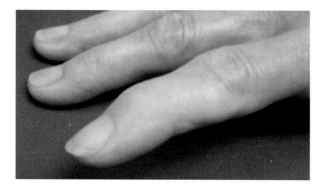

    A. Bouchard's nodes
    B. Heinz nodes
    C. Heberden's nodes
    D. Boutonniere nodes

44. Which of the following is a vitamin D deficiency resulting in abnormalities in the shape and structure of bones?

    A. Rickets
    B. Scurvy
    C. Bulimia
    D. Beriberi

45. Which of the following is the name of the maneuver, shown below, that is used to test for DeQuervain's tenosynovitis?

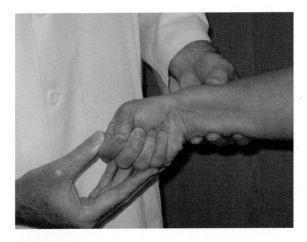

A. Allen's test
B. Tinel's test
C. Phalen's test
D. Finkelstein's test

46. A 70-year-old female presents having slipped on the ice in front of her home, falling onto her outstretched palm. She complains of pain and decreased range of motion of her wrist. Her radiograph is shown below. Which of the following is the most likely diagnosis?

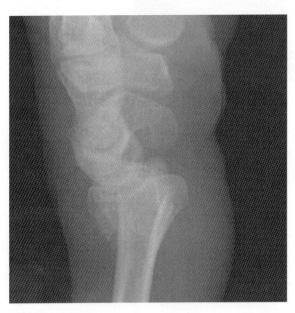

A. Colles' fracture
B. Smith's fracture
C. Scaphoid fracture
D. Boxer's fracture

ANSWERS

1. **The correct answer is D.** Anatomic snuffbox tenderness after a fall is considered a fracture until proven otherwise. The scaphoid is the most commonly fractured carpal bone, and initial radiographs can prove to be negative up to 15% of the time. The clinician should take care to obtain navicular or scaphoid views of the patient's wrist. Immediate immobilization and referral to an orthopedic specialist is the most appropriate management. Repeat radiographs, an MRI, or a bone scan are all possible radiographic options for these patients on follow-up.

2. **The correct answer is D.** The glenohumeral joint is the most commonly dislocated major joint in the body. Anterior dislocations account for over 95% of all shoulder dislocations. The mechanism for this injury may be surprisingly minor, and the recurrence rate is high in young patients with this condition. A fractured clavicle is possible, but in such a case, the patient can usually move the shoulder. Calcific tendonitis is not a traumatic one-time injury. Biceps tendon rupture is usually a disease of mature adults, and complaints often are felt further down the arm.

3. **The correct answer is B.** Posterior shoulder dislocations are uncommon, but classic seizure injuries. Anterior dislocations are much more common, but not commonly seen after seizures. Scapular fractures are rare, and the diagnosis of clavicular fractures is much less challenging. The clinician should note that frequently, there is a delay in the diagnosis of posterior shoulder dislocations.

4. **The correct answer is D.** The clavicle is the most commonly fractured bone of childhood. A direct blow to the shoulder often fractures the clavicle. Posterior shoulder dislocations are rare, but are commonly seen in patients who have suffered seizures or electric shock. The rotator-cuff muscles are the supraspinatus, infraspinatus, subscapularis, and teres minor. Rotator-cuff injuries generally result from degenerative changes with age and occur less likely secondary to trauma or a sports injury. Humeral fractures have swelling down the arm, not near the clavicle. This patient also has suffered an acromioclavicular (AC) separation due to his injuries.

5. **The correct answer is B.** The biceps tendon frequently tears in older patients, especially after a resisted contraction of the biceps itself. Over 90% occur proximally, almost exclusively involving the long head. Often the ecchymosis will be quite impressive and be present over much of the upper arm. A lump may be present in the mid-humerus area as this area's muscle generally contracts following rupture. It is unusual to have ecchymosis in the arm with the other injuries. A fall was not involved, which would be a more common mechanism with the other injuries.

6. **The correct answer is D.** Avascular necrosis is not common with this injury, but it is common with navicular or scaphoid fractures and lunate fractures in the carpus. The concern with these fractures is the possibility of rotational deformities. The fifth metacarpal is the most commonly fractured metacarpal.

7. **The correct answer is C.** The most common fracture at the elbow is a radial head fracture. Commonly, the patient has tenderness and pain and is unable to fully extend or supinate the elbow. Olecranon bursitis is commonly confused with cellulitis and is not a fracture.

8. **The correct answer is B.** The nerve supply to the hand is complex. The ulnar nerve is responsible for abduction and adduction of the fingers. The radial nerve is responsible for wrist extension and thumb extension. The radial nerve does provide sensation to much of the skin on the dorsum of the hand. The median nerve clearly provides the sensory and motor function to the thenar eminence.

9. **The correct answer is D.** Patients older than 50 and younger than 18 having complaints of back pain are cause for concern. A history of ovarian cancer should raise concern about metastatic disease. Back pain in an IV drug abuser with a temperature should also cause concern about an infectious cause.

10. **The correct answer is D.** Prostatitis, abdominal aortic aneurysm, and osteoarthritis are all possible reasons for low back pain in an 80-year-old patient. Osteopenia (low bone mass) is typically asymptomatic.

11. **The correct answer is B.** There is no popliteal reflex, and all of the other answers represent important parts of the neurologic exam in a patient with low back pain.

12. **The correct answer is D.** Hip pain is not necessarily a part of cauda equina syndrome. All of the other answers are clearly part of the syndrome. It is important to identify cauda equina syndrome, because it is a surgical emergency.

13. **The correct answer is C.** Hip fracture is the most likely diagnosis. Patients present with the leg in an externally rotated and shortened fashion. Hip dislocations are much less common. Pelvic fractures do not cause shortening of the limb, and the other problems are present at the knee, not the hip.

14. **The correct answer is A.** Quadriceps tendon ruptures most often occur in patients older than 40 years of age. They are common with jumping activities. Knee dislocations are uncommon. Achilles tendon ruptures occur more distally. Chondromalacia patella is a more chronic problem.

15. **The correct answer is D.** Anterior cruciate injuries are common. The patients often are young, and the injuries frequently occur as a result of twisting, rotational injuries. Patients usually develop an immediate joint effusion and have a positive Lachman's test along with laxity on the anterior drawer test.

16. **The correct answer is D.** Trauma to the outside of the knee often causes medial collateral ligament (MCL) injuries. They typically present as described in the question. Lateral collateral ligament (LCL) injuries are lateral injuries. Patellar dislocations do not cause laxity on ligamentous testing of the knees.

17. **The correct answer is D.** Osgood-Schlatter disease is common in adolescents. They often present with symptoms after running, jumping, or squatting activities. All of the other diagnoses are rarely bilateral, except for chondromalacia, which does not cause tenderness and swelling at the tibial tubercles.

18. **The correct answer is A.** An ankle sprain can happen this way, but it will not cause the palpable defect of the Achilles. Peroneal tendonitis does not cause any degree of ecchymosis.

19. **The correct answer is A.** Lateral ankle sprains are the most common. A sprain of the deltoid ligament is a sprain of the medial ankle ligaments. If it were a tibial fracture, the patient would be unable to walk.

20. **The correct answer is C.** Nursemaid's elbow is the most common elbow injury in young children. Treatment almost always includes closed reduction in the office or emergency department. All of the other injuries would probably present with swelling. All of the fractures would have radiographic evidence of injury.

21. **The correct answer is D.** This patient has probably ruptured his Achilles tendon. Thompson's test evaluates the integrity of the Achilles tendon. To do this test, the patient hangs his or her lower legs off the end of the exam table while lying in the prone position. The examiner squeezes the calf while observing for passive plantar flexion. The result is posi-

tive if there is no movement of the foot. This would indicate an Achilles tendon rupture. Homans' test is an early sign indicating venous thrombosis of the deep veins of the calf. Current literature suggests that performing a Homans' test may actually cause the clot to dislodge and place the patient at increased risk, and several texts recommend against performing this test. Diagnosis of deep vein thrombosis bases primarily on physical exam, Doppler ultrasound, and a positive D-dimer. When the foot is passively dorsiflexed, the patient has pain produced in the calf. Tailor's test is positive when pain is elicited along the sartorius muscle of the thigh as one actively flexes, abducts, and laterally rotates the thigh. This occurs with an injury to the sartorius muscle. The sartorius muscle is the longest in the body and enables the crossing of the legs in the "tailor's position." Thomas' test is used to check for flexion contracture of the hip. The clinician flexes the patient's hip as the patient lays in the supine position. This causes the lumbar spine to flatten, which stabilizes the pelvis. Further flexion can then only originate in the hip joint. The normal limit for hip flexion is approximately 135°. Inability to extend the leg straight without arching the thoracic spine constitutes a fixed flexion contracture. The extent of a flexion contracture can be determined by estimating the angle between the table and the patient's leg.

22. **The correct answer is A.** Phalen's test evaluates for carpal tunnel syndrome. The patient holds both forearms perpendicular to the ground, flexes both wrists, and then holds them against each other for 30 seconds. Patients who experience numbness or tingling in the distribution of the median nerve have a positive result. Finkelstein's test evaluates for De Quervain's tenosynovitis of the wrist. The performance of this test entails flexing and ulnarly deviating the wrist while the thumb is grasped into flexion. Pain at the dorsoradial aspect of the wrist indicates tenosynovitis of the first dorsal compartment (abductor pollicis longus and extensor brevis) tendons. Froment's test evaluates for weakness or paralysis of the flexor pollicis brevis and impairment of the conduction of the median nerve supplying muscles to the thenar eminence. In attempting to grasp a playing card between the thumb and base of the index finger, the flexor pollicis longus takes over from the weakened pollicis brevis so that the thumb collapses into flexion at the interphalangeal joint. Grip strength can be diminished in both cervical radiculopathy or carpal tunnel.

23. **The correct answer is A.** Avascular necrosis refers to diminished blood supply causing eventual death of areas of tissue or bone, in this case, the femoral head. This traumatic dislocation of the patient's hip might compromise the blood supply of the vessels of the ligamentum teres through the fovea centralis and the retinaculum of Weitbrecht leading to the femoral head, eventually causing bone death and collapse of the subchondral bone. Trochanteric bursitis is inflammation of the bursa (a padlike sac lined with a synovial membrane that contains fluid that reduces friction between a tendon and a bone) overlying the proximal femoral thick process projecting upward externally to the union of the neck and shaft of the femur (hip). A fatigue fracture is a fine hairline fracture that develops from repetitive microtrauma, such as distance running. Fibromyositis is chronic pain in muscles and soft tissues surrounding joints.

24. **The correct answer is B.** Mallet finger deformities occur due to disruption of the terminal extensor tendon at the distal interphalangeal joint, causing an active extension deficit. Boutonnière deformity can occur as a result of progressively worsening arthritis or secondary to an acute trauma. The cause is due to damage of the central slip, which is vital to the extensor mechanism of the proximal interphalangeal (PIP) joint. It results in a fixed flexed PIP joint and a hyperextended distal interphalangeal joint (DIP) joint. Dupuytren's contracture results from a nodular thickening and contraction of the palmar fascia, causing an inability to extend the finger. Trigger finger refers to the first annular pulley in the volar palm of the hand, which may become thickened and stenotic from chronic inflammation and irritation. Motion of the tendon is limited, and the finger may snap or lock during flexion or may be unable to actively extend the finger.

25. **The correct answer is B.** Smith's fracture is a displaced volarly angulated (apex dorsally) extra-articular fracture of the distal radius (wrist). Potential complications with this fracture presentation include median nerve damage and radial artery damage. A displaced fracture needs anatomical realignment. It should not be casted as is. Colles' fracture is a displaced dorsally angulated (apex volar) extra-articular fracture of the distal radius (wrist). Again, a displaced fracture needs anatomical realignment. The treatment plan should not solely be a bulky dressing until the swelling subsides and then a long arm cast; the fact that the fracture is displaced and needs to be reduced must be addressed.

26. **The correct answer is A.** Dupuytren's disease is a nodular thickening and contraction of the palmer fascia. It causes hard nodules near the distal palmar crease, which eventually result in contracture of the finger at the metacarpal phalangeal joint. It most commonly affects men older than age 50 and has a dominant genetic component involving people of Northern European descent, which is why it is sometimes referred to as "Viking disease." Carpal tunnel syndrome is median nerve compression (entrapment) at the wrist; it is most common among middle aged and pregnant women. Trigger finger results when the first annular pulley in the volar palm of the hand becomes thickened and stenotic from chronic inflammation and irritation. Motion of the tendon is limited, and the finger may snap or lock during flexion or may be unable to extend actively. De Quervain's tenosynovitis is swelling or stenosis of the sheath that surrounds the abductor pollicis longus and the extensor pollicis brevis tendons on the thumb side of the wrist. The inflammation thickens the tendon sheath and constricts the tendon as it glides in the sheath. This can cause pain. Often precipitated by repetitive use of the thumb, it is more common in middle-aged women.

27. **The correct answer is C.** A torus fracture is a compression fracture of the cortex occurring 2 to 3 cm proximal to the physis. It is most common in the distal radius of a child. A fatigue fracture is a fine hairlike fracture that develops from repetitive microtrauma, such as distance running. The term *impacted fracture* may be applied to a fracture in which the ends of the bones are wedged together (and shortened). An epiphyseal fracture is a growth-plate fracture. It can be classified according to an injury pattern (Salter-Harris classification).

28. **The correct answer is C.** A compartment syndrome involves increased interstitial pressure within a closed fascial compartment. It can obstruct microcirculation to the nerves and muscles lying within the involved space, causing tissue necrosis that usually becomes irreversible after 4 to 6 hours. The term *occult fracture* describes a suspected fracture that is not visible on radiograph (e.g., stress fractures or fatigue fractures). The Achilles tendon is a band of tissue that connects the heel bone to the calf muscle. Tear of this tendon would cause obvious functional deficits to the patient's plantar flexion capability. A torn Achilles tendon will result in a positive Thompson's test. The formation of a blood clot within one or more veins in the deep venous system of the upper or lower extremities refers to a deep vein thrombosis.

29. **The correct answer is B.** The correct answer is the use of short half-life radiopharmaceutical agents to visualize bones. A bone scan would show *increased*, not decreased, uptake in an area of concern, such as a fracture, osteomyelitis, or metastases.

30. **The correct answer is A.** A Jones fracture is a fracture located at the base of the fifth metatarsal at the junction of the diaphysis and metaphysis. A torus fracture is a compression fracture of the cortex occurring 2 to 3 cm proximal to the physis and is most common in the distal radius of a child. A Bennett's fracture is an oblique intra-articular fracture occurring at the base of the first metacarpal. A Smith's fracture is a displaced volarly angulated (apex dorsally) extra-articular fracture of the distal radius.

31. The correct answer is D. Podagra, more commonly referred to as gout, most commonly affects the joints of the foot or of the great toe. Pogoniasis is excessive growth of the beard or growth of a beard in a woman. Podobromidrosis is offensive perspiration of the feet. Tophyperidrosis is excessive sweating in local areas.

32. The correct answer is C. A compound fracture is an open fracture. Any break in the skin that communicates with the hematoma and injured tissue surrounding a fracture permits bacterial contamination of the wound. Prompt surgical debridement is required. The patient should also receive antibiotics and a tetanus update. None of the other answers is acceptable.

33. The correct answer is B. The term *occult fracture* is sometimes used to refer to a fracture that does not appear on radiograph (e.g., a stress fracture or a fatigue fracture). A greenstick fracture is an incomplete fracture in a bone of a child. With a greenstick fracture, one cortex is broken and the other cortex and periosteum remain intact on the compression side of the fracture. A fatigue fracture is a fine hairlike fracture that develops from repetitive microtrauma, such as distance running. A pathologic fracture is an occurrence of a fracture secondary to underlying pathology (e.g., metastatic bone lesion).

34. The correct answer is B. Erythema migrans is the rash related to Lyme disease, which usually presents followi ng a bite from an infected tick. The rash has an inflamed annular border and moves away from the site. It eventually becomes a large, bluish-red area with a firm border. Neurologic symptoms of Bell's palsy (unilateral facial paralysis affecting the seventh cranial nerve) can develop in a patient with Lyme disease. Arthralgia and arthritis occur in up to 80% of untreated patients with Lyme disease. The knee is the most commonly affected joint. Lyme disease received its name from the town of Lyme, Connecticut, in 1975 after several children developed a mysterious arthritis of unknown cause that was subsequently found to be caused by the spirochete *Borrelia burgdorferi*. Erythema multiforme is a macular eruption with dark red papules, wheals, vesicles, and bullae. It typically occurs on the extremities, including the palms and the soles. It appears in successive eruptions for short durations. The eruption may appear in separate concentric rings called target lesions. The cause is presumed to be an immune reaction to antigens, such as viruses or mycobacteria, or as a side effect to certain drugs. Stevens-Johnson syndrome is a severe form of erythema multiforme in which there are bullae on the oral mucosa, pharynx, conjunctiva, and anal area. The rash does not relate to Lyme disease.

35. The correct answer is D. Salter classification:

Salter I: Fracture at the level of the growth plate

Salter II: Fracture above the level of the growth plate

Salter III: Fracture below the level of the growth plate

Salter IV: Fracture that traverses through the growth plate from the metaphysis to the epiphysis

Salter V: Fracture that crushes the growth plate

36. The correct answer is C. The apprehension sign evaluates for chronic shoulder dislocation (instability). Please note the picture below. The clinician should abduct and externally rotate the patient's arm to a position where it might easily dislocate. If the patient is experiencing impending dislocation, the patient will have a noticeable look of apprehension and will resist further motion. To perform this test, the examiner should place the patient's arm at 90° abduction and then externally rotate the shoulder. The sulcus sign tests for inferior shoulder laxity. The clinician should apply traction in an inferior direction with the arm relaxed at the patient's side. This maneuver causes inferior subluxation of the humeral head and a widening of the sulcus between the humerus and the acromion in a person with inferior shoulder laxity. The jerk test evaluates posterior capsule instability. The patient's arm is placed in 90° of flexion and maximum internal rotation with the elbow flexed at 90°. The arm is then adducted across the body in the horizontal plane while pushing the humerus in a posterior direction. The test is positive if a posterior subluxation or dislocation occurs. The impingement sign is as follows: With the patient seated, depress the scapula with one hand while elevating the arm with the other. This maneuver compresses the greater tuberosity against the anterior acromion and elicits discomfort in patients who have impingement syndrome.

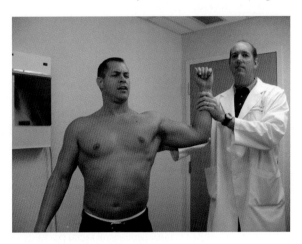

37. **The correct answer is B.** A boxer's fracture is a fracture of the fifth metacarpal neck with volar displacement of the metacarpal head. It is typically caused by direct impact on the metacarpal head with the hand in a clenched fist position. The term *Salter fracture* describes a growth-plate injury in a child.

38. **The correct answer is B.** Lachman's test evaluates the anterior cruciate ligament (ACL) for deficiency. With the thigh supported and thigh muscle relaxed, flex the knee to 15°. Grasp the distal femur from the lateral side with one hand and the proximal tibia from the medial side with the other hand. Initiate a shucking motion by pulling anteriorly on the tibia while pushing posteriorly on the femur. Focus on the amount of bony transla-tion of the tibia relative to the femur. Increased anterior translation indicates a tear of the ACL. The straight-leg raise tests for competency of the quadriceps and patella tendon. If a patient is unable to perform a straight-leg elevation while lying in the supine position, the integrity of either extensor mechanism is in question. McMurray's test evaluates for meniscal tears. For a questionable medial meniscus tear, flex the knee of a patient who is lying in the supine position. With the knee flexed, externally rotate the tibia on the femur. Gradually extend the knee. If this maneuver elicits a click or pain, the clinician should be suspicious of a posterior horn medial meniscus tear. The posterior drawer test helps to elicit posterior cruciate ligament (PCL) deficiencies. With the patient supine, flex the knee to 90°. With a PCL injury, the tibia is in a posterior position relative to the femur.

39. **The correct answer is A.** The straight-leg raise evaluates the competency of the quad-riceps and patella tendon. If a patient is unable to perform a straight-leg elevation while lying in the supine position, the integrity of either extensor mechanism is in question. Lachman's test evaluates the anterior cruciate ligament (ACL) deficiency. With the thigh supported and thigh muscle relaxed, flex the knee to 25°. Grasp the distal femur from the lateral side with one hand and the proximal tibia from the medial side with the other hand. Initiate a shucking motion by pulling anteriorly on the tibia while pushing posteriorly on the femur. Focus on the amount of bony translation of the tibia relative to the femur. Increased anterior translation indicates a tear of the ACL. The valgus stress test evaluates the competency of the medial collateral ligament (MCL). Stabilizing the lateral lower thigh with one hand (above the knee), use the other hand placed on the

inner lower leg to apply a valgus force onto the knee stressing the medial collateral ligament. If there is a laxity (or gapping) appreciated, one could clinically assess that there is a tear to the MCL. McMurray's test evaluates for meniscal tears. For a questionable medial meniscus tear, flex the knee of a patient who is lying in the supine position. With the knee flexed, externally rotate the tibia on the femur. Gradually extend the knee. If this maneuver elicits a click or pain, the clinician should be suspicious of a posterior horn medial meniscus tear.

40. **The correct answer is D.** Morton neuroma is a perineural fibrosis of the common digital nerve as it passes between the metatarsal heads. The fibrosis is secondary to repetitive irritation of the nerve. The condition is most common between the third and fourth toes (web space). It has a female to male ratio of 5:1. A plantar callus is hardened skin located at the bottom of the foot, typically as a response to excessive pressure over a bony prominence. Plantar fasciitis is the most common cause of heel pain in adults. The etiology is probably a degenerative tear of part of the fascial origin from the calcaneus, followed by a tendinosis-type reaction. It affects women twice as often then men and is more common in overweight persons. A hammer toe is a flexion deformity of the proximal interphalangeal (PIP) joint with no significant deformity of the distal interphalangeal (DIP) or metacarpophalangeal (MP) joints. A callus (corn) can develop on the dorsum of the PIP joint due to increased pressure and demonstrates accentuation of the skin lines.

41. **The correct answer is A.** Sever's disease, also known as calcaneal apophysitis, most commonly affects active prepubertal children and presents with pain in the posterior aspect of the heel following play and sports activities. Kienbock's disease is osteochondrosis of the lunate bone of the wrist. Freiberg's infraction is osteochondritis of the head of the second metatarsal bone of the foot. Charcot-Marie-Tooth is a form of progressive neural atrophy of muscles supplied by the peroneal nerves. It presents as progressive weakness of the muscles of the feet. Muscles atrophy, reflexes are lost, foot drop develops, and cutaneous sensations are lost. The disease usually develops in childhood and is more common in males.

42. **The correct answer is B.** Osgood-Schlatter disease (OSD) results from repetitive injury and small avulsion injuries at the patellar tendon insertion into the secondary ossification center of the tibial tuberosity. Gaucher disease is a chronic disorder of lipid metabolism caused by a deficiency of the enzyme beta-glucocerebrosidase. Legg-Calve-Perthe's disease is an idiopathic avascular necrosis of the hip epiphysis of the femoral head and its associated complications in a growing child. Reiter syndrome is a syndrome consisting of urethritis, arthritis, and conjunctivitis. It occurs mainly in young men. *Chlamydia trachomatis* is the organism most frequently isolated.

43. **The correct answer is C.** Heberden's nodes are hard nodules or enlargements of the tubercles of the distal interphalangeal joints typically associated with osteoarthritis. Bouchard's nodes are bony enlargements or nodules located at the proximal interphalangeal joints; they are typically associated with rheumatoid arthritis. Heinz nodes are a fictitious diagnosis (although a Heinz body is a granule in red blood cells causing damage to the hemoglobin molecules). Boutonnière nodes are another fictitious diagnosis (although Boutonnière deformity is a contracture of hand musculature marked by PIP joint flexion and DIP joint hyperextension).

44. **The correct answer is A.** Rickets is a vitamin D deficiency in children that results in inadequate deposition of lime salts in developing cartilage and newly formed bone, causing abnormalities in the shape and structure of bones. Scurvy results from a vitamin C deficiency, usually due to a dietary lack of fruits and vegetables. It presents with hemorrhagic manifestations and the abnormal formation of bones and teeth. Bulimia nervosa is a disorder marked by episodes of binge eating followed by self-induced

vomiting and diarrhea, excessive exercise, strict dieting or fasting, and an exaggerated concern about body shape and weight. Beriberi results from a thiamine deficiency. This disease presents with peripheral neurologic, cerebral, and cardiovascular abnormalities. Early deficiency produces fatigue, irritation, poor memory, and sleep disturbances. It is endemic in Asia and the Philippines due to a diet high in polished rice that has lost all thiamine content through the milling process.

45. **The correct answer is D.** Finkelstein's test evaluates for De Quervain's tenosynovitis of the wrist. The practitioner flexes and ulnarly deviates the wrist while the thumb is grasped into flexion. Pain at the dorsoradial aspect of the wrist indicates tenosynovitis of the first dorsal compartment (abductor pollicis longus and extensor brevis) tendons. Allen's test evaluates blood supply to the hand. The patient first opens and closes his fist several times. With the patient's fist closed, the clinician applies pressure to the radial and ulnar arteries in order to occlude them. When the patient opens his or her hand, the examiner releases pressure from one of the arteries and the hand should flush immediately. If the hand does not flush or reacts slowly, then the assumption is that one of the arteries is partially or completely occluded. Phalen's test evaluates carpal tunnel syndrome. The patient holds both forearms perpendicular to the ground, then flexes both wrists, while holding them against each other for 30 seconds. Patients who experience numbness or tingling in the distribution of the median nerve have a positive result. Tinel's sign also evaluates carpal tunnel syndrome. A cutaneous tingling sensation occurs when the clinician taps directly on the damaged nerve trunk (over the volar retinaculum).

46. **The correct answer is A.** Colles' fracture is a displaced dorsally angulated (apex volar) extra-articular fracture of the distal radius (wrist). Smith's fracture is a displaced volarly angulated (apex dorsally) extra-articular fracture of the distal radius (wrist). Potential complications with this fracture presentation include median nerve damage and radial artery damage. A displaced fracture needs anatomical realignment. A scaphoid fracture typically presents with pain over the anatomical snuffbox and usually follows a forced abduction of the thumb. A boxer's fracture is aptly named due to the fact it usually follows an injury in which the patient strikes an object (such as a wall or a mandible) and sustains a fracture of the fifth metacarpal.

REFERENCES

Deyo, R. A., and Weinstein, J. N. (2001). "Low back pain." *The New England Journal of Medicine* 344(5): 363–370.

Greene, W. (2001). *Essentials of Musculoskeletal Care*, 2nd ed. American Academy of Orthopedic Surgeons, Rosemont, IL.

Hoppenfeld, S. (1976). *Physical Examination of the Spine and Extremities*. Elsevier Publishing, Philadelphia, PA.

Kessel, L., and Boundy, U. (1988). *Diagnostic Picture Tests in Orthopaedics*. Wolfe Medical Publications, London.

Kozin, S., and Berlet, A. (1997). *Handbook of Common Orthopedic Fractures*, 3rd ed. Medical Surveillance Publishers, Portland, OR.

Marx, J. A., Hockberger, R. S., and Walls, R. M. (2002). *Rosen's Emergency Medicine: Concepts and Clinical Practice*, 5th ed. Mosby, St. Louis, MO.

Netter, F. (1990). "Musculoskeletal system: Part II." *The Ciba Collection of Medical Illustrations*, *Volume 8*. Novartis Publication, Cambridge, MA.

Rockwood, Jr., C., and Green, D. (2008). *Rockwood and Green Fractures in Adults*, 6th ed. Lippincott Williams and Wilkins, Philadelphia, PA.

Rouzier, P. (1999). *The Sports Medicine Patient Advisor*. Sports Medicine Press, Amherst, MA.

Saunders, C., and Ho, M. (1992). *Current Emergency Diagnosis and Treatment*, 4th ed. McGraw-Hill Medical Publishing, New York.

Skinner, H. B. (2006). *Current Diagnosis and Treatment in Orthopedics*, 4th ed. McGraw-Hill Medical Publishing, New York.

Tintinalli, J. E., Kelen, G. D., and Stapczynski, J. S. (2004). *Emergency Medicine: A Comprehensive Study Guide*, 6th ed. McGraw-Hill Publishing, New York.

Ufberg, J., and McNamara, R. (2004). Management of common dislocations. In Roberts, J. R., Hedges, J. R., eds. *Clinical Procedures in Emergency Medicine*, 4th ed, pp. 969–975. WB Saunders Company, Philadelphia, PA.

Venes, D. (2005). *Taber's Cyclopedic Medical Dictionary*, 20th ed. F. A. Davis Company. Philadelphia, PA.

Weinstein, S., and Buckwalter, J. (1994). *Turek's Orthopaedics*, 5th ed. Lippincott, Williams and Wilkins, Philadelphia, PA.

Rheumatology

Nicole M. Orzechowski, DO

1. Which of the following is *not* indicated for the treatment of symptomatic osteoarthritis of the hip?

   A. acetaminophen
   B. Physical therapy
   C. Intra-articular hyaluronic acid
   D. Total hip arthroplasty

2. A 65-year-old male presents for evaluation of right knee pain. The pain has been present intermittently for the last 3 years, but it seems to be getting worse. He describes 5 to 10 minutes of morning stiffness. The pain increases as the day goes on and is particularly bad when he walks down stairs. He takes acetaminophen with good relief. The physical examination reveals a well-developed male in no acute distress. He is overweight. Examination of the right knee shows hypertrophic changes and crepitus. There is no effusion or increased warmth. You obtain a radiograph shown below. Which of the following would *not* be a reasonable treatment/action?

   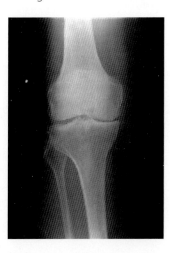

   A. Physical therapy for quadriceps strengthening
   B. Intra-articular corticosteroid injection
   C. Total knee arthroplasty
   D. Weight loss

3. A 67-year-old female presents for evaluation of bilateral hand pain and stiffness of several years' duration. The pain in her hands worsens as the day goes on. She notices that her fingers are starting to "bend" near the fingertips. She thinks they swell occasionally. Her rheumatoid factor is 50 IU/ml, and her cyclic citrullinated peptide antibody (CCP-Ab) is negative. Her erythrocyte sedimentation rate (ESR) and C-reactive protein (CRP) are within normal limits. Radiographs of her right hand are shown below. Which of the following is the most likely diagnosis?

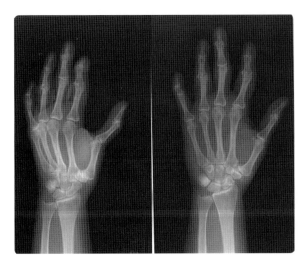

A. Rheumatoid arthritis
B. Gouty arthritis
C. Osteoarthritis
D. Psoriatic arthritis

4. A 70-year-old male with hypertension and chronic renal insufficiency presents to the emergency department with an acute, painful, red and swollen right great toe that awoke him from sleep at 5 A.M. He is unable to walk on it. He denies a history of a previous occurrence. Examination reveals marked swelling and erythema of the right great toe. It is exquisitely tender to palpation. Aspiration of the first metatarsophalangeal (MTP) joint yields one drop of yellow fluid. Polarized microscopy of this fluid is below. Which of the following is *not* an appropriate treatment option for this acute episode?

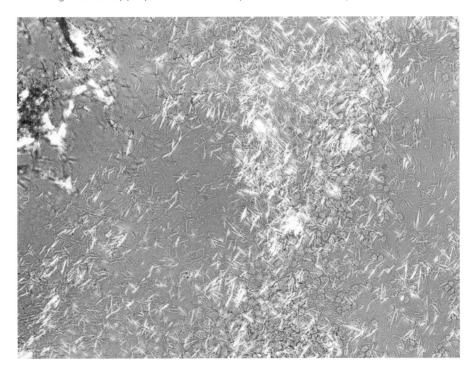

A. Oral prednisone
B. Intra-articular corticosteroid
C. allopurinol
D. indomethacin

5. A 40-year-old male presents with multiple joint complaints. He states that he feels like he is "80 years old." In the morning, he feels stiff all over for 20 to 30 minutes. He has not noticed any joint swelling. The joints that bother him the most are his shoulders, knees, hips, wrists, and metacarpophalangeal (MCP) joints. Initial workup includes negative rheumatoid factor (RF), Cyclic Citrullinated Peptide antibody (CCP-Ab), and antinuclear antibody (ANA). Erythrocyte sedimentation rate (ESR), C-reactive protein (CRP), and complete blood count (CBC) are within normal ranges. On examination, you note Heberden's and Bouchard's nodes and his knees show hypertrophic changes. There is no evidence of synovitis in the upper or lower extremity joints. Radiographs of his knee are shown below. Which of the following is the most likely diagnosis?

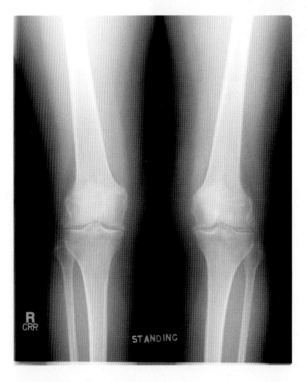

A. Gout
B. Rheumatoid arthritis
C. Ankylosing spondylitis
D. Calcium pyrophosphate deposition disease (CPPD)

6. Which of the following is *not* typically associated with polyarticular CPPD crystal deposition disease?

A. Hyperparathyroidism
B. Hemochromatosis
C. Hyperthyroidism
D. Trauma or surgery

7. An 85-year-old farmer presents for evaluation of bilateral hand pain and stiffness. He states his hands have been bothering him for years and that he manages the pain with acetaminophen and topical analgesics. He has noticed some "lumps" that developed over the last few months. His bilateral radiographs are shown below. Which of the following is the most likely diagnosis?

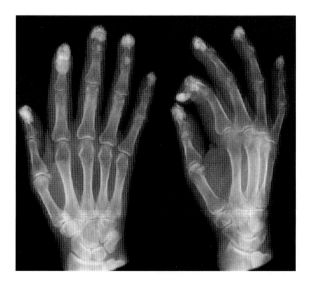

A. Rheumatoid arthritis
B. Osteoarthritis
C. Gouty arthritis
D. Pseudogout

8. Which of the following medications is the most appropriate for the management of chronic tophaceous gout?

A. prednisone
B. indomethacin
C. allopurinol adjusted for the patient's creatinine clearance
D. colchicine

9. A 50-year-old male comes to you for evaluation of acute right knee swelling that has been going on for 2 days. It is painful, and he has difficulty walking. He does not remember any recent trauma and denies fever. He takes no medications on a regular basis. You aspirate his knee and remove 30 ml of yellow, slightly cloudy fluid. Polarized microscopy of his aspirate is shown below. Which of the following is the most appropriate communication to the patient?

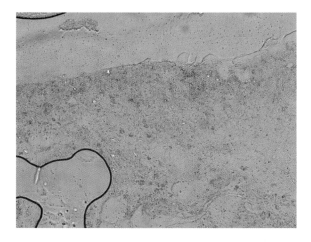

A. "This looks like gout, but infection still needs to be ruled out."
B. "This looks like pseudogout, but infection still needs to be ruled out."
C. "This looks like hemarthrosis. Are you sure there has been no trauma to your knee?"
D. "The synovial fluid looks normal."

10. A 50-year-old female presents with a 2-week history of right hip pain. She describes the pain as achy, and rubs her lateral thigh when she describes the pain. The pain wakes her at night when she rolls onto her right side. Flexion/extension and internal/external rotation of the right hip are unremarkable to passive and active range of motion. Her radiograph is shown below. Which of the following is true regarding therapy for this patient?

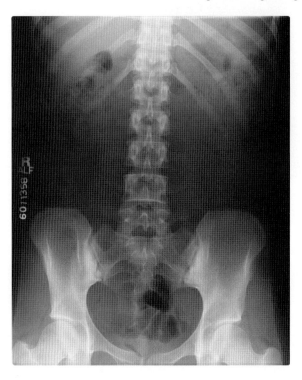

A. Heat and passive stretching do not work in the acute phase.
B. She should have underlying gait abnormalities corrected.
C. First-line therapy includes corticosteroid injection.
D. The patient will need opioids for pain relief.

11. A 55-year-old male presents for evaluation of right shoulder pain that has lasted 1 month. He does not remember any trauma or overuse. During the day, he has been using a sling for comfort. He describes a generalized mild ache that is always present, but his main complaint is shoulder stiffness. On exam, the patient can abduct the right arm to 45°, flex to 30°, and extend to 20°. Additionally, he has very little internal and external rotation of the right shoulder. The left shoulder moves without difficulty. Which of the following is the most likely diagnosis based upon his examination?

A. Adhesive capsulitis (frozen shoulder)
B. Rotator-cuff tendonitis
C. Rotator-cuff tear
D. Biceps tendonitis

12. A 45-year-old female presents for evaluation of left shoulder pain. She states that her shoulder aches at night and she cannot lie upon it. On exam, she is able to abduct her left arm painlessly from 0° to 45°. From about 45° to 120° she experiences pain, but from 120° to 180° it goes away. Which of the following is the most likely diagnosis?

A. Biceps tendonitis
B. Frozen shoulder
C. Acromioclavicular separation
D. Rotator-cuff impingement/subacromial bursitis

13. A 25-year-old construction worker presents for evaluation of acute low back pain that started today. He reached down, lifted a 50-pound bag of concrete, and immediately felt sharp pain in his low back. The pain goes across his entire low back, but not down his legs. He states that sitting relieves his pain. Your examination reveals a young man in mild distress secondary to pain. The straight-leg raise is negative bilaterally. Reflexes and strength are unremarkable bilaterally. There is no loss of bowel or bladder function and no saddle anesthesia. Which of the following is the most appropriate next step?

   A. MRI of lumbar spine
   B. Radiograph of the lumbar spine
   C. Epidural steroid injection
   D. Heat, NSAIDs, and a short course of muscle relaxants

14. A 30-year-old male pipefitter is evaluated for acute low back pain. He states he bent over at work and developed an acute, stabbing right-sided low back pain that radiated into his right buttock, posterior thigh, lateral leg, and dorsum of his foot. He denies any sensory loss, including saddle anesthesia. The straight-leg raise is positive on the right. Reflexes in the lower extremities are unremarkable (+4/5). Pain limits strength testing in the lower extremities, however his strength appears grossly normal and symmetric bilaterally. The rectal exam is noncontributory. Which of the following statements is *false* regarding the management of this patient?

   A. MRI results are significant only when they correlate with the patient's exam findings and clinical symptoms.
   B. Physical therapy, NSAIDs, and epidural corticosteroids are helpful in managing pain during an acute episode.
   C. Thirty percent of these patients typically require surgical decompression.
   D. When impingement has been present for 8 weeks or longer, electromyography (EMG) and nerve conduction study (NCS) tests may document abnormal nerve function.

15. A 52-year-old female waitress complains of bilateral foot pain. She notes that the pain is worse when she first gets out of bed in the morning. She describes the pain as being close to the heel. She has had the pain for 3 months. She tried to alleviate the pain by purchasing new shoes and placing over-the-counter heel cups in them. This only resulted in mild improvement. On exam, there is tenderness to palpation in the bilateral heels near the insertion of the plantar fascia when the feet are dorsiflexed. Which of the following is *not* likely contributing to this patient's condition?

   A. Prolonged standing
   B. Use of improper shoes
   C. Obesity
   D. Pes cavus

16. A 45-year-old woman presents with complaints of fatigue and widespread pain that has been going on for years. She admits to poor sleep, and her hands feel swollen. Prior investigations revealed "normal" or "negative" levels for the following: complete blood count (CBC); erythrocyte sedimentation rate (ESR); liver and kidney function tests; thyroid-stimulating hormone (TSH); electrolytes, calcium, magnesium, vitamin D, antinuclear antibody (ANA), rheumatoid factor (RF), and muscle enzymes. She is up-to-date with preventive medical services. The physical examination is noncontributory except for the presence of 14 to 18 generalized tender points. Which of the following would *not* be helpful in the treatment of this patient?

   A. NSAIDs
   B. tricyclic antidepressants (TCAs)
   C. cyclobenzaprine
   D. duloxetine

17. A 72-year-old female with a 35-year history of rheumatoid arthritis scheduled to undergo an elective total knee arthroplasty presents to your office for her preoperative evaluation. She swims 15 laps per day at her local gym and denies exertional chest discomfort or dyspnea. She has hypertension controlled with hydrochlorothiazide. She has been on oral methotrexate 15 mg weekly for the last 10 years. Today, she mentions that she occasionally has neck pain that radiates into the base of her skull. She also has tingling in both of her hands on occasion. She understands from her orthopedist that this was likely due to carpal tunnel syndrome. Which of the following preoperative evaluations is *most* important in this patient?

    A. dobutamine stress echocardiogram
    B. Complete blood count (CBC)
    C. Cervical spine radiograph with flexion and extension views
    D. Electrocardiogram (ECG)

Questions 18 and 19 refer to the same patient.

18. A 65-year-old female's rheumatologist diagnosed her with rheumatoid arthritis 6 months ago and placed her on 15 mg of methotrexate twice weekly. Over the last 2 months, she noticed an insidious onset of dyspnea on exertion. She now has difficulty walking one flight of stairs, whereas 6 months ago she could easily climb 4 to 5 flights without difficulty. She has also experienced a dry cough. She denies fevers, chills, and chest pain. On examination, her resting O$_2$ saturation is 91%. Her cardiac examination is non-contributory. Her lung examination revealed bibasilar crackles. Which of the following is the *least* likely cause of this patient's dyspnea?

    A. methotrexate-induced lung injury
    B. Interstitial lung disease
    C. Atypical pneumonia
    D. Pulmonary embolism

19. Which of the following is the most appropriate next step for the patient in question 18?

    A. Obtain a CT angiogram of the chest.
    B. Prescribe a methylprednisolone dose pack.
    C. Halt the methotrexate, obtain a chest radiograph, and prescribe empiric antibiotics.
    D. Prescribe 40 mg of furosemide by mouth daily.

20. A 27-year-old female received the diagnosis of rheumatoid arthritis 9 months ago. For the last 4 months, she has been taking 25 mg of methotrexate by subcutaneous injection, hydroxychloroquine 200 mg twice daily by mouth, and 10 mg of prednisone by mouth daily. Despite these medications, she reports 1 to 2 hours of morning stiffness and difficulty sleeping secondary to pain. She has difficulty working because of hand stiffness and pain. On examination, you note synovitis in her bilateral second, third, and fourth metacarpophalangeal (MCP) joints, proximal interphalangeal (PIP) joints, and bilateral wrists. Which of the following would be the most appropriate next step?

    A. Increase prednisone to 20 mg daily.
    B. Add leflunomide.
    C. Start etanercept 50 mg subcutaneously weekly.
    D. Wait an additional 4 weeks for the current medications to take effect.

21. Which of the following statements regarding rheumatoid arthritis and pregnancy is true?

    A. Only 10% of women will have a flare up of their disease within the first 3 months of delivery.
    B. The majority of women will have improvement of their symptoms during pregnancy.
    C. Women with rheumatoid arthritis are much more likely to experience fetal loss compared with the general population.
    D. NSAIDs generally are safe to use.

22. Which of the following is the safest treatment option for pregnant women with symptomatic rheumatoid arthritis?

   A. Low-dose prednisone
   B. azathioprine
   C. methotrexate
   D. cyclosporine

23. A 45-year-old male newly diagnosed with rheumatoid arthritis comes to see you for severe mouth pain that developed 2 days ago. He thought he was developing a "canker sore," but it quickly worsened. He has not been able to eat or drink for 24 hours secondary to pain. An image of his hard palate is shown below. Which of the following medications likely caused this reaction?

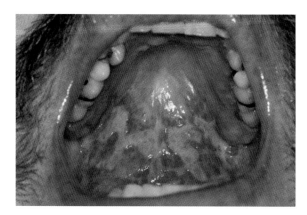

   A. hydroxychloroquine
   B. prednisone
   C. methotrexate
   D. etanercept

24. A 27-year-old female with a history of systemic lupus erythematosus (SLE) for 7 years presents for evaluation of widespread pain and fatigue. These symptoms have been present for 6 months. Her SLE has manifested in the past as a malar rash, leukopenia, arthralgias, and pleuritic chest pain. She has never had kidney involvement. She is currently taking hydroxychloroquine 200 mg twice a day. She has tried naproxen for the pain, and it has not helped. The following are her most recent lab values: hemoglobin, 13 mg/dL; white blood cell, 6,500/mm³; platelets, 350,000/mm³; erythrocyte sedimentation rate (ESR), 5 mm/hr; and C-reactive protein (CRP), 0.1 mg/dl. Her liver and kidney function tests, and urinalysis, are within normal parameters. Which of the following is the most appropriate next step?

   A. Prescribe prednisone 60 mg per day, tapered over the next 6 months to 1 year.
   B. Add methotrexate.
   C. Start fluoxetine for depression.
   D. Initiate therapies for fibromyalgia.

25. Which of the following statements is *false* regarding Raynaud's phenomenon?

   A. Up to 15% of the general population has symptoms of Raynaud's phenomenon.
   B. Symptoms are usually severe and are associated with ischemic tissue damage.
   C. Primary Raynaud's typically occurs between the ages of 15 and 25.
   D. More than 90% of patients with systemic sclerosis have Raynaud's phenomenon.

26. A 35-year-old female with systemic lupus erythematosus (SLE) since age 20 presents for evaluation of left hip pain that started abruptly 2 weeks ago. It is aggravated with ambulation and relieved with rest. She rates the pain as an 8 on a pain scale of 1 to 10. She has tried acetaminophen and ibuprofen with little relief. For the last 10 years, she has required varying doses of prednisone for control of her SLE, and the lowest dose she has been able to tolerate is 5 mg per day. You highly suspect osteonecrosis of the hip. Which of the following is the test of choice for identifying the early stages of osteonecrosis?

    A. Plain film
    B. CT
    C. Bone scan
    D. MRI

27. A 70-year-old female presents with a week of severe headache. She tried acetaminophen, with no relief. She describes severe pain in her temples and notes that it hurts even to comb her hair in those areas. She describes generalized fatigue and states that she just does not feel well. Examination reveals thickened and tender temporal arteries. Her erythrocyte sedimentation rate (ESR) is 120 mm/hr. Which of the following is the most appropriate next step?

    A. Temporal artery biopsy
    B. Head CT
    C. prednisone 60 mg per day and referral to ophthalmology for a temporal artery biopsy
    D. CT angiogram of the chest

28. A 35-year-old male presents with back pain and stiffness of 3 years. He is particularly stiff in the morning; however, he gets better as the day progresses. He notices that if he sits for too long it is difficult to move again. His lumbar spine and pelvis radiograph is shown below. Which of the following is the *least* likely diagnosis?

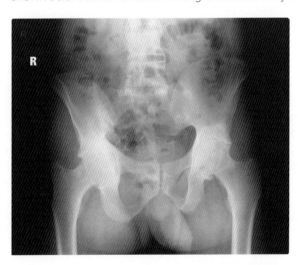

    A. Psoriatic arthritis
    B. Ankylosing spondylitis
    C. Rheumatoid arthritis
    D. Enteropathic arthropathy

29. Which of the following does *not* suggest psoriatic arthritis?

    A. "Sausage digits"

    B. Nail pitting

    C. Absence of rheumatoid factor (RF)

    D. Symmetric joint involvement

30. A 25-year-old female presents to your office with a 2-day history of a painful and swollen left knee. She denies trauma. She also denies fevers and chills or any preceding infectious illness. She cannot ambulate well secondary to pain. Examination of the left knee shows a fluid wave and the patella is ballottable. The left knee is warm compared to the right. Her range of motion limits to 15° of flexion and 10° of extension. Which of the following is the most appropriate next step?

    A. Obtain a knee radiograph.

    B. Aspirate the knee with synovial fluid analysis for cell count, crystals, gram stain, and culture.

    C. Check serum rheumatoid factor (RF).

    D. Prescribe a 1-week course of naproxen sodium and follow-up.

31. Which of the following is true regarding Lyme arthritis?

    A. It occurs early in the disease course.

    B. It is usually monoarticular, affecting the knee.

    C. Musculoskeletal complaints rarely occur in the disease.

    D. Laboratory tests are sensitive early in the disease.

32. An 80-year-old female nursing home patient with rheumatoid arthritis presents to the emergency department for an acute onset of left knee swelling, warmth, and fever. She received treatment last week for left-leg cellulitis with a 7-day course of dicloxicillin. She is currently unable to bear weight on her left leg. Passive range of motion of the left knee elicits exquisite tenderness. There is a tense knee effusion with mild erythema and increased warmth. Which of the following results from her synovial fluid analysis is *most* consistent with septic bacterial arthritis?

    A. 30,000 WBC/mm^3 and >85% lymphocytes

    B. 1,500 WBC/mm^3

    C. 95,000 WBC/mm^3 and >85% polymorphonuclear leukocytes (PMNs)

    D. 10,000 WBC/mm^3 and >10% monocytes

ANSWERS

  1. The correct answer is C. Intra-articular hyaluronic acid is FDA approved for symptomatic knee osteoarthritis only. All of the other choices are reasonable.

  2. The correct answer is C. This patient has osteoarthritis (OA) of the right knee with the medial compartment narrowing on radiograph. The aim of treatment for symptomatic knee OA is maintaining/improving joint function and limiting pain. Quadriceps weakness is a common finding in patients with knee OA, with research suggesting it is a side effect of disuse. Seeing a physical therapist for evaluation and treatment of this problem can increase the patient's functional ability. Intra-articular corticosteroids provide short-term pain relief. Patients who have pain unresponsive to medical therapy along with significant impairment in functional status when performing activities of daily living may require total knee arthroplasty. Weight loss has been shown to decrease the symptoms of knee OA.

  3. The correct answer is C. Elevated rheumatoid factor (RF) is nonspecific and typically occurs in up to 15% of healthy patients over the age of 65. Osteoarthritis, however, presents as shown in the radiograph. Psoriatic and gouty arthritis present with clinical pictures related to the psoriasis or gout. In this case, the patient did not present this way.

4. **The correct answer is C.** It is inappropriate to start allopurinol (a uric-acid–lowering agent) during an acute gouty attack, because it can worsen the condition. Chronic uric-acid–lowering therapy is appropriate treatment for tophaceous gout or when a patient has two or more disabling attacks per year. The goal serum uric acid level is below 6 mg/dl.

5. **The correct answer is D.** This patient has accelerated osteoarthritis (OA). Calcium pyrophosphate dehydrate deposition (CPPD) crystal deposition causes an acceleration of joint/cartilage destruction, causing accelerated OA. Ankylosing spondylitis typically presents in the spine. Rheumatoid arthritis would have a positive rheumatoid factor (IgM antibodies), as well as large numbers of lymphocytes in the synovial tissue.

6. **The correct answer is C.** Calcium pyrophosphate dehydrate deposition (CPPD) typically presents with inflammation in one or more joints lasting for several days to 2 weeks. Most commonly, CPPD is associated with hyperparathyroidism, hemochromatosis, hypothyroidism, amyloidosis, hypomagnesemia, trauma/surgery, and hypophosphatemia. Hyperthyroidism is not typically associated with this condition.

7. **The correct answer is C.** The "lumps" this patient describes are most likely tophi, which develop in chronic tophaceous gout. They can predispose the patient to gouty arthritis. This stage of gout usually begins after approximately 10 years of gout. The first attack often involves a sudden onset of painful arthritis, usually in the first metatarsophalangeal (MTP) joint, but also may occur in the ankle, knee, finger, wrist, or elbow. Chronic gouty arthritis (which this patient likely has) is notable for tophaceous deposits, deformity of the joint, constant pain, and swelling. Tophi typically appear in imaging studies once calcified. The other conditions do not present with the tophi noted in the question.

8. **The correct answer is C.** Allopurinol is the agent of choice for those patients who have urate overproduction, tophus formation, nephrolithiasis, or other contraindications to urosuric therapy. The other medications listed are appropriate for acute gouty attacks, not for a chronic condition such as that described in the question.

9. **The correct answer is B.** Pseudogout (also known as calcium pyrophosphate dehydrate deposition disease, CPPD) is most often accompanied by chondrocalcinosis of the affected joints. Identification of calcium pyrophosphate crystals in the aspirate is diagnostic. On microscopy, the crystals are rhomboid shaped versus the needlelike shape of gouty crystals. In all cases, the clinician should still rule out infection.

10. **The correct answer is B.** This patient describes a typical picture of trochanteric bursitis. The appropriate treatment for this condition includes injections for pain refractory to NSAIDs, along with heat and stretching exercises for 6 to 8 weeks. However, there should be correction of any underlying gait abnormalities before treatment can be successful.

11. **The correct answer is A.** Greater than 50% reduction in range of motion in all planes compared to the good shoulder suggests frozen shoulder. This descriptive term describes a stiffened glenohumoral joint that has lost significant range of motion. Classically, frozen shoulder has three phases: (1) a painful range-of-motion loss along with daily achy pain, (2) progressive stiffness, and (3) a supple phase that can last a month to 3 years. Rotator-cuff tendinitis is pain with overhead motion and can result from an impingement syndrome. A rotator-cuff tear most often results from an impingement syndrome that awakens the patient at night and results in gradual loss of strength. Biceps tendinitis results in pain whenever the biceps tendon shortens.

12. **The correct answer is D.** Impingement of the subacromial bursa and supraspinatus tendon between the greater tuberosity of the humerus, the acromioclavicular (AC) joint, and the coracoid ligaments causes pain as the shoulder moves through the arc.

The pain increases at night, especially when the patient lies upon it. Again, greater than 50% reduction in range of motion in all planes compared to the good shoulder suggests a frozen shoulder. This term describes a stiffened glenohumoral joint that has lost significant range of motion. Classically, frozen shoulder has three phases: (1) painful freezing with daily achy pain, (2) progressive stiffness, and (3) a supple phase that can last a month to 3 years. An acromioclavicular joint separation would present typically following a direct downward blow to the tip of the shoulder. The patient usually presents holding the arm close to the side.

13. **The correct answer is D.** This is a typical acute low back muscle strain without the usual red flags of concern, such as loss of bowel or bladder function, saddle anesthesia, or radiculopathy. Therefore, invasive treatments such as steroid injections or expensive testing would be inappropriate at this time. Conservative treatment is warranted until, or if, the situation changes.

14. **The correct answer is C.** A, B, and D are all correct in this likely case of disk herniation. The signs and symptoms, along with the mechanism of injury, are all consistent with this diagnosis. Historically, these patients required surgical decompression. However, approximately one-half of all patients with disk herniation recover within 1 month and greater than 95% recover in 6 months. The practitioner should also note that the rate of surgical treatment is much higher in the United States than in other countries. In one study, surgically treated patients had better results at 1 year than those treated conservatively; however, the two cohorts showed nearly equal results in terms of function at 4 and 10 years.

15. **The correct answer is D.** This patient has plantar fasciitis, which is the most common form of heel pain. Contributing factors include dorsiflexion of the toes, increased stress due to obesity, improper footwear, and prolonged standing. Pes cavus, or cavus foot deformity, is characterized by an abnormal elevation of the longitudinal arch, with resulting decrease in the plantar–weight-bearing area. This does not typically contribute to plantar fasciitis, however.

16. **The correct answer is A.** This patient has obvious fibromyalgia. The patient requires reassurance and education that fibromyalgia is not a psychiatric disorder, deforming, or life threatening. Medications that improve sleep are the most effective treatment. NSAIDs and corticosteroids have not proven to be as effective when prescribed as single agents, although in one study, ibuprofen did enhance the effectiveness of alprazolam.

17. **The correct answer is C.** Although it is entirely possible this patient has carpal tunnel syndrome, the diligent practitioner must rule out other, more serious problems. The patient requires testing to rule out a cervical cause for her extremity pain. The patient shows no signs or symptoms of cardiac problems, thus an ECG and stress echocardiogram would not be the *most important* preoperative tests. Although an ECG is important in the preoperative workup of a 72-year-old patient, in light of the choices it is not the most important. She also does not present with signs and symptoms of an infection. Again, although a complete blood count (CBC) is important in the routine preoperative workup of a patient, it is not the best choice in this case.

18. **The correct answer is D.** Patients with rheumatoid arthritis may present with various lung diseases and injuries, such as interstitial lung disease, atypical pneumonia, and/or methotrexate-induced injury. The signs and symptoms of a pulmonary embolism are usually more dramatic, including, at the very least, markedly reduced oxygen saturation. Therefore, the patient likely does not have a pulmonary embolism.

19. **The correct answer is C.** Based on the patient's history; she could have a lung injury and/or atypical pneumonia. A CT scan is unnecessary in this case, because a chest radiograph will most likely yield appropriate diagnostic results. The prudent clinician should stop the methotrexate immediately, obtain a diagnostic chest radiograph, and

begin empiric antibiotics until s/he confirms a definitive diagnosis. Furosemide is typically indicated for treatment of exacerbations of congestive heart failure.

20. **The correct answer is C.** Some studies have indicated the relative safety of low-dose steroids (5 mg/day or less). Treatment with 20 mg/day of prednisone for the short term has proven effective in some studies. Because this patient is on 10 mg/day already, an increase would not be prudent. The patient is on one of the least toxic of the DMARDs (disease modifying anti-rheumatic drugs). Placing the patient on another DMARD, such as leflunomide, would be dangerous in terms of toxicity. The patient is having difficulty with her daily activities, so waiting would not be helpful in this case. Etanercept is an injectable drug that blocks tumor necrosis factor alpha (TNF alpha). It has FDA approval for use in the treatment of rheumatoid arthritis, ankylosing spondylitis, and psoriatic arthritis. TNF alpha is a protein produced during the inflammatory response. TNF alpha promotes inflammation and its associated fever and signs (pain, tenderness, and swelling). Etanercept binds to TNF alpha, thereby removing the TNF alpha molecules from joints and blood, which reduces inflammation. It is relatively safe and acts in a different pathway, making it the appropriate choice in this situation.

21. **The correct answer is B.** Most women do have improvement of symptoms during pregnancy. Women with rheumatoid arthritis (RA) do not suffer fetal loss at any greater rate than those without. The exact number of women who flare during pregnancy is nebulous at best. The use of nonsteroidal anti-inflammatory drugs (NSAIDs) during pregnancy has been proven ineffective. NSAID use, especially in the third trimester, is contraindicated as they can cause premature closure of the patent ductus arteriosus (PDA).

22. **The correct answer is A.** Low-dose prednisone is the safest alternative of the medications listed. The others are either toxic and/or teratogenic.

23. **The correct answer is C.** Methotrexate is an effective medication in the treatment of rheumatoid arthritis (RA), but it does have side effects, including, but not limited to, gastrointestinal problems, interstitial lung disease, and atypical pneumonia. Cold or canker sores are also untoward manifestations to its use, especially in immunocompromised patients. The other medications listed have a lower profile of adverse effects.

24. **The correct answer is D.** Approximately one-quarter of patients with connective tissue disorders develop fibromyalgia, as appears to have happened in this case. Initiation of therapy for fibromyalgia is the most appropriate step in this case.

25. **The correct answer is B.** Patients with Raynaud's phenomenon do not typically have ischemic tissue damage. All of the other statements are true.

26. **The correct answer is D.** In cases of osteonecrosis, an MRI offers the best diagnostic yield, especially in patients with connective tissue disorders. Plain films are useful in advanced stages, but not in the early stages of the disease. MRI is both sensitive and specific for the diagnosis, and CT does not offer any advantage over MRI.

27. **The correct answer is C.** This patient probably has temporal arteritis. In order to prevent blindness, therapy should begin immediately, even before the diagnosis is definitive.

28. **The correct answer is C.** Of the choices, only rheumatoid arthritis spares the spine and sacroiliac joints.

29. **The correct answer is D.** The classic presentation of psoriatic arthritis includes a large joint (sausage digits), oligoarthritis, and a history of psoriasis. Nail pitting is possible, and there is no rheumatoid factor. Symmetric joint involvement is not a usual presentation of psoriatic arthritis. Note these findings in the picture below.

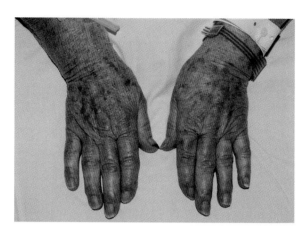

30. **The correct answer is B.** Aspiration and fluid analysis should be the first test in the evaluation of any acute monoarticular arthritis. The purpose is to rule out joint infection, which is a true medical emergency. Gram-positive organisms within a joint can destroy the cartilage within days. In any patient with monoarticular arthritis, assume infection until proven otherwise.

31. **The correct answer is B.** The arthritis of Lyme disease is most often monoarticular and usually affects the knee. However, it occurs late in the disease (stage III). Musculoskeletal complaints are frequent with Lyme disease (approximately 60% of patients), and laboratory tests frequently are insensitive early in the disease.

32. **The correct answer is C.** Blood cultures are positive in approximately 50% of patients. Leukocyte counts of the synovial fluid typically exceed 50,000/mm^3 and often up to 100,000/mm^3, with 90% or more PMNs. The glucose count is usually low.

REFERENCES

Carpenter, C. C. J., Griggs, R. C., and Benjamin, I. J. (2007). *Cecil Essentials of Medicine*, 7th ed. Saunders Elsevier, Philadelphia, PA.

Klippel, J. H. (1998). *Rheumatology*, 2nd ed. Elsevier, Philadelphia, PA.

Klippel, J. H. (2001). *Primer on the Rheumatic Diseases*, 12th ed. The Arthritis Foundation, 216. 4, Atlanta, GA.

McPhee, S. J., Papadakis, M. A., and Tierney, L. M. (2007). *Current Medical Diagnosis and Treatment*, 47th ed. McGraw-Hill Medical Publishers, New York.

Skinner, H. B. (2003). *Current Diagnosis and Treatment in Orthopedics*, 3rd ed. McGraw-Hill Medical Publishing, New York.

10

Neurology

Barry Korn, DO, DPM, DAAPM

1. A 42-year-old male presents complaining of frequent headaches that started about 2 weeks ago. The headaches start around 9 P.M. each day. The headaches are located over the right temporal area as well as around the right eye and last approximately 20 minutes. He also reports nasal congestion and lacrimation on the right side. The patient states that he feels agitated and "cannot sit still" during the headache episode. Which of the following is the most likely diagnosis?

   A. Migraine
   B. Tension headache
   C. Trigeminal neuralgia
   D. Cluster headache

2. A 28-year-old male presents with a sudden onset of right facial weakness. He notes an "uncomfortable" feeling around his right ear and is increasingly sensitive to sound. His right eye seems to have a decrease in tear production. Physical examination reveals an impaired ability to wrinkle the right side of the forehead. You also note a drooping of the right brow and corner of the mouth. Closure of the right eye is impaired. The symptoms have been present for 5 days. Which of the following best describes this scenario?

   A. Transient ischemic attack
   B. Trigeminal neuralgia
   C. Middle cerebral artery infarction
   D. Bell's palsy

3. A 68-year-old male presents with a resting tremor in both hands. The tremor has a pill-rolling type of movement. The patient also exhibits bradykinesia and cogwheel rigidity. Handwriting analysis demonstrates micrographia. Which of the following best describes this patient's condition?

   A. Multiple sclerosis
   B. Parkinson's disease
   C. Huntington's disease
   D. Lacunar infarction

4. A 50-year-old female noticed a tremor in her hands when pouring water into a cup and eating with utensils. She has difficulty dressing herself. The patient also notes that her tremor improves after drinking wine. She further states that her head has been "shaking." Examination reveals increased tremor with finger-to-nose testing. Which of the following is the best explanation of this patient's problem?

   A. Essential tremor
   B. Parkinson's disease
   C. Anxiety disorder
   D. Petit mal seizure

5. A 46-year-old male presents to the emergency department complaining of a burning sensation in a bandlike distribution on the left side of his chest. He also states that the area occasionally itches. Diagnostic studies reveal an unremarkable ECG with normal cardiac enzymes. There is no rash noted on physical examination. The emergency staff discharged the patient with ibuprofen for pain. Five days later, the patient returns to the emergency department complaining that a "rash" has developed in the same area as his pain. Your examination reveals an erythematous papular rash with grouped vesicles in the same area of distribution as the pain (shown below). Which of the following is the most likely diagnosis?

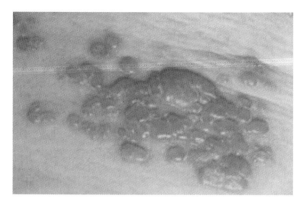

   A. Allergic dermatitis
   B. Herpes zoster
   C. Pustular psoriasis
   D. Complex regional pain syndrome

6. A 10-year-old female's mother brings her to your office. The mother states her daughter's schoolwork has deteriorated and that her daughter frequently "stares into space." These staring episodes come without warning and last approximately 10 seconds. You are able to provoke an episode by having the patient hyperventilate. Which of the following is the most likely diagnosis?

   A. Grand mal seizure
   B. Absence seizure
   C. Metabolic seizure
   D. Attention-deficit disorder

7. A 65-year-old male presents to the emergency department complaining of the "worst headache of his life." He reports some slight headaches over the past week prior to this event. He also has nausea and vomiting. Ophthalmologic examination reveals sub-hyaloid hemorrhages and a third-nerve palsy. Which of the following should be the first diagnostic test you order?

   A. MRI of the brain without contrast
   B. Lumbar puncture
   C. CT of the brain without contrast
   D. Carotid ultrasound

8. Which of the following is the most likely diagnosis for the patient in question 7?

   A. Epidural hematoma
   B. Subarachnoid hemorrhage
   C. Migraine headache
   D. Cluster headache

9. A 47-year-old female patient presents with a history of lancing pain around her left maxillary area that lasts only a few seconds. The patient notes these attacks are frequent and confined to the left maxillary area. Mild sensory stimuli, such as applying makeup, may initiate the attacks. She notes these attacks occur spontaneously. Which of the following is the most likely diagnosis?

   A. Trigeminal neuralgia
   B. Partial complex seizure
   C. Transient ischemic attack
   D. Absence seizure

10. Which of the following is the hallmark pathologic lesion of multiple sclerosis?

    A. Lewy bodies
    B. Barr bodies
    C. Heinz bodies
    D. Demyelinated plaques

11. A patient presents with a restriction in head mobility. The head has assumed an abnormal posture of rotation to the right, along with backward deviation. The patient notes that the symptoms began with initial neck stiffness. The patient also reports associated neck and shoulder pain. Which of the following is the most likely diagnosis?

    A. Parkinson's disease
    B. Partial complex seizure
    C. Cervical dystonia
    D. Chorea

12. Which of the following is a typical neurologic manifestation of vitamin B_{12} deficiency?

    A. Demyelination of the posterior and lateral columns
    B. Plaques in the medulla
    C. Lesions in the dorsal root ganglion
    D. Lesions of the anterior motor cell

13. A patient presents with right shoulder girdle pain extending to the arm and forearm. The patient notes numbness and paresthesia in the central portion of the right hand and the third digit. The patient has a herniated disc. Which of the following anatomic levels is most likely affected?

    A. C4
    B. C5
    C. C6
    D. C7

14. Which of the following is usually *not* a major concern regarding the emergency care of headaches?

    A. Headache in a 35-year-old male
    B. Sudden onset of headache
    C. Increased headache frequency and severity
    D. Headache with fever and stiff neck

15. Which of the following is *not* a risk factor for stroke?

    A. History of hypertension
    B. Diabetes mellitus
    C. Previous stroke
    D. Age of 50 years or younger

16. Which of the following does *not* indicate an infarction of the middle cerebral artery?

    A. Ipsilateral hemiparesis

    B. Deviation of head and eyes toward the lesion side

    C. Contralateral hemianesthesia

    D. Aphasia

17. Which of the following refers to a brief episode of neurologic dysfunction typically lasting less than 1 hour caused by focal brain ischemia?

    A. Reversible ischemic neurologic dysfunction

    B. Stroke in progress

    C. Transient ischemic attack

    D. Partial complex seizure

18. A 32-year-old female presents with daily headaches. Past attempts at prophylactic headache medication treatments have all failed. She takes daily headache medication, including butalbital. She is a frequent visitor to the Emergency Department for her headaches. Which of the following best describes this patient's headache?

    A. Classic migraine

    B. Drug-rebound headache

    C. Cluster headache

    D. Tension headache

19. Which of the following is *not* a clinical sign of amyotrophic lateral sclerosis (Lou Gehrig's disease)?

    A. Symmetric muscle weakness

    B. Hyperreflexia

    C. Fasciculations

    D. Muscle atrophy

20. Which of the following statements is *false*?

    A. Postural tremor affects a body part that maintains position against gravity.

    B. Isometric tremor is muscle contraction against a stationary object.

    C. Kinetic tremor occurs with involuntary movement.

    D. Intention tremor occurs during visually guarded movement toward an object.

21. Which of the following terms describes when a person has more than one seizure and does not recover between the seizures?

    A. Status epilepticus

    B. Grand mal seizure

    C. Absence seizure

    D. Myoclonic seizure

22. Which of the following terms refers to repetitive, stereotyped motor movements that are exaggerations of normal movements?

    A. Tremor

    B. Chorea

    C. Dystonia

    D. Tic

23. Which of the following is *not* typically associated with Wernicke's encephalopathy?

    A. Nystagmus

    B. Gaze palsies

    C. Gait ataxia

    D. Folate deficiency

24. Which of the following is *not* usually a precipitating cause of carpal tunnel syndrome?

    A. Injury to the radial nerve
    B. Diabetes mellitus
    C. Thyroid disease
    D. Systemic lupus erythematosus (SLE)

25. A 64-year-old male presents with cognitive impairment. He recently suffered a thromboembolic cerebrovascular accident. He is now socially impaired and cannot perform his occupational duties. Which of the following is the most likely clinical diagnosis?

    A. Poststroke dementia
    B. Alzheimer's disease
    C. Lewy body disease
    D. Wernicke-Korsakoff syndrome

26. Which of the following evaluations is *not* usually associated with the Glasgow Coma Scale?

    A. Evaluate eye opening
    B. Evaluate best verbal response
    C. Evaluate best motor response
    D. Evaluate best sensory response

27. Which of the following is the most appropriate test to distinguish between an ischemic stroke and a hemorrhagic stroke?

    A. Lumbar puncture
    B. Brain CT
    C. Brain MRI
    D. Electroencephalography (EEG)

28. Which of the following is the most malignant of all the astrocytomas?

    A. Glioblastoma multiforme
    B. Meningioma
    C. Oligodendroglioma
    D. Ependymoma

29. Which of the following is *false* concerning giant cell arteritis?

    A. It is more common in women.
    B. Average age of onset is 50.
    C. Headache is the most common symptom.
    D. Pain occurs with gentle stroking of the patient's hair.

30. Which of the following is *not* a pain-sensitive structure in the head?

    A. Brain
    B. Scalp
    C. Carotid arteries
    D. Meninges

31. A 42-year-old male presents with numbness in the bottom of his right foot. Examination reveals a positive Tinel's sign over the right posterior tibial nerve. Vascular examination is noncontributory. He denies back pain. Which of the following is the most likely diagnosis?

    A. Diabetic neuropathy
    B. Tarsal tunnel syndrome
    C. Complex regional pain syndrome
    D. Neuroma

32. A patient presents with hearing loss, balance problems, tinnitus, and vertigo. An MRI study of the brain reveals a mass at the cerebellopontine angle. Which of the following is the most likely diagnosis?

   A. Acoustic neuroma
   B. Menière's disease
   C. Trigeminal neuralgia
   D. Multiple sclerosis

33. A 24-year-old male presents with a complaint of dizziness. The episodes of dizziness last several seconds and are provoked by changes in head position, such as rolling out of bed and bending over. He is not suffering from hearing loss or tinnitus. Which of the following is the most likely diagnosis?

   A. Menière's disease
   B. Benign positional vertigo
   C. Vestibular neuritis
   D. Migraine

34. A 24-year-old female presents to the emergency department with fever, neck stiffness, and mental-status changes. Following appropriate diagnostic decisions, you perform a lumbar puncture. Which of the following agent(s) is/are the most likely organism(s) explaining this patient's condition?

   A. *Neisseria meningitidis* and *Streptococcus pneumoniae*
   B. *Pseudomonas aeruginosa* and *Escherichia coli*
   C. *Haemophilus influenzae*
   D. *Staphylococcus aureus*

35. Which of the following is the most common cause of primary dementia?

   A. Parkinson's disease
   B. Huntington's chorea
   C. Alzheimer's disease
   D. Multiple sclerosis

36. On clinical examination, a patient is having difficulty repeating the phrase "no ifs, ands, or buts." The patient is able to comprehend written and spoken language, but is frustrated with his difficulty in speech. Which of the following terms describes this clinical condition?

   A. Broca's aphasia
   B. Wernicke's aphasia
   C. Dementia
   D. Alzheimer's disease

37. Which of the following does the physical examination procedure shown below best assess?

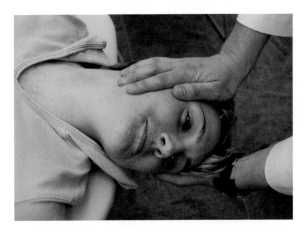

- **A.** Dementia
- **B.** Level of consciousness
- **C.** Vertigo
- **D.** Memory

38. Which of the following medications typically aborts an impending migraine headache?

- **A.** Amitriptyline
- **B.** Nortriptyline
- **C.** Valproic acid
- **D.** Sumatriptan

39. A patient presents to the emergency department following a witnessed tonic-clonic seizure. Examination of the patient's mouth reveals the physical findings as shown in the picture. Which of the following antiseizure medications is the most likely cause of this oral condition?

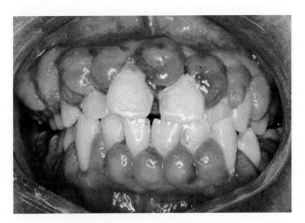

- **A.** Carbamazepine
- **B.** Gabapentin
- **C.** Valproic acid
- **D.** Phenytoin

ANSWERS

1. **The correct answer is D.** As the name implies, cluster headaches are "clusters" of head-aches that occur over time—as in this case, with daily headaches beginning around 9 P.M. for 2 weeks. Frequently, there are pain-free periods. They are usually located (and begin) temporally, and patients often note sinus or nasal congestion and excessive eye tearing. There may also be redness of the eye(s). Many patients report an increased cor-relation with alcohol consumption. Increased anxiety is a frequent component. These headaches occur more often in middle-aged men. Cluster headaches are also known as migrainous neuralgia, but this is the only thing they have in common with migraines. Migraines frequently present in women. They frequently are generalized and typically lateralize to one area. They begin in adolescence, and often feature visual disturbances, such as photophobia, flashing lights (photopsia), or field defects/geometric patterns. Migraine patients may present with aphasia, numbness, increased clumsiness, and focal-ized weakness. Tension headaches typically are vague and nonspecific and often follow periods of high stress, fatigue, or noise, or any combination therewith. They are most often located in the neck and back of the head. Trigeminal neuralgia (tic douloureux) is facial pain along the distribution of the trigeminal nerve and occurs more often in women. It commonly arises on one side of the mouth and radiates toward the ear.

2. **The correct answer is D.** Bell's palsy is characterized as noted in the question, but perhaps the most significant clue to the condition is found on physical examination. Neurologic testing reveals the findings as described, which confirms the diagnosis. It often occurs in patients who have Lyme disease. Transient ischemic attacks (TIA), or "little strokes," present with an acute onset of a focal or clinical deficit that resolves in 24 hours. Because this patient's deficit has been present for 5 days, he has not had a TIA. Trigeminal neuralgia (tic douloureux) presents with intermittent facial pain along the distribution of the trigeminal nerve (occurring almost exclusively in the maxillary and mandibular branches) and, again, occurs more often in women. The pain commonly arises on one side of the mouth with radiation toward the ear. It is usually described as sharp, stabbing electric shocks. Cerebral infarctions (irrespective of the location) are frequent precursors to a TIA or stroke. Middle cerebral infarctions often lead to contralateral hemiplegia with associated sensory loss and perhaps a homonymous hemianopsia. This patient does not exhibit these symptoms.

3. **The correct answer is B.** This is the classic presentation of Parkinson's disease. Mul-tiple sclerosis patients are usually under the age of 55 and most commonly present with weakness, paresthesia, or anesthesia of a limb. They may have spastic paraparesis, diplopia, or urinary symptoms. Huntington's disease is a gradual and progressive disease that frequently presents after the age of 30 and before 50. Early presentation is usually restlessness or other abnormal movements along with intellectual changes characterized by irritability, moodiness, and antisocial behavior. Physical movements typically progress to choreiform movements and dystonic posturing. The intellectual or behavioral changes inevitably progress to dementia. Lacunar infarctions are small lesions that frequently lead to TIA or stroke. These patients present with sensory or motor deficits, including ipsilateral ataxia, clumsiness, or hemiparesis.

4. **The correct answer is A.** Essential tremor is frequently confused with Parkinson's disease and is much more common. Essential tremor usually presents as a trembling up-and-down movement of the hands associated with doing something such as drinking water or sewing. It affects the ability to perform fine-motor skills. It is a gradually progressive condition. Essential tremor may affect the head, whereas the tremor of Parkinson's does not. Essential tremor does not usually present with a stooped posture, shuffling gait, or memory problems, as in Parkinson's disease. Parkinson's disease usually presents with a resting pill-rolling type of tremor in both hands, along with bradykinesia and cogwheel rigidity. The tremors of Parkinson's frequently occur at rest, with the patient's hands

located at his or her sides. Anxiety disorders are psychiatric disorders frequently characterized by tension, fear, an inability to concentrate, and general apprehension. Acute attacks are usually associated with tachypnea. Petit mal seizures typically present as an *abrupt* onset characterized by loss of consciousness. They may also have other atonic or clonic components, such as postural tone loss.

5. **The correct answer is B.** Herpes zoster (shingles) usually presents in adults. Pain frequently presents before the rash appears (as in this case). Lesions follow a nerve-root distribution, which can vary depending on the nerve root. Frequently, this is in a single dermatome. The skin lesions resemble those of varicella (chickenpox), beginning as a maculopapular rash that develops into vesicles and pustules. Allergic dermatitis usually occurs after contact with an allergen and most often occurs at the point of contact. Although it presents with a maculopapular rash, the presentation can vary from patient to patient and is not normally in a dermatomal distribution. Pustular psoriasis typically presents with pustules and silvery scales on bright red, well-demarcated plaques and may have itching associated with it. Complex regional pain syndrome, or reflex sympathetic dystrophy, is a rare disorder of the extremities characterized by diffuse pain usually localized to an arm, leg, hand, or foot. Typically, there is swelling of the affected extremity along with limited range of motion and temperature changes.

6. **The correct answer is B.** Absence seizures most often start in childhood and last until the patient is in his or her 20s. Frequently, the patient is unaware of the seizure activity. A loss of consciousness (which may manifest as the "staring into space," as noted in the question) typically characterizes these seizures. Patients may lose postural tone or suffer enuresis. In some cases, hyperventilation can provoke the seizure. Tonic-clonic movements following loss of consciousness along with associated rigidity characterize grand mal seizures. Metabolic seizures can be caused by withdrawal from alcohol or drugs or from other causes, such as uremic disorders or hyper-or hypoglycemia. Attention-deficit disorder does not include loss of consciousness or triggering of episodes with hyperventilation. The disorder is not limited to timed episodes, although children with attention-deficit disorder do have frequent problems with schoolwork.

7. **The correct answer is C.** This patient's presentation strongly suggests a subarachnoid hemorrhage (SAH). The clinician should obtain a CT scan without contrast immediately to confirm the presence of a SAH and certainly within the first 24 hours. In the presence of a suspected bleed, contrast is contraindicated. Lumbar puncture is acceptable to identify the presence of a SAH in patients with suspected bleeding but who have *normal CT findings*. Lumbar puncture is most sensitive within 12 hours of the SAH. Magnetic resonance imaging (MRI) is not the diagnostic test of choice, because CT is faster and more sensitive in detecting a bleed. Carotid arteriography is useful because these patients usually have multiple aneurysms; however, carotid ultrasound would generally not be helpful.

8. **The correct answer is B.** Subarachnoid hemorrhage (SAH) presents as a sudden, severe headache often characterized as "the worst headache of my life." Subarachnoid hemorrhage (SAH) causes up to 10% of strokes. SAH usually occurs as a result of the rupture of an arteriovenous (AV) malformation or aneurysm. The sudden, severe headache is a characteristic clinical picture and may be followed by severe nausea and vomiting. Fundoscopic examination can reveal hemorrhages, as noted, and the neurologic examination can present as everything from nerve palsies to nuchal rigidity and other signs of meningeal irritation. In many cases, patients are often confused with meningitis cases. Epidural hematoma may present with headaches, although not usually described as in the question, along with neurologic deficits, such as confusion, somnolence, and seizures. Migraines are more common in women and are more general in nature and tend to lateralize. They also can begin in adolescence and often feature visual disturbances,

such as photophobia, flashing lights (photopsia), or field defects/geometric patterns. Migraine patients may also present with aphasia, numbness, increased clumsiness, and focalized weakness. As the name signifies, cluster headaches are frequently "clusters" of headaches that occur over time. Frequently, there are pain-free periods. Cluster headaches are usually located (and begin) temporally, and patients often note sinus or nasal congestion and excessive tearing. There may also be redness of the eye(s). Many patients report an increased correlation with alcohol consumption. Increased anxiety is a frequent component. These headaches are more common in middle-aged men.

9. **The correct answer is A.** Trigeminal neuralgia, or tic douloureux, typically occurs in middle-aged and older women. Patients present with sudden lancinating pains along the distribution of the trigeminal nerve. Attacks frequently begin on one side of the mouth and move toward the ear, but not always. Attacks occur and remit spontaneously. As the disorder progresses, however, the frequency of the attacks increases. Touch may trigger the pain as in this case by the application of makeup. Transient ischemic attacks (TIA), or "little strokes," present with an acute onset of a focal or clinical deficit that resolves in 24 hours. Although TIAs may occur spontaneously, they do not usually manifest so specifically as along the trigeminal nerve. Both of the seizures noted have noticeable loss of consciousness associated with them and do not usually present as a pain syndrome.

10. **The correct answer is D.** Multiple sclerosis presents pathologically with focal areas of demyelination scattered throughout the white matter of the brain/spinal cord and optic nerves. Lewy bodies are pathologically associated with Alzheimer's patients. Barr bodies are the inactive X chromosome in female mammals and the inactive Z chromosome in male mammals. Heinz bodies are small red blood cell inclusions that represent denatured hemoglobin seen in certain forms of anemia, such as thalassemia and G6PD deficiency.

11. **The correct answer is C.** Cervical dystonia involves a fixed, abnormal position of the neck. It is usually painful and associated with muscle spasm. Although there is no definitive cure for dystonia, treatment includes physical therapy, anticholinergics, benzodiazepines, baclofen, and botulinim toxin injections. A resting tremor, cogwheel rigidity, and bradykinesia best characterize Parkinson's disease. Partial complex seizures manifest with impaired consciousness and "automatic movements," such as screaming, disrobing, and kicking. Chorea is an abnormal involuntary movement disorder.

12. **The correct answer is A.** Pernicious anemia is the most common cause of vitamin B_{12} deficiency. Neurologic manifestations include dementia, depression, ataxia, and neuropathy (due to demyelination of the posterior and lateral columns). Plaques in the brain may indicate a demyelinating disorder, such as multiple sclerosis. Vitamin B_{12} deficiency does not cause lesions in the dorsal root ganglions and anterior motor cells.

13. **The correct answer is D.** Sensory disturbance of a C7 lesion may produce disturbance in the region of the middle finger. C5 sensory deficits typically involve the thumb side. C4 lesions do not usually manifest as sensory deficits in the upper extremity.

14. **The correct answer is A.** Red flags to consider in headache evaluation include onset after age 50, increasing frequency and severity of headache, presence of papilledema, headache secondary to trauma, and headache with signs of systemic illness.

15. **The correct answer is D.** Prior stroke or transient ischemic attack (TIA), hypertension, cigarette smoking, diabetes mellitus, atrial fibrillation, and arterial disease are all risk factors for stroke. The risk factor for stroke doubles for each decade after age 55.

16. **The correct answer is A.** Middle cerebral artery infarct leads to contralateral hemiparesis. Ischemic injury to the dominant hemisphere leads to aphasia.

17. **The correct answer is C.** This is by definition a transient ischemic attack (TIA). Reversible ischemic neurologic dysfunction is a cerebral infarction lasting longer than 24 hours but less than 72 hours. Partial complex seizure is commonly associated with impaired consciousness as well as variable motor and behavior activities arising from a single brain area.

18. **The correct answer is B.** Classic migraine (also called *migraine with aura*) lasts 4 to 72 hours and frequently is accompanied by an aura. Cluster headache is a painful, unilateral headache lasting 15 minutes to 3 hours. These headaches are associated with autonomic signs such as ptosis, conjunctival injection, lacrimation, and rhinorrhea. Tension headaches typically last 4 to 6 hours and patients often describe a feeling of pressure or a tight band around the head. In this case, the history indicates this patient takes butalbital. By itself, this is simply a phenobarbital. However, most preparations to treat migraines with butalbital as an ingredient also contain caffeine and perhaps acetaminophen. Caffeine withdrawal typically causes vasodilation and thus a rebound headache.

19. **The correct answer is A.** Asymmetric muscular weakness along with atrophy, fasciculations, and hyperreflexia typically occur in patients with amyotrophic lateral sclerosis (ALS).

20. **The correct answer is C.** Kinetic tremor occurs with voluntary movement. All of the other statements are true.

21. **The correct answer is A.** Grand mal seizures result in loss of consciousness and are associated with generalized muscle spasms. Absence seizures are brief episodes of staring and are usually limited to childhood. Rapid, brief contractions on both sides of the body characterize myoclonic seizures. They do not result in loss of consciousness.

22. **The correct answer is D.** Tics are a stereotypical involuntary repetitive movement. Simple tics may manifest as eye blinking and repetitive throat clearing, whereas complex tics involve distinct movements that employ several muscle groups. Tics, coprolalia (uttering swear words), and echolalia (repeating words or phrases of others) may be part of Tourette's syndrome. A tremor is an involuntary, rhythmic muscular movement of a body part. Chorea is an involuntary, irregular movement that is random in direction. Dystonia is a sustained muscle contraction that usually presents with an abnormal posture.

23. **The correct answer is D.** This condition is due to thiamine deficiency, most commonly found in alcoholics. The oculomotor signs are a result of involvement of the oculomotor, abducens, and vestibular nuclei.

24. **The correct answer is A.** Carpal tunnel syndrome involves injury to the median nerve. All of the other listed choices may (and frequently do) appear in patients with carpal tunnel syndrome.

25. **The correct answer is A.** By definition, any dementia that occurs following a recent stroke is poststroke dementia (PSD). Research indicates that the prevalence of PSD will likely increase in the future. In community-based studies, the prevalence of PSD in stroke survivors is about 30% and the incidence of new-onset dementia after stroke increases from 7% after 1 year to 48% after 25 years. In other words, having a stroke doubles the risk of dementia. Patient-related variables associated with an increased risk of PSD include increasing age, prestroke cognitive decline (without dementia), low education level, dependency before stroke, atrial fibrillation, diabetes mellitus, and myocardial infarction (especially if significant post–myocardial-infarction sequelae exist). Furthermore, patients may present with epileptic seizures, sepsis, transient ischemic attacks (TIA) or silent cerebral infarcts, cardiac arrhythmias, congestive heart failure, global and medial temporal lobe atrophy, and white-matter changes. Poststroke dementia may lead to

Alzheimer's, but it is not usually the first dementia seen in poststroke patients. These patients have high mortality rates and are likely functionally impaired. Lewy body disease is a disease of essentially unknown etiology caused by the buildup of Lewy bodies in the brain. Research has linked it to multisystem atrophy and Parkinson's disease. These buildups cause progressive neurologic impairment, ultimately leading to dementia. Unfortunately, postmortem examination is where we make the diagnosis. The term Wernicke's encephalopathy describes the symptom complex of ophthalmoplegia, ataxia, and an acute state of confusion. If persistent learning and memory deficits are present, the symptom complex is termed Wernicke-Korsakoff syndrome. A deficiency of thiamine (vitamin B_1) is responsible for the symptom complex manifested in Wernicke-Korsakoff syndrome, and any condition resulting in a poor nutritional state places patients at risk. However, the most common etiology of Wernicke-Korsakoff syndrome is heavy alcohol consumption. Patients frequently present with gait disturbances and memory changes, which is unlike the pure dementia states.

26. **The correct answer is D.** Simply put, *coma* is defined as not opening the eyes, not obeying commands, and not uttering understandable words. The elements of the Glasgow Coma Scale are as follows (for adults):

Eye Opening	E
Spontaneous	4
To speech	3
To pain	2
No response	1
Best Motor Response	**M**
To verbal command:	
Obeys	6
To painful stimulus:	
Localizes pain	5
Flexion-withdrawal	4
Flexion-abnormal	3
Extension	2
No response	1
Best Verbal Response	**V**
Oriented and converses	5
Disoriented and converses	4
Inappropriate words	3
Incomprehensible sounds	2
No response	1

E + M + V = 3 to 15

The Glasgow Coma Scale provides a score in the range of 3–15; patients with scores of 3–8 are usually said to be in a coma. The total score is the sum of the scores in three categories.

Less than or equal to 8 = coma.

Greater than or equal to 9 = not in coma.

The critical score is 8: Less than or equal to 8 at 6 hours has a 50% mortality rate.

9 to 11 = moderate severity.

Greater than or equal to 12 = minor injury.

For children under 5, the verbal response criteria are adjusted as follows:

Score	2 to 5 years	0 to 23 months
5	Appropriate words or phrases	Smiles or coos appropriately
4	Inappropriate words	Cries and consolable
3	Persistent cries and/or screams	Persistent inappropriate crying &/or screaming
2	Grunts	Grunts or is agitated or restless
1	No response	No response

27. **The correct answer is B.** Historically CT scans have been put forth as superior to MRI in detection of hemorrhagic stroke. Many texts and tests still hold this to be true. However, a growing body of evidence indicates that MRI is just as effective in detecting hemorrhagic stroke. We urge the clinician to evaluate the literature on this subject. An electroencephalogram (EEG) is best in evaluating seizure and other brain activity, but not the presence or absence of ischemia or hemorrhage in the brain. The practitioner should not use lumbar puncture in order to determine a bleed, because this could cause cerebral infarction and/or herniation.

28. **The correct answer is A.** Astrocytomas are the most common primary brain tumor. According to the World Health Organization's classification, the most malignant grades are anaplastic astrocytoma (AA; grade III) and glioblastoma multiforme (GBM; grade IV), with glioblastoma multiforme being the most common malignant brain tumor in adults. The CT scan is the diagnostic test of choice, and as you can see from the images below, contrast makes the tumor more visible (see pictures below with and without contrast). Other types include low-grade astrocytomas; oligodendrogliomas (which vary in grade but are not as dangerous as anaplastic astrocytoma or glioblastoma multiforme); and the rare ependymoma (originating from ependymal cells), which is usually low grade. Meningiomas are not in the astrocytoma class and are relatively benign. See CT.

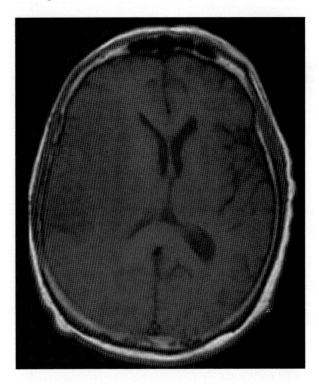

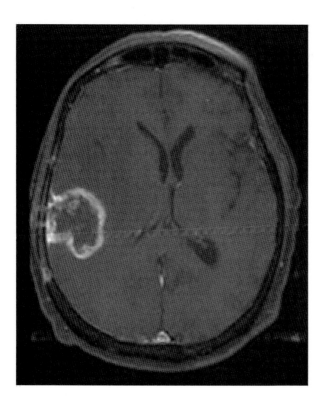

29. **The correct answer is D.** Giant cell arteritis (GCA), sometimes called temporal arteritis or granulomatous arteritis, is a systemic inflammatory vasculitis of unknown etiology that affects medium- and large-sized arteries. It is a disease of elderly persons, with an average age of onset of 50 years. Permanent visual impairment may occur in as many as 60% of patients. Women are two to four times more likely to have the disease. The hallmark symptom of GCA is new-onset localized headache, usually localized to the temporal or occipital area. Scalp tenderness accompanies the headache, especially over the temporal region; however, gentle pressure frequently induced the pain as well. The pain (usually from hypersensitivity or hyperesthesia) that arises from gentle stroking of a patient's hair is more common in migraines. Other symptoms of GCA include temporal tenderness or pulselessness, jaw claudication, facial pain, earache, toothache, tongue and palate pain, and odynophagia. Pulselessness and/or tenderness along the course of the temporal artery may occur, along with bruits in the cranial or carotid areas.

30. **The correct answer is A.** The brain itself has no sensory nerve endings or receptors. Mass effects in the brain usually cause pain by exerting pressure on surrounding structures. Nociception is the process whereby receptors throughout the body detect painful stimuli and transmit the information along a nerve via the spinal cord to the brain.

31. **The correct answer is B.** This patient has tarsal tunnel syndrome, which is analogous to carpel tunnel syndrome in the wrist. Overuse or any repetitive activity that creates inflammation and swelling along the posterior tibial nerve can result in tarsal tunnel syndrome. The patient usually presents with pain and paresthesias along the medial aspect of the ankle, radiating distally, although there may be occasional proximal radiation. Diabetic neuropathy presents with a variety of symptoms, which could include pain and paresthesia, but most likely will result in anesthesia that frequently occurs in a stocking and glove pattern and is not limited to one nerve root. Complex regional pain syndrome, also known as reflex sympathetic dystrophy or causalgia, usually presents with continuous, intense pain after an injury of some type. The pain often is out of proportion to the severity of the injury and typically worsens over time. In most cases, a whole limb is affected, and it presents with changes in the color and temperature of the skin over

the affected limb or body part, accompanied by intense, burning pain; skin sensitivity; sweating; and swelling. The cause of complex regional pain syndrome is unknown, but research suggests an immune-response component. The most common neuroma is a Morton neuroma. Because it is located at the base of the third and fourth toes, it is sometimes known as an intermetatarsal neuroma. Irritation of the neuroma could lead to swelling of the affected nerve and possible permanent damage. Typically, patients present with pain and paresthesia or anesthesia of the foot and toes. Patients also report the sensation of something in their shoes, such as a rolled-up sock.

32. **The correct answer is A.** An acoustic neuroma, also known as a vestibular schwannoma, is a slow-growing benign tumor of the eighth cranial nerve. Patients present with tinnitus and hearing loss in the affected ear, along with vertigo. Less commonly, patients may present with headache, difficulty in understanding speech (which seems out of proportion to the hearing loss), transient visual abnormalities, and pain in the face or affected ear. Menière's disease presents with the triad of hearing loss, tinnitus, and vertigo, but does not demonstrate a mass effect on MRI. Trigeminal neuralgia typically presents with pain along the distribution of the trigeminal nerve. Multiple sclerosis is a chronic, demyelinating disease of the central nervous system. Patients present with global symptoms depending on the area of the brain affected.

33. **The correct answer is B.** This patient has benign positional vertigo (BPV). This is the most common cause of dizziness reported in adults, occurring in up to 40% of adults with a complaint of dizziness. Research suggests that BPV occurs due to the presence of otoliths typically composed of calcium carbonate. These otoliths inappropriately displace into the semicircular canals of the vestibular labyrinth of the inner ear. They typically attach to hair cells on a membrane inside the utricle and saccule. Because the otoliths are denser than the surrounding endolymph, vertical head movement causes the otoliths to tilt the hair cells (which give us our sense of positional space, regardless of whether our eyes are open). If the otoliths displace from the hair cells, they can free-float within the posterior semicircular canal, causing the symptoms described in the question. Menière's disease is a disorder of the inner ear probably related to an abnormality in fluid flow through the ear. The symptoms of Menière's disease are episodic rotational vertigo hearing loss, tinnitus, and a sensation of fullness in the affected ear. The tinnitus and fullness may precipitate an attack or conversely, constantly be present. Early on, the patient may experience low-pitched hearing loss; however, this eventually develops into a fixed hearing loss over time that affects all sound pitches. Vertigo is the usual reason that patients present to their practitioners. An acute, sustained dysfunction of the peripheral vestibular system with secondary nausea, vomiting, and vertigo best describes vestibular neuritis, or neuronitis. Because this condition is not clearly inflammatory in nature, neurologists often refer to it as vestibular neuropathy. The etiology is unknown, although the prevailing opinion is that many cases are due to reactivation of a latent herpes simplex virus type I in the vestibular ganglia. Most patients recover spontaneously within a few weeks. However, some patients have recurrent attacks with rapid head movements for years after the onset of symptoms. Patients typically complain of an abrupt onset of severe, debilitating vertigo (usually spinning), with associated unsteadiness, nausea, and vomiting. The vertigo increases with head movement, especially rapid head movements. Migraines present with pain, usually following a visual or auditory disturbance, along with photophobia. Dizziness is variable among patients.

34. **The correct answer is A.** One of three types of bacteria typically is the most common cause of bacterial meningitis. These include: *Haemophilus influenzae* type b (Hib), *Neisseria meningitidis*, and *Streptococcus pneumoniae*. Before the 1990s, Hib was the leading cause of bacterial meningitis, but new vaccines administered to children as part of their routine immunizations have reduced the occurrence of serious Hib disease. Today, *Neisseria meningitidis* and *Streptococcus pneumoniae* are the leading causes of bacterial meningitis.

35. **The correct answer is C.** The most common causes of primary dementia in the United States are vascular dementia and Alzheimer's disease. Huntington's disease, an inherited neurologic disease, can cause dementia, but it is not the most common cause. Huntington's disease causes behavioral changes and chorea. The usual age of onset of Huntington's disease is between 40 and 60 years. Parkinson's disease is a progressive neurologic disease affecting movement and muscle control. Symptoms of Parkinson's disease include tremors, balance problems, difficulty walking, and a rigid posture. Parkinson's disease destroys the brain's nerve cells that are responsible for muscle control. Up to 20% of patients in advanced stages of Parkinson's disease develop some degree of dementia. However, the dementia of Parkinson's disease is not the most common cause of primary dementia. Multiple sclerosis is a disease resulting in plaque formation in areas of the brain and spinal cord. It causes a variety of symptoms depending on the location of the plaques. Multiple sclerosis is also not the most common cause of primary dementia.

36. **The correct answer is A.** Broca's aphasia (named after Paul Broca), also known as expressive aphasia, is due to a lesion in the Broca's area of the brain (the lower part of the left frontal lobe). It is one of the main language areas in the cerebral cortex, because it controls the motor aspects of speech. Persons with Broca's aphasia can usually understand what words mean, but have trouble performing the motor, or output, aspects of speech. Thus, other names for this disorder are expressive and motor aphasia. Depending on the severity of the lesion to Broca's area, symptoms can range from the mildest type (cortical dysarthria), with intact comprehension and the ability to communicate through writing, to a complete loss of the ability to speak aloud. Fluent, but meaningless, speech and severe impairment of the ability to understand written or spoken words characterize Wernicke's aphasia. It is also known as fluent and sensory aphasia. Memory impairment and impairment in another area of thinking, such as the ability to organize thoughts and reason, the ability to use language, or the ability to see accurately (unrelated to eye disease) best describe dementia and Alzheimer's disease in particular. These impairments are severe enough to cause a decline in the patient's usual level of functioning.

37. **The correct answer is C.** To perform the Dix-Hallpike maneuver, the patient initially sits upright. The examiner should warn the patient that vertigo may occur as a result of the maneuver. The examiner turns the patient's head 30° to 45° toward the side that is tested. The patient focuses on the examiner's eyes or forehead with his or her eyes open. Then, as the examiner supports the patient's head, the patient quickly lies supine (within 2 seconds), allowing the neck to hyperextend slightly and hang off the edge of the examining table 20° to 30° past the horizontal. After a 2- to 20-second latent period, the onset of torsional upbeat or horizontal nystagmus denotes a positive test for benign paroxysmal positional vertigo (BPV). The episode can last 20 to 40 seconds. Nystagmus changes direction when the patient sits upright again. To assess certain dementias and memory the practitioner uses the Mini-Mental, or Mental, State Exams. Level of consciousness is best assessed using the practitioner's own skills of observation and physical examination.

38. **The correct answer is D.** Sumatriptan is currently recommended as an abortive or preventative measure for patients with impending migraine headaches. The patient typically self-administers the medication at the first perceived sign of migraine (such as visual prodromes).

39. **The correct answer is D.** Phenytoin's side effects for connective tissue include facial feature coarsening, lip enlargement, hypertrichosis, Peyronie's disease (an abnormal curvature of the penis secondary to the formation of fibrous plaques), and gingival hyperplasia. None of the remaining medications is a cause of hyperplasia.

REFERENCES

Fauci, A. S., Braunwald, E., Kasper, D. L., Hauser, S. L., Longo, D. L., Jameson, J. L., and Loscalzo, J. (2008). *Harrison's Textbook of Internal Medicine*, 17th ed. McGraw-Hill Medical Publishing, New York.

Goetz, C. G., and Pappert, E. J. (2007) *Textbook of Clinical Neurology*, 3rd ed. Saunders Elsevier Publishing, Philadelphia, PA.

Goldmann, L., and Ausiello, D. (2008). *Cecil Medicine*, 23rd ed. Saunders Elsevier, Philadelphia, PA.

Ropper, A. H., and Brown, R. H. (2005). *Adams and Victor's Principles of Neurology*, 8th ed. McGraw-Hill, New York.

Tierney, L. M., Jr., McPhee, S. J., and Papadakis, M. A. (2008). *Current Medical Diagnosis and Treatment*. The McGraw-Hill Companies, Inc., New York.

General Practice

Tabassum Salam, MD, FACP
Irwin Wolfert, MD

1. An 80-year-old male nursing home resident presents to the emergency department for evaluation. He has become increasingly confused over the past day, and he has a low body temperature. He has a history of a stroke. His only current medication is a daily aspirin. His electrolytes are within normal limits, and his leukocyte count is 14,000/mm³. The chest radiograph shows a small interstitial infiltrate in the left lower lung field. You decide to start antibiotic therapy. Which of the following organisms would probably *not* cause this patient's condition and therefore not require antibiotic coverage?

    A. *Aspergillus fumigatus*
    B. *Enterobacter* species
    C. Anaerobic bacteria
    D. *Pseudomonas aeruginosa*

2. A 72-year-old woman presents with complaints of dyspnea on exertion and palpitations for the past 2 hours. The palpitations started suddenly and are still present. She is not on any medication and has no other medical problems. On physical examination, her blood pressure is 130/80 mmHg and her pulse is irregular. Her electrocardiogram is shown below. Which of the following best describes her heart rhythm?

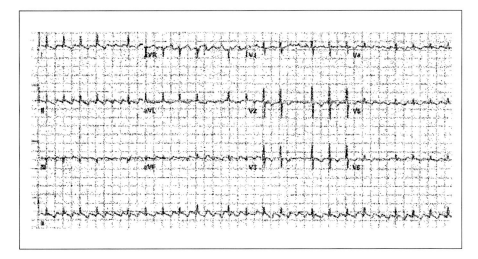

    A. Atrial fibrillation
    B. Atrial flutter
    C. Atrial tachycardia
    D. Ventricular tachycardia

3. You discharge an 82-year-old woman from the hospital in October, where she received treatment for an exacerbation of chronic obstructive pulmonary disease (COPD). Her only other medical problems are hypertension and a history of tobacco use. She quit smoking 3 years ago. She received a pneumococcal vaccine 7 years ago. She received the influenza vaccine 1 year ago. Which of the following vaccines is/are now indicated in this patient?

 A. Pneumococcal and influenza vaccines
 B. Pneumococcal vaccine
 C. Influenza vaccine
 D. There is no indication for vaccination.

4. A 64-year-old male presents with hypertension and a 10-year history of type 2 diabetes. He is overweight. His blood pressure is 156/92 mmHg, his hemoglobin A_1C is 7.9%, and his serum creatinine is 1.2 mg/dL. Which of the following medications should you prescribe as part of his first-line antihypertensive regimen?

 A. metoprolol
 B. amlodipine
 C. clonidine
 D. ramipril

5. A 37-year-old woman presents for evaluation of her cholesterol levels. Her weight and body mass index (BMI) are within normal range, and she does not complain of chest pain with exercise. However, she has a strong family history of early coronary disease. On physical examination, she has cutaneous infiltrates above both eyes and large painless lumps on both Achilles tendons. Her lab results are as follows:

Fasting plasma glucose: 92 mg/dL

Total cholesterol: 460 mg/dL

Triglycerides: 110 mg/dL

High-density lipoprotein cholesterol: 55 mg/dL

Low-density lipoprotein cholesterol: 375 mg/dL

Which of the following would be the most appropriate next step in the treatment of this patient?

 A. Statin therapy
 B. Repeat lipid profile in 6 months
 C. Suspect lab error and repeat the blood work
 D. Begin a bile-acid sequestrant

6. A 65-year-old female undergoes a total right hip replacement. Three weeks later, she complains that her left leg has become warm and swollen. Doppler ultrasound of her lower extremities shows proximal deep venous thrombosis of her left leg. You elect treatment with heparin and warfarin. How long should you continue the warfarin?

 A. 4 weeks
 B. 2 months
 C. 6 months
 D. For the rest of her life

7. A 76-year-old man presents complaining of 6 months of epigastric pain with meals. He does not experience pain on swallowing. He has not had any weight loss. Initially, he took over-the-counter antacids and H$_2$ blockers with relief. However, lately these medications no longer relieve his epigastric abdominal pain. Physical examination is unremarkable. His hemoglobin is 11.2 g/dL. Which of the following is the most effective next step in the management of the patient?

   A. CT scan of the abdomen
   B. Serologic testing for *Helicobacter pylori*
   C. Radionuclide gastric-emptying study
   D. Upper endoscopy

8. A 34-year-old woman presents to the emergency department complaining of having vomited blood 1 hour ago. She was at a retirement party and had vomited a "large" amount of bright red blood. On physical examination, her heart rate is 102 bpm and regular. Her blood pressure is 95/60 mmHg, left arm, supine. Her labs are as follows:

   Serum sodium: 136 mEq/L

   Serum potassium: 2.9 mEq/L

   Serum chloride: 86 mEq/L

   Serum bicarbonate: 34 mEq/L

   Serum blood urea nitrogen: 21 mg/dL

   Serum creatinine: 0.9 mg/dL

   The patient undergoes upper endoscopy, which reveals erosive esophagitis without active bleeding and a fresh Mallory-Weiss tear with an adherent clot. Which of the following is the most likely cause?

   A. NSAID–induced esophagitis
   B. *Staphylococcus aureus* toxin ingestion
   C. *Bacillus cereus* toxin ingestion
   D. Bulimia

9. A 73-year-old woman presents complaining that for the past 3 months her abdomen has been distended and she has gained 12 pounds. She has a history of hepatitis C. On physical examination, she has mild abdominal distention with shifting dullness. She also has peripheral edema. An abdominal ultrasound shows moderate ascites and splenomegaly. You perform a paracentesis. The ascitic fluid polymorphonuclear leukocyte count is 150/mm^3, and albumin is 1.2 g/dL. Serum albumin is 2.6 g/dL. Which of the following is the most likely cause of her ascites?

   A. Spontaneous bacterial peritonitis
   B. Portal hypertension
   C. Ovarian cancer
   D. Peritoneal carcinomatosis

10. A 26-year-old man presents complaining of shortness of breath for the past 5 days. He was diagnosed with stage III Hodgkin's disease 10 years ago, which was treated with multiple chemotherapy agents and radiation therapy. He does not take any medications at present. His blood work shows the following:

    Hemoglobin: 8.5 g/dL

    White blood cell count: 2,300/mm^3

    Platelet count: 64,000/mm^3

    Which of the following is the most likely cause of these results?

    A. Relapsed Hodgkin's disease
    B. Secondary myelodysplastic syndrome
    C. Anemia of chronic disease
    D. Drug-induced bone marrow suppression

11. A 41-year-old woman presents for evaluation of a lump in her left breast. She first felt it 6 weeks ago. On palpation, there is a firm 6-mm mass in the left upper outer quadrant that is minimally tender and not freely mobile. The patient undergoes bilateral mammography, and the results are unremarkable. Which of the following is the best course of action?

    A. Schedule patient for a repeat physical examination after 3 months.
    B. Perform a fine-needle aspiration.
    C. Order a repeat mammogram with specialized views.
    D. No further evaluation is necessary.

12. A 42-year-old woman works in a nursing home. A few weeks ago some residents of the nursing home developed bloody diarrhea and acute abdominal pain. She developed the same symptoms, but gradually improved without treatment. A few weeks later, she presents with diffuse musculoskeletal pain in the neck, right wrist, left knee, and low back. She has marked swelling, warmth, and limited motion of the right wrist and left knee. Which of the following is the most likely diagnosis?

    A. Fibromyalgia
    B. Rheumatoid arthritis
    C. Disseminated *Neisseria gonorrhoeae* infection
    D. Reactive arthritis

13. A 69-year-old woman undergoes bone density scanning with dual absorptiometry. Her scores are as follows:

Spine: T score, −2.6; Z score, −1.3

Hip: T score, −1.5; Z score, −0.9

Which of the following is the most likely diagnosis?

    A. Normal bone mass
    B. Osteopenia
    C. Osteomalacia
    D. Osteoporosis

14. An obese 62-year-old man comes in for a visit to discuss his type 2 diabetes, He first received his diagnosis 4 years ago at which time his first hemoglobin A_1C was 7.2%. He initially managed his diabetes by changing his diet and increasing his physical activity. Two years ago, his hemoglobin A_1C rose to 8.2%, therefore he began taking glyburide 10 mg daily. His hemoglobin A_1C subsequently fell to 6.9%. Over the past year, the patient has gained 12 pounds. His most recent hemoglobin A_1C is 7.9%. His creatinine is 1.6 mg/dL, and his hemoglobin is 14.2 g/dL. In addition to suggesting weight loss and exercise, what is the next best intervention to make?

    A. Change glyburide to glipizide.
    B. Add metformin to glyburide.
    C. Increase glyburide to 20 mg daily.
    D. Add pioglitazone.

15. A 39-year-old man is hospitalized with *Pneumocystis jiroveci (carinii)* pneumonia. He is HIV positive with a CD4 count of 50 cells/μL. He begins IV trimethoprim-sulfamethoxazole. However, he deteriorates rapidly requiring intubation and mechanical ventilation. His arterial blood gas shows a PaO_2 of 72 mmHg on 60% oxygen and a positive end-expiratory pressure (PEEP) of 7.5 mmHg. Which of the following is the most appropriate next step?

    A. Change the trimethoprim-sulfamethoxazole to IV pentamidine.
    B. Add azithromycin.
    C. Add prednisone.
    D. Add IV pentamidine.

16. You evaluate a 42-year-old woman of Italian descent during a routine annual examination. She is feeling well and her examination is unremarkable. Her blood work reveals the following:

Hematocrit: 35%

Mean corpuscular volume: 63 fL

White blood cell count: 6,700/mm³

Reticulocyte count: 0.7%

Platelet count: 270,000/mm³

Which of the following tests would best confirm the diagnosis?
- **A.** Serum iron-binding capacity and serum ferritin level
- **B.** Measurement of hemoglobin A_2
- **C.** Peripheral blood smear
- **D.** Glucose-6-phosphate dehydrogenase screen

17. An 82-year-old man complains of morning stiffness, especially in his hips and shoulders. He does not have headaches, jaw claudication, or changes in vision. He has mild crepitus of the knees, but no frank effusions or synovitis. His hematocrit is 28%, and his erythrocyte sedimentation rate (ESR) is 116 mm/hr. Which of the following would be the most appropriate next step?
- **A.** Start ibuprofen.
- **B.** Get a chest radiograph.
- **C.** Start prednisone.
- **D.** Send the patient for a temporal artery biopsy.

18. A 27-year-old male admits to the hospital in January. He complains of shortness of breath and a persistent cough that has lasted for 3 weeks. He is HIV positive with a CD4 count of 350/uL. A chest radiograph reveals bibasilar infiltrates and a right-sided pleural effusion. His pulse oximetry on room air is 93%. He undergoes fiberoptic bronchoscopy, which reveals a violaceous lesion on the mucosa of the mainstem bronchus. The lesion is raised and 0.8 cm in diameter. You obtain samples of bronchoalveolar lavage, and the results are pending. Which of the following is the most likely diagnosis?
- **A.** Immune thrombocytopenic purpura (AITP)
- **B.** Leukocytoclastic vasculitis
- **C.** Kaposi's sarcoma
- **D.** Disseminated herpes simplex

19. A 60-year-old woman has chronic hepatitis C due to a remote blood transfusion. A liver biopsy reveals cirrhosis. An endoscopy shows large, distal esophageal varices. Which of the following is the most appropriate next step?
- **A.** Band ligation of esophageal varices
- **B.** Dietary protein restriction
- **C.** Nonselective β-blocker
- **D.** Daily norfloxacin

20. A 72-year-old man undergoes a resection of an adenocarcinoma of the transverse colon. There is adequate resection and nodal dissection. There are no lymph node metastases, and there is no other organ invasion. Which of the following tests should he undergo in 1 year?
- **A.** Colonoscopy
- **B.** Liver enzyme levels
- **C.** CT scan of the abdomen
- **D.** Fecal occult blood testing

21. A 72-year-old man is brought to the emergency department because of 5 days of fever, lethargy, and progressive confusion. He recently went to the dentist for regular periodontal care. He has a temperature of 101.0°F, papilledema, mild left-sided weakness, and a "stiff" neck. Which of the following is the most likely diagnosis?

   A. Bacterial meningitis
   B. Viral meningitis
   C. Brain tumor
   D. Pyogenic brain abscess

22. A 39-year-old woman presents with 8 days of chills and complaints of pain on urination. The physical exam is unremarkable. Blood count, serum electrolytes, and renal function are all within normal laboratory parameters. Her urinalysis reveals the following:

pH: 6.4

Blood: 2+

Protein: Trace

Glucose: Trace

Erythrocytes: 5–10 per hpf

Leukocytes: 40–50 per hpf

Leukocyte esterase: Positive

The urine culture grows *Proteus mirabilis* >100,000 col/cc. An abdominal radiograph reveals an irregular calcified object measuring 2 × 4 cm overlying the left renal shadow. An IV pyelogram shows a branched, calcified calculus in the upper one-half of the left renal collecting system. Which of the following is the likely cause of this patient's urinary stones?

   A. Calcium oxalate
   B. Calcium phosphate and oxalate
   C. Uric acid
   D. Triple phosphate (struvite)

23. A 35-year-old woman with a long history of IV heroin use is brought to the Emergency Department by a friend. She is comatose and cyanotic. The friend reports that the patient appeared well when he saw her the previous night. She has a temperature of 36.6°C; a pulse rate of 116 bpm; a respiratory rate of 8 breaths per minute; and a blood pressure of 90/60 mmHg, right arm, semi-supine. She has constricted pupils, bilateral rales, and marked cyanosis of her fingertips. The chest radiograph shows bilateral infiltrates. Her ECG shows sinus tachycardia without ST-segment changes. Her pulse oximetry reveals an oxygen saturation of 50%. Which of the following is the most appropriate immediate treatment for this patient?

   A. IV naloxone
   B. IV furosemide
   C. IV flumazenil
   D. IV digitalis

24. A 68-year-old man with a 14-year history of heavy alcohol use has severe abdominal pain exacerbated by meals. Refer to the abdominal radiograph below. Which of the following is the most likely cause of the abnormalities noted in the radiograph?

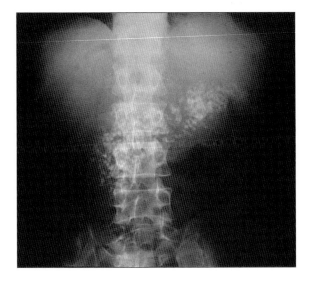

A. Cholelithiasis
B. Chronic pancreatitis
C. Duodenal ulcer
D. Nephrolithiasis

25. A 17-year-old female complains of 3 days of urinary frequency and dysuria. She is not sexually active and has otherwise been well. The urinalysis reveals 10–15 WBCs/hpf and 20–30 RBCs/hpf. Which of the following is the most appropriate treatment option for this patient?

A. A single dose of ciprofloxacin
B. 3 days of trimethoprim-sulfamethoxazole
C. 7 days of trimethoprim-sulfamethoxazole
D. 7 days of nitrofurantoin

26. You recently diagnosed your patient, a 42-year-old male, with essential hypertension. He exhibits no signs or symptoms of end-organ damage. His blood pressure readings have consistently been in the following range: 162–168/92–96 mmHg. According to JNC-7, which of the following would be the most appropriate initial management?

A. Treatment with a diuretic
B. Lifestyle modification alone
C. Treatment with a beta blocker
D. Treatment with an ACE inhibitor/diuretic combination

27. A 72-year-old female presents complaining of a 2-week history of intermittent palpitations. She has no history of heart or lung disease. She denies chest pain, dyspnea, or syncope. An ECG reveals atrial fibrillation with a ventricular rate between 100 and 110 beats per minute. In addition to a laboratory evaluation, which of the following actions is most appropriate?

A. Prescribe digoxin and warfarin.
B. Arrange for urgent cardioversion.
C. Prescribe a β-blocker and warfarin.
D. Prescribe aspirin and digoxin.

28. A 47-year-old female treated with warfarin for a deep vein thrombosis presents to the emergency department with a pulmonary embolism. Her INR values have consistently been between 2 and 3. Which of the following is the most appropriate management of this patient?

   A. Increase her warfarin to achieve an INR between 3 and 4.
   B. Begin low molecular weight heparin.
   C. Add aspirin to her warfarin.
   D. Insert an inferior vena cava filter.

29. A 64-year-old male with a past medical history of hypertension and a stroke has a low-density lipoprotein (LDL) cholesterol level of 118 mg/dL. His current medication regimen includes simvastatin 40 mg daily. Which of the following would be the most appropriate treatment for this patient?

   A. Add ezetimibe 10 mg to his regimen.
   B. Add niacin to his regimen.
   C. Increase his simvastatin dosage to 80 mg.
   D. Switch his medication from simvastatin to lovastatin, 40 mg.

30. An 8-year-old female presents with a 24-hour history of nausea and diarrhea. Her mother describes her stools as watery without obvious blood. The child has not vomited and has been afebrile. She denies abdominal pain. Her examination is unremarkable. Which of the following is the most likely cause of her diarrhea?

   A. *Clostridium difficile*
   B. Rotavirus
   C. Staphylococcal food poisoning
   D. *Giardia lamblia*

31. Which of the following is typical of infection with the hepatitis C virus?

   A. Acute course of abdominal pain and jaundice
   B. Persistent elevation of liver function tests
   C. Chronic infection in 80% of infected patients
   D. Commonly transmitted via sexual activity

32. An 80-year-old female with New York Heart Association (NYHA) Class II heart failure presents to the emergency department with a 4-day history of increasing dyspnea on exertion. She does not appear to be in distress, and her vital signs are normal. Her pulse oximetry is 94% on room air. Examination reveals an S4 gallop and a few crackles at her lung bases. There is no leg edema. Electrocardiogram and chest radiographic studies are consistent with left ventricular enlargement, but no acute processes are noted. Troponin and CK-MB levels are normal. Adjustment of which of the following medications would provide the greatest symptomatic relief for the patient?

   A. lisinopril
   B. furosemide
   C. digoxin
   D. metoprolol

33. Which of the following typically is not associated with metabolic syndrome?

   A. Increased waist circumference
   B. Fasting blood glucose >110 mg/dL
   C. Low-density lipoprotein (LDL) cholesterol >130 mg/dL
   D. Blood pressure ≥130/85 mmHg

34. A 10-year-old male with asthma has successfully used ihis albuterol inhaler 4 to 5 days a week to control episodes of bronchospasm. Which of the following therapeutic options is *not* consistent with current recommended guidelines?

A. Adding inhaled cromolyn
B. Adding inhaled corticosteroids
C. Adding an oral leukotriene antagonist
D. Maintaining the current regimen

35. A 71-year-old female has osteoporosis of her lumbar spine and hip. Which of the following would not be an appropriate recommendation for this patient?

A. raloxifene
B. alendronate
C. Calcium supplementation
D. Vitamin D supplementation

36. You admit an 82-year-old male to the hospital. You obtain a chest radiograph shown below. Which of the following antibiotic regimens is the most appropriate treatment?

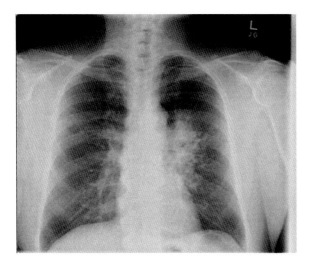

A. cephalexin plus clarithromycin
B. levofloxacin
C. ampicillin plus gentamicin
D. ciprofloxacin

37. According to the American Academy of Pediatrics (AAP), when considering a period of observation versus medication for otitis media, which of the following clinical items indicates a need for antibiotic treatment?

A. Fever of 102.5°F
B. Erythematous tympanic membrane
C. Mild otalgia
D. Associated cervical lymphadenopathy

38. A 61-year-old female with no significant past medical history presents with a 24-hour history of pain in the right preauricular area that radiates toward the right eye. She denies upper respiratory symptoms or visual changes. Examination is unremarkable except for a small vesicle on the tip of her nose. Which of the following is the most appropriate action?

A. carbamazepine therapy
B. Referral to an otolaryngologist
C. Referral to an ophthalmologist
D. A tapering course of oral corticosteroids

39. A 13-year-old female presents to your office with her mother. For the past 8 months, she has been experiencing moderate-to-severe monthly, right temporal headaches accompanied by nausea but no vomiting. The headaches worsen with physical activity. After an appropriate evaluation, which of the following would be the best therapeutic option?

A. Daily propanolol
B. sumitriptan, as needed
C. acetaminophen/butalbital/caffeine, as needed
D. Daily topiramate

40. Which of the following agents is *not* associated with a potential cognitive impairment in the elderly?

A. amitriptyline
B. diphenhydramine
C. hydrochlorothiazide
D. prednisone

41. A 50-year-old male complains of a 3-year history of productive cough and shortness of breath while climbing stairs. He has smoked two packs of cigarettes daily since the age of 25. Which of the following tests would be most useful in establishing a diagnosis of COPD?

A. Pulmonary function testing
B. Chest radiography
C. Exercise stress test
D. Arterial blood gas analysis

42. A 24-year-old female is unable to donate blood due to "anemia." A complete blood count confirms a hemoglobin value of 10.8 g/dL (normal is 12.3–15.2 g/dL) with a mean corpuscular volume of 69 fL (normal is 80–96 fL). Further testing reveals the following:

Serum ferritin: 85 μg/mL (normal is 40–200 μg/mL)

Total iron-binding capacity: 322 μg/dL (normal is 300–360 μg/dL)

Serum iron: 128 μg/dL (normal is 60–150 μg/dL)

Which of the following is the most likely cause of her anemia?

A. Iron deficiency
B. Glucose-6-phosphate dehydrogenase deficiency anemia
C. Anemia of chronic disease
D. β-thalassemia minor

43. Which of the following is *not* usually associated with gastroesophageal reflux disease (GERD)?

A. Hoarseness
B. Cough
C. Odynophagia
D. Chest pain

44. A 36-year-old male complains of severe pain in his left great toe in the absence of trauma. He has also experienced nausea and a low-grade fever. Which of the following medications would *not* be an appropriate treatment for this condition?

A. colchicine
B. allopurinol
C. prednisone
D. ibuprofen

ANSWERS

1. **The correct answer is A.** This patient is at risk for nosocomial pneumonia because he lives in a nursing home. *Pseudomonas* and *Enterobacter* often cause nosocomial pneumonias. The patient has suffered a stroke in the past; hence, he may be at risk for aspiration. Patients who aspirate may develop pneumonia with anaerobic agents. *Aspergillus* is not a common pneumonia-causing organism in nursing home residents; it usually affects severely immunocompromised individuals. It is a fungus commonly seen on decaying vegetation. Treatment of pulmonary aspergillus infection may include oral or inhaled corticosteroids or antifungal medications such as amphotericin B. Surgery may be indicated in cases of advanced aspergilloma.

2. **The correct answer is B.** The ECG shows an irregular ventricular rate. A sawtooth pattern is present in leads II, III, and AVF. This pattern is characteristic of atrial flutter. There is variable conduction of the flutter waves, leading to an irregular rhythm.

3. **The correct answer is C.** The patient should receive only the influenza vaccine in the fall, as long as she does not have an allergy to eggs. The patient is at high risk of developing life-threatening pulmonary infections due to her COPD. She only needs to receive the pneumococcal vaccine once over the age of 65. There is no role for a booster dose of the pneumococcal vaccine except in severely immunocompromised patients.

4. **The correct answer is D.** The HOPE trial showed that diabetic patients benefit from the addition of an angiotensin-converting enzyme (ACE) inhibitor to reduce the overall incidence of vascular events. ACE inhibitors slow the progression of renal disease in patients with diabetes and proteinuria.

5. **The correct answer is A.** The patient has xanthelasma and tendinous xanthomata. She also has a significant family history of coronary disease. She has a very elevated LDL cholesterol. She probably has heterozygous familial hypercholesterolemia and is at risk of developing her first myocardial infarction in her 40s. Hence, the clinician should begin treatment to reduce her LDL cholesterol. The most effective initial treatment is a statin.

6. **The correct answer is C.** In this patient, the cause of the deep vein thrombosis is very likely the recent joint replacement surgery and the subsequent immobility. Hence, treatment with warfarin for 3 to 6 months is adequate. Treatment for fewer than 3 months will lead to a higher recurrence risk. Lifetime treatment will put her at high risk for bleeding complications.

7. **The correct answer is D.** This patient has two warning signs for a possible gastric malignancy or a complication of a gastric ulcer: (1) he is presenting with new symptoms over the age of 50 and (2) he is slightly anemic. He should thus undergo early upper endoscopy with biopsies. Other alarm symptoms are anorexia, weight loss, dysphagia, gross or occult gastrointestinal bleeding, and barium x-ray findings suspicious for cancer.

8. **The correct answer is D.** The patient's blood work shows hypochloremia, hypokalemia, and a high bicarbonate level. These findings are consistent with repeated vomiting, not just an acute 1-hour history of vomiting. The endoscopy findings of esophagitis and the Mallory-Weiss tear are most consistent with bulimia. There should not be any endoscopic changes with bacterial–toxin-mediated gastroenteritis. NSAID–related esophagitis would cause chronic changes on endoscopy, but not the electrolyte changes.

9. **The correct answer is B.** The serum-to-ascites albumin gradient (SAAG) is $2.6 - 1.2 = 1.4$. A SAAG greater than 1.1 denotes portal hypertension. All the other conditions listed are inflammatory and neoplastic disorders that present with a SAAG of less than 1.1.

10. **The correct answer is B.** Up to 5% of survivors of Hodgkin's lymphoma treated with chemotherapy and radiation therapy usually develop secondary myelodysplastic syndrome or leukemia within 3 to 11 years of treatment.

11. **The correct answer is B.** This mass remains fixed on exam—a concerning feature of malignancy. The mass has also been present for more than one menstrual cycle. Mammograms have a false negative rate of 25% in premenopausal women. A practitioner skilled in fine-needle aspiration should sample a persistent palpable mass.

12. **The correct answer is D.** The patient probably had an enteric infection a few weeks ago, possibly with *Shigella flexneri*, *Salmonella*, *Campylobacter*, or *Yersinia*. She now has reactive arthritis. Disseminated *Neisseria gonorrhoeae* infection usually causes an acute, migratory arthritis or a septic arthritis of one joint (e.g., a knee). The presentation of rheumatoid arthritis usually involves the small peripheral joints in a symmetric manner.

13. **The correct answer is D.** World Health Organization (WHO) criterion for osteoporosis is a T score at or below −2.5 at either the spine or the hip.

14. **The correct answer is D.** The ideal goal for the hemoglobin A_1C level is less than 7%. At this level, the risks of microvascular and macrovascular complications decrease. Substituting one sulfonylurea for another will not improve glycemic control. This patient already receives the maximum dosage of glyburide. Metformin can be used synergistically with glyburide; however, it should not be prescribed to patients with a creatinine greater than 1.5 mg/dL. Thiazolidinediones also work synergistically with sulfonylureas.

15. **The correct answer is C.** This patient should receive adjunctive corticosteroid therapy for his *Pneumocystis jiroveci (carinii)* pneumonia. Past research indicates this improves morbidity and mortality in patients with hypoxemia. There is no need to change the antibiotic therapy.

16. **The correct answer is B.** This patient has the β-thalassemia trait. This causes mild anemia with profound microcytosis. She will have an elevated level of hemoglobin A2. The microcytosis is not as pronounced in mild anemia. In order to have an MCV of 63 in iron deficiency anemia, the corresponding hematocrit would be in the low 20% range.

17. **The correct answer is C.** This patient has polymyalgia rheumatica. The classic symptoms are limb-girdle stiffness, anemia, and an elevated sedimentation rate (ESR). He will probably show marked improvement after a short course of prednisone. He does not have symptoms of temporal arteritis (i.e., visual loss, headache, scalp tenderness, or beading of the temporal arteries). Hence, there is no need for a temporal artery biopsy at this time.

18. **The correct answer is C.** The raised, purple endobronchial lesion is Kaposi's sarcoma. It can occur at any CD4 cell count. Kaposi's sarcoma can cause diffuse pulmonary infiltrates and pleural effusions. It has also been linked oncogenically to human herpes virus −8.

19. **The correct answer is C.** Nonselective β-blockers can prevent initial variceal hemorrhage. Prophylactic band ligation of esophageal varices has not proven useful in preventing initial variceal bleeds.

20. **The correct answer is A.** The patient has had a curative resection of his colon cancer. The best surveillance test will be a colonoscopy. The CT scan and liver enzyme tests would be too nonspecific.

21. **The correct answer is D.** In light of the patient's recent dental procedures, the fever, nuchal rigidity, altered mental status, and papilledema make a brain abscess the likely diagnosis. Diagnosis will require neurologic imaging. An MRI is superior to a CT scan of the brain in this situation.

22. **The correct answer is D.** Struvite stones occur in the setting of infection with *Proteus mirabilis*. *Proteus* is a urea-splitting organism, thus producing NH₃ and raising the pH of the urine. It causes staghorn calculi.

23. **The correct answer is A.** This patient has heroin-induced pulmonary edema. She will improve rapidly after administration of IV naloxone and oxygen. Flumazenil is appropriate for reversal of the respiratory suppression caused by the benzodiazepines.

24. **The correct answer is B.** The presence of calcifications in the pancreas on plain film of the abdomen is characteristic of chronic pancreatitis.

25. **The correct answer is B.** This patient has uncomplicated cystitis, probably caused by *Escherichia coli*. A 3-day course of trimethoprim-sulfamethoxazole should be highly effective in treating this. If she does not show improvement within 48 hours, she may need to change medications to a fluoroquinolone, due to the possible development of trimethoprim-sulfamethoxazole-resistant strains.

26. **The correct answer is D.** The patient has stage 2 hypertension. JNC 7 recommends that initial treatment should include two pharmaceutic agents.

27. **The correct answer is C.** The patient presents with hemodynamically stable atrial fibrillation. She does not require urgent cardioversion; however, consideration of this in the future is not out of the question. In order to reduce stroke risk (her age and hypertension place her at a higher risk), she requires anticoagulation with warfarin. A β-blocker is the agent of choice for rate control.

28. **The correct answer is D.** The patient is adequately anticoagulated on warfarin. Increasing her INR or adding heparin or aspirin would not necessarily provide further benefit. Placement of a filter may prevent further emboli.

29. **The correct answer is A.** The patient has vascular disease; therefore, his LDL goal is less than 100 mg/dL. Doubling his simvastatin dosage would only improve his LDL by 6% (rule of sixes). Adding ezetimbe would likely reduce his LDL by 20 to 25%. Niacin is not a potent drug for LDL reduction, and lovastatin is a weak statin drug.

30. **The correct answer is B.** The most common cause of an acute onset of noninflammatory diarrhea in this age group is rotavirus. Patients with *Clostridium difficile* typically present with tenesmus and may be febrile. *Staphylococcus* generally presents with vomiting and may lack diarrhea. *Giardia* is less common than rotavirus and typically produces symptoms (bloating, foul-smelling stools, and weight loss) that wax and wane over time.

31. **The correct answer is C.** All patients with hepatitis C do not experience an acute illness. Liver function tests often fluctuate throughout the course of the disease. Transmission via sexual activity is thought to be a rare event.

32. **The correct answer is B.** The patient's presentation is consistent with a mild flare of her congestive heart failure (CHF). Examination and lab features do not support other causes of dyspnea (acute myocardial infarction, pneumonia, pulmonary embolism). Lisinopril and metoprolol may be indicated for the chronic management of cardiomyopathy, but do not resolve acute symptoms. Digoxin use in CHF patients generally reserves for those with coexistent atrial fibrillation. Diuretics are the drugs of choice for symptomatic relief of acute dyspnea.

33. **The correct answer is C.** Metabolic syndrome occurs when the patient has a constellation of any three of the following conditions: abdominal obesity, triglycerides ≥150 mg/dL, HDL cholesterol ≤40 mg/dL for men or ≤50 mg/dL for women, fasting glucose ≥110 mg/dL, and hypertension.

34. The correct answer is D. The patient has mild persistent asthma, characterized by symptoms greater than twice weekly. The National Asthma Education and Prevention Program Expert Panel recommends the use of an anti-inflammatory agent in all patients with persistent asthma. These agents include inhaled corticosteroids, cromolyn, nedocromil, and leukotriene antagonists.

35. The correct answer is A. All patients with osteoporosis should receive calcium and vitamin D supplementation. Raloxifene is most appropriate for patients with osteoporosis involving the spine but not the hip. Alendronate is best used for patients with involvement of both the spine and the hip.

36. The correct answer is B. The chest radiograph shows a hilar pneumonia. Empiric treatment for community-acquired pneumonia includes any of the following antibiotics: macrolides (clarithromycin or azithromycin), doxycycline, or an antipneumococcal fluoroquinolone. If the patient requires hospitalization (non-ICU), then the following medications should be ordered: a macrolide plus an extended-spectrum beta lactam (ceftriaxone or cefotaxime) or an antipneumococcal fluoroquinolone. Ciprofloxacin does not have sufficient antipneumococcal activity.

37. The correct answer is A. The AAP guidelines suggest the option of observation versus initiation of antibiotics in children older 2 years of age with mild illness associated with acute otitis media (AOM). Mild illness is mild otalgia and fever above 39°C (102.2°F).

38. The correct answer is C. The patient is exhibiting symptoms consistent with neuropathic facial pain. Vesicle formation on the tip of the nose (Hutchinson's sign) is suggestive of herpes zoster ophthalmicus. Involvement of the nasociliary nerve dermatomes warrants prompt evaluation by an ophthalmologist, which could prevent scarring of the cornea. Tegretol is useful for trigeminal neuralgia, another facial neuralgia syndrome. Other eye complications could include keratitis, scleritis, episcleritis—some of which could lead to blindness. Oral corticosteroids have a controversial role in the management of herpes zoster virus infections.

39. The correct answer is B. The patient fulfills the International Headache Society criteria for migraines: recurrent headaches with (1) two of the following: unilateral location, pulsating quality, moderate-to-severe intensity, aggravation by physical activity; and (2) one of the following: nausea or vomiting, photophobia, or phonophobia. Because this patient only suffers from headaches on a monthly basis, abortive therapy would be her treatment of choice. The drugs of choice for abortive therapy are the triptans. Acetaminophen/butalbital/caffeine has sedative side effects and abuse potential. Propanolol and topiramate are useful for prophylaxis. The practitioner should consider these if headaches occur more than four times a month or are not controlled with abortive therapy.

40. The correct answer is C. The anticholinergic side effects of the tricyclic antidepressants and classic antihistamines cause sedation and cognitive impairment in the elderly. Corticosteroids may cause delirium in the elderly.

41. The correct answer is A. The patient has accumulated a 50-pack-year history of tobacco use. This places him at risk for chronic obstructive pulmonary disease (COPD). The criteria for diagnosis of chronic bronchitis include a productive cough exhibited for at least 3 months per year over 2 consecutive years and dyspnea on exertion. Air-flow obstruction is the hallmark of COPD. The diagnosis may be confirmed by demonstrating FEV1 and FEV1/FVC ratio less than 70% of predicted normal values. The chest radiograph is not sensitive or specific for COPD. It may demonstrate bullae, hyperlucencies, hyperinflation, and flattened diaphragms. Arterial blood gases play a role in evaluating patients with COPD exacerbations. They assess alveolar ventilation and acid-base status, but are not sensitive in making the diagnosis.

42. **The correct answer is D.** The differential diagnosis for microcytic anemia includes iron deficiency, thalassemia, and anemia of chronic disease. Only the minor thalassemias present with normal serum iron and total iron-binding capacity levels.

43. **The correct answer is C.** Atypical symptoms of GERD include chest pain, cough, laryngitis, cough, and wheezing. Odynophagia or dysphagia would warrant additional diagnostic studies such as barium swallow to rule out stricture or possible malignancy.

44. **The correct answer is B.** The patient has signs and symptoms of acute gouty arthritis. Nonsteroidal anti-inflammatory drugs (NSAIDs) are the agents of choice for treatment, with corticosteroids as an alternative. Colchicine is effective, although it can produce severe diarrhea. Allopurinol is useful in reducing attacks of chronic gout. However, it may promote an acute attack when initiated; therefore it should not be prescribed during or shortly following an acute flare.

REFERENCES

Fauci, A. S., Braunwald, E., Kasper, D. L., Hauser, S. L., Longo, D. L., Jameson, J. L., and Loscalzo, J. (2008). *Harrison's Textbook of Internal Medicine*, 17th ed. McGraw-Hill Medical Publishing, New York.

Goldmann, L., and Ausiello, D. (2008). *Cecil Medicine*, 23rd ed. Saunders Elsevier Publishing, Philadelphia, PA.

McPhee, S. J., Papadakis, M. A., and Tierney, L. M. (2008). *Current Medical Diagnosis and Treatment*, 47th ed. McGraw-Hill Publishers, New York.

Infectious Disease

Robert Bettiker, MD

1. A 22-year-old woman is complaining of a cough. Her radiograph shows multiple patchy infiltrates, and the culture grows *Aspergillus*. She has a history of a *Staphylococcus aureus* liver abscess, several *S. aureus* skin infections, frequent dental infections, and an episode of spinal osteomyelitis with *Chromobacterium violaceum*. Which of the following is the most likely diagnosis?

   A. X-linked agammaglobulinemia (XLA)
   B. Job's syndrome (hyperimmunoglobulin E syndrome)
   C. Chronic granulomatous disease (CGD)
   D. Selective IgA deficiency

2. An elderly woman with mild dementia has a rapid plasma reagin (RPR) titer of 1:8. Her lumbar puncture is VDRL positive. Her puncture also shows mildly elevated protein and a white blood cell (WBC) count of 10 with 85% lymphocytes. You start her on intravenous penicillin G for suspected neurosyphilis. Which of the following signs or symptoms are *least* likely to result from an adverse reaction to penicillin?

   A. Maculopapular rash across the trunk
   B. Increasing creatinine
   C. Neutropenia
   D. Ataxia

3. A mother of a toddler who attends day care presents complaining of her child's runny nose. She asks if an antibiotic will clear up the child's symptoms more quickly. Which of the following is most likely indicative of bacterial infection in this child?

   A. Bright red pharynx
   B. Vesicles on the soft palate
   C. 10-day duration of symptoms
   D. Fever

4. An 82-year-old mildly demented woman living in a nursing home has had repeated positive urine cultures for *Klebsiella oxytoca* over the past year. She is always afebrile and does not complain of dysuria. She has had multiple rounds of oral antibiotics, most recently a 2-week course of trimethoprim-sulfamethoxazole followed by 2 weeks of ciprofloxacin. Currently, her urinalysis has 0–5 white blood cells, no red blood cells, and greater than 100,000 CFU (colony forming units) of *K. oxytoca*. Which of the following would be the most appropriate next step for this patient?

   A. Nothing. Asymptomatic bacteriuria in a female nursing home resident does not require treatment.
   B. Perform an ultrasound of the kidneys to evaluate for pyelonephritis.
   C. Order a cystoscopy to evaluate for transitional cell carcinoma of the bladder.
   D. Prescribe chronic suppressive antibiotic therapy.

5. A 29-year-old prison inmate presents to the emergency department complaining of weakness for 3 days that has acutely worsened. He thought that he had caught some "viral bug," but now feels weak and short of breath. He complains of a large boil on his thigh and says that several of the inmates have similar lesions. His vital signs are as follows: temperature, 38°C (100.4°F); pulse, 122 bpm; blood pressure, 77/38 mmHg; and respiratory rate of 28 breaths per minute. He appears ill, but the rest of his physical exam is noncontributory except for a draining 3-cm skin abscess on his left thigh. His laboratory values are as follows:

White blood cell count: 15,375/mm^3

Differential: 85% neutrophils, 9% lymphocytes, 6% monocytes

Hgb/Hct: 10.5g/dL, 30%

Platelets: 110,000/mm^3

Albumin: 3.1 g/dl

Total protein: 6.3 g/dl

ALT: 93 IU

Total bilirubin: 0.9 mg/dl

AST: 88 IU

Creatinine: 2.3 mg/dl

Gram stain of draining fluid from the skin lesion showed moderate white blood cells with gram-positive cocci in clusters. Which of the following would *not* be appropriate treatment for this patient?

A. Administration of high-dose steroids

B. Administration of vancomycin

C. Administration of drotrecogin alpha (activated protein C), if hypotension remains after hydration

D. Insertion of a urinary catheter

6. A 63-year-old woman with a known history of cholelithiasis presents with 1 day of right upper quadrant pain, fever, weakness, nausea, and vomiting. She is febrile to 38.6°C, has a regular pulse of 122 bpm, blood pressure of 148/90 mmHg, and a respiratory rate of 22 breaths per minute and regular. On physical examination, she appears ill and has right upper quadrant tenderness without guarding. The rectal and pelvic exams are noncontributory. She has a leukocytosis of 18,500/mm^3, with a differential of 80% polymorphonuclear cells and 10% bands. Liver ultrasound shows a thickened gallbladder wall with a stone in the common bile duct. Which of the following actions is most appropriate in treating this patient?

A. Remove the stone.

B. Prescribe broad-spectrum antibiotics that have activity against enteric gram-negative rods, *Enterococcus* spp., and anaerobes.

C. Immediately order a radionuclide cholescintigraphy (hepato-iminodiacetic acid [HIDA] scan).

D. Administer ursodiol to dissolve the stone.

7. A 45-year-old man who has had a fever for 6 weeks reports to your office. He is tired and achy, but otherwise the review of symptoms is negative. He reports no sick contacts. On physical examination, his temperature is 100.3°F; his heart rate is 96 bpm and regular; his respiratory rate is 16 breaths per minute and regular; and his blood pressure is 150/96 mmHg left arm, sitting. He is not in acute distress. He is anicteric, and his mouth is moist with poor dentition. His lungs are clear. The heart has a regular rhythm with a II/VI holosystolic murmur at the apex. His abdomen is obese and soft with normoactive bowel sounds. His extremities have no edema. Two days later, an orthopantogram shows no odontogenic abscess, but blood cultures are growing *Streptococcus mutans*. Which of the following physical signs is *not* typically attributable to the underlying infection?

    A. Retinal hemorrhage
    B. Small, nodulelike hemorrhages on his palms
    C. Tiny linear hemorrhages under the fingernails
    D. Heme-positive stool

8. A coworker brings a 45-year-old man to your office due to his increasing confusion. The man is somnolent, but easily aroused; however, he does not answer questions appropriately. He complains of a headache and notes that the light hurts his eyes. On physical examination, his temperature is 38.9°C, his heart rate is 115 bpm and regular, and his blood pressure is 128/78 mmHg. His eyes are anicteric with no papilledema, and his neck has marked decreased flexion. You auscultate crackles at the right lung base. His heart reveals no murmurs. His abdomen is soft, and no skin rash is noted. Which of the following statements is most correct regarding this patient?

    A. The most likely etiologic agent is *Streptococcus pneumoniae*.
    B. You should administer ampicillin plus gentamicin.
    C. You should not administer steroids except in the pediatric population.
    D. The coworker should receive a prophylactic course of rifampin or ciprofloxacin.

9. A 55-year-old man with a history of diabetes had extensive surgery and radiation therapy 2 months ago to treat an oral cancer. He is now complaining of swelling in his jaw over the past several weeks. A 5-day course of amoxicillin had no effect. The patient is now anxious about his appearance, because there is a small amount of drainage from a dimple in the center of the swelling. A CT scan shows only soft-tissue swelling and no evidence of recurrent cancer. An oral surgeon incises the area and notes small yellowish granules. Gram stain and culture are both negative. Which of the following is the most appropriate course of action for this patient?

    A. Nothing. The patient has osteoradionecrosis of the jaw due to his radiation therapy.
    B. Prescribe amoxicillin for several months.
    C. Return the patient to the operating room for extensive debridement.
    D. Send a biopsy for silver stain to verify a *Mucor* spp. infection.

10. A 17-year-old high school football player is complaining of "super pimples" on his groin and upper thighs. They are hard, red, and painful. He notes they often rupture and drain, leaving scars. Several of his teammates have similar lesions. He took a course of amoxicillin, which had no impact. He is afebrile and has no systemic symptoms. Which of the following actions would *not* be appropriate regarding this patient?

    A. Incision and drainage of the lesions
    B. Oral cephalexin
    C. Washing the locker room showers with a dilute bleach solution
    D. Washing towels and washcloths after each use

11. A few hours after attending an afternoon family picnic, 10 people have nausea and vomiting. Some of them also have diarrhea. One afflicted person is pregnant. Which of the following is the most correct statement regarding this situation?

   A. Stool culture will make the diagnosis of a *Bacillus cereus* food-poisoning outbreak.
   B. *Staphylococcus aureus* in contaminated potato salad is the most likely culprit.
   C. Viral culture of stool will most likely be positive for Norovirus.
   D. The stools of those afflicted will probably culture *Listeria monocytogenes*.

12. A healthy 72-year-old woman had her hip replaced 9 months ago and now presents with 1 month of increasing pain. Hip radiographs show some resorption of bone near the prosthesis. Hip-aspirate cultures grow coagulase-negative *Staphylococcus*. Which of the following is the most appropriate course of action?

   A. Intravenous vancomycin plus rifampin; consult orthopedics if symptoms do not improve in 10 to 14 days.
   B. Complete joint removal, antibiotic spacer placement, and intravenous vancomycin for 3 months.
   C. Lifelong minocycline plus rifampin to treat chronic osteomyelitis.
   D. Send another hip-aspirate culture, because coagulase negative *Staphylococcus* is often a skin contaminant, and consult orthopedics for prosthesis removal.

13. A 16-year-old girl presents with lower abdominal pain and a fever that has lasted 3 days. She has nausea, but no vomiting. Her mother is concerned about appendicitis, because it "runs in the family." The girl denies sexual intercourse and a β-HcG is negative. She is febrile to 38.2°C and has diffuse lower abdominal pain without guarding. On bimanual exam, there is tenderness noted when you press on the cervix. Which of the following is the most appropriate course of action?

   A. Admit the patient to the hospital, start intravenous ampicillin/sulbactam, and consult surgery.
   B. Give ceftriaxone intramuscularly, prescribe doxycycline, and follow-up in 3 days.
   C. Recommend fluids for acute gastroenteritis.
   D. Perform a pelvic ultrasound to rule out an ovarian cyst.

14. A 32-year-old elementary school teacher comes to you with a red, teary eye. She denies photophobia and vision changes. Two of the children in her class went home with similar symptoms. Which of the following is the most correct statement regarding this patient?

   A. She is highly contagious and should avoid close personal contact for approximately 2 weeks.
   B. Untreated infection can lead to corneal scarring.
   C. Broad-spectrum antibiotic eyedrops will shorten the duration of symptoms.
   D. Spread of infection to the other eye is uncommon.

15. A 45-year-old man comes to you after his wife told him that he had "yellow" eyes. He complains of 1 week of malaise, nausea, and diarrhea. His urine is dark, so he has been drinking extra fluids because he thought that he was dehydrated. One month previously, he traveled because of business and engaged in extramarital sex at that time. He has some right upper quadrant tenderness with hepatomegaly. Labs are as follows:

ALT: 3,470 IU/L

AST: 3,180 IU/L

Total bilirubin: 5.3 μmol/L

Creatinine: 1.1 mg/dl

Hepatitis B surface antibody: Positive

Hepatitis B surface antigen: Negative

Hepatitis B core IgM: Negative

Hepatitis A IgM: Positive

Hepatitis C antibody: Negative

Which of the following statements is *not* true regarding this patient?

A. The patient could contract this illness either sexually or by eating contaminated food.

B. The wife should receive hepatitis A immune globulin if she is not already immune.

C. This patient should receive HIV screening.

D. This illness may become a chronic infection.

16. A 21-year-old college student presents complaining of fever, malaise, sore throat, and a rash of 2 weeks' duration. She thinks that she picked up mononucleosis, but the university's student health clinic found her to have a negative monospot test. The patient's boyfriend had a similar illness 4 months ago. Her past medical history is significant for a torn anterior cruciate ligament (ACL) repair due to a sports injury. She has no known drug allergies, and her medications include oral contraceptives, along with an occasional ibuprofen for knee pain. She has "social" alcohol intake and a family history of arthritis. On physical examination, there is mild conjunctival injection, palatal ulcers without tonsillar exudates, diffuse adenopathy in the anterior and posterior cervical chains, as well as bilateral axillary lymphadenopathy. Her lungs are clear, and her heart does not murmur. Her abdomen is soft, without masses or organomegaly. She is not experiencing joint swellings. There is a blanching macular-papular rash on her trunk. Her labs are as follows:

Monospot: Negative (per the university clinic)

White blood cell count: 3,500/mm³

Differential: 80% neutrophils, 9% lymphocytes, 10% monocytes, 1% eosinophils

Hgb/Hct: 10 g/dl, 30%

Platelets: 102,000/mm³

Albumin: 3.2 g/dl

Total protein: 9 g/dl

ALT: 124 IU/L

Total bilirubin: 0.9 μmol/l

AST: 118 IU/L

HIV antibody: Negative

Which of the following is the most correct diagnosis?

A. The clinician should prescribe oral acyclovir as the patient has primary herpes simplex virus type 1 (HSV-1) infection.

B. The patient has monospot-negative mononucleosis, and the clinician should submit Epstein-Barr virus titers.

C. The patient has a parvovirus B19 infection and should have parvovirus (IgG and IgM) submitted.

D. The patient has acute HIV syndrome and should have an HIV PCR (viral load) submitted.

17. As part of your hospital's bioterrorism response team, you must come up with a smallpox vaccination and treatment plan. Which of the following statements regarding smallpox is *not* correct?

A. Suspected patients will require respiratory droplet precautions, because the disease spreads via respiratory droplets, similar to *Neisseria meningitidis* and the influenza virus.

B. The disease varies from varicella (chickenpox) in that smallpox lesions are all in the same stage, whereas varicella lesions are in different stages of macular rash, vesicles, ulceration, and crusting.

C. Treatment of suspected infection should consist of moderate to high doses of anti-retroviral medications.

D. Smallpox has an incubation period of approximately 7 to 14 days.

18. A 26-year-old male presents complaining of painful ulcerations on the shaft of his penis that occur every 4 to 5 months. They start out as small fluid-filled "bumps" that eventually break down. Which of the following statements is *not* correct regarding this patient?

A. He is contagious and can pass on the infection even between episodes.

B. Acyclovir may abort or shorten the duration of an episode if taken at the first sign of an outbreak.

C. A bacterial culture will usually yield the diagnosis in about 48 hours.

D. Episodes can be associated with stress or immunosuppression.

19. A 28-year-old amateur drummer is complaining of sore wrists and hands. The pain began about 1 week ago and interferes with his playing. He has had some tactile fevers. On physical examination, his temperature is 37.2°C. You note a faint macular, blanching rash across his trunk, and the patient volunteers that his daughter had a bright red rash on her cheeks about two weeks ago. Which of the following is the most likely diagnosis?

A. Adult-onset Still's disease

B. Gonococcal tenosynovitis

C. Reiter's syndrome (Reactive arthritis [ReA])

D. Parvovirus B19 infection

20. A nursing home asks you for advice regarding an influenza outbreak. Ten residents have confirmed influenza, half of whom had received the influenza vaccine. The nursing home wants to bring the epidemic under control, but is concerned about the costs of anti-influenza drugs. Which of the following would be the most appropriate action in this situation?

A. Administer rimantadine to those unvaccinated residents.

B. Administer amantadine to all nursing home residents, regardless of vaccination status.

C. Administer oseltamivir to all nursing home residents and unvaccinated staff.

D. Administer zanamivir to all nursing home residents and staff, regardless of vaccination status.

21. You admit a 45-year-old woman to the intensive care unit whereupon you find it necessary to intubate her. During the previous week, she was in New Mexico cleaning out her summer home and setting traps for mice. Upon return, her family states that she was coughing and complaining of some shortness of breath. She then progressed to severe respiratory distress and EMS transported her to the emergency department. Her laboratory values are as follows:

    White blood cell count: 13,000/mm³

    Differential: 78% PMNs, 5% bands, 4% monocytes, 7% lymphocytes, 5% atypical lymphocytes

    Hemoglobin/hematocrit: 16.5 g/dl, 50%

    Platelets: 108,000/mm³

    ALT: 55 IU

    AST: 60 IU

    The chest radiograph shows significant bilateral pulmonary edema. Which of the following is the most likely diagnosis?

    A. Influenza
    B. Community-acquired methicillin-resistant *Staphylococcus aureus* (CA-MRSA) pneumonia
    C. Respiratory syncytial virus
    D. Hantavirus pulmonary syndrome

22. You admit a 24-year-old woman to the intensive care unit for respiratory distress. One week ago, she visited the emergency department for cough and fever. Her diagnosis at that time was community-acquired pneumonia; the emergency room staff prescribed a macrolide, and then discharged her to home. According to her mother, she improved over the next few days, but then started to feel worse. She had increasing cough and dyspnea and complained that her eyes hurt. She returned to the emergency department when she could not open her eyes and was short of breath at rest. Physical examination reveals the following: temperature, 37°C; heart rate, 108 bpm and regular; respiratory rate, 31 breaths per minute; and blood pressure, 112/68 mmHg. A pulse oximeter shows 90% oxygen saturation. She has injected conjunctivae and multiple ulcers in her mouth and nose. She is tachypneic, but her lungs are otherwise clear. Furthermore, she has small erythematous targetlike lesions on the palms of her hands and soles of her feet. A genitourinary exam shows ulcers in the vagina and perirectal area. Which of the following is the most likely diagnosis?

    A. Acute HIV syndrome
    B. Erythema multiforme due to *Mycoplasma pneumoniae* infection
    C. *Staphylococcus aureus* superinfection
    D. Acute varicella (chickenpox)

23. An avid 67-year-old female golfer presents complaining of a swollen and painful right knee. She has seen many deer on her favorite golf course in central New Jersey. She suspects Lyme disease, but she does not recall a tick bite or a rash. When asked about other joints, she states that her wrists are sore but that it is just "arthritis." Which of the following statements is *not* correct regarding this patient?

    A. The symptoms are consistent with tertiary Lyme disease, and the patient will require IV antibiotic therapy.
    B. Up to 30% of all Lyme cases do not have the characteristic "target lesion" rash of erythema migrans chronicum.
    C. Even though you can drain the knee for symptomatic relief, swelling may reoccur even if there is eradication of the infection.
    D. The Lyme blood test may remain positive for years after successfully treating the infection.

24. A 67-year-old man with severe rheumatoid arthritis, currently managed with methotrexate and prednisone, saw a rheumatologist for initiation of injections of infliximab, a tumor necrosis factor (TNF)-alpha inhibitor. The rheumatologist performed a PPD test and read it as 11 mm of induration. The patient has no known tuberculosis exposures. He is not experiencing fevers, weight loss, or cough. Which of the following statements is most correct regarding this patient?

   A. The PPD test is negative, and you refer the patient back to the rheumatologist "cleared" for infliximab injections.
   B. Order a chest x-ray. If it is negative for active tuberculosis, begin treatment for latent tuberculosis infection.
   C. The PPD is positive, but the patient is too old to undergo isoniazid therapy for latent tuberculosis infection.
   D. Begin four-drug therapy (isoniazid, rifampin, pyrazinamide, and ethambutol) along with vitamin B_6 for active tuberculosis infection and allow the infliximab injections to begin.

25. A microbiology laboratory technician presents with pneumonia. Her sputum culture grew yeast at 37°C. She is convinced that she caught the pneumonia while working on fungal cultures. On several occasions, the exhaust fan over the fungal-culture station was inoperative. Which of the following organisms is the most likely culprit?

   A. *Sporothrix schenckii*
   B. *Candida albicans*
   C. *Aspergillus fumigatus*
   D. *Histoplasma capsulatum*

26. A physician assistant student tired of his microbiology lectures and decided to go hiking in the Pine Barrens of southern New Jersey. He received multiple scrapes from brushing up against the bushes and pine trees. Several weeks later, he noted a small papule on the dorsum of his left hand that grew larger and ulcerated. He further noted two additional papules forming in a line further up his forearm. A biopsy showed no pathogens, but a fungal culture at 25°C grew a mold after 4 days. One of his fellow students (who went to all of the microbiology lectures) correctly diagnosed it as which of the following?

   A. Sporotrichosis
   B. Chromoblastomycosis
   C. Histoplasmosis
   D. Blastomycosis

27. Two weeks after a hiking trip in the Andes Mountains, a 26-year-old male complains of bloating, flatulence, and greasy, foul-smelling stools. His girlfriend, who also went on the trip, denies symptoms. Which of the following is the most likely diagnosis?

   A. Enterotoxigenic *Escherichia coli* (ETEC)
   B. *Giardia lamblia*
   C. *Campylobacter jejuni*
   D. *Entamoeba histolytica*

28. On the night before returning home from spring break, a 21-year-old college student engages in a party on a beach in the Caribbean. He eats a lot of seafood, becomes extremely intoxicated, abrades his knee after a fall on a wooden pier, and has sexual relations with another partygoer. On the plane ride home, he develops nausea, vomiting, diarrhea, and abdominal cramping, which he attributes to a hangover. He presents to your office 1 week later because he now has numbness of his lips and throat, headache, blurred vision, and sharp pains down his legs. He appears anxious and complains that he is afraid that his "teeth are going to fall out." Which of the following is the most correct statement regarding this patient?

A. He has acute HIV and should have an HIV antibody test and an HIV viral load run.

B. He has food poisoning from *Vibrio parahaemolyticus*, and you should prescribe a quinolone.

C. He has primary genital herpes infection (HSV-2) and you should prescribe acyclovir.

D. He has ciguatera, and there is little that you can offer him.

29. A 2-year-old boy has had fever; bilateral conjunctival injection; cracked lips, which occasionally bleed; a red tongue; and an erythematous oropharynx for 2 weeks. He has a 2-cm, mildly tender, right submandibular lymph node. The mother is anxious, because the palms of his hands are now peeling. Which of the following would be the most appropriate treatment for this patient?

A. Amoxicillin

B. Aspirin

C. Clindamycin

D. Steroid cream for the hands and lips

30. One week after undergoing a bone marrow transplant for leukemia, your neutropenic patient spikes a fever to 103°F (39°C). You draw blood cultures and start vancomycin, ceftazidime, and tobramycin. Three days later the patient is still having fevers, and her condition is worsening. Blood cultures are negative, but chest radiography shows a right upper lobe infiltrate. You perform a bronchoalveolar lavage (BAL), and examine the fluid via microscopy. Which of the following would you most likely expect to see to explain the cause of the pneumonia?

A. Gram-positive cocci

B. Gram-negative bacilli

C. Branching, septate hyphae

D. Viral inclusion bodies in white cells under cytologic examination

ANSWERS

1. The correct answer is C. This patient has chronic granulomatous disease (CGD). CGD is a hereditary disease characterized by an inability of phagocytes to make hydrogen peroxide and other oxidants. Because of this defect, patients with CGD have an increased susceptibility to bacterial and fungal infections. The condition is also associated with an excessive accumulation of immune cells into granulomatous aggregates (hence the name of the disease) at sites of infection or other inflammation. The hallmark of this disease is early onset of severe recurrent bacterial and fungal infections. Most patients present with the disease during the first 5 years of life. The most commonly involved organs are those that serve as barriers against the entry of microorganisms from the environment, such as the skin, lungs, gastrointestinal tract, lymph nodes, liver, and spleen. The common clinical presentation includes skin infections, lung abscesses and pneumonia, suppurative lymphadenitis, enteral diarrhea, perianal or perirectal abscesses, and hepatic or splenic abscesses. Patients may also progress or present with septicemia or osteomyelitis. Fungal infections present in approximately 20% of patients, with *Aspergillus* pneumonia as the most common presentation. X-linked agammaglobulinemia (XLA), or Bruton's agammaglobulinemia, is present at birth. Low or completely absent levels of immunoglobulins in the bloodstream characterize this condition. Symptoms of immunoglobulin deficiency, which include frequent ear and sinus infections, pneumonia, and gastroenteritis, appear after the infant is 6 months old. Certain viruses, such as hepatitis and polioviruses, can also pose a threat. Children with XLA grow slowly, have small tonsils and lymph nodes, and may develop chronic skin infections. Hyperimmunoglobulin E (hyper-IgE or HIE) syndrome is a rare immunodeficiency disorder. The most common findings are recurrent skin abscesses, pneumonia with pneumatocele development, and high serum levels of IgE. Facial, dental, and skeletal features are also associated with this syndrome. Moderate-to-severe papular, pruritic eczematous lesions are typically located in the flexural areas, the area behind the ears, and the area around the hairline. Furunculosis and cellulitis may also be present. Pneumonia with complicating pneumatocele development and empyema may be present, although these are less common in children who are receiving prophylactic antibiotics. Recurrent bacterial arthritis and *staphylococcal osteomyelitis* may occur at fracture sites. Frequent long bone, rib, and pelvic fractures are also prominent features of Job's syndrome and occur in persons of all ages. These fractures usually occur with an absence of pain. Approximately one-third of patients have scoliosis of at least 20° curvature. Selective IgA deficiency is a complete absence of IgA. These patients usually present with a variety of infections not limited to any one area (including, skin, bone, lung, or other infections).

2. **The correct answer is D.** All of the other items mentioned, albeit rare, may be complications of penicillin therapy. Jarisch-Herxheimer reaction includes fever, chills, myalgias, and rash exacerbations secondary to endotoxin release by the organism in response to treatment.

3. **The correct answer is C.** A bright red pharynx or vesicles on the soft palate can be viral or bacterial in origin. Similarly, fever can be of a known or unknown origin. However, 10 days of symptoms probably indicates a bacterial infection, because viral infections of this nature usually resolve in less time.

4. **The correct answer is A.** Asymptomatic bacteriuria in a nursing home patient does not usually require treatment; therefore, all of the other choices are inappropriate.

5. **The correct answer is A.** High-dose steroids are ineffective in cases such as this one. If the patient remains hypotensive after receiving IV fluids, then drotrecogin alfa is appropriate therapy. A urinary catheter may be useful in monitoring volume status and renal function, especially in the face of acute renal insufficiency.

6. **The correct answer is A.** Although one certainly should consider antibiotics in this situation and consider a HIDA scan, removal of the obstruction offers the greatest chance of curing the patient. Ursodiol's effect is far too slow to help this patient.

7. **The correct answer is D.** All of the other choices are classic findings of subacute bacterial endocarditis.

8. **The correct answer is A.** This patient probably has community-acquired bacterial meningitis. The most likely etiologic agent is *Streptococcus pneumoniae*. The standard therapy for patients with this condition is vancomycin plus cefotaxime or ceftriaxone. Adjunctive steroid usage is appropriate in adults and children.

9. **The correct answer is B.** This patient has an actinomycosis infection. Actinomycosis is a chronic bacterial infection attributed to *Actinomyces* spp., most commonly *A. israelii*. This gram-positive, anaerobic organism is part of the normal flora of the human oropharynx, gastrointestinal tract, and female genital tract. Actinomycetes are usually nonvirulent in nature, but a disruption of the protective mucosal barrier and alteration

of the resident microbial flora play a crucial role in infection (as probably is the case secondary to this patient's therapy). Infections most commonly occur in the cervicofacial, abdominopelvic, and thoracic regions. Documentation exists of central nervous system (CNS) involvement and it could spread secondary to hematogenous spread or by direct extension. Cervicofacial actinomycosis, also known as lumpy jaw, is the most common variant encountered and accounts for 55% of cases. Poor dental hygiene, dental disease, and dental procedures are common predisposing factors. These patients may present with palpable nodularity, soft-tissue swelling, and fibrosis involving the submandibular or perimandibular region. The most helpful diagnostic feature is the presence of sulfur granules (the yellowish granules discovered upon incision of his swelling). The clinician may occasionally observe sulfur granules clinically as 1-mm yellow grains that resemble sand. Histologically, they contain numerous intertwined filamentous gram-positive bacteria. Historically, treatment of actinomycosis was high-dose penicillin administered over a prolonged period. Typically, appropriate therapy consisted of intravenous penicillin for a 2 to 6 week course, followed by a 6 to 12 month course of oral penicillin or amoxicillin. Recent literature, however, has shown short-term therapy to be effective. In the case of a patient with a penicillin allergy, suitable alternatives include one of the tetracyclines, erythromycin, clindamycin, or a cephalosporin. Because of the potential for relapse of infection, the clinician should follow these patients closely in order to detect any recurrence. None of the other choices is appropriate, because he needs antimicrobial treatment. Extensive debridement will not solve the problem without appropriate antibiotic treatment. Furthermore, the etiologic agent is not *Mucor* spp.

10. **The correct answer is B.** This is most likely community-acquired methicillin-resistant *Staphylococcus aureus* (CA-MRSA). All of the measures mentioned are appropriate in this situation, except oral treatment with cephalexin. This patient will probably require parenteral antibiotics, such as oxacillin or nafcillin. The oral treatment of choice for MRSA is trimethoprim-sulfamethoxazole.

11. **The correct answer is B.** Preformed toxins can act within a few hours. Only *Bacillus cereus* and *Staphylococcus aureus* make preformed toxins, and neither of them will be evident in the stool.

12. **The correct answer is B.** This patient needs complete removal of the infected joint and IV vancomycin for at least 3 months. Simply removing the infected joint and replacing it with another prosthesis will only lead to a probable recurrence of infection, hence the need for antibiotic spacer placement. Waiting for a response to antimicrobial therapy without removing the offending prosthesis will likely be unsuccessful. Similarly, this is why lifelong treatment for osteomyelitis will be unsuccessful. The patient's symptoms clearly point to an infection of coagulase-negative *Staphylococcus*.

13. **The correct answer is B.** This patient obviously has pelvic inflammatory disease (PID). There is no need for admission to the hospital at this time and she does not have gastroenteritis, thus a simple increase of fluids would be inappropriate. Although appendicitis may "run" in this patient's family, there is no strong indicator that this is her problem. An ovarian cyst is also unlikely. The clinician must consider all factors when determining treatment, including the possibility that the history might not be entirely accurate.

14. **The correct answer is A.** This patient has conjunctivitis ("pink-eye"), which is highly contagious. The interesting fact about conjunctivitis is that whether bacterial or viral, it is usually self-limited, lasting from 10 days to 2 weeks. Typically, the infection begins in one eye and rapidly spreads to the other. Untreated infections rarely lead to corneal scarring. Broad-spectrum antibiotics may shorten the duration of symptoms if the infection is of bacterial origin.

15. **The correct answer is D.** This patient has hepatitis A, contracted by sexual contact or by eating contaminated food. The patient's wife should also receive the hepatitis A immune globulin if she proves not to be immune. The patient's lab results also indicate a previous exposure or immunity to hepatitis B. Screening for HIV in this patient is appropriate at this time. Hepatitis A does not usually progress to chronic infection.

16. **The correct answer is D.** Unfortunately, this patient has an acute HIV syndrome. The laboratory results do not support any of the other choices, and there is no reason to suspect that a repeat monospot will produce different results. The name "acute HIV syndrome" refers to the early stage of HIV infection, when a patient first receives infection with HIV. Patients typically present with fever; malaise; lymphadenopathy; pharyngitis, with or without tonsillitis; joint and muscle aches; diarrhea; and a generalized blanching rash. The symptoms of acute HIV syndrome usually last for about 14 days after HIV exposure. The signs and symptoms of HIV infection may resemble mononucleosis (mono), tonsillitis, or the flu. The truncal blanching rash does not sound indicative of a herpes simplex virus infection. Of course, the patient's boyfriend should receive HIV testing as well, because the history does not indicate the use of preventative measures.

17. **The correct answer is C.** Smallpox is an airborne pathogen akin to varicella (chickenpox) or tuberculosis. All of the other answers are appropriate preparations for an outbreak.

18. **The correct answer is C.** Herpes simplex virus 2 requires viral culture techniques to grow. Viral shedding occurs even in the absence of an outbreak. Multiple studies have shown that antiherpes therapies can shorten or stop an outbreak if taken during the prodrome phase. Initial infections may be systemic and manifest as an aseptic meningitis. Stress or immunosuppression can precipitate an outbreak.

19. **The correct answer is D.** Research first identified human parvovirus B19 in 1975. Human parvovirus B19 is the cause of fifth disease in children and adults. A petechial rash similar to the skin lesions seen in erythema multiforme characterizes the disease. This rash occurs in a "stocking and glove" distribution in the pattern of a lacelike or reticular rash covering the trunk. Another finding is a characteristic reddening of the cheeks, referred to as the "slapped-cheek" sign. Other symptoms include a systemic lupuslike syndrome of arthritis, edema, mucosal ulcers of the mouth and/or genital tract, uveitis, fever, joint pain, muscle weakness, and purpura or bruising of the lower extremities. The disease can occur in adults who are exposed to children with fifth disease. In 1916, Hans Reiter described the classic triad of arthritis, nongonococcal urethritis, and conjunctivitis, historically known as Reiter's syndrome but now most commonly referred to as reactive arthritis (ReA). It refers to acute, nonpurulent arthritis complicating an infection elsewhere in the body. It falls under the disease category of seronegative spondyloarthropathies, which include ankylosing spondylitis, psoriatic arthritis, the arthropathy of associated inflammatory bowel disease, juvenile-onset ankylosing spondylitis, and juvenile chronic arthritis. Gonococcal tenosynovitis is a gonococcal arthritis in which tenosynovitis is the most common sign. It occurs three times more in women than in men, and usually in pregnant or menstruating women. It presents with 1 to 4 days of migratory polyarthralgias typically initially involving the wrist, knee, ankle, or elbow, then progressing to the tenosynovitis type. Still's disease is a form of arthritis characterized by high spiking fevers and an evanescent salmon-colored rash. Still's disease is a type of juvenile rheumatoid arthritis (JRA), also known as systemic-onset JRA. Still's disease first described in children, and also occurs much less commonly in adults (adult-onset Still's disease). The cause of Still's disease is unknown. Symptoms typically include joint inflammation, high fevers, gland swelling, and internal organ involvement.

20. **The correct answer is C.** Nursing home residents tend to have a poor response to the vaccine and are at high risk of complications from influenza. Unvaccinated staff should receive prophylaxis as well.

21. **The correct answer is D.** This patient has hantavirus pulmonary syndrome (HPS). Hantaviruses, first discovered in 1993 in the southwestern United States, are RNA zoonotic viruses transmitted to humans from rodent hosts. Hantavirus pulmonary syndrome (HPS) presents as a febrile prodrome typically followed by acute respiratory failure and then death due to circulatory collapse. The basic pathophysiologic lesion of HPS is an increase in capillary permeability following endothelial damage. The increased capillary permeability gives rise to widespread protein-rich edema, which leads to hemorrhage and eventual lung necrosis. Severe cases of HPS present clinically as noncardiogenic pulmonary edema. The pathophysiology of the pulmonary findings is pulmonary capillary leak syndrome. The heart is not directly affected. Hypoxia also contributes to the state of shock in these patients. Physical findings, reported in 80 to 90% of patients, include fever, tachypnea, tachycardia, and rales. The chest radiograph typically shows a pattern of noncardiac pulmonary edema. The pulmonary capillary leak may show radiographically as peribronchial cuffing or Kerley B lines, and pleural effusions are common. Respiratory syncytial virus (RSV) infection, which manifests primarily as bronchiolitis and/or viral pneumonia, is the leading cause of lower respiratory tract infection in infants and young children, with a peak incidence between 2 to 8 months. The disease is characterized by cough, coryza, wheezing, rales, low-grade fever (<101°F), and decreased oral intake. Usually a family history of asthma and/or atopy exists. Methicillin-resistant *Staphylococcus aureus* (MRSA) pneumonia presents as rapid-onset pneumonia with progression to significant illness. The history of exposure to mice droppings in a presumably remote area (New Mexico summer home) would tend to discount this as a cause. Although influenza can be a cause of upper respiratory symptoms and eventual pneumonia, it more often occurs in the fall and is rarely so insidious.

22. **The correct answer is B.** Erythema multiforme major, also known as Stevens-Johnson syndrome (SJS), is often confused in the literature. SJS is a mucocutaneous disorder. Stevens and Johnson first described the disorder in 1922 as a condition with febrile erosive stomatitis, severe conjunctivitis, and disseminated cutaneous eruption. Flat, atypical lesions, described as irregular purpuric macules, may feature occasional blistering and typically begin on the face and trunk. Most patients also have extensive mucosal involvement. Medication usage attributes to more than 50% of all cases. Unlike erythema multiforme or erythema multiforme minor, this is a serious, potentially life-threatening illness. A diagnosis of erythema multiforme major applies to patients who also display oral mucosal involvement. This is similar to that described by Stevens and Johnson. As many as one-half of patients with herpes-associated erythema multiforme present with oral ulcers. These ulcers appear as a variant of erythema multiforme, rather than Stevens-Johnson syndrome (SJS). Because SJS and erythema multiforme have different precipitating factors and different clinical patterns, the terms erythema multiforme major and erythema multiforme minor are rapidly becoming archaic terms. Bullous erythema multiforme now replaces the term erythema multiforme with mucosal involvement. Stevens-Johnson syndrome is a separate clinical entity. Patient history may include the presence of influenza flulike prodrome consisting of fever, cough, and malaise; patients may also present with mucocutaneous eruptions that are usually symmetric and that extend from the face and torso to the trunk and proximal extremities. Oral or nasal ulceration as well as painful micturition secondary to genitourinary tract ulceration may also be present. Patients may also have photophobia, burning eyes, or visual impairment secondary to ocular ulceration. Ulceration of the gastrointestinal tract can lead to profuse diarrhea. If there is tracheobronchial involvement, then the patient may have shortness of breath. SJS may follow a recent or current herpes simplex virus or *Mycoplasma pneumoniae* infection, which may cause erythema multiforme. Frequently, this syndrome follows medication usage. The physical examination may show discrete, irregular, flat, dark red, purpuric macules over the face and trunk, progressing rapidly to involve the abdomen, back, and proximal extremities. The clinician should note that mucous membrane involvement frequently appears in 90% of patients. The most com-

mon sites affected, in order of frequency, are the oropharynx, conjunctivae, genitalia, anus, tracheobronchial tree, esophagus, and bowel. Acute varicella, or chickenpox, is a generalized infection caused by the varicella zoster virus. A blistery rash, poetically described as a "dew drop on a rose petal base," characterizes this condition. It occurs most frequently in children between the ages of 5 and 8. Less than 20 percent of all cases in the United States affect people over the age of 15. The lesions are not generally located in the mucous membranes, as described in this patient. Acute HIV syndrome is the early stage of HIV infection that follows the initial infection with the HIV virus. Patients typically present with fever, malaise, lymphadenopathy, pharyngitis with or without tonsillitis, joint and muscle aches, diarrhea, and a generalized blanching rash. The symptoms of acute HIV syndrome usually last about 14 days after HIV exposure. The signs and symptoms of HIV infection may resemble mononucleosis (mono), tonsillitis, or the flu

23. **The correct answer is A.** If this is Lyme disease, it is indeed tertiary Lyme disease; however, only CNS Lyme and Lyme myocarditis (both components of tertiary Lyme disease) require IV treatment. A vaginal culture or a knee aspirate could help to rule out gonorrhea as a cause of the patient's arthritis.

24. **The correct answer is B.** This one is a bit tricky. Tumor-necrosis factor-alpha antagonists are associated with tuberculosis infection, thus the clinician should rule out the diagnosis of latent tuberculosis before initiation of therapy. Immunosuppressed persons, including those on prednisone, are at higher risk of developing tuberculosis. A PPD result of greater than 10 mm is positive for a patient on chronic corticosteroid use. Isoniazid therapy is as toxic as in the past and therefore practitioners may administer it to patients of any age with latent tuberculosis infection.

25. **The correct answer is D.** *Sporothrix schenckii* causes skin infections by direct inoculation under the skin. *Candida albicans* rarely, if ever, causes pneumonia. *Aspergillus fumigatus* can cause pneumonia, but only in immunocompromised hosts, and it never grows as a yeast. *Histoplasma capsulatum* can cause pneumonia in normal hosts and grows as a yeast at 37°C.

26. **The correct answer is A.** The patient has sporotrichosis, a subacute or chronic infection caused by the soil fungus *Sporothrix schenckii*. The characteristic infection involves suppurating subcutaneous nodules that progress proximally along lymphatic channels (lymphocutaneous sporotrichosis). It can progress to a rare primary pulmonary infection (pulmonary sporotrichosis) or symptoms and signs related to direct inoculation into tendons, bursae, or joints. Immunocompromised patients (i.e., AIDS patients) may present with a disseminated infection consisting of widespread cutaneous lesions and involvement of multiple visceral organs. The prognosis for complete recovery after antimicrobial therapy is excellent. Chromoblastomycosis is a chronic fungal infection of the skin and the subcutaneous tissue caused by traumatic inoculation of a specific group of dematiaceous fungi (usually *Fonsecaea pedrosoi*, *Phialophora verrucosa*, *Cladosporium carrionii*, or *Fonsecaea compacta*) through the skin. The disease usually appears at the site of a previous, often unnoticed or unremembered, trauma to the skin. After several years, a small, raised, erythematous, asymptomatic papule develops. As the lesion develops over years, it assumes a scaly and infiltrated aspect. The timing of this patient's symptoms makes this an unlikely cause for his problems. Most individuals infected with histoplasmosis are asymptomatic. It is an inhaled disease, and those who develop clinical manifestations are usually immunocompromised. Other patients who typically present with acute pulmonary symptoms have probably received exposure to a high quantity of inoculums. If symptoms develop, onset occurs 3 to 14 days after exposure and usually consists of fever, headache, malaise, myalgia, abdominal pain, and chills. Blastomycosis occurs because of the endemic dimorphic fungi *Blastomyces dermatitidis*. The disease is endemic in the southeastern and south central United States, along the Mississippi and Ohio Rivers. Outbreaks have been associated with occupational or recreational activities

around streams or rivers with high content of moist soil enriched with organic debris and/or rotting wood. The infection occurs via inhalation of the conidia, which transform into the yeast form once in the lungs. After 30 to 45 days, an acute pulmonary disease indistinguishable from a bacterial pneumonia may occur. However, at least 50% of primary infections are asymptomatic.

27. **The correct answer is B.** Giardiasis is the most prevalent protozoal infection of the human intestine. *Giardia lamblia* is one of the most common causative agents of epidemic and endemic diarrheal illness throughout the world. It continues to be the most frequently identified water-borne intestinal pathogen in the United States. *Giardia lamblia* may be in as many as 80% of raw water supplies from lakes, streams, and ponds and in as many as 15% of filtered water samples. Approximately one-half of patients infected with *G. lamblia* may present with symptoms, including acute watery diarrhea progressing to chronic diarrhea, and chronic diarrhea with malabsorption and weight loss. Abdominal cramping with acute diarrhea is the most common symptom, occurring in 90% of symptomatic subjects. Abdominal cramping, bloating, and flatulence occur in 70 to 75% of symptomatic patients. Physical findings other than weight loss and those related to fluid loss are rarely present. Enterotoxic *Escherichia coli* (i.e., traveler's diarrhea) usually occurs in persons from industrialized countries who visit tropical or subtropical regions. It typically presents with abdominal cramps and frequent, explosive bowel movements appearing 1 to 2 days after exposure to contaminated food or water. The *E. coli* enterotoxin acts on the gastrointestinal mucosa, leading to an outpouring of copious fluid from the small bowel. Symptoms are self-limited, usually lasting only 3 to 4 days. The clinician should monitor patients closely, because large fluid loss can result in dehydration. *Campylobacter jejuni* is now the leading cause of food poisoning in the United States; it most often spreads by contact with raw or undercooked poultry. Symptoms tend to start 2 to 5 days after exposure and typically last a week. Symptoms resemble viral gastroenteritis (diarrhea, fever, abdominal pain, cramping, nausea, and vomiting); however persons infected with *C. jejuni*, typically present with fever and bloody diarrhea. Most patients improve within 5 days without specific treatment. Amebiasis, an infection caused by the protozoal organism *Entamoeba histolytica*, causes amebic colitis and liver abscess. In developed countries, infection occurs primarily among travelers to endemic regions, recent immigrants from endemic regions, homosexual males, immunosuppressed persons, and institutionalized individuals. Transmission usually occurs by food-borne exposure, particularly when food handlers are shedding cysts or food is cultivated in feces-contaminated soil, fertilizer, or water. Less common means of transmission include contaminated water, oral and anal sexual practices, and direct rectal inoculation through colonic irrigation devices. Patients with amebic colitis typically present with a history of several weeks of abdominal pain, diarrhea, and bloody stools. The timing of this patient's symptoms makes this diagnosis unlikely.

28. **The correct answer is D.** Ciguatera poisoning is the most common nonbacterial, fish-borne poisoning in the United States. It occurs following consumption of reef fish that feed on certain algae typically found in coral reef systems. Previously, ciguatera poisoning was a significant concern in tropical areas for centuries as it is confined to coral reef fish in water between the latitudes of 35 degrees north and 35 degrees south. However, with our current modern world travel and rapid transportation, many warm-water fish are available in markets throughout the world, therefore the clinician may see cases of ciguatera poisoning in any location. Most of these outbreaks in the United States occur in Florida and Hawaii, although tourists may develop symptoms after returning home. *Gambierdiscus toxicus* is the dinoflagellate most notably responsible for production of ciguatoxin, although recent research identifies other species. The species of fish most frequently implicated include barracuda, grouper, red snapper, amberjack, eel, sea bass, and Spanish mackerel. Fish larger than 2 kg contain significant amounts of toxin. Ingestion of the fish produces the toxic effects. GI symptoms often are the first to appear, may

last 1 to 2 days, and include nausea/vomiting, diarrhea, or abdominal pain. If neurologic symptoms occur, they have an unusual presentation. The symptoms may begin from a few hours to 3 days following the meal. They may persist, lasting weeks to months consisting of painful extremity paresthesias, circumoral and lingual paresthesias, and, interestingly enough, a temperature reversal—that is, cold objects feel hot and hot objects feel cold to the patient. This is a classic finding of the poisoning. Patients also feel as though their teeth have loosened. Other complaints include arthralgia and myalgias, pruritus, weakness, vertigo or ataxia. The patients may progress to full-blown respiratory paralysis and coma. The physical examination may reveal dehydration secondary to nausea/vomiting or diarrhea. The patient may exhibit signs of shock with hypotension secondary to bradycardia and fluid loss, vasodilation and myocardial depression. The treatment is largely symptom driven and supportive. The prognosis is generally excellent as most patients fully recover. Of course, the clinician should advise these patients to avoid any fish or shellfish products, as well as nuts and alcoholic beverages. During the acute or recovery phases of this poisoning, opiates and barbiturates may exacerbate the symptoms. The clinician should not prescribe these medications. *Vibrio parahaemolyticus* is a possibility, but it does not have a neurologic component. Primary herpes simplex virus-2 (HSV-2) can cause a systemic illness, but the incubation period is too short and it has no gastrointestinal component. Acute HIV might account for all of these symptoms, but, again, the incubation period is too short.

29. **The correct answer is B.** This child has Kawasaki disease. Kawasaki disease is most common among children of Japanese and Korean descent, but it can affect a person from any ethnic group. The first phase of Kawasaki disease, which can last for up to 2 weeks, usually involves a persistent fever higher than 104°F (39°C) that lasts for at least 5 days. Patients also present with severe erythematous eyes; a maculopapular rash on the stomach, chest, and genitals; red, dry, cracked lips; a swollen tongue with a white coating and large red lesions; a sore, irritated throat; swollen palms of the hands and soles of the feet with a purple-red color; and lymphadenopathy. During the second phase, which usually begins within 2 weeks of when the fever started, the skin on the hands and feet may begin to peel away in large pieces. The child also may experience diarrhea, vomiting, joint pain, or abdominal pain. Treatment usually consists of intravenous doses of gamma globulin and should ideally begin within 10 days of fever onset. The child should also receive a high dose of aspirin to reduce the risk of potential myocardial problems. The other treatments are inappropriate for this condition.

30. **The correct answer is C.** The patient should be doing much better on the vancomycin if the pneumonia is due to a gram-positive cocci, such as *Staphylococcus aureus*. Likewise, ceftazidime or tobramycin should cover even resistant gram-negative bacteria, such as *Pseudomonas aeruginosa*. Clearly, this patient is at risk of developing *Aspergillus* pneumonia. Viral inclusion bodies may be present during a cytomegalovirus (CMV) infection, but CMV infections generally do not occur until 4 weeks or later in a transplant patient. The same is true for *Pneumocystis jiroveci* (formally *Pneumocystis carinii*).

REFERENCES

Advisory Council for the Elimination of Tuberculosis. (1995). "Screening for tuberculosis and tuberculosis infection in high-risk populations recommendations of the Advisory Council for the Elimination of Tuberculosis." *Morbidity and Mortality Weekly Report* 44(RR-11): 18–34.

American Thoracic Society (ATC)/Centers for Disease Control Standing Committee on Latent Tuberculosis Infection. (2000). "Targeted tuberculin testing and treatment of latent tuberculosis infection." *Morbidity and Mortality Weekly Report* 49(RR-06): 1–54.

Bernard, G. R., Vincent, J. L., Laterre, P. F., LaRosa, S. P., Dhainaut, J. F., Lopez-Rodriguez, A., Steingrub, J. S., Garber, G. E., Helterbrand, J. D., Ely, E. W., and Fisher, C. J. Jr., (2001). "Efficacy and safety of recombinant human-activated protein C for severe sepsis." *New England Journal of Medicine* 344(10): 699–709.

Bisno, A. L. (2001). "Acute pharyngitis." *New England Journal of Medicine* 344: 205–211.

Carpenter, H. A. (1998). "Bacterial and parasitic cholangitis." *Mayo Clinic Proceedings* 73(5): 473–478.

"Ciguatera Fish Poisoning—Texas, 1998, and South Carolina, 2004." (2006). *Morbidity and Mortality Weekly Report* 55(34): 935–937.

Cleri, D. J., Porwancher, R. B., Ricketti, A. J., Ramos-Bonner, L. S., and Vernaleo, J. R. (2006). "Smallpox as a bioterrorist weapon: Myth or menace?" *Infectious Disease Clinics of North America* 20(2): 329–357, ix.

Craig, A. S., and Schaffner, W. (2004). "Prevention of hepatitis A with the hepatitis A vaccine." *New England Journal of Medicine* 350(5): 476.

Crane, J. K. (1999). "Preformed bacterial toxins." *Clinics in Laboratory Medicine* 19(3): 583–599.

Couch, R. B. (2000). "Prevention and treatment of influenza." *New England Journal of Medicine* 343(24): 1778–1787.

Daum, R. S. (2007). "Skin and soft-tissue infections caused by methicillin-resistant *Staphylococcus aureus.*" *New England Journal of Medicine* 357(4): 380–390.

Duchin, J. S., Koster, F. T., and Peters, C. J. (1994). "Hantavirus pulmonary syndrome: A clinical description of 17 patients with a newly recognized disease." *New England Journal of Medicine* 330(14): 949–955.

Falcini, F. (2006). "Kawasaki disease." *Current Opinion in Rheumatology* 18(1): 33–38.

Garner, J. S., and the Hospital Infection Control Practices Advisory Committee. (1996). "Guideline for isolation precautions in hospitals." *Infection Control and Hospital Epidemiology* 17(1): 53–80.

Gruchalla, R. S., and Pirmohamed, M. (2006). "Antibiotic allergy." *New England Journal of Medicine* 354(6): 601–609.

Hospital Infection Control Practices Advisory Committee. (1996). "Guideline for isolation precautions in hospitals. Part II. Recommendations for isolation precautions in hospitals. Hospital Infection Control Practices Advisory Committee." *American Journal of Infection Control* 24(1): 32–52.

Irwin, R. S., and Madison, J. M. (2000). "The diagnosis and treatment of cough." *New England Journal of Medicine* 343(23): 1715–1721.

Kahn, J. O., and Walker, B. D. (1998). "Acute Human Immunodeficiency Virus Type 1 Infection." *New England Journal of Medicine* 339(1): 33–39.

Kauffman, C. A. (1999). "Sporotrichosis." *Clinical Infectious Diseases* 29(2): 231–236; quiz 237.

Keane, J., Gershon, S., Wise, R. P., Mirabile-Levens, E., Kasznica, J., Schwieterman, W. D., Siegel, J. N., and Braun, M. M. (2001). "Tuberculosis associated with infliximab, a tumor necrosis factor alpha-neutralizing agent." *New England Journal of Medicine* 345(15): 1098–1104.

Kimberlin, D. W., and Rouse, D. J. (2004). "Genital herpes." *New England Journal of Medicine* 350(19): 1970–1977.

Leibowitz, H. M. (2000). "The red eye." *New England Journal of Medicine* 343(5):345–351.

Lekstrom-Himes, J. A., and Gallin, J. I. (2000). "Immunodeficiency diseases caused by defects in phagocytes." *New England Journal of Medicine* 343(23): 1703–1714.

Marr, K. A., Carter, R. A., and Boeckh, M. (2002). "Invasive aspergillosis in allogeneic stem cell transplant recipients: Changes in epidemiology and risk factors." *Blood* 100(13): 4358–4366.

McCormack, W. M. (1994). "Pelvic inflammatory disease." *New England Journal of Medicine* 330(2): 115–119.

Musher, D. M., and Musher, B. L. (2004). "Contagious acute gastrointestinal infections." *New England Journal of Medicine* 351(23): 2417–2427.

Mylonakis, E., and Calderwood, S. B. (2001). "Infective endocarditis in adults." *New England Journal of Medicine* 345(18): 1318–1330.

Nicolle, L. E. (2001). "Urinary tract infections in long-term-care facilities." *Infection Control and Hospital Epidemiology* 22(3): 167–175.

Pinals, R. S. (1994). "Polyarthritis and fever." *New England Journal of Medicine* 330(11): 769–776.

Ramos-e-Silva, M., Vasconcelos, C., Carneiro, S., and Cestari, T. (2007). "Sporotrichosis." *Clinics in Dermatology* 25(2): 181–187.

Russell, J. A. (2006). "Management of sepsis." *New England Journal of Medicine* 355(16): 1699–1713.

Satou, G. M., Giamelli, J., and Gewitz, M. H. (2007). "Kawasaki disease: Diagnosis, management, and long-term implications." *Cardiology in Review* 15(4): 163–169.

Sharkawy, A. A. (2007). "Cervicofacial actinomycosis and mandibular osteomyelitis." *Infectious Disease Clinics of North America* 21(2): 543–556, viii.

Steere, A. C. (2001). "Lyme disease." *New England Journal of Medicine* 345(2): 115–125.

Thielman, N. M., and Guerrant, R. L. (2004). "Acute infectious diarrhea." *New England Journal of Medicine* 350(1): 38–47.

Van-Burik, J., and Weisdorf, D. (2005). "Infections in recipients of hematopoietic stem cell transplantation." In Mandell, G. L., Bennett, J. E., and Dolin, R., eds., *Principles and Practices of Infectious Diseases*, 6th ed., Elsevier, Philadelphia, PA, p. 3489.

Van de Beek, D., de Gans, J., Tunkel, A. R., and Wijdicks, E. F. M. (2006). "Community-acquired bacterial meningitis in adults." *New England Journal of Medicine* 354(1):44–53.

Westphalm, J. F., and Brogard, J. M. (1999). "Biliary tract infections: A guide to drug treatment." *Drugs* 57(1): 81–91.

Young, N. S., and Brown, K. E. (2004). "Parvovirus B19." *New England Journal of Medicine* 350(6): 586–597.

Zimmerli, W., Trampuz, A., and Ochsner, P. E. (2004). "Prosthetic-joint infections." *New England Journal of Medicine* 351(16): 1645–1654.

Pharmacology

Tep Kang, PharmD, BCPS

1. Patients should avoid alcohol when taking which of the following medications?
   - **A.** ampicillin
   - **B.** metronidazole
   - **C.** erythromycin
   - **D.** doxycycline

2. Which of the following medications typically causes an elevated anticoagulant effect of warfarin when administered concomitantly?
   - **A.** trimethoprim-sulfamethoxazole
   - **B.** acetaminophen
   - **C.** enalapril
   - **D.** diltiazem

3. Which of the following medications can cause hyperkalemia?
   - **A.** esomeprazole
   - **B.** ranitidine
   - **C.** enalapril
   - **D.** albuterol

4. Patients should avoid dairy products when taking which of the following medications?
   - **A.** ciprofloxacin
   - **B.** acetaminophen
   - **C.** propranolol
   - **D.** amiodarone

5. Patients should avoid prolonged exposure to the sun when taking which of the following medications?
   - **A.** cephalexin
   - **B.** doxycycline
   - **C.** oxycodone
   - **D.** lisinopril

6. One milligram (mg) of injectable hydromorphone is equal to approximately how many micrograms (µg) of injectable fentanyl?
   - **A.** 10
   - **B.** 50
   - **C.** 100
   - **D.** 150

7. Which of the following antipsychotic agents causes few or no extrapyramidal side effects?

   A. haloperidol
   B. ziprasidone
   C. fluphenazine
   D. perphenazine

8. Which of the following antihypertensive agents can cause cyanide intoxication?

   A. nitroprusside
   B. nicardipine
   C. hydralazine
   D. esmolol

9. Five milligrams of prednisone is equivalent to approximately how many milligrams of hydrocortisone?

   A. 5
   B. 10
   C. 15
   D. 20

10. Which of the following medications does not typically alter gastric pH?

   A. sucralfate
   B. cimetidine
   C. pantoprazole
   D. esomeprazole

11. Which of the following medications is generally safe to administer during pregnancy when managing patients with hyperthyroidism?

   A. propylthiouracil
   B. levothyroxine
   C. methimazole
   D. anodized iodide

12. One gram of lipid yields how many kilocalories?

   A. 4
   B. 5
   C. 7
   D. 9

13. Deficiency of which of the following fat-soluble vitamins is associated with bleeding?

   A. Vitamin A
   B. Vitamin D
   C. Vitamin E
   D. Vitamin K

14. Which of the following chemotherapeutic agents can cause hemorrhagic cystitis?

   A. busulfan
   B. ifosfamide
   C. cisplatin
   D. vincristine

15. Which of the following medications is the first-line therapy for treatment of *Clostridium difficile*?

   A. vancomycin
   B. clindamycin
   C. levofloxacin
   D. ampicillin

16. Which of the following medications contains the highest amount of elemental iron?

   A. ferrous sulfate
   B. ferrous gluconate
   C. ferrous fumarate
   D. ferrous sulfate (exsiccated)

17. Which of the following insulins has the longest duration of effect?

   A. aspart
   B. lispro
   C. glulisine
   D. glargine

18. Which of the following cholesterol-lowering agents can cause flushing upon administration?

   A. niacin
   B. atorvastatin
   C. clofibrate
   D. lovastatin

19. Which of the following agents causes neuroleptic malignant syndrome?

   A. fluoxetine
   B. haloperidol
   C. amitriptyline
   D. nortriptyline

20. Patients should follow strict dietary restrictions (avoid the use of aged cheeses) in order to avoid hypertensive crisis when taking which of the following antidepressant drugs?

   A. paroxetine
   B. fluoxetine
   C. sertraline
   D. phenelzine

21. A neighbor discovers a white male unresponsive at his home. He was lying on the floor holding an empty bottle of alprazolam in his hand. Which of the following is the antidote of choice for alprazolam overdose?

   A. protamine
   B. flumazenil
   C. naloxone
   D. *n*-acetylcysteine

22. Which of the following is the drug of choice for the management of *Pneumocystis jiroveci* (*carinii*) pneumonia (PCP) in HIV-infected individuals?

   A. ciprofloxacin
   B. pyrimethamine
   C. rifabutin
   D. trimethoprim-sulfamethoxazole

23. Which of the following medications causes lactic acidosis?

   A. glyburide
   B. glipizide
   C. metformin
   D. repaglinide

24. Which of the following antiepileptic medications can cause hyponatremia?

    A. phenytoin
    B. carbamazepine
    C. levetiracetam
    D. valproic acid

25. Which of the following antiarrhythmic drugs could cause systemic lupus erythematosus (SLE)?

    A. amiodarone
    B. mexiletine
    C. procainamide
    D. quinidine

ANSWERS

1. **The correct answer is B.** Metronidazole inhibits the liver enzyme aldehyde dehydrogenase, which is responsible for metabolizing alcohol. This enzyme inhibition causes acetaldehyde to accumulate. Excessive acetaldehyde causes facial flushing, throbbing headache, nausea and vomiting, tachycardia, dizziness, hypotension, and blurred vision. This reaction is a disulfiram-like reaction. Ampicillin, erythromycin, and doxycycline do not inhibit alcohol dehydrogenase.

2. **The correct answer is A.** Trimethoprim-sulfamethoxazole inhibits the hepatic enzyme pathway cytochrome P-450, which is responsible for clearing warfarin. If the enzyme is inhibited, less warfarin clears and more warfarin is available to cause a pharmacologic effect. Acetaminophen, enalapril, and diltiazem do not inhibit the same hepatic enzyme that is responsible for clearing warfarin.

3. **The correct answer is C.** Enalapril is an antihypertensive agent belonging to the angiotension-converting enzyme inhibitor (ACE-I) class. ACE inhibitors can cause hyperkalemia. Esomeprazole and ranitidine do not cause hyperkalemia. Albuterol causes hypokalemia, not hyperkalemia.

4. **The correct answer is A.** Ciprofloxacin is a fluoroquinolone antimicrobial agent. This class of drugs forms a complex with dairy products, thus preventing the drug from being absorbed in adequate amounts. Acetaminophen, propanolol, and amiodarone do not interact with dairy products.

5. **The correct answer is B.** Doxycycline is an antimicrobial agent that causes photosensitivity to the skin. Prolonged exposure to the sun while taking doxycycline could cause excessive sunburn. Cephalexin, oxycodone, and lisinopril do not cause such an effect.

6. **The correct answer is C.** The equivalent of 1 mg of hydromorphone is approximately 100 μg of fentanyl.

7. **The correct answer is B.** Ziprasidone is a second-generation and/or atypical antipsychotic agent. These newer agents cause few or no acutely occurring extrapyramidal side effects. Haloperidol, fluphenazine, and perphenazine are first-generation and/or typical antipsychotic agents with higher incidences of extrapyramidal side effects.

8. **The correct answer is A.** Because nitroprusside is metabolized into cyanide and then to thiocyanate, which is eliminated by the kidneys, serum thiocyanate levels should be monitored when infusions are continued longer than 72 hours. Nicardipine, hydralazine, and esmolol do not produce cyanide as a byproduct of their metabolism.

9. **The correct answer is D.** This is a straightforward conversion problem. Essentially, hydrocortisone is four times stronger than prednisone, therefore, 5 mg of prednisone equals 20 mg of hydrocortisone.

10. **The correct answer is A.** Sucralfate is a combination drug consisting of a sugar molecule bound to aluminum. Sucralfate works by coating the surface of the gastrointestinal tract without altering the gastric pH. Cimetidine, pantoprazole, and esomeprazole all work by inhibiting acid secretion, therefore altering the gastric pH.

11. **The correct answer is A.** Propylthiouracil crosses the placental membranes only one-tenth as well as methimazole. Methimazole readily crosses the placenta and appears in breast milk. Levothyroxine is the appropriate medication for the management of hypothyroidism, not hyperthyroidism.

12. **The correct answer is D.** One gram of lipid, dextrose, and protein yield 9, 4, and 4 kilocalories, respectively.

13. **The correct answer is D.** Certain clotting factors and anticoagulants depend on vitamin K. Vitamin K deficiency causes coagulopathy, whereas vitamin A deficiency leads to night blindness. Vitamin D deficiency leads to osteomalacia, and vitamin E deficiency leads to hemolysis.

14. **The correct answer is B.** Ifosfamide causes hemorrhagic cystitis. Busulfan can cause skin hyperpigmentation. Cisplatin is nephrotoxic. Vincristine causes peripheral neuropathy.

15. **The correct answer is A.** Vancomycin is the preferred agent for the treatment of *Clostridium difficile*. Clindamycin, levofloxacin, and ampicillin do not have any activity against this pathogen.

16. **The correct answer is C.** Ferrous sulfate, ferrous gluconate, ferrous fumarate, and ferrous sulfate (exsiccated) contain 20%, 12%, 33%, and 30% of elemental iron, respectively.

17. **The correct answer is D.** Aspart, lispro, and glulisine are rapid-acting insulins, with a duration of effect of approximately 3 to 5 hours. The duration of effect of glargine is approximately 22 to 24 hours.

18. **The correct answer is A.** Niacin causes flushing upon administration. Low-dose aspirin taken daily with niacin reduces the incidence of this adverse side effect. Atorvastatin and lovastatin can cause liver toxicity, whereas clofibrate causes cholesterol gallstones.

19. **The correct answer is B.** Neuroleptic malignant syndrome is associated with the use of antipsychotic agents. The syndrome is manifested as hyperthermia, catatonia, altered level of consciousness, autonomic dysfunction, and rigidity. Fluoxetine, amitriptyline, and nortriptyline are antidepressants and do not typically cause this syndrome.

20. **The correct answer is D.** Phenelzine is a monoamine-oxidase inhibitor (MAO-I). Monoamine oxidase, an enzyme, is responsible for eliminating neurotransmitters such as norepinephrine, serotonin, tyramine, and so on. By inhibiting the enzyme, the body is unable to clear these neurotransmitters. High levels of these neurotransmitters can cause hypertensive crisis. Aged cheese contains high levels of tyramine. Paroxetine, sertraline, and fluoxetine are selective serotonergic reuptake inhibitors. They do not inhibit the monoamine oxidase.

21. **The correct answer is B.** Alprazolam is a benzodiazepine. The antidote for a benzodiazepine is flumazenil. Flumazenil antagonizes the actions of benzodiazepines on the central nervous system. The drug competitively inhibits the activity at the benzodiazepine recognition site on the GABA/benzodiazepine receptor complex. Protamine is an antidote for heparin overdose, naloxone for opioid overdose, and *n*-acetylcysteine for acetaminophen overdose.

22. The correct answer is D. *Pneumocystis jiroveci* (*carinii*) pneumonia (PJP, formally PCP) has a mortality of nearly 100% if left untreated. Trimethoprim-sulfamethoxazole is the regimen of choice for the treatment and prophylaxis of PJP in patients with and without HIV infection. Ciprofloxacin, pyrimethamine, and rifabutin are not effective in the treatment of PJP.

23. The correct answer is C. Metformin causes lactic acidosis in approximately 3 cases per 100,000 patient years. Metformin therapy should not be administered in any disease state that may increase lactic acid production (hypoperfusion) or decrease lactic acid removal (renal failure). Glyburide, glipizide, and repaglinide cause hypoglycemia, not lactic acidosis.

24. The correct answer is B. Carbamazepine causes hyponatremia. Phenytoin could cause hematologic disorders. Levetiracetam can cause sedation, and valproic acid causes hepatic failure.

25. The correct answer is C. Procainamide may be a causative factor in systemic lupus erythematosus (SLE). Amiodarone may cause pulmonary fibrosis. Mexiletine could cause psychosis, and quinidine may cause cinchonism (also known as quininism, or poisoning from cinchona or its alkaloids).

REFERENCES

Arcangelo, V., and Peterson, A. (2006). *Pharmacotherapeutics for advanced practice: A practical approach*, 2nd ed. Lippincott, Williams and Wilkins, Philadelphia, PA.

Dipiro, J., Talbert, R. L., Yee, G. C., Matzke, G. R., and Wells, B. G. (2005). *Pharmacotherapy: A pathophysiologic approach*, 6th ed. McGraw-Hill Companies, New York.

Hardman, J., Hardman, J. G., Limbird, L. E., and Gilman, A. G. (2001). *Goodman and Gilman's the pharmacological basis of therapeutics*, 10th ed. McGraw-Hill Companies, New York.

CHAPTER 14

Physical Diagnosis

Donna M. Agnew, MT (ASCP), MSPAS, PA-C

1. Which of the following is *not* an expected physical exam finding associated with Cushing's syndrome?

   A. Abdominal striae
   B. Buffalo hump
   C. Moon facies
   D. Hypotension

2. A 33-year-old female presents to the emergency department shortly after sustaining a facial contusion. When testing her extraocular movements, you note that the patient is unable to look down and to the right with her left eye. Which of the following muscles is most likely adversely affected?

   A. Left inferior oblique
   B. Left inferior rectus
   C. Left superior oblique
   D. Left superior rectus

3. On routine physical examination of a 24-year-old male, you note persistence of lumbar lordosis when the patient bends forward to touch his toes. There is no evident muscle spasm. Which of the following conditions best describes these findings?

   A. Ankylosing spondylitis
   B. Listing associated with herniated disc
   C. Scoliosis
   D. Spondylolisthesis

4. A 33-year-old left-hand dominant female presents complaining of worsening left elbow pain over the past 2 weeks. She admits to painting recently, but denies any history of known trauma. On inspection, there is no erythema, edema, nodules, or tophi. Localized tenderness with palpation is present in the area shown below. Extension of the wrist against resistance exacerbates her pain. The patient demonstrates full passive and active range of motion, with +2/+4 deep tendon reflexes and intact sensation. Which of the following conditions is the most likely diagnosis?

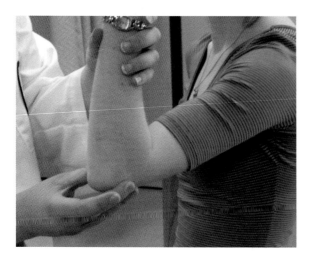

    A. Lateral epicondylitis
    B. Medial epicondylitis
    C. Olecranon bursitis
    D. Ulnar neuropathy

5. Which of the following tests should a clinician perform prior to drawing an arterial blood gas specimen on a patient in acute respiratory distress?

    A. Allen's test
    B. Appley's test
    C. Asterixis
    D. Tinel's test

6. Your patient has chronic obstructive pulmonary disease (COPD). Which of the following physical exam findings would unlikely be present?

    A. Decreased tactile fremitus
    B. Diffuse hyperresonant percussion notes
    C. Diminished breath sounds
    D. Elevated diaphragmatic levels

7. Which of the following statements is *least* consistent with the murmur of aortic stenosis?

    A. The clinician would best hear this murmur with the patient seated and leaning forward.
    B. It is a loud, medium-pitched crescendo–decrescendo systolic murmur.
    C. Radiation may be to the carotids or down the left sternal border.
    D. Valsalva strain increases the intensity of the murmur.

8. Which of the following sensations would most likely be lost or impaired in patients with peripheral neuropathy?

    A. Graphesthesia
    B. Stereognosis
    C. Two-point discrimination
    D. Vibration

9. A 73-year-old poorly controlled diabetic female admits to a constant dribbling of urine and a decreased force of urinary stream. She denies fever, dysuria, hematuria, nausea, vomiting, or flank pain. On abdominal exam, the bladder is enlarged and mildly tender. A preliminary dipstick in the office is negative for leukocyte esterase, nitrites, glucose, ketones, and protein. Which of the following is the most likely diagnosis?

   A. Asymptomatic urinary tract infection
   B. Overflow incontinence
   C. Stress incontinence
   D. Urge incontinence

10. A left-hand dominant male mechanic presents complaining of left volar wrist pain and paresthesias, primarily in his left thumb, index and middle fingers, that awaken him at night. He notes diminished grip strength. Considerable weakness is noted when the patient attempts to abduct his left thumb against resistance (as shown below). Which of the following is the most likely diagnosis?

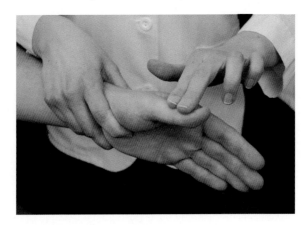

   A. Carpal tunnel syndrome
   B. De Quervain's tenosynovitis
   C. Ganglion cyst
   D. Osteoarthritis

11. Which of the following signs would you most likely find in a patient with Graves' disease?

   A. Bradycardia
   B. Delayed deep tendon reflexes
   C. Lid lag
   D. Queen Anne's sign

12. A patient complains of localized anterior shoulder pain with the maneuver shown below. This response suggests inflammation or arthritis in which of the following anatomic sites?

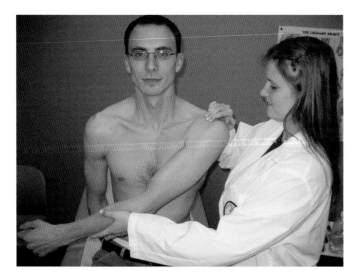

    A. Acromioclavicular joint
    B. Coracoid process
    C. Glenohumeral joint
    D. Sternoclavicular joint

13. A patient who complains of left shoulder pain rotates her forearm medially against resistance (shown below). Which of the following rotator cuff muscles does this physical maneuver best assess?

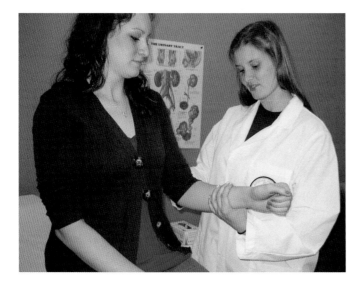

    A. Infraspinatus
    B. Subscapularis
    C. Supraspinatus
    D. Teres minor

14. A 19-year-old female presents to the student health center complaining of fever, a diffuse petechial rash, and neck stiffness for 1 day. On physical examination, the patient flexes her hips and knees with the maneuver shown below. This response denotes meningeal inflammation and indicates that which of the following is positive?

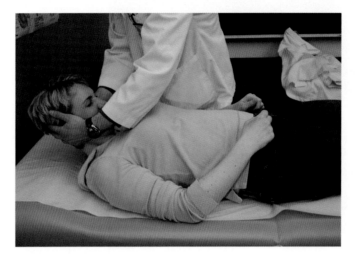

   A. Brudzinski's sign
   B. Kernig's sign
   C. Thomas' test
   D. Thompson's test

15. On funduscopic exam of a septic 23-year-old patient who admits to current IV drug abuse, you visualize cotton wool spots surrounded by an arteriole bleed. Which of the following best define these retinal bleeds?

   A. Janeway lesions
   B. Osler nodes
   C. Roth spots
   D. Splinter hemorrhages

16. A 69-year-old right-hand dominant diabetic patient presents complaining of an increasing flexor contracture of his right ring finger over the past 6 months, as shown below. Which of the following is the most likely diagnosis?

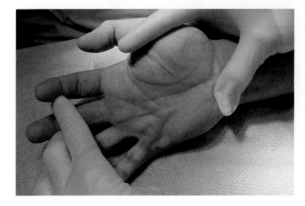

   A. Boutonnière deformity
   B. Dupuytren's contracture
   C. Swan neck deformity
   D. Trigger finger

17. Which of the following structures is most likely torn when the maneuver shown below demonstrates significant forward movement of the tibia greater than 5 mm?

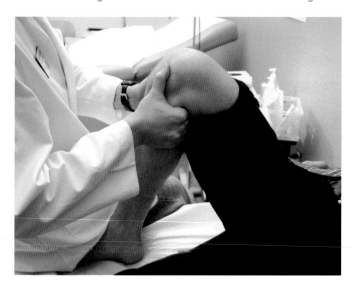

  A. Anterior cruciate ligament
  B. Medial collateral ligament
  C. Medial meniscus
  D. Posterior cruciate ligament

18. Which of the following cranial nerves does the exam technique shown below assess?

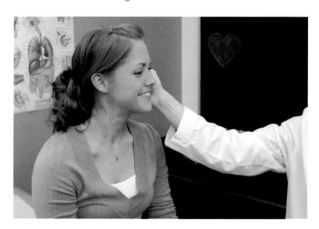

  A. V (trigeminal)
  B. VII (facial)
  C. X (vagus)
  D. XI (spinal accessory)

19. A 42-year-old female presents with acute onset of right upper quadrant abdominal pain. She describes the pain to be a constant, gnawing pain, with intermittent radiation to the right scapula. She notes an associated low-grade fever, anorexia, and nausea and a single episode of vomiting that produced only a small amount of bilious liquid. You suspect acute cholecystitis, as confirmed by which of the following examination techniques shown below?

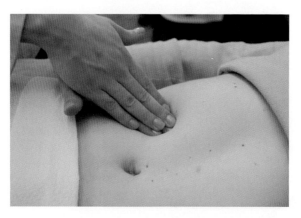

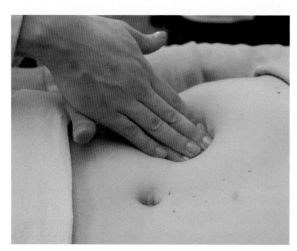

    A. Fist percussion of the liver
    B. Hepatojugular reflux
    C. Murphy's sign
    D. Obturator sign

20. On routine inspection, you note an annular area of alopecia on a patient's left parietal scalp. The hair shafts are broken at variable lengths, and there is no scalp erythema or scaling. Which of the following is the most likely diagnosis?

    A. Alopecia areata
    B. Psoriasis
    C. Tinea capitis
    D. Trichotillomania

21. Which of the following oral manifestations is typically associated with phenytoin therapy?

    A. Atrophic glossitis
    B. Fordyce granules
    C. Gingival hyperplasia
    D. Tooth attrition

22. A 53-year-old male landscaper presents with acute onset of right groin pain radiating into the right scrotum. He notes exacerbation of his pain with defecation and heavy lifting. He denies any gross hematuria, dysuria, penile discharge, or lesions. On genital examination, there is a bulging of the right scrotum. With the examiner's finger in the inguinal canal, a protrusion is felt on the examiner's fingertip when the patient coughs. Which of the following is the most likely diagnosis?

    A. Direct inguinal hernia
    B. Femoral hernia
    C. Indirect inguinal hernia
    D. Varicocele

23. On digital rectal examination, a patient's prostate is symmetric, moderately enlarged, and smooth, without nodules or tenderness. There is obliteration of the medial sulcus. Which of the following conditions most likely presents in this fashion?

    A. Acute prostatitis
    B. Benign prostatic hypertrophy
    C. Normal prostate gland
    D. Prostate cancer

24. Which of the following conditions usually elicits a red reflex response?

    A. Artificial eye
    B. Cataract
    C. Glaucoma
    D. Retinoblastoma

25. Which of the following murmurs produces a characteristic opening snap following S2 and an accentuated S1?

    A. Aortic stenosis
    B. Mitral valve prolapse
    C. Mitral stenosis
    D. Pulmonic stensosis

26. Which of the following stool colors or consistencies would a patient with an intestinal malabsorption syndrome most likely present?

    A. Acholic stools
    B. Black, tarry stools
    C. Thin, pencil-like stools
    D. Yellow, greasy, frothy stools

27. Which of the following would most likely account for a falsely increased liver span measured in the right midclavicular line?

    A. Congestive heart failure
    B. Colonic gas
    C. Perforated peptic ulcer
    D. Ruptured bullae in the right lung base

28. Which of the following characteristic nail changes is usually seen in patients with a history of psoriatic arthritis?

    A. Beau's lines
    B. Clubbing
    C. Pitting
    D. Terry's nails

29. On routine physical examination of an adolescent female, you note enlargement of the breast and areola as a single mound with no distinction in contour of the two. Which Tanner stage of breast development does this finding best represent?

A. 2
B. 3
C. 4
D. 5

30. Which of the following sensory discriminatory functions is impaired in a patient who cannot properly identify an item such as a key when it is placed in his or her hand?

A. Extinction
B. Graphesthesia
C. Proprioception
D. Stereognosis

31. Which of the following physical examination findings is most likely in a patient with long-standing ulnar neuropathy?

A. Atrophy of the hypothenar eminence
B. Depression of the thenar eminence
C. Furrowing between the metacarpals
D. Subluxation and ulnar deviation of the fingers

32. Which of the following anatomic sites best distinguishes yellowing due to carotenemia versus bilirubin?

A. Alae nasi
B. Frenulum of the tongue
C. Palmar creases
D. Sclerae

33. Your patient has asterixis. In which of the following conditions would this most likely occur?

A. Hyperthyroidism
B. Metabolic encephalopathy
C. Parkinson's disease
D. Huntington's chorea

34. Which of the following does *not* indicate anorexia or bulimia nervosa on physical exam?

A. Bilateral parotid or submandibular enlargement
B. Calloused index finger
C. Erosion of incisor tooth enamel
D. Geographic tongue

35. Examination of a patient with right anterior shoulder pain reveals localized tenderness with palpation of the anatomic site shown below. His pain worsens when he attempts to supinate his forearm against resistance with his arm at his side and his elbow flexed at 90°. Which of the following is the most likely diagnosis?

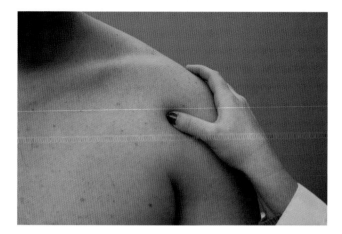

    A. Bicipital tendonitis
    B. Deltoid tendonitis
    C. Subacromial bursitis
    D. Supraspinatus tendonitis

36. Which of the following is consistent with a sensorineural hearing loss?

    A. The patient's hearing seems to improve in noisy surroundings.
    B. It may result from otosclerosis of the ossicles.
    C. With Rinne testing, air conduction is greater than bone conduction.
    D. With Weber testing, the sound lateralizes to the impaired ear.

37. A patient complains of left foot pain, which he describes as a burning ache with intermittent numbness of the third and fourth toes with increased ambulation. On specialized examination (shown below), there is localized tenderness on the plantar surface of the third and fourth metacarpal heads. Which of the following is the most likely diagnosis?

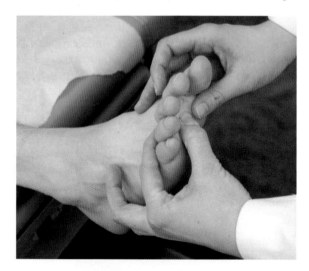

    A. Gouty arthritis
    B. Hammer toes
    C. Morton neuroma
    D. Plantar fasciitis

38. You prescribe a phenothiazine antiemetic for symptomatic relief of intractable vomiting in a patient with acute gastroenteritis. Shortly after taking the medication, she experiences rhythmic facial grimacing and repetitive mouth openings and tongue protrusions. Which of the following terms best describes this complication?

A. Athetosis
B. Chorea
C. Dystonia
D. Tardive dyskinesia

39. Which of the following is the most appropriate test for hip laxity and instability in an infant?

A. Babinski response
B. Barlow's test
C. Galeazzi's test
D. Ortolani's test

40. During a routine examination of an 8-week-old infant, you place the infant supine while supporting the head, back, and neck. You quickly lower the infant's body about 2 feet and notice abduction and extension of his arms, opening of his hands, and flexion of his legs in response to this maneuver. Which of the following infant reflexes does this best describe?

A. Asymmetric tonic neck reflex
B. Galant reflex
C. Moro reflex
D. Parachute reflex

ANSWERS

1. **The correct answer is D.** Signs and symptoms associated with Cushing's syndrome include central obesity with muscle wasting and atrophy of the limbs; hypertension; "moon facies"; "buffalo hump"; supraclavicular fat pads; hirsutism; purpura; striae; telangiectasias; acne; and limb atrophy. Hypotension is seen in adrenal insufficiency and hypocortisolism associated with Addison's disease.

2. **The correct answer is C.** Hint: Draw a line in the direction of gaze. The arrow points to the muscle responsible for each eye's movement in that direction. See the figure shown below. For instance, when looking down and to the right, the muscle responsible for the right eye is the inferior rectus. The superior oblique is responsible for the left eye. Remember: Cranial nerve innervations are lateral rectus, CN VI (abducens) and the superior oblique, CN IV (trochlear). Cranial nerve III (oculomotor) innervates the remainder of the extraocular muscles. A helpful mnemonic for remembering the innervation is LR_6SO_4 and all the rest are III.

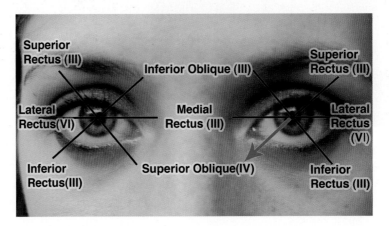

3. **The correct answer is A.** Ankylosing spondylitis leads to the loss of normal lumbar concavity and spine mobility. Lateral flexion is often the first movement lost. Palpation bilaterally over the sacroiliac joints may elicit tenderness. Disk herniation would be accompanied by radicular symptoms or perhaps sciatic nerve tenderness. Scoliosis will demonstrate a deviated spine and a thoracic deformity. With spondylolisthesis, one would expect to palpate a vertebral "step off," indicating the slippage of one vertebra upon another.

4. **The correct answer is A.** Lateral epicondylitis, or "tennis elbow," is tenderness of the extensor muscle tendons at their insertion at the lateral epicondyle. It is an overuse syndrome resulting from repetitive extension and supination/pronation of the forearm. Treatment options include NSAIDs, nonarticular braces, and resistance exercises; surgical intervention is reserved for refractory cases. Medial epicondylitis, or "golfer's elbow," results from repetitive wrist flexion. Examination demonstrates pain with palpation of the medial epicondyle and with flexion of the wrist against resistance. With olecranon bursitis, there is usually moderate edema superficial to the olecranon process. After carpal tunnel syndrome, ulnar compression is the second most common neuropathy of the upper extremity. The practitioner may note numbness and tingling of the medial palm, distally at the fourth digit and at the medial aspect of the fourth digit. Hypothenar atrophy may also occur with long-standing ulnar neuropathy.

5. **The correct answer is A.** Allen's test (shown below) ensures the patency of the ulnar artery and radial arteries prior to puncture of the radial artery for arterial blood gas specimen collection. Appley's test evaluates for a meniscal tear of the knee. This test is not performed as often (if at all) as in the past, as it has not demonstrated the same diagnostic yield as the McMurray test. This test occurs with the patient prone and the examiner flexing the knee and externally rotating the tibial plateau on the condyles. This maneuver causes compression of the menisci and elicits pain. Asterixis (arms extended with wrists in extension, "stopping traffic") is positive in hepatic encephalopathy. Tinel's sign (test) is percussion over the volar wrist that produces a tingling sensation or pain over the distribution of the median nerve in patients with carpal tunnel syndrome. The picture depicts the first phase of the Allen's test (radial atery patency).

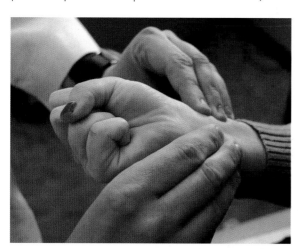

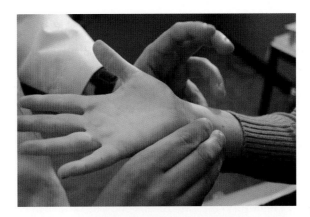

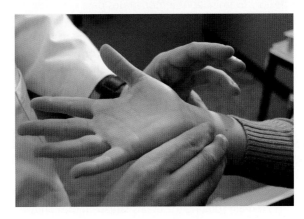

6. **The correct answer is D.** In chronic obstructive pulmonary disease (COPD), the lungs are generally hyperinflated, leading to diminished or absent breath sounds, flattened diaphragms, decreased tactile fremitus, and hyperresonance to percussion.

7. **The correct answer is D.** During the strain phase of valsalva, there is decreased venous return to the heart, resulting in decreased left ventricular blood volume. Less blood passing through a stenotic aortic valve subsequently diminishes the murmur.

8. **The correct answer is D.** Loss of vibratory sense is usually the earliest indication of peripheral neuropathy. Impaired graphesthesia, stereognosis, and two-point discrimination suggest a lesion in the sensory cortex. Graphesthesia translates from Greek as "writing perception" and is the patient's ability to identify a character traced on the palm of his or her hand. Stereognosis refers to the patient's ability to recognize objects placed in his or her hand solely by touch while the eyes are closed.

9. **The correct answer is B.** An asymptomatic urinary tract infection is unlikely with a negative urine dipstick result. Overflow incontinence occurs because of the inability of the bladder to fully empty. This presents with a palpable bladder on exam along with dribbling of small amounts of urine. It occurs secondary to a neurogenic bladder, weak detrusor and sphincter muscles, or urethral obstruction of urinary flow. Stress incontinence is due to weakness in the pelvic floor muscles, which causes urine to leak when abdominal pressure increases, such as with coughing, sneezing, or exercise. Urge incontinence is due to detrusor overactivity and causes the patient to experience involuntary loss of urine at the first sensation of the need to urinate. Pharmacologic treatment of urge incontinence includes the blockade of muscarinic receptors, which serve to reduce detrusor activity.

10. **The correct answer is A.** Tests for carpal tunnel syndrome include Phalen's test (wrists actively held in full flexion, see below); Tinel's test (percussion of the medial nerve along its course at the volar wrist, see below); and thumb abduction against resistance. The thumb abduction maneuver tests the strength of the abductor pollicis brevis muscle, innervated solely by the median nerve. Ganglion cysts typically appear on the dorsum of the wrist. They become more prominent with wrist flexion and are often asymptomatic. De Quervain's tenosynovitis produces a positive Finkelstein's test, which is pain elicited when a patient flexes the thumb in a closed fist and the hand is deviated in the ulnar direction.

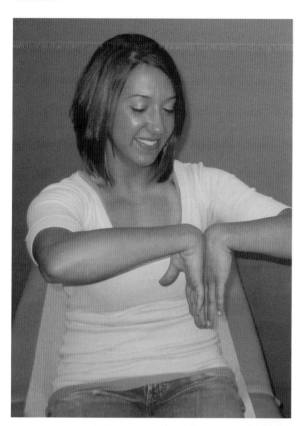

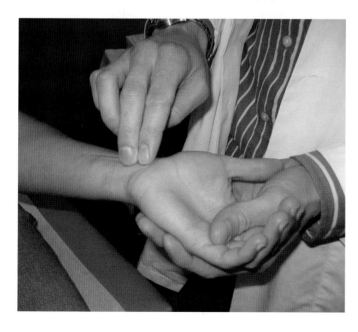

11. **The correct answer is C.** Lid lag is a physical manifestation of hyperthyroidism. Bradycardia, delayed deep tendon reflexes, and Queen Anne's sign (loss of the lateral aspect of the eyebrows) are findings consistent with hypothyroidism.

12. **The correct answer is A.** Pain with adduction of the arm constitutes a positive "crossover test" and indicates inflammation or degenerative changes in the acromioclavicular joint.

13. **The correct answer is B.** To assess for subscapularis integrity, the patient rotates the forearm medially against resistance. Having the patient abduct the forearm against resistance assesses the supraspinatus. When the patient rotates the forearm laterally against resistance, then the clinician evaluates the infraspinatus and teres minor muscles.

14. **The correct answer is A.** Involuntary flexion of the hips and knees in response to neck flexion constitutes a positive Brudzinski's sign. Another test for meningeal inflammation is Kernig's sign (shown below). With this test, the patient is placed with both the hip and knee flexed and, upon extension of the knee, pain and increased resistance is elicited. Thomas' test evaluates for a fixed flexion deformity of the hip. Thompson's test assesses Achilles tendon function indicated by plantar flexion of the foot in response to palpation of the posterior calf.

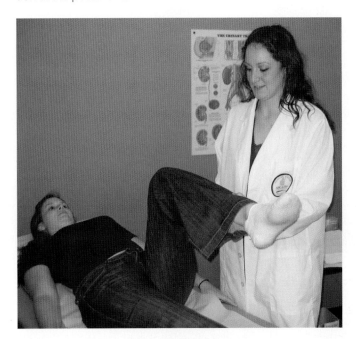

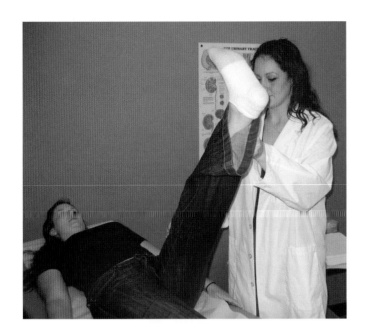

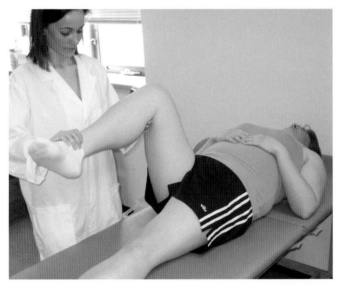

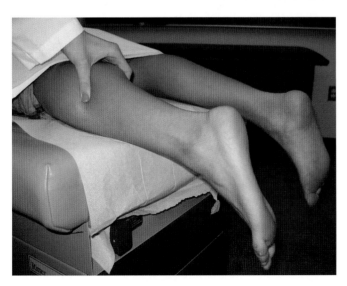

15. **The correct answer is C.** Infective endocarditis typically presents with Janeway lesions (painless erythematous macules on the palms and soles), Osler nodes (small, tender nodules on the palms, soles, and finger pads), Roth spots (although not specific to endocarditis), splinter hemorrhages, and petechiae.

16. **The correct answer is B.** Dupuytren's contracture results from a progressive plaque formation along the flexor tendon, which ultimately results in the formation of a fibrous cord. Boutonnière and swan-neck deformities frequently occur in chronic rheumatoid arthritis. Trigger finger is caused by a nodule at the head of the metacarpals, which makes the finger get "caught" in the flexed position and "pop" into extension.

17. **The correct answer is A.** Forward laxity with the anterior drawer test is indicative of an anterior cruciate ligament (ACL) tear. Lachman's test (shown below) also checks the integrity of the ACL. The valgus or abduction stress test assesses the medial collateral ligament (MCL). A meniscal injury is best identified with McMurray's test.

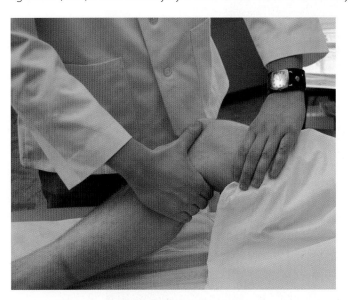

18. **The correct answer is D.** Cranial nerve XI (spinal accessory nerve) innervates both the sternocleidomastoid and the trapezius muscles. Turning the head against resistance evaluates the motor strength of the sternocleidomastoid muscles; shrugging the shoulders against resistance tests the strength of the trapezii. Palpating the patient's temporal and masseter muscles while the patient clenches his or her teeth evaluates cranial nerve V (trigeminal nerve). Maneuvers that assess cranial nerve VII (facial nerve) include asking the patient to: raise both eyebrows, frown, smile, show upper and lower teeth, puff out the cheeks, and to keep eyes tightly closed while the examiner attempts to open them. Asking the patient to say "ahh" and watching for the symmetric rise of the uvula best evaluates cranial nerve X (vagus nerve).

19. **The correct answer is C.** The exam technique in which the patient abruptly halts inspiration while the examiner palpates deeply into the right upper quadrant constitutes a positive Murphy's sign. This is typically indicative of acute cholecystitis. Pain with rotation of the leg both laterally and medially with both the hip and the knee flexed to 90° denotes a positive obturator sign. This usually denotes peritonitis and may occur in such conditions as a ruptured appendix or a pelvic abscess. Fist percussion of the liver elicits generalized liver tenderness. Hepatojugular reflux evaluates for portal circulation congestion.

20. **The correct answer is D.** Hair twisting or pulling, as seen in trichotillomania, results in broken hair shafts of varying lengths. Alopecia areata usually presents with a well-

demarcated area of complete hair loss. Psoriasis generally presents as a dry, scaly plaque formation. Tinea demonstrates xerotic scaling with well-demarcated borders. With tinea infections, the hair shafts appear "mowed down" close to the scalp, also known as "black dot alopecia."

21. **The correct answer is C.** Phenytoin therapy can cause gingival hyperplasia (shown below). Atrophic glossitis presents with a tender, smooth, shiny tongue and may be a result of an iron, vitamin B_{12}, folic acid, riboflavin, niacin, or pyridoxine deficiency. It may also be secondary to chemotherapeutic agents. Fordyce granules are small, yellow spots seen on the buccal or labial mucosa and represent normal sebaceous glands. Repetitive chewing or grinding of the teeth (bruxism) results in an erosion of the enamel and exposure of the tan dentin of the tooth.

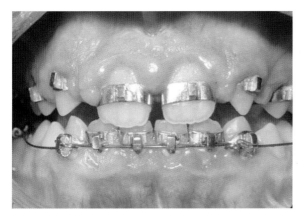

Courtesy of Dr. Joel Jaspan

22. **The correct answer is C.** An indirect hernia extends down the inguinal canal and often protrudes into the scrotum, placing pressure on the examiner's fingertip when the patient strains in valsalva. A direct hernia rarely courses into the scrotum; it puts pressure on the medial aspect the examiner's finger, because it protrudes anteriorly. With a femoral hernia, the inguinal canal remains empty, and it never extends into the scrotum. A varicocele represents a varicosity around the spermatic cord. It typically reduces when the patient is in the supine position and/or with scrotal elevation.

23. **The correct answer is B.** In benign prostatic hypertrophy, the medial sulcus is often not discernable. In acute prostatitis, there may be an enlarged gland, which would be warm and tender on palpation. In a "normal" prostate gland, the medial sulcus is palpable between the two lateral lobes. Cancer of the prostate usually presents with a firm nodularity that leads to an irregular contour.

24. **The correct answer is C.** Glaucoma does not produce opacities that would interfere with producing the normal red reflex response.

25. **The correct answer is C.** Mitral stenosis is a diastolic murmur that occurs between S2 and S1. It has a characteristic opening snap. Aortic stenosis and pulmonic stenosis are systolic murmurs, occurring between S1and S2. With mitral valve prolapse, the practitioner may auscultate a floppy valve during diastole and may also be heard as a click.

26. **The correct answer is D.** Steatorrhea, yellow-grey foamy stools that float in the commode, typically occur in malabsorption. Acholic stools, seen in acute hepatitis and in biliary obstruction, lack bile and, as a result, appear light in color. Black, tarry stool, or melena, usually occurs as a result of an upper gastrointestinal bleed, most often proximal to the ligament of Treitz. Pencil-thin stools usually represent an "apple core" obstructing lesion of the sigmoid colon.

27. **The correct answer is A.** Fluid accumulation associated with coronary heart failure would produce dullness to percussion, leading to a falsely increased liver span. Colonic gas, perforated viscus, and ruptured bullae would produce tympany over the right thorax and upper quadrant of the abdomen, falsely decreasing the estimated size of the liver.

28. **The correct answer is C.** Nail pitting, onycholysis, nail thickening, and "oil spot" lesions are characteristics of psoriasis. Beau's lines are transverse depressions in the nails that generally form subsequent to a severe acute illness. Clubbing may be indicative of chronic hypoxia, cirrhosis, coronary artery disease, or carcinoma of the lung. Terry's nails may be demonstrated in a variety of chronic disease states, including diabetes, congestive heart failure, and cirrhosis.

29. **The correct answer is B.**
Tanner 1: A raised nipple only
Tanner 2: Breast bud elevation of the areola
Tanner 3: Enlargement of the breast and areola as a single mound
Tanner 4: Areola forms a secondary mound
Tanner 5: A more pigmented recessed areola and part of the general breast contour with projection of the nipple

30. **The correct answer is D.** This best describes stereognosis. With extinction, the patient (with closed eyes) identifies places the examiner touches, pointing to the locations of simultaneous bilateral stimuli. Graphesthesia is the technique whereby a patient identifies a number or letter traced on the palm of his or her hand. Propioception evaluates body positioning and coordination and is a good reflection of a patient's cerebellar function.

31. **The correct answer is A.** Hypothenar atrophy suggests ulnar nerve dysfunction, whereas thenar atrophy suggests a median nerve disorder. Furrowing between the metacarpals is due to atrophy of the interosseus muscles. This may occur with aging or chronic rheumatoid arthritis. Subluxation, bogginess of metacarpophalangeal joints, and ulnar deviation of the fingers commonly present in patients with rheumatoid arthritis. Also remember that Heberden's nodes occur at distal interphalangeal joints and Bouchard's nodes present at proximal interphalangeal (PIP) joints in osteoarthritis (degenerative joint disease). Flexion of the PIP and hyperextension of the DIP in Boutonnière deformity and hyperextension of the PIP with flexion of the DIP in swan-neck deformity also occur in chronic rheumatoid arthritis.

32. **The correct answer is D.** Carotenemia is a benign yellow discoloration of the skin due to the ingestion of yellow fruits and vegetables and, unlike jaundice it does not affect the sclerae.

33. **The correct answer is B.** Asterixis, also known as liver flap, is the irregular flapping of the patient's hands when asked to "stop traffic" with arms and hands extended and fingers spread apart. Rhythmic flapping occurs due to episodic loss of extensor muscle tone. It is typically associated with hepatic encephalopathy, cerebrovascular disease, uremia, and severe pulmonary insufficiency. Hyperthyoidism may produce a resting tremor, whereas Parkinson's disease is associated with a pill-rolling, resting tremor. Choreiform movements are generally brief, jerky, and unpredictable.

34. **The correct answer is D.** Geographic tongue is a benign condition characterized by an irregular pattern of smooth areas void of papillae interspersed with normal rough-coated areas. Repetitive self-induced vomiting can produce a calloused index finger. Regurgitated stomach contents can physically erode tooth enamel, especially the posterior aspect of the incisors. Parotid and submandibular enlargement occurs secondary to hyperstimulation. Other signs and symptoms of anorexia include amenorrhea, bradycardia, hypotension, hypothermia, and increased lanugo body hair.

35. The correct answer is A. These are the classic examination findings seen in a patient with bicipital tendonitis.

36. The correct answer is C. Answers A, B, and D occur in conductive hearing loss. With a sensorineuronal hearing loss, the sound would lateralize to the unaffected ear on Weber testing (shown below, see first image), and air conduction would be greater than bone conduction on Rinne testing (shown below, see second two images).

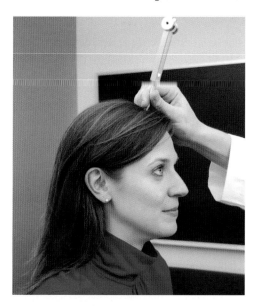

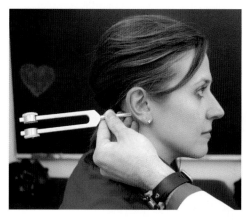

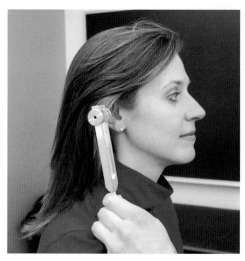

37. The correct answer is C. These are the classic history and physical examination findings in a patient with Morton neuroma. Gout typically presents in the first metatarsophalangeal (MTP) joint, with marked inflammation secondary to deposition of uric acid crystals. Hammer toe presents with hyperextension of the MTP and flexion of the proximal interphalangeal joint, usually involving the second toe. The pain of plantar fasciitis is most severe in the morning with the first few steps taken upon arising from bed and improves with ambulation. The pain associated with plantar fasciitis may be reproduced with palpation of the medial heel at the site of its insertion.

38. The correct answer is D. Tardive dyskinesia is rhythmic, repetitive movement that usually involves the face and mouth. It can be an adverse side effect of psychotropic drugs. Athetosis, seen in conditions such as cerebral palsy, is a slow, writhing movement that involves the face and extremities. Chorea movement is jerky, unpredictable, and does not usually repeat. Dystonia may also result from drugs, such as phenothiazines, but it usually involves larger portions of the body, such as the trunk.

39. The correct answer is B. Barlow's test evaluates an intact hip for laxity and hip instability. With this test, the infant is positioned supine with the hips flexed to 90°. The clinician then adducts the hip and places downward pressure to sublux the hip posteriorly. An Ortolani maneuver also positions the patient supine with knees flexed 90°. The hip is then abducted (remember "**o**ut" for **O**rtolani), with upward pressure placed laterally on the greater trochanter (shown below). A positive Ortolani presents as a palpable clunk as the posteriorly dislocated hip relocates back into the acetabulum. Asymmetric skin folds may provide another clue to a unilateral hip dislocation. The left hip most often displaces because the most common fetal lie in utero adducts the left hip directly against the mother's lumbosacral spine. A positive Babinski response presents by dorsiflexion of the big toe and fanning of the other toes in response to plantar stimulation. It is a normal response from infancy up to age 2 years. The Galeazzi, or Alice, test checks for any variation in knee heights while the infant is supine with knees flexed. This indirectly assesses for a femoral length discrepancy.

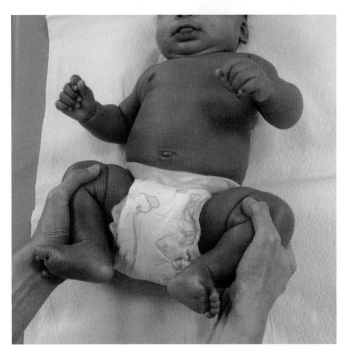

40. The correct answer is C. This correctly describes the Moro, or startle reflex, which a clinician can elicit in an infant from birth up to 4 months of age. The asymmetric tonic neck reflex usually lasts up to 2 months of age. To demonstrate the asymmetric tonic neck reflex, the examiner places the baby in a supine position and then turns the baby's head to one side. The arms and legs ipsilateral to the side the head is turned extend, whereas the arm and leg on the opposite side flex. With Galant's reflex, the examiner supports the baby in the prone position and then strokes one side of the back about 1 centimeter lateral of midline, causing the baby to curve his or her trunk in the direction of the stimulation. With the parachute maneuver, the examiner holds the baby prone and then lowers the baby's head, prompting the infant to extend his or her arms and legs out like a parachute. This reflex usually does not occur until 8 months or so of age. Other primitive reflexes include rooting, palmar grasp (shown below), plantar grasp (shown below), and stepping (shown on next page). The depiction shows the stepping motion of the child; however, this examination should occur with the leg raising up to a higher surface.

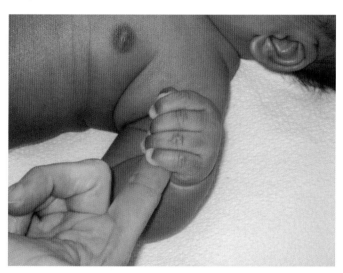

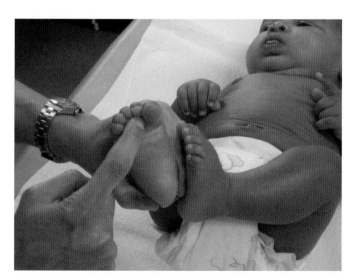

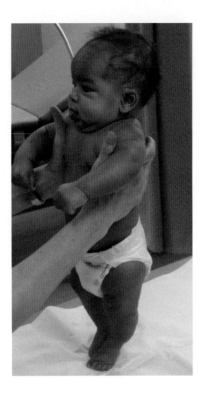

REFERENCES

Bencardino, J. T., and Rosenberg, Z. S. (2006). "Entrapment neuropathies of the shoulder and elbow in the athlete." *Clinics in Sports Medicine* 25(3): 465–487.

Bickley, L. S., and Szilagyi, P. G. (2007). *Bates' guide to physical examination*, 9th ed. Lippincott Williams & Wilkins, Philadelphia, PA.

Hanson, E. H., and Neuhauser, T. S. (2003). *The complete history and physical exam guide.* Elsevier Science, Philadelphia, PA.

Johnson, G. W., Cadwallader K., Scheffel, S. B., and, Epperly, T. D. (2007). "Treatment of lateral epicondylitis." *American Family Physician* 76(6): 843–848.

LeBlond, R. F., DeGowin, R. L., and Brown, D. D. (2004). *DeGowin's diagnostic evaluation*, 8th ed. McGraw Hill, New York.

Pavonello, R., De Martino, M. C., De Leo, M., Lombardi, G., and Colao, A. (2008). "Cushing's syndrome." *Endocrinology and Metabolism Clinics* 37(1): 135–149.

Seidel, H. M., Ball, J. W., Dains, J. E., and Benedict, G. W. (2006). *Mosby's guide to physical examination*, 6th ed. Mosby Elsevier, St. Louis.

Smith, P. P., McCrery, R. J., and Appell, R. A. (2006). "Current trends in the evaluation and management of female urinary incontinence." *Canadian Medical Association Journal* 175(10): 1233–1240.

Storer, S. K., and Skaggs, D. L. (2006). "Developmental dysplasia of the hip." *American Family Physician* 74(8): 1310–1316.

Radiology

Melissa Kohler Justice, PA-C, MHS

1. A 40-year-old man presented complaining of left elbow pain after he fell on the ice onto his outstretched hands. The radiologist reported a fracture and displacement of anterior and posterior fat pads. Based on the radiologist's report and the patient's radiograph, shown below, which of the following is the most likely diagnosis?

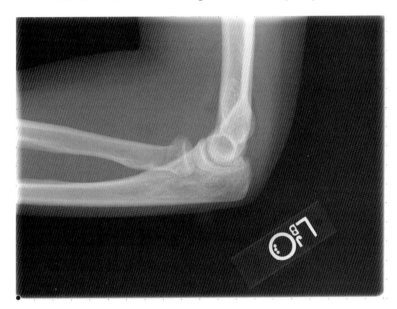

   A. Colles' fracture
   B. Nursemaid's elbow
   C. Radial head fracture
   D. Smith's fracture

2. A 17-year-old male presents complaining that he has been coughing up copious amounts of purulent sputum "ever since he can remember." He is dyspneic, and you can hear him wheeze while he is speaking. He says that he recently "caught a cold" and that his symptoms have worsened. A chest radiograph shows linear atelectasis ("tram lines") and dilated, thickened bronchial markings. To confirm your diagnosis, you have the patient get a chest CT, which is shown below. Which of the following is the most likely diagnosis?

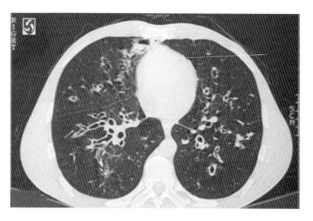

A. Acute bronchitis
B. Streptococcal pneumonia
C. Bronchiectasis
D. *Bordetella pertussis* infection

3. A 14-year-old male presents complaining of a headache. His blood pressure is 150/96 mmHg. On physical examination, you palpate strong brachial artery pulses and weak femoral pulses, bilaterally. You obtain an ECG, which depicts left ventricular hypertrophy. The patient's chest radiograph is shown below. What finding on the radiograph is most diagnostic in confirming your suspicions?

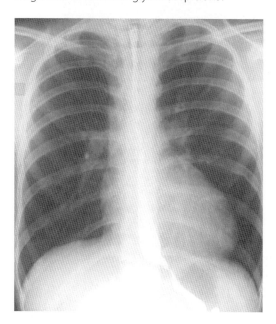

A. Rib notching
B. Right-sided aortic arch
C. Subclavian artery occlusion
D. Main pulmonary artery dilation

4. A 64-year-old contractor who has worked in demolition of old buildings for the last 40 years presents for a routine physical exam. You hear end-inspiratory crackles on auscultation, and note that he is dyspneic and cyanotic at rest. The patient is a nonsmoker and reports that he is "always trying to catch his breath." You obtain a chest radiograph, shown below. Which of the following is the patient *not* likely to exhibit on the film?

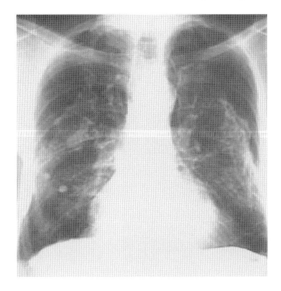

   A. Calcified plaques
   B. Thickened pleura
   C. Interstitial fibrosis
   D. Cavitary lesions

5. An 18-year-old male says that he has had a swollen right testicle "for a while now." He says that it does not hurt and that it is almost normal size in the morning after sleeping through the night. On physical examination, you note that the right scrotum feels like a "bag of worms." You order an ultrasound of his scrotum, which is shown below. The radiologist reports abnormal dilatation and tortuosity of the pampiniform venous plexus within the spermatic cord. Which of the following is the most likely diagnosis?

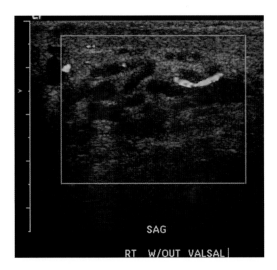

   A. Hydrocele
   B. Varicocele
   C. Testicular torsion
   D. Epididymitis

6. A very tall, 62-year-old male presents with chest pain and vague back pain. He said his voice has become hoarse over the last few months and he has noticed increasing difficulty with swallowing. His primary care provider has been treating his hypercholesterolemia and hypertension. He is s/p 2-vessel CABG three years ago. You immediately obtain a chest radiograph, which is shown below. Which of the following is the most likely diagnosis?

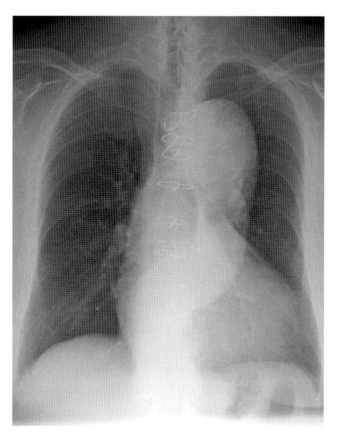

A. Pulmonary embolism
B. Thoracic aortic aneurysm
C. Tension pneumothorax
D. Coarctation of the aorta

7. A tall, 62-year-old male presents to the emergency department complaining of a sudden, severe pain in his chest and back that he describes as a "tearing sensation." The patient has a past medical history of uncontrolled hypertension. He recently stopped smoking after a 40-pack-year history. On physical examination, the patient is diaphoretic, pale, and tachycardic. His blood pressure in his right arm is 189/112 mmHg and 168/102 mmHg in the left. His ECG showed ST-segment depression, inferiorly. The imaging shown below confirms which of the following diagnoses?

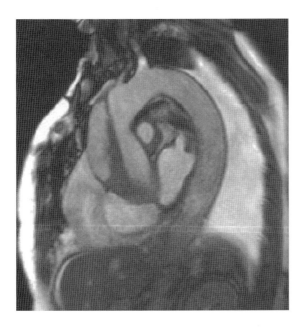

A. Descending thoracic aortic aneurysm
B. Acute myocardial infarction
C. Ascending aortic dissection
D. Cardiac tamponade

8. A 6-year-old boy presents with acute onset of high fever, sore throat, muffled voice, and drooling. He says he "can't swallow." You immediately order a lateral soft-tissue radiograph of the patient's neck, which is shown below. Which of the following is the most likely diagnosis?

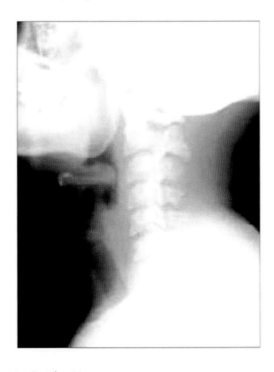

A. Epiglottitis
B. Peritonsillar abscess
C. Laryngotracheobronchitis
D. Bronchiolitis

9. A 70-year-old woman is 2 days postop following a total hip replacement. The patient suddenly develops dyspnea, tachypnea, and pleuritic chest pain. Her blood pressure is 89/45 mmHg, and her oxygen saturation level dropped to 80% on room air. You hemodynamically stabilize the patient and then obtain an ECG, which shows right ventricular strain. You order a CT angiogram with IV contrast; the results are shown below. Which of the following is the most likely diagnosis?

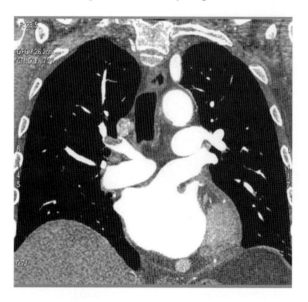

   A. Aortic dissection
   B. Pulmonary embolism
   C. Acute myocardial infarction
   D. Cardiac tamponade

10. A 12-year-old boy presents with an acutely tender and swollen scrotum. The patient said that he was playing at recess when the pain suddenly began. On physical examination, you note an asymmetrical high-riding testis on the affected side with a "bell-clapper" deformity. Which of the following is the best study to expedite and confirm your diagnosis?

   A. Pelvic CT
   B. Ultrasound with Doppler
   C. Radionucleotide imaging
   D. Kidney, ureter, and bladder flat-plate radiograph

11. Which of the following should be the first line of treatment based on the diagnosis in question 10?

   A. Rest, ice, scrotal elevation, and NSAIDs
   B. ceftriaxone and doxycycline for 10 days
   C. Urinalysis with Gram stain and culture. Wait for results before treatment
   D. Immediate surgical consultation and exploration

12. A 32-year-old female colleague confides in you that she experienced vertigo over the past few months and has had a painful tingling, spastic sensation in her hands that resolved spontaneously. She then describes what sounds like optic neuritis, explaining that it has been happening frequently, and afterward her eyesight diminishes for several hours. She also complains about a "band of tightness" around her waist. Obviously concerned for your colleague, you recommend that she see her primary care provider as soon as possible for evaluation and treatment. Which test is the most sensitive for confirming the likely diagnosis?

A. CT scan
B. Brain MRI
C. Evoked potentials
D. Evaluation of cerebrospinal fluid

13. A 45-year-old female presents to the emergency department with an acute onset 8 hours ago of nausea, vomiting, and abdominal pain. The patient's past surgical history is significant for a total abdominal hysterectomy 2 years ago. The patient describes her abdominal pain as "crampy," and it comes and goes every 5 minutes. She says she is unable to pass flatus. On physical examination, you note abdominal distention; high-pitched, hyperactive bowel sounds on auscultation. There are no palpable hernias. You order a flat-plate obstruction series, which is shown below. Which of the following is the most likely diagnosis?

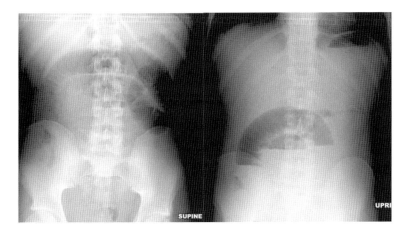

A. Ileus
B. Gastroenteritis
C. Small-bowel obstruction
D. Colonic obstruction

14. A 32-year-old overweight female presents complaining of severe "heartburn" as she rubs her epigastric region. She said she has had worsening work-related stress lately. She says she feels burning in her chest several hours after she eats, and the burning awakens her from sleep. She denies regurgitation, dysphagia, or unexplained weight loss. She states that antacids and food help lessen the discomfort. Which of the following is the most likely diagnosis?

A. Duodenal ulcer
B. Cholelithiasis
C. Gastroesophageal reflux disease (GERD)
D. Stable angina

15. Based on the diagnosis in question 14, which of the following would *not* be helpful in evaluating this patient's condition?

A. Noninvasive testing for *Helicobacter pylori*, followed by antibiotics if infection is found
B. Several trials with different antisecretory medications
C. Upper endoscopy with *Helicobacter pylori* testing
D. Upper GI study with barium swallow

16. A nonambulatory elderly patient is admitted to the hospital for gastrointestinal bleeding. She has a history of anticoagulation treatment at the nursing home with warfarin for recurrent deep vein thrombosis, documented on bilateral lower extremity ultrasound. Her coagulopathy is reversed, and her gastrointestinal bleed has been localized and treated. However, now that she is no longer a candidate for anticoagulation therapy, which of the following is the best treatment to prevent a possible pulmonary embolism?

  A. Inferior vena cava filter placement
  B. Sequential compression devices
  C. Elevation of affected limb and symptomatic relief of peripheral edema
  D. Nothing can be done for this patient

17. Using the Salter-Harris classification for pediatric fractures, which of the following is the best classification for the fracture shown?

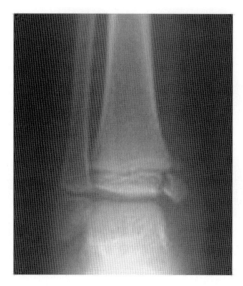

  A. Salter II
  B. Salter III
  C. Salter IV
  D. Salter V

18. A 17-year-old female presents reporting that she felt a painless lump in her right breast for the first time last month. The patient noticed that the lump did not change in size with her menstrual cycle. The patient has no family history of breast cancer. Which of the following is the best first step in managing this patient?

  A. Unilateral screening mammogram with additional views
  B. Ultrasound of the breast to determine if it is a simple cyst, complex cyst, or solid mass
  C. Surgical consult with a breast surgeon for surgical excision
  D. Order a unilateral breast MRI

19. Which of the following is *not* true regarding screening mammography in the United States?

  A. Screening reduces population mortality by 30% in women over the age of 50.
  B. Mammographic screening is a proven method for early breast cancer detection and diagnosis.
  C. Screening mammograms should be performed periodically, every 1 to 3 years, to detect preclinical asymptomatic breast cancer.
  D. The recommended age to begin screening mammograms is 40.

20. A 70-year-old male presents to the emergency department brought by his wife because he suddenly lost feeling in his left arm 1 hour ago. The wife noticed that he was unable to speak clearly and that the left side of his face was drooping. Which of the following should be the first imaging study you order?

    A. MRA of the brain with gadolinium

    B. Ultrasound of the carotid arteries

    C. Head CT without contrast

    D. Cerebral angiography

21. Which of the following are *not* typical signs of increased pulmonary venous hypertension on a chest radiograph?

    A. Kerley A and B lines

    B. Cephalization

    C. Perihilar alveolar edema

    D. Right ventricular hypertrophy

22. A thin, 35-year-old man presents with a 3-year history of dysphagia. The patient relates to you that when he eats solid food he almost always has to regurgitate it to relieve the retrosternal pain that follows. You order a chest radiograph, which shows a vastly dilated esophagus behind the heart. No other masses are noted. You then order a barium swallow study. The results are shown below. The radiologist notes a dilated esophagus, a rather long segment of spasm, and a "bird's beak" appearance of the distal esophagus. Which of the following is the most likely diagnosis?

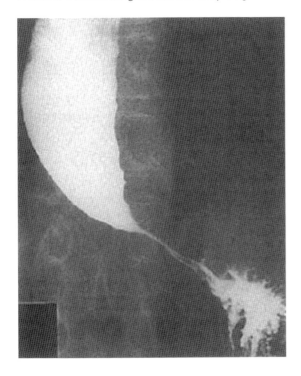

    A. Esophageal stricture from reflux esophagitis

    B. Achalasia

    C. Hiatal hernia

    D. Schatzki's rings

23. A radiograph (shown below) of an elderly woman's hand obtained to "assess morning stiffness" shows polyarticular erosive changes to the metacarpophalangeal and proximal interphalangeal joints with joint space narrowing, sparing the distal interphalangeal joints. There is periarticular soft-tissue inflammation around the affected joints, with a boutonnière deformity of the middle finger. Which of the following is the most likely diagnosis?

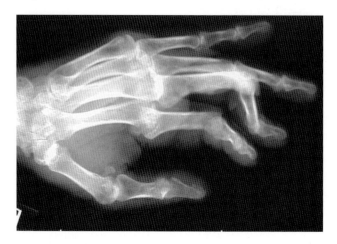

A. Osteoarthritis
B. Gout
C. Infectious arthritis
D. Rheumatoid arthritis

24. A 55-year-old male who has been training for a marathon presents to the Emergency Department hunched over and complaining of acute onset of right-sided low back pain and nausea. He said when the pain is bad, it is a "10 out of 10," but after 20 minutes, the pain is back down to a "4 out of 10." He said the pain started several hours ago after a 17-mile run. He feels like he has to urinate, but has difficulty beginning the flow. He said he finally came to the emergency department when he noticed blood in his urine. On physical examination, you note point tenderness of his right flank. The patient is febrile; however, his other vital signs are unremarkable. You order appropriate labs and start him on IV fluids. You manage his pain with ketorolac tromethamine. Which of the following is the best imaging study to confirm your diagnosis and rule out any other pathology?

A. Abdominal ultrasound
B. Flat-plate kidney-ureter-bladder (KUB) radiograph
C. Noncontrast abdominal CT
D. MRI of the lumbar region

25. A 64-year-old woman presents complaining of increasing shortness of breath and weight loss over the last few weeks. She has dyspnea on exertion and at times has a nonproductive cough. You are concerned because of her history of left breast cancer, diagnosed and treated 7 years ago. You order an immediate chest radiograph, which is shown below. Which of the following is the best way to manage this patient's condition?

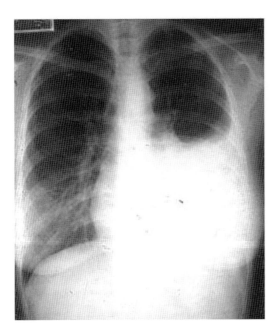

A. Obtain chest CT scan, followed by ultrasound-guided diagnostic thoracentesis
B. Surgical consult for chest tube placement for chemical pleurodesis
C. Diuretic therapy and a nebulizer breathing treatment
D. A consult with a pulmonologist for a bronchoscopy

26. You drain an effusion from a 66-year-old female's chest. The effusion was discovered when the patient presented with 3 weeks of dyspnea on exertion along with a nonproductive cough. The patient has a history of breast carcinoma, diagnosed and treated approximately 8 years ago. The aspirate that you drained from the patient's thorax is yellow-brown, cloudy, and thick. How would you describe this effusion?

   A. Hemothorax
   B. Exudative effusion
   C. Chylothorax
   D. Transudative effusion

27. Which of the following statements about malignant pleural effusions (MPE) is *not* true?

   A. The effusions tend to be significant in size, recur despite frequent aspiration, and are associated with extensive lung and systemic metastasis.
   B. Lung, breast, ovary, and lymphoma cancers account for the majority of cases of MPE.
   C. The majority of patients with MPE have incurable disease, so the treatment is generally palliative.
   D. Effusions occurring in lung and liver cancer generally occur on the same side of the body as the primary lesion.

28. A 46-year-old male presents with recurrent epigastric pain radiating to his back along with nausea and vomiting 20 minutes after eating. He states this has happened in the past, but it "went away" when he sat up and leaned forward. He says he drinks "about a case" of beer per day, and he has noticed having "clay-colored" stools lately. All of the following lab values are essentially normal: complete blood count (CBC), liver function tests (LFTs), and electrolytes. Abdominal ultrasound showed calcifications in the epigastrium. The abdominal CT shown below confirms which of the following diagnoses?

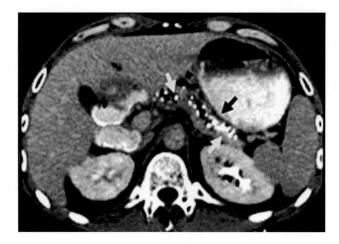

A. Peptic ulcer disease
B. Chronic pancreatitis
C. Acute cholecystitis
D. Subacute appendicitis

29. You discover a 1.5-cm solitary pulmonary nodule incidentally on a patient's chest CT. The patient used to smoke "a lot," but stopped 15 years ago. He recently had a negative PPD test. After taking a thorough history, you are concerned that this patient might have lung carcinoma. Which of the following is the first step in this patient's workup?

    A. Follow-up in 6 months with a repeat chest CT and look for any changes.
    B. Obtain a PET/CT to try to differentiate a benign nodule from a malignant nodule and assess for other areas of suspicion.
    C. Perform percutaneous biopsy of the nodule.
    D. Consult a thoracic surgeon for lung wedge resection using video-assisted thoracoscopy surgery (VATS).

30. A small, 2-year-old child is having his fifth lower respiratory *Pseudomonas* infection in a year. He has a chronic, productive cough, and his mother performs nightly chest percussions to break up the secretions. Inhalers do not help his wheezing. He takes enzymes to treat his fat and protein malabsorption. His chest radiograph (shown below) shows bilateral hyperinflation, perihilar interstitial markings compatible with bronchiectasis, mucus plugging, and recurrent pneumonitis. Which of the following is the most likely diagnosis?

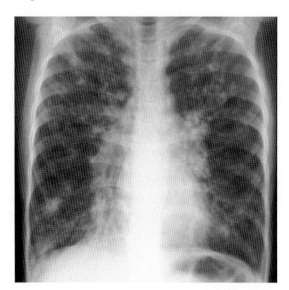

A. Cystic fibrosis
B. Bronchiolitis obliterans
C. Bronchial atresia
D. Bacterial pneumonia

31. A newly enlisted soldier presents complaining of pain in his foot that started after several months of marching. He says it hurts the most when he is standing and is relieved somewhat when he is nonweight bearing. He denies any trauma. On physical examination, he can pinpoint the most tender spot. Otherwise, the examination is unremarkable. Plain film radiographs were noncontributory. Which of the following imaging options is the *least sensitive* in assessing this patient's current condition?

A. Triple-phase radioisotopic bone scan
B. MRI of the foot
C. CT scan of the lower extremity
D. Color Doppler studies of the affected extremity

32. A patient suffers from the injury shown in the following radiograph. Which of the following structures are most likely to be injured?

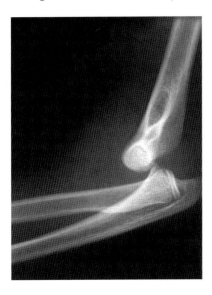

A. Radial artery and median nerve
B. Brachial artery and ulnar nerve
C. Brachial artery and median nerve
D. Radial artery and radial nerve

33. An elderly woman with a known history of osteoporosis presents complaining of sudden, acute back pain after bending over to tie her shoe. She says it hurts to sit or move, and she feels the pain on both sides of her back which radiates anteriorly into her abdomen. She denies any radiating pain into her lower extremities. She is hemodynamically stable. Once you have treated her pain, which of the following should you first obtain to confirm your diagnosis?

A. Lumbar CT
B. Plain radiographs of dorsolumbar spine
C. Lumbar MRI
D. Triple-phase radionucleide bone scan

34. A 78-year-old man presents with severe, periumbilical abdominal pain with nausea and vomiting. The patient has a known history of coronary artery disease with rate-controlled atrial fibrillation and claudication. He is hemodynamically stable, but his blood work shows leukocytosis. The abdominal radiograph you ordered (shown below) demonstrates distended, fixed, dilated loops of the small bowel with wall thickening (arrow) and separation of the bowel loops. Which of the following do you need to quickly confirm your diagnosis?

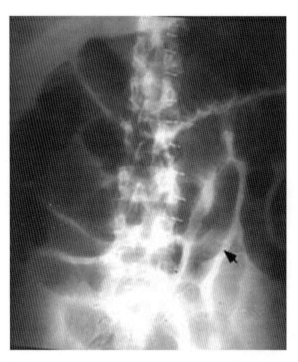

  A. Doppler-flow ultrasonography
  B. Barium study of the upper gastrointestinal tract and small bowel follow-through
  C. CT angiography of mesentery
  D. Upper endoscopy

35. A male patient presents with an acute onset of severe right upper quadrant abdominal pain of over 4 hours. The patient is febrile and has leukocytosis. He splints on inspiration when you press on the right upper quadrant. Which of the following is the best initial study to order?

  A. CT of the chest, abdomen, and pelvis
  B. Abdominal ultrasound
  C. Cholescintigraphy (HIDA scan)
  D. Endoscopic retrograde cholangiopancreatography (ERCP)

36. A 17-year-old female with a family history of a first-degree relative with a berry aneurysm suddenly loses consciousness after experiencing the "worst headache of her life." Which of the following would *not* help you confirm your diagnosis?

  A. Lumbar puncture with cerebrospinal fluid (CSF) analysis
  B. Cerebral angiography
  C. Noncontrast head CT
  D. Transcranial ultrasound

37. Which of the following does *not* put patients at high risk for developing contrast-induced nephropathy?

   A. Concurrent intravenous hydration with normal saline
   B. Cardiovascular disease
   C. Several large doses of intravenous contrast media administered within a short time interval
   D. Diabetes mellitus with renal insufficiency

38. A gynecologist finds an adnexal mass during a routine physical exam in an asymptomatic patient. What of the following imaging modalities are *not* sensitive in the evaluation and characterization of primary ovarian masses?

   A. Transvaginal Doppler ultrasound
   B. Positron emission tomography (PET)
   C. Computed tomography (CT)
   D. Magnetic resonance imaging (MRI)

39. A 70-year-old male presents to the emergency department with fever; nausea and vomiting; acute, constant left lower abdominal pain; and rectal bleeding. On physical examination, he has decreased bowel sounds and rebound tenderness, along with guarding of the affected side. His blood work is significant for leukocytosis. Which of the following should you obtain to confirm your diagnosis and rule out complications of this acute condition?

   A. CT of abdomen and pelvis
   B. Ultrasound of abdomen and pelvis
   C. Barium contrast enema
   D. Technetium Tc 99m–labeled red blood cell scan

40. A 91-year-old woman presents from the nursing home because she is dyspneic and has pleuritic chest pain. Her escort does not know when it started, but knows that she has been like this for a few hours. Once you determine that she is hemodynamically stable, you obtain a radiograph of her chest, which is read as "indeterminate" because of the patient's positioning and skin folds. You then order a chest CT (shown). Which of the following is the most likely diagnosis?

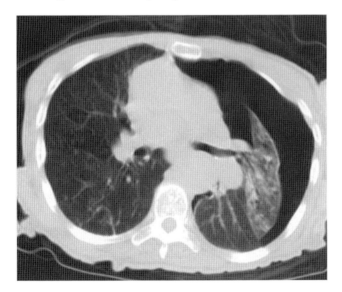

   A. Empyema
   B. Subcutaneous emphysema
   C. Tension pneumothorax
   D. Pericardial effusion

41. A young man present to the emergency department with hematemesis. While obtaining his history, you calculate that he has vomited around 300 cc of bright red blood in the last few hours. The physical examination was negative for acute abdominal distention or focal tenderness. Once you have determined that the patient is hemodynamically stable, which of the following would you recommend to determine the source of the bleeding?

    A. 99mTc pertechnate–labeled autologous red blood cell scan
    B. Diagnostic upper endoscopy
    C. Upper GI barium study
    D. Double-contrast enteroclysis

42. A 32-year-old white male presents to your clinic with inflammatory back pain that radiates to his buttocks. He also complains of arthritis in his hips and shoulders. These pains are worse in the morning and improve as the day progresses. However, his fatigue and anorexia remain constant. On physical examination, you notice the absence of the lumbar lordosis. His labs show an elevated erythrocyte sedimentation rate (ESR) and positive HLA-B27. The lumbar radiographs (shown) receive a reading by radiology as "bilateral sacroiliitis (not shown) and formation of marginal syndesmorphytes from ossification of the annulus fibrosus in the lumbar spine, creating a 'bamboo spine.'" Which of the following is the most likely diagnosis?

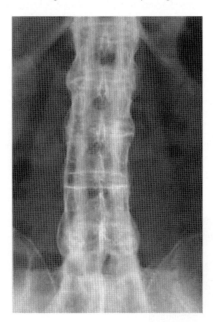

    A. Osteitis condensans
    B. Degenerative spondylolisthesis
    C. Ankylosis spondylitis
    D. Spondylolysis

43. Your patient just completed a CT scan with intravenous contrast injection when she begins to complain that she feels "itchy" and "slightly flushed." You notice that she has developed hives on her neck and along her arm where she had the injection. She denies any difficulty in breathing at this time. The patient denies having any known allergies or any history of anaphylaxis or asthma. Which of the following is the best approach to take with this patient?

A. Monitor the patient's vital signs. Administer 25 to 50 mg IV diphenhydramine and observe any improvement or progression of symptoms.

B. Advise the patient that the reaction is self-limiting and discharge the patient home.

C. Monitor the patient's vital signs. Start IV hydration and administer 16 mg methyl-prenisolone orally. Observe any improvement or progression of symptoms.

D. Call a "code" and start Basic Life Support.

44. Which of the following is the best management for a woman with a new, nonpalpable, pleomorphic cluster of breast calcifications discovered on mammogram?

A. Follow-up with a repeat mammogram in 6 months and compare findings.

B. Order additional views and/or ultrasound (if warranted), consult a breast surgeon for evaluation, order an image-guided diagnostic core, and perform surgical excision if the abnormality is atypical or malignant.

C. Order unilateral breast MRI of affected side to assess for extent of disease to determine whether a mastectomy is warranted.

D. Consult a breast surgeon for a sentinel node biopsy and surgical excision of the mammographic abnormality.

45. A patient well known to you presents with new unilateral lower extremity edema and erythema. He denies any trauma to the leg or any intense exercise that might have torn or otherwise injured a muscle. He has no history of cancer or clotting abnormality. However, his leg became swollen and tight yesterday after a long, cramped flight across the country. Which of the following should you order to quickly confirm your diagnosis?

A. MR venography

B. Contrast venography

C. Impedance plethysmography

D. Compression duplex venous ultrasonography

46. A new mother urgently brings in her 6-week-old son who has been "spitting up everything" from the bottle yet still seems hungry after feeding. He has not gained weight in 2 weeks, has projectile nonbilious vomiting, and exhibits persistent hunger. On physical examination, you feel a firm, mobile mass, or "palpable olive," in his right upper abdominal quadrant. You note the baby to be dehydrated and emaciated. An abdominal ultrasound shows a "target sign," exaggerated peristalsis, an elongated pylorus with thickened muscle, and an "antral nipple sign." Which of the following is the most likely diagnosis?

A. Gastroesophageal reflux

B. Gastroenteritis

C. Hiatal hernia

D. Infantile pyloric stenosis

47. A urologist consults you urgently requesting an interventional radiology study for his patient. He unsuccessfully attempted an inpatient cystoscopy on a patient with an obstruction from a ureteral tumor. The preoperative IVP (intravenous pyelogram) indicated a dilated right renal pelvis and collecting system. The patient has persistent, acute right flank pain, leukocytosis, and is febrile. Which of the following is the most appropriate first action?

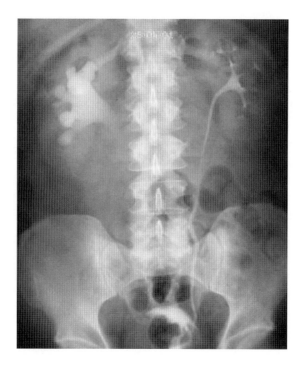

A. Consult surgery for a possible nephrectomy.
B. Place a percutaneous nephrostomy tube using fluoroscopic guidance.
C. Obtain a renal radioisotope scintigraphy scan with furosemide to assess bilateral renal function.
D. Begin prophylactic antibiotics.

48. A 57-year-old African drum maker presents with complaints of worsening flu-like symptoms 5 days after receiving an animal-hide shipment from Africa. Two days ago he felt myalgias and fever. However, he has become much sicker. He is dyspneic, hypoxemic, diaphoretic, and exhibiting stridor. You immediately obtain serologic testing to confirm your diagnosis. The patient is HIV negative. The chest radiograph (shown below) shows widening of the mediastinum and a small left-sided pleural effusion. Which of the following is the most likely diagnosis?

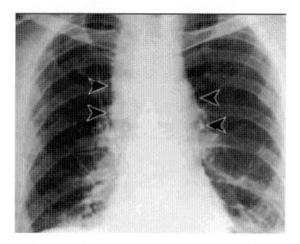

A. Inhalation anthrax
B. Community-acquired pneumonia
C. Influenza
D. Histoplasmosis

ANSWERS

1. **The correct answer is C.** With this type of injury, the "fat pads" often give the "sail sign" on radiograph. Colles' fracture is a fracture of the distal radius and ulna, with dorsal displacement and volar angulation. Smith's fracture is same location as a Colles' fracture, but with volar displacement and dorsal angulation. Nursemaid's elbow is a radial head subluxation.

2. **The correct answer is C.** The clinical picture and chest radiograph indicates bronchiectasis. Pneumonia would show as peripheral pneumonic infiltrates, and the patient would have cough, fever, tachypnea, tachycardia, and sputum production. Patients with acute bronchitis have cough and sputum production for 10 to 20 days and often have bronchospasm (asthmatic component) with self-limiting bronchial inflammation. *Bordetella pertussis* is whooping cough and is incorrect.

3. **The correct answer is A.** Rib notching is a sign of coarctation of the aorta. It increases with age. The posterior one-third of the third through eighth ribs are notched due to enlarged collateral intercostal arteries.

4. **The correct answer is D.** The first three options are definitive for asbestosis and interstitial lung disease, especially pleural plaques. In addition, the hazy "ground glass" appearance on the radiograph is a hallmark of asbestosis. Disease processes that cause cavitary lung lesions include tuberculosis; sarcoidosis; neoplasms; other fungal infections, such as histoplasmosis and coccidioidomycosis; cystic fibrosis; and invasive aspergillosis.

5. **The correct answer is B.** The diagnosis of varicocele primarily hinges on the clinical picture and the venous plexus "bag of worms" on ultrasound. On ultrasound, a hydrocele looks more like a cystic scrotal mass, and the practitioner should also see if the mass transilluminates. This patient does not present with urgent pain, ruling out torsion.

6. **The correct answer is B.** The chest radiograph shows an enlarged nonruptured thoracic descending aorta that is hard to miss, which rules out the other options. Additionally, the clinical picture supports the diagnosis.

7. **The correct answer is C.** The CT imaging defines the extent of the injury. The patient said he felt a "tearing" pain, which is a common description of the onset of the dissection. The most specific finding is the different blood pressures in each upper extremity. Pulsus paradoxus is more indicative of cardiac tamponade.

8. **The correct answer is A.** This is a true medical emergency. The diagnostic "thumb sign" on lateral radiograph along with the typical clinical picture confirms this diagnosis. If you lay the patient supine, it will likely compromise his airway. Laryngotracheobronchitis—viral croup—also has a barking cough, but shows a "steeple" sign on lateral radiograph. Bronchiolitis is a respiratory syncytial virus (RSV) infection, more of a bronchopneumonia in infants. A midline or unilateral swelling of the posterior pharyngeal wall on physical exam confirms the diagnosis of peritonsillar abscess.

9. **The correct answer is B.** The imaging confirms a thrombus in the pulmonary artery and rules out a dissection. The signs and symptoms are classic for pulmonary embolism (PE), but can also indicate acute myocardial infarction or cardiac tamponade. Tamponade, however, classically includes an elevated heart rate, jugular venous distention, and pulsus paradoxus. Clinical suspicion and the ECG findings lead toward obtaining the proper imaging to confirm a pulmonary embolism.

10. **The correct answer is B.** This is a true medical emergency. To quickly and inexpensively confirm the diagnosis, ultrasound is the best modality. Radionucleotide imaging, a flat

radiograph, or pelvic CT would not necessarily result in the diagnosis and are expensive choices. Ultrasound quickly and accurately confirms diagnostically what you know clinically.

11. **The correct answer is D.** As described in the answer to question 10, this is a true medical emergency. The duration of testicular ischemia will predict the clinical outcome. Empiric antibiotics cover infectious epididymitis; NSAIDs, rest, and ice treat noninfectious epididymitis.

12. **The correct answer is B.** All of the answer options are reasonable for predicting the evolution of multiple sclerosis, but MRI is the most sensitive and specific. CT scanning is the least sensitive.

13. **The correct answer is C.** The most frequent causes of small-bowel obstruction (SBO) are postop adhesions and hernias. This patient has had a hysterectomy, which is a common surgical history for patients with SBO, and the physical exam showed no hernias. The patient is dehydrated, which furthers her problem of electrolyte imbalances. The radiograph confirms the obstruction, because the loops of small bowel proximal to the obstruction are dilated and fluid filled. Distally, there is decompression of the large bowel, so the answer is definitely not D. An ileus normally occurs in recent postoperative patients and has absent bowel sounds. In an ileus, there is usually dilation of both the small and large bowels.

14. **The correct answer is A.** This presentation is classic for a duodenal ulcer, when acid is secreted in the absence of a food buffer. The patient exhibits an ulcer-like pattern of dyspepsia. The patient denies any dysphagia or regurgitation, such as the acidic watery brash that is classic for gastroesophageal reflux disease (GERD). She does not present with symptoms of gallbladder problems or angina.

15. **The correct answer is B.** Only a single, short-term trial of an empiric "antiulcer" medication would be appropriate in this situation. If symptoms do not respond within a few weeks, then the patient should be worked up with any of the other three options, depending on clinical suspicion.

16. **The correct answer is A.** This woman cannot receive further anticoagulation, so the clinician should place an inferior vena cava filter in order to prevent an embolism from entering the pulmonary artery (pulmonary embolism). This filter *does not* prevent deep vein thrombosis from forming. Preventive techniques include compression devices and ambulation.

17. **The correct answer is C.** This is a Salter IV fracture because the fracture is "T"hrough the metaphysis, physis, and epiphysis. *Salter* stands for Slipped, Above, Lower than, Through, and Everything (or a crush-type injury).

18. **The correct answer is B.** In women younger than 35 years of age, ultrasound is the most appropriate imaging modality to examine a breast lump in order to determine if it is solid or cystic, rather than exposing a young woman to radiation. In a patient this age, drainage of a cyst should only occur if the cyst is painful.

19. **The correct answer is C.** In the United States, screening mammograms are performed yearly to detect preclinical symptomatic breast cancer.

20. **The correct answer is C.** According to advanced cardiac life support (ACLS) guidelines, non-contrast head CT is necessary to quickly differentiate between potential ischemic versus hemorrhagic stroke and rule out other pathologic processes that could mimic stroke.

21. The correct answer is D. Pulmonary venous hypertension is caused by *left* ventricular failure, not right ventricular hypertrophy.

22. The correct answer is B. This clinical scenario appears to be achalasia, but carcinoma is always a concern. Carcinoma would look more like a "rat's tail" than a "bird's beak" of the distal esophagus. Reflux esophagitis causes esophageal strictures but these usually have an asymmetric appearance with puckering of one wall of the stricture due to eccentric scarring. Schatzki's rings are thin, smooth mucosal structures that occur at the gastroesophageal junction.

23. The correct answer is D. Patients with rheumatoid arthritis (RA) typically present with metacarpophalangeal and proximal interphalangeal joint involvement, inflammatory erosive soft warm tender joint swelling, and morning stiffness. A patient with osteoarthritis (OA) presents with distal interphalangeal joint involvement, hard bony joint swelling, joints that stiffen with use, and joint space narrowing from bone remodeling.

24. The correct answer is C. To make the diagnosis and to rule out other possibilities for flank pain and hematuria, CT is the preferred image modality. Ultrasound is often helpful, but can miss smaller stones. Uric acid stones are not visible on the KUB flatplate (abdominal radiograph). There is no indication for MRI.

25. The correct answer is A. CT is the best imaging modality to obtain detail about the nature of a pleural effusion and the extent of lung and pleural involvement. An ultrasound proves useful for accurate guidance of the thoracentesis. The pleural fluid should then undergo cytologic analysis for a definitive diagnosis.

26. The correct answer is B. This is the classic appearance of an exudative effusion. A hemothorax is bloody. A chylothorax is whitish, pale, and cloudy from lymph drainage. A transudate is serous and clear, usually without pus.

27. The correct answer is A. Effusions occurring in lung and breast carcinoma occur on the same side of the body as the primary cancer, whereas liver metastases usually have bilateral effusions, but not every time, thus this is a true statement. The effusions do tend to be significant in size and recurrent, but this varies from patient to patient. Furthermore, they are not always associated with extensive lung metastasis.

28. The correct answer is B. The patient's history (i.e., longstanding alcohol use) is the first clue. CT confirms the diagnosis, clearly outlining the pancreas and the calcifications within. The clay-colored stools are due to the lack of bilirubin as a result of probable biliary obstruction.

29. The correct answer is B. Primarily, the goal is to differentiate immediately between a benign lesion and a malignant lesion. Positron emission tomography (PET)/computed tomography (CT) prove useful now for this purpose. Because of the size of the lesion (1.5 cm), a PET/CT is most appropriate. The lesion is too large to just watch and evaluate its growth over 6 months. Once the clinician(s) evaluates the PET/CT results, a biopsy would be appropriate provided clinical suspicion deems that the benefits outweigh the risks of the procedure.

30. The correct answer is A. The patient's clinical picture and radiographic findings support this diagnosis. The only other key not included in the clinical scenario is the mention of a sweat chloride test (the classic diagnostic clue). Bronchial atresia has overexpanded segments and characteristic finger-like opacities lateral to the hilum with mucous plugs distal to the atretic lumen.

31. The correct answer is C. The radioisotope bone scan and MRI are more sensitive than CT in assessing the extent of bone strain or silent stress reactions (i.e., periosteal and marrow edema) before the strain evolves into a fracture. The CT picks up stress fractures once they appear in the bone, but not early on in the stress reaction.

32. **The correct answer is B.** Elbow dislocations are usually due to hyperextension and occur posteriorly, thus affecting the brachial artery. The most commonly injured nerve is the ulnar nerve, followed by the median nerve. Therefore, the clinician should be most concerned with these areas.

33. **The correct answer is B.** This woman has suffered a vertebral compression fracture. Plain dorsolumbar radiographs should be the first imaging performed to confirm the diagnosis. If a neurologic abnormality is present and surgical intervention becomes necessary, then the practitioner should order a CT or an MRI.

34. **The correct answer is C.** The correct diagnosis is acute mesenteric ischemia. The gold standard in making this diagnosis is mesenteric angiography, especially CT angiography, which requires less IV contrast and is noninvasive. These patients should not have intraluminal barium studies. Abdominal ultrasound would be technically limited in this patient.

35. **The correct answer is B.** Ultrasound is usually the first test obtained to confirm this diagnosis, because it is inexpensive, sensitive, and specific in determining gallbladder wall thickening as well as the presence of gallstones. A "sonographic Murphy's sign" can also prove useful in confirming the diagnosis. The HIDA scan is usually ordered if the ultrasound is equivocal. Endoscopic retrograde cholangiopancreatography (ERCP) is invasive, requires sedation, and should only be done once the presence and location of the stones have been confirmed.

36. **The correct answer is D.** This patient has a subarachnoid hemorrhage (SAH). Transcranial ultrasound is only useful for detecting vasospasm, which begins several days after an aneurysm ruptures. A negative head CT and cebrospinal fluid test effectively eliminate the diagnosis of SAH. Cerebral angiography is essential in ruling out an aneurysm.

37. **The correct answer is A.** IV hydration is the primary recommendation for extracellular volume expansion. It actually helps reduce the incidence of contrast-induced renal failure. The other options place the patient in danger of nephropathy.

38. **The correct answer is B.** Positron emission tomography (PET) is not diagnostic for primary ovarian cancer, but it is helpful in staging ovarian cancer metastasis. All of the other modalities are more sensitive in diagnosing and categorizing ovarian metastases; however, even they have their limitations. The least sensitive is still the PET scan, but the clinician should not expect the best results from the other modalities either.

39. **The correct answer is A.** The CT scan is the preferred test because it can confirm the diagnosis and exclude other abdominal and pelvic diseases/disorders. Prior to obtaining the CT, barium enemas used to be the primary method of diagnosing these patients. However, barium enemas do not distinguish between colon cancer and diverticulitis as well as the CT does. With barium enemas, you should be concerned with the risk of a perforated bowel and extravasation of contrast into the peritoneum. Ultrasound can be helpful, but it is not very sensitive, and it is operator dependent. A nuclear medicine scan could be helpful in finding the bleed, but it has a limited role in the diagnosis of diverticulitis.

40. **The correct answer is C.** This is a tension pneumothorax, as indicated by the mediastinal shift across the midline to the contralateral side. Empyema would have an opacified appearance and appear dense in the thorax, as opposed to air in the pneumothorax, which appears black. Subcutaneous emphysema is trapped air in the soft tissues outside the thoracic space, not inside. That said, this picture does not definitely diagnose the tension

pneumothorax beyond a reasonable doubt. Therefore, it is imperative that the clinician use all the tools at his/her disposal (history, physical examination, chest radiograph) to confirm the diagnosis.

41. **The correct answer is B.** Endoscopy is highly sensitive and specific for locating upper gastrointestinal (GI) bleeds. This diagnostic procedure could prove useful for treatment and hemostasis as well. An upper GI barium study in this setting will interfere with further studies and therefore is not an appropriate diagnostic study. The tagged red blood cell study only localizes bleeding to an area in the abdomen. Enteroclysis is performed by passing a tube into proximal small bowel and is not appropriate in this situation.

42. **The correct answer is C.** This patient clearly has ankylosing spondylitis. This diagnosis is due to several facts: 100% of these patients have sacroiliitis; HLA-B27 is positive in 90 to 95% of these patients; finally, the patient's inflammatory back pain with the "bamboo spine" radiograph finding. The other choices do not apply to this clinical and radiographic picture.

43. **The correct answer is A.** Hives and other symptoms constitute a mild hypersensitivity reaction. Diphenhydramine is normally enough to counteract this allergic response to IV contrast. Oral steroids will not help acutely. Parenteral steroids can prove useful in full-blown anaphylaxis; however, this is not the case with the patient in this problem.

44. **The correct answer is B.** In a woman with new pleomorphic (different shapes and sizes —therefore, more suspicious) breast calcifications on mammography, further imaging is necessary to evaluate with magnified views. Most practitioners would say these new calcifications warrant biopsy via the least invasive and most breast-conserving method available. A mastectomy is far too aggressive at this stage in the absence of a firm diagnosis. Sentinel node biopsy is a nuclear medicine study to evaluate if an infiltrating breast cancer has metastasized to the ipsilateral lymph nodes. Again, before performing a sentinel node biopsy, the clinician should have a definite diagnosis in hand.

45. **The correct answer is D.** This patient has a deep vein thrombosis (DVT) in a lower extremity. Ultrasound is noninvasive, inexpensive, has high patient compliance, and is highly accurate in the diagnosis of DVT. The others are options if the ultrasound is inconclusive or if the ultrasound findings do not correlate with a strong clinical suspicion.

46. **The correct answer is D.** This infant has infantile pyloric stenosis. The "palpable olive" rules out gastroesophageal reflux disease (GERD). Gastroenteritis is not the answer as it is usually a diagnosis of exclusion and far more prevalent in adults. A hiatal hernia does not present in this fashion.

47. **The correct answer is B.** The patient initially presented with a right hydronephrosis that progressed into a pyelonephritis following a failed cystoscopy. It requires drainage to decompress the kidney and provide an outlet for the infection. The other choices would not be appropriate in this situation. D is actually correct, but only in the face of Gram stain and culture to identify the pathogen. It is inappropriate to prescribe prophylactic antibiotics in the face of not having a definite identification of the offending organism, especially in this time of resistant pathogens. Ideally, the surgical consult will appropriately make this identification. However, it would be prudent to Gram stain and culture, if appropriate, in anticipation of appropriate antimicrobial therapy.

48. **The correct choice is A.** This patient has inhalation anthrax. The three major anthrax syndromes are inhalation, cutaneous (most common), and gastrointestinal. The widening mediastinum (from hemorrhagic mediastinitis) and pleural effusion on chest radiograph are classic findings, which indicate anthrax when paired with the patient's clinical history. Histoplasmosis can cause pneumonia with mediastinal lymphadenopathy on chest radiography, but the disease progression is different.

REFERENCES

American Heart Association. (2005). *Guidelines for cardiopulmonary resuscitation and emergency cardiac care.* American Heart Association, Dallas, Texas.

Berg, W. A., and Birdwell, R. L. (2006). *Diagnostic imaging of the breast.* Harcourt Publishers, Elsevier Group, Philadelphia, PA.

Chen, M. Y. M., Pope, T. L., Jr., and Ott, D. J. (eds.). (2004). *Basic radiology.* Lange Medical Books. McGraw-Hill Companies, New York.

Gay, S. B., and Woodcock, R. B. (2003). *Radiology review manual,* 5th ed. Lippincott, Wilkins and Williams, Philadelphia, PA.

Kasper, D., Braunwald, E., Fauci, A., Hauser, S., Longo, D., Jameson, J., and Isselbacher, K. (eds.). (2007). *Harrison's internal medicine,* 16th ed. McGraw-Hill Companies, New York.

McPhee, S., and Papadakis, M. (2007). *Current medical diagnosis and treatment.* McGraw-Hill Medical, New York.

Laboratory Medicine

Donna M. Agnew, MT (ASCP), MSPAS, PA-C

1. Which of the following would *not* account for a serum potassium level of 6.3 mEq/L?

    A. Acute renal insufficiency
    B. Hyperaldosteronism
    C. Metabolic acidosis
    D. Prolonged tourniquet application during venipuncture

2. A 37-year-old female presents for routine follow-up care for hypothyroidism. She admits to increasing fatigue and a 10-pound weight gain over the past 3 months. Her current dose of levothyroxine is 0.05 mg po daily. Her thyroid-stimulating hormone (TSH) level is 6.9 mIU/L. Which of the following would be the most appropriate next step in the management of this patient?

    A. Continue the current dose and recheck TSH in 6 to 8 weeks.
    B. Decrease the dose to 0.025 mg po daily and recheck TSH in 6 to 8 weeks.
    C. Increase the dose to 0.075 mg po daily and recheck TSH in 6 to 8 weeks.
    D. Maintain the current dose and order a free T_4 to validate the elevated TSH.

3. Narcotics elevate serum lipase levels through which of the following mechanisms?

    A. They damage the pancreatic acinar cells.
    B. They stimulate excretion of the enzyme by the salivary glands.
    C. They reduce renal excretion of the enzyme.
    D. They cause contraction of the sphincter of Oddi.

4. Which of the following assays best assesses the liver's synthesizing ability?

    A. Albumin and prothrombin time (PT)
    B. Aspartate aminotransferase (AST) and alanine aminotransferase (ALT)
    C. Bilirubin and lactate dehydrogenase (LDH)
    D. Gamma glutamyl transpeptidase (GGT) and alkaline phosphatase (ALP)

5. Which of the following helminth infections can result in vitamin B_{12} deficiency?

    A. Fish tapeworm (*Diphyllobothrium latum*)
    B. Pinworm (*Enterobius vermicularis*)
    C. Roundworm (*Ascaris lumbricoides*)
    D. Whipworm (*Trichuris trichiura*)

6. On inspection, you note slightly raised, well-circumscribed, yellow plaques along the nasal aspects of a patient's eyelids bilaterally. Which of the following laboratory tests would best assist in confirming a diagnosis?

    A. Fasting plasma glucose
    B. Fasting lipid panel
    C. Serum thyroid-stimulating hormone (TSH)
    D. Serum uric acid

7. Which of the following best evaluates in vivo platelet function?
   A. Bleeding time
   B. Platelet count
   C. Mean platelet volume
   D. Prothrombin time

8. A 33-year-old male job applicant submits a urine toxicology screen as part of a pre-employment physical. The results are positive for a *cannabis* metabolite, which triggers a review of his disclosed medications. Which of the following medications could produce a false positive initial screening for *cannabis*?
   A. labetolol 50 mg po daily for hypertension
   B. ibuprofen 400 mg po qid prn for shoulder tendonitis
   C. ranitidine 150 mg po bid for gastroesophageal reflux disease (GERD)
   D. sertraline 50 mg po daily for depression

9. Which of the following conditions would most likely result in an elevated direct bilirubin?
   A. Biliary tract obstruction
   B. Gilbert's syndrome
   C. Neonatal jaundice
   D. Sickle-cell crisis

10. Which of the following tests for syphilis, once positive, will remain positive for the life of the patient, irrespective of treatment?
    A. DFA-TP
    B. FTA-ABS
    C. RPR
    D. VDRL

11. A 73-year-old female with a 4-year history of congestive heart failure (CHF) presents to your clinic complaining of headache, generalized muscle weakness, yellow vision, and persistent nausea and constipation over the past 48 hours. Prior to the past two days' complaints she reports being asymptomatic for the past 2 years on a regiment of digoxin, furosemide, and a long-acting nitrate. She denies recent weight changes, shortness of breath, cough, orthopnea, paroxysmal nocturnal dyspnea (PND), edema, or chest pain. Which of the following tests will provide the most crucial diagnostic information regarding this patient?
    A. BNP (brain natriuretic peptide)
    B. Serum digoxin
    C. Serum potassium
    D. Serum thyroid-stimulating hormone (TSH)

12. Which of the following statements regarding serum ferritin levels is *false*?
    A. Ferritin levels represent available iron stores in the body.
    B. A plasma ferritin level below 10 ng/ml is considered diagnostic of iron deficiency anemia.
    C. Subsequent to decreases in hemoglobin, decreased ferritin levels are late indicators of iron deficiency anemia.
    D. In acute inflammatory conditions, there may be elevations as ferritin is an acute-phase reactant protein.

13. A urine dipstick shows 1+ blood, but microscopic examination of the same specimen shows only 3 RBCs/hpf (shown below). Which of the following explanations does *not* account for this discrepancy?

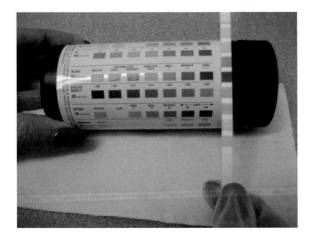

- **A.** Cleansing with a povidone–iodine antiseptic prior to sample collection
- **B.** Free hemoglobin from lysed red blood cells seen in cases of severe hemolysis
- **C.** Ingestion of high doses of vitamin C
- **D.** Myoglobin resulting from muscle trauma, myocardial infarction, or infection

14. Which of the following would result in a decreased erythrocyte sedimentation rate (ESR)?

- **A.** Acute myocardial infarction
- **B.** Multiple myeloma
- **C.** Polymyalgia rheumatica
- **D.** Sickle-cell anemia

15. Which of the following types of urinary casts is highly suggestive of acute glomerulo-nephritis?

- **A.** Broad, waxy cast
- **B.** Hyaline cast
- **C.** Red blood cell cast
- **D.** White blood cell cast

16. Lymphocytosis is the hallmark of which acute bacterial infection?

- **A.** Cellulitis (*Staphylococcus aureus*)
- **B.** Pharyngitis (*Streptococcus pyogenes* [Group A β-hemolytic])
- **C.** Vaginitis (*Chlamydia trachomatis*)
- **D.** Whooping cough (*Bordetella pertussis*)

17. A 71-year-old with a history of arrhythmias well controlled on procainamide presents for routine follow-up. He complains of worsening arthralgias, myalgias, and generalized "flulike" symptoms. Diagnostic laboratory tests reveal a positive antinuclear antibody (ANA) titer of 1:320 with a peripheral (rim) pattern. What additional lab test, if positive, would confirm your suspicion of a drug-induced lupus?

- **A.** Anti-ds DNA
- **B.** Anti-Smith antibodies
- **C.** Antihistone antibodies
- **D.** Anti-SSA antibodies; anti-SSB antibodies

18. Which of the following leukemias commonly show smudge cells (shown below) on peripheral blood smears?

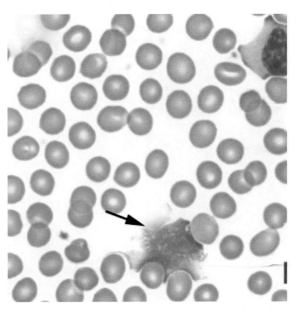

Permission granted by Donald Innes, M.D., Department of Pathology, University of Virginia Health Sciences Center

   A. Acute lymphoblastic leukemia (ALL)
   B. Acute myelogenous leukemia (AML)
   C. Chronic lymphocytic leukemia (CLL)
   D. Chronic myelogenous leukemia (CML)

19. Which of the following components of a routine lipid panel represents a calculated, not a directly measured, value?

   A. High-density lipoprotein (HDL)
   B. Low-density lipoprotein (LDL)
   C. Total cholesterol
   D. Triglycerides

20. Which of the following conditions commonly demonstrate basophilic stippling as shown in the peripheral smear below?

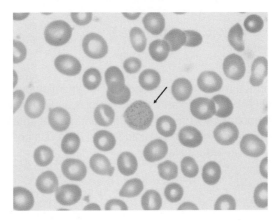

   A. Aplastic anemia
   B. Heavy metal poisoning
   C. Iron deficiency anemia
   D. Polycythemia vera

21. You admit your patient to the hospital with a diagnosis of urosepsis. His complete blood count (CBC) reveals the following results: white blood cell, 18,000/mm³; red blood cell, 3.22×10^5 mm³; hemoglobin, 13.1 g/dL; hematocrit, 39.6%; platelets, 242,000/mm³; with a differential of 87% neutrophils, 4% bands, 1% metamyelocytes, 7% lymphocytes, and 1% monocytes. Which of the following best represents these laboratory findings?

   A. Left shift
   B. Leukemoid reaction
   C. Reversed differential
   D. Right shift

22. Which of the following laboratory findings match incorrectly?

   A. Spherocyte; increased mean cell hemoglobin concentration (MCHC) and osmotic fragility
   B. Rouleaux formation; stacking of red blood cells seen in multiple myeloma
   C. RDW (red cell distribution width); degree of poikilocytosis
   D. Howell-Jolly bodies; red blood cell inclusion of DNA remnants in postsplenectomy patients

23. A 72-year-old patient presents to the emergency department complaining of generalized muscle weakness over the past 2 to 3 days. Her past medical history is significant for hypertension × 25 years, which, until recently, was well controlled with a β-blocker. Her primary care physician added an ACE inhibitor approximately 2 weeks ago. You obtain an electrocardiogram (ECG). Based on the precordial lead changes shown below, which of the following electrolyte imbalances would most likely cause such an ECG change?

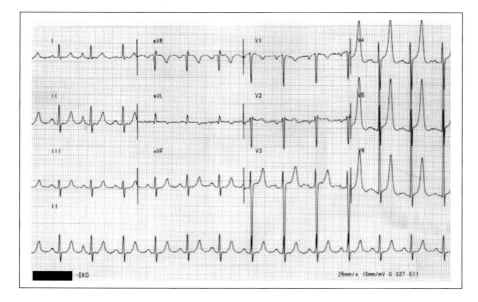

   A. Chloride
   B. Carbon dioxide
   C. Potassium
   D. Sodium

24. A 43-year-old preschool teacher presents complaining of abdominal bloating and cramping for the past 3 weeks. She notes more frequent, softer, greasy stools, for the past week. She denies any ill contacts, recent travel, sushi or shellfish ingestion, nausea, vomiting, hematochezia, or melena. Her stool culture reveals normal flora. Two of the three specimens submitted for ova and parasites are positive for the trophozoite shown below. Which of the following parasites is the most likely cause of her symptoms?

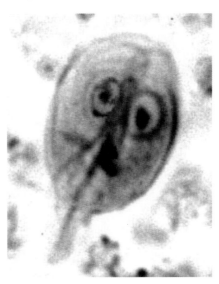

A. *Ascaris lumbricoides*
B. *Balantidium coli*
C. *Dientamoeba fragilis*
D. *Giardia lamblia*

25. A 23-year-old male presents complaining of a persistent cough following a recent upper respiratory infection. He admits to night sweats and a swollen, nontender cervical lymph node. You order a lymph node biopsy when treatment with an antibiotic and anti-inflammatory medication does not resolve his problem. The lymph node biopsy reveals the cell shown below. This cell is pathognomonic for which of the following?

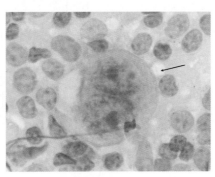

A. Burkitt's lymphoma
B. Hairy cell leukemia
C. Hodgkin's lymphoma
D. Non-Hodgkin's lymphoma

26. Using the following basic metabolic profile, calculate the correct anion gap: glucose, 156 mg/dL; BUN, 12 mg/dL; creatinine, 0.8 mg/dL; sodium, 142 mEq/L; potassium, 3.7 mEq/L; chloride, 102 mEq/L; bicarbonate, 24 mmol/L.

A. 12
B. 14
C. 15
D. 16

27. A patient presents acutely to the emergency department with symptoms of fever, headache, and nuchal rigidity. Which of the following lumbar puncture findings most strongly support your diagnosis of viral or aseptic meningitis?

A. Decreased glucose
B. Increased opening pressure
C. Increased protein
D. Lymphocyte predominance

28. A 29-year-old female presents complaining of exquisite calf swelling and tenderness for the past day after returning from a trip to Australia. Doppler ultrasound confirms your suspicion of deep vein thrombosis. You admit the patient to the hospital for anticoagulation therapy, consisting of a bolus followed by a continuous intravenous drip of heparin. When should you obtain the initial partial thromboplastin time (PTT) to evaluate her response to therapy?

A. In 3 hours
B. In 6 hours
C. At 7 A.M. the following morning
D. 12 hours after the initial bolus

29. A patient with a history of chronic atrial fibrillation currently takes a 5 mg daily dose of warfarin. Routine monthly monitoring yields an international normalized ratio (INR) of 3.6. Which of the following is the most appropriate next step in the management of this patient?

A. Decrease the warfarin dose to 4 mg po daily and recheck the PT/INR in 1 week.
B. Hold dosing for 1 week and then resume 5 mg po daily and recheck the PT/INR in 1 week.
C. If there is no evidence of bleeding, maintain the current dose and recheck the PT/INR in 1 week.
D. Question the patient about ingestion of leafy green vegetables.

30. Which of the following conditions does not utilize alpha-fetoprotein (AFP) as a serologic marker of disease?

A. Germ cell tumors
B. Hepatocellular carcinoma
C. Neural tube defects
D. Prostate cancer

31. Which of the following conditions in a patient's family history warrant obtaining alpha-1 antitrypsin levels?

A. Coronary artery disease
B. Emphysema
C. Leukemia
D. Pancreatic cancer

32. Which of the following laboratory tests best represents the amount of endogenous insulin produced by a diabetic patient currently on 70/30 NPH/R injectable insulin?

A. C-peptide
B. Insulin assay
C. Glucagon
D. Glycosylated hemoglobin

33. Which of the following serologic markers for hepatitis B virus is indicative of active viral replication along with a high degree of infectivity?

A. HBsAg
B. HBeAg
C. HBcAg
D. IgM anti-BcAB

34. Which of the following laboratory values best represents the most common electrolyte imbalance found in hospitalized patients?

   A. Potassium of 3.2 mEq/L
   B. Potassium of 6.7 mEq/L
   C. Sodium of 147 mEq/L
   D. Sodium of 129 mEq/L

35. Which of the following is *least* diagnostic for multiple myeloma in a 73-year-old patient who presents with bone pain?

   A. Bence-Jones protein in the urine
   B. Bone marrow plasmocytosis greater than 30%
   C. Monoclonal IgG spike on serum protein electrophoresis (SPEP)
   D. Rouleaux formation on peripheral smear

36. A 42-year-old female presents with complaints of excessive thirst, which she attributes to her tricyclic antidepressant medication. Upon further questioning, she describes urinary symptoms of frequency and nocturia over the past 6 months, significantly disrupting her sleep. She has a remote history of head trauma secondary to a motor vehicle accident (completely rehabilitated) at age 17. Which of the following laboratory values is most suggestive of a diagnosis of central diabetes insipidus?

   A. Decreased antidiuretic hormone (ADH)
   B. Decreased urine specific gravity
   C. Decreased serum aldosterone
   D. Increased fasting plasma glucose

37. You treat a G3P1102 preeclamptic female at 39 weeks gestation with magnesium sulfate anhydrous (MgSO4). Shortly after administration of the drug, the patient complains of a warm, flushing sensation and has two episodes of clear bilious vomiting. Her serum magnesium level is 5.7 mEq/L. Which of the following would be the most appropriate next step in the management of this patient until the safe delivery of the fetus?

   A. Administer IV calcium gluconate.
   B. Hydrate with IV fluid ½ normal saline (0.45%)
   C. Prescribe 60 mg furosemide IV
   D. Recommend hemodialysis

38. You evaluate an 11-year-old girl to determine the etiology of her jaundice and splenomegaly. Laboratory studies reveal a hemoglobin of 9 g/dL with an increased mean cell hemoglobin concentration (MCHC), increased osmotic fragility, normal aspartate aminotransferase (AST), normal alanine aminotransferase (ALT), negative acute hepatitis profile, and a negative direct antiglobulin test. Which of the following red blood cell morphologies is most likely to appear on a peripheral smear?

   A. Codocyte (target cell)
   B. Ovalocyte
   C. Spherocyte
   D. Schistocyte

39. A 57-year-old male with macrocytic anemia and decreased serum B_{12} levels undergoes a Schilling's test for evaluation of pernicious anemia. He demonstrated decreased urinary excretion of radiolabeled B_{12} in all three stages of testing as listed below:

Stage 1: Oral administration of radiolabeled B_{12} followed by intramuscular B_{12}

Stage 2: Administration of intrinsic factor

Stage 3: Administration of an antibiotic

Which of the following best explains these laboratory results assuming the patient has normal renal function?

A. This represents a normal Schilling's test, and folic acid deficiency may be the cause of his macrocytic anemia.

B. This most likely represents a malabsorption syndrome that will require parenteral vitamin B_{12} therapy.

C. This is indicative of bacterial overgrowth in the distal ileum and requires a longer course of antibiotic therapy.

D. This confirms your suspicion of pernicious anemia and warrants a hematology referral.

40. A 23-year-old male landscaper presents complaining of lumbar back pain associated with morning stiffness for the past 6 months. He notes improvement of his symptoms with stretching, movement, and exercise. He denies any history of trauma, nephrolithiasis, or incontinence. Radiographic films reveal evidence of bilateral sacroiliitis. Which of the following laboratory tests, if positive, would support a preliminary diagnosis of ankylosing spondylitis?

A. Antinuclear antigen (ANA)

B. HLA-B27

C. Rheumatoid factor (RF)

D. C-reactive protein (CRP)

ANSWERS

1. **The correct answer is B.** Aldosterone enhances sodium reabsorption and potassium excretion. Hyperaldosteronism results in decreased serum potassium levels due to an accelerated potassium secretion by the kidney. Acute renal insufficiency or failure would limit potassium excretion by the kidneys. Metabolic acidosis causes hydrogen ions to enter into the cell in exchange for potassium ions. The net effect is the redistribution of potassium from the intracellular space to the extracellular space, causing serum potassium levels to rise. Prolonged tourniquet application and repeated fist clenching during venipuncture results in pseudohyperkalemia. These maneuvers cause lysis of the red blood cells and subsequent leakage of potassium out of the cell. If the specimen is centrifuged prior to complete clot formation, red blood cell damage could occur.

2. **The correct answer is C.** This patient exhibits symptoms of worsening hypothyroidism (increased fatigue and weight gain) and an increased thyroid-stimulating hormone (TSH) level (normal is 0.5–5.0 mU/L). Proper management includes increasing her dose of levothyroxine (synthetic T_4) and rechecking her TSH level in 6 to 8 weeks. Regulation of the thyroid hormones—T_4 and T_3—depends on the following physiologic steps:

- The hypothalamus releases thyroid-releasing hormone, which exerts an effect on the anterior pituitary gland to release TSH.

- Thyroid stimulating hormone (TSH) causes the thyroid gland to release more T_4 than T_3. These hormones circulate in the bloodstream, bound primarily to thyroid-binding globulin (TBG). Total T_4 and T_3 levels rise when TBG is elevated, such as when there is increased estrogen (e.g., pregnancy, oral contraception, and hormone replacement therapy). In these situations, it is better to evaluate free unbound thyroid hormone than total levels.

- Thyroid stimulating hormone (TSH) is the most sensitive and specific test to evaluate thyroid function. In hypothyroidism, because of a negative feedback system, you would expect to see low levels of T_4 and T_3 and increased TSH. In hyperthyroidism, you would expect to see elevated levels of T_4 and T_3 with low or negligible TSH levels. Thyroid stimulating hormone releases in a pulsatile fashion from the pituitary gland, but does not fluctuate daily, as do T_4 or T_3 levels.

Note: When reviewing TSH levels on patients on thyroid replacement therapy (assuming that they are not on suppression therapy), adjust the thyroid medication in the same direction as the TSH. For example, if there is an elevated TSH, then increase the dose; if there is a decreased TSH, then decrease the dose.

3. **The correct answer is D.** Plasma levels of amylase and lipase may be elevated up to 24 hours after administration of opiate analgesics due to increased biliary pressure caused by sphincter of Oddi spasm. Drugs that specifically alter lipase levels include codeine, meperidine, morphine, indomethacin, and anticholinergic medications. In cases of acute pancreatitis, meperidine should be used (provided the patient is not allergic) for pain management, because it causes less sphincteric spasm than morphine.

4. **The correct answer is A.** Albumin and all of the clotting factors, with the exception of Factor VIII (antihemolytic factor manufactured by platelets), synthesize in the liver. Aspartate aminotransferase (AST), alanine aminotransferase (ALT), gamma glutamyl transpepetidase (GGT), lactate dehydrogenase (LDH), and alkaline phosphatase (ALP) are indicators of liver inflammation. ALP is not specific for the liver, because it comes from both the liver and the bone. Only a fractionated ALP would distinguish a bone from liver source.

5. **The correct answer is A.** Infection with *Diphyllobothrium latum*, the fish tapeworm, presents with intermittent abdominal cramping and distention, diarrhea, and flatulence. Research indicates the tapeworm competes for vitamin B_{12} and interferes with its absorption from the small intestines. This leads to vitamin B_{12} deficiency in the host, which in some cases can progress to a megaloblastic or pernicious anemia. Enterobiasis, or pinworm infection, is the most common helminth infection in the United States. The most common presenting symptom is perianal pruritus (pruritus ani). This is because the adult female migrates nocturnally to the anus to deposit her eggs. Direct visualization of eggs on cellulose acetate tape makes the identification and confirms the diagnosis. *Ascaris lumbricoides* is the largest nematode to cause intestinal infection. Larvae in the soil penetrate the skin of human hosts and travel to the lungs via the bloodstream and lymphatic system. The host coughs up and swallows the larvae, where they mature further in the small intestines. Detection of eggs in the stool or passage of adult worms rectally confirms the diagnosis. *Trichuris trichiura* is referred to as a "whipworm," because the anterior two-thirds of the adult worm is long and threadlike and tapers off the thick, posterior portion. In some cases, this nematode can actually cause prolapse of the rectum. Infection occurs with ingestion of embryonated eggs. The eggs hatch in the duodenum, and adult worms migrate to the cecum. Identification of the classic "football-shaped" eggs containing bipolar plugs in stool samples confirms the diagnosis.

6. **The correct answer is B.** Although xanthelasmas are not specific for lipid disorders, they are often associated with them. These yellow eyelid deposits have no direct correlation with diabetes, thyroid dysfunction, or gout. Diabetes carries an increased risk for retinopathy. Thyroid dysfunction may present with periorbital edema, or Queen Anne's sign (absence of the lateral third of the eyebrows) as seen in hypothyroidism. Lid lag, lid retraction, or exophthalmos is typically characteristic of hyperthyroidism. Hyperuricemia may cause gouty tophi, which frequently form on the external ear.

7. **The correct answer is A.** Bleeding time best evaluates in vivo platelet function. The Ivy method of testing involves the placement of a blood-pressure cuff on a patient inflated to and maintained throughout the test at 40 mmHg. The clinician should then make a standardized incision of 1-mm thickness on the flexor surface of the patient's forearm. The bleeding is blotted with a filter paper at 30-second intervals. Measurement of the

bleeding time begins from the time of incision placement and continues until the patient has ceased bleeding. Normal ranges are from 1 to 9 minutes. Quantitative platelet counts may be normal, but platelets may not function properly to provide hemostasis. Prothrombin time (PT) measures the extrinsic pathway, whereas the thrombin time (TT) measures the fibrinogen-to-fibrin final reactions in the common pathway of the coagulation cascade. Neither PT nor TT directly measures platelet function.

8. **The correct answer is B.** On initial screening, NSAIDs such as ibuprofen may produce a false positive for *cannabis*. Labetolol and ranitidine can cause a false positive screen for amphetamines and methamphetamines. Sertraline causes a false positive for PCP. Even ingestion of poppy seeds can cause a false positive for opiates in screening toxicology. Whenever a false positive is suspected on initial drug screening, it is prudent to obtain a confirmatory test.

9. **The correct answer is A.** Bilirubin is the final product of heme degradation. Following this degradation, bilirubin conjugates with glucaronic acid within the liver into a more water-soluble form prior to excretion by the kidneys. Conjugated bilirubin is another term for direct bilirubin. In biliary tract obstruction, conjugated bilirubin does not release into the bile and therefore direct bilirubin levels increase. Gilbert's disease is a benign inherited disorder in which there is reduced activity of glucuronyltranferase, the enzyme that facilitates the conjugation of bilirubin. This condition results in increased levels of unconjugated, or indirect, bilirubin. Neonatal physiologic jaundice results from the inability of an immature liver to conjugate bilirubin, resulting in an increase in indirect bilirubin. In sickle-cell crisis, increased hemolysis overcomes the ability of the liver to conjugate bilirubin, leading to increased indirect bilirubin levels.

10. **The correct answer is B.** Immunologic testing for syphilis consists of the detection of antibodies to the spirochete *Treponema pallidum*. The nontreponemal tests such as RPR and VDRL detect a nonspecific antibody called reagin, used primarily for screening. The treponemal tests detect antibodies directed against the organism itself. The FTA-ABS (fluorescent treponemal antibody-absorption) test is a highly specific and sensitive confirmatory treponemal test for the diagnosis of syphilis. It is the first serologic marker to become positive in primary syphilis, approximately 4 to 6 weeks after inoculation. Treponemal tests such as FTA-ABS remain positive for a patient's lifetime, regardless of treatment. The DFA-TP (direct fluorescence antibody for *Treponema pallidum*) depends on the presence of the organism directly isolated from a lesion.

11. **The correct answer is B.** Potassium loss from diuretic use increases a patient's risk for digoxin toxicity. Symptoms and signs of digoxin toxicity include confusion, headache, palpitations, nausea, vomiting, diarrhea, and visual changes, such as blurred vision, scotoma, halos around bright lights, and changes in color perception.

12. **The correct answer is C.** Decreased ferritin levels are *early* indicators of iron deficiency anemia. The body initially depletes iron stores before a significant decrease in hemoglobin levels is recognized. It is for this reason that iron supplementation is continued for months after the hemoglobin levels have normalized in order to replenish these iron stores.

13. **The correct answer is C.** Ingestion of high doses of vitamin C may cause a false negative urine dipstick for blood, because the test depends on a pseudoperoxidase reaction. A positive dipstick *indicates the presence of blood* or, more specifically, heme, free hemoglobin, and free myoglobin. Interference with povidone–iodine may also cause a false positive on a dipstick without the microscopic presence of red blood cells.

14. **The correct answer is D.** The erythrocyte sedimentation rate (ESR) is the rate at which red blood cells settle in a saline solution in 1 hour, measured in millimeters. In conditions

associated with inflammation (polymyalgia rheumatica), infection, neoplasm (multiple myeloma), tissue necrosis, or infarction (acute MI), increased proteins, primarily fibrinogen, are found in the plasma. These proteins, in turn, cause the red blood cells to stack closely, becoming heavier and settling faster, as demonstrated by an increased sedimentation rate. In sickle-cell anemia, the morphology of the red blood cells inhibits the settling or stacking of the red blood cells, leading to a decreased sedimentation rate.

15. **The correct answer is C.** Red blood cell casts are associated with acute glomerulonephritis. Broad, waxy casts represent stasis of the large collecting tubules and present in chronic renal failure. Hyaline casts are in concentrated urine and may be associated with fever, diuretic use, or following strenuous exercise. White blood cell casts occur in conditions of inflammation or infection, such as interstitial nephritis or pyelonephritis. Pigmented granular casts occur in conditions of acute tubular necrosis.

16. **The correct answer is D.** *Bordetella pertussis*, an aerobic coccobacillary organism, is the causative agent of whooping cough. It produces an acute infection of the upper respiratory tract in young children, usually younger than age 2. After an incubation period of 1 to 3 weeks, the patient enters the catarrhal stage, characterized by coryza, lacrimation, and a cough, which initially is worse at night. The paroxysmal stage follows, characterized by intermittent episodes of rapid consecutive coughs concluding with a high-pitched inspiratory "whoop." A convalescent period follows the paroyxmal stage, where the patient gets some relief from the severity and frequency of the cough. Nasopharyngeal culture using Bordet-Gengou media or identification of the organism by PCR assays makes the diagnosis. White blood cell counts average in the 20,000/mm^3 range in the catarrhal stage with a predominance of lymphocytes. Counts surge to nearly 50,000/mm^3 during the paroxysmal stage. Immunization and disease do not confer lasting immunity to pertussis. The Tdap vaccine, as a one-time booster for patients ages 11 through 64, can be useful to increase waning antibody titers to pertussis. Treatment of infected patients and prophylaxis of close contacts include erythromycin, azithromycin, clarithromycin, and trimethoprim-sulfamethoxazole.

17. **The correct answer is C.** Systemic lupus erythematosus (SLE) is an autoimmune disease characterized by diffuse inflammation and immune complex deposition. Initial laboratory testing includes an ANA (antinuclear antibody), which is positive in greater than 95% of patients and often coincides with the onset of symptoms. Additional serologic tests include anti-dsDNA and anti-Smith, which are highly specific for the disease. Anti-dsDNA titers fluctuate and correspond to disease activity and may signal a lupus flare. Histones are arginine- and lysine-rich proteins found in cells complexed with DNA. Although antihistone antibodies occur in approximately 30 to 60% of patients with lupus, they appear in nearly 95% of patients with drug-induced lupus. Research identifies nearly 40 drugs as causing a lupus-like syndrome, with hydralazine, procainamide, and quinidine being the most common. Patients with drug-induced lupus generally do not demonstrate the central nervous system (CNS) and kidney manifestations generally seen in SLE. Theories regarding the pathophysiology of drug-induced lupus include drug interference with enzymes that alter gene suppression and drug-immune complexes that activate the immune response. Symptoms generally resolve upon discontinuation of the offending drug.

18. **The correct answer is C.** Smudge cells are small, fragile lymphocytes easily destroyed during peripheral smear preparation. Although these cells are not specific to chronic lymphocytic leukemia (CLL), they occur in greater frequency in CLL than in any other condition.

19. **The correct answer is B.** A lipid profile measures total cholesterol, low-density lipoproteins (LDL), high-density lipoproteins (HDL), and triglycerides. The use of formulas such as the Friedewald Formula provides laboratory determination of LDL cholesterol.

$$LDL = total\ cholesterol - HDL - (triglycerides/5)$$

The LDL calculation has validity only if the fasting triglyceride level is less than 400 mg/dl. Errors in LDL estimation may occur with a triglyceride level between 250–400 mg/dl.

20. **The correct answer is B.** Coarse bluish-purple–staining granules within the cytoplasm of red blood cells describe basophilic stippling. These granules represent precipitated RNA, specifically ribosomal protein. They frequently occur in heavy metal poisonings, such as lead poisoning, thalassemias, and liver disease.

21. **The correct answer is A.** A myeloid left shift refers to the presence of increased numbers of immature neutrophils circulating in the peripheral blood, such as bands, metamyelocytes, myelocytes, and promyelocytes. The clinician should remember that neutrophils are the first line of defense in response to a bacterial infection. As neutrophils in the functional and storage pools deplete, the bone marrow releases more of these immature cells to compensate for the loss. In leukemoid reactions, there is profound leukocytosis, with counts exceeding 25,000/mm^3 in response to trauma or infection. In leukemoid reactions, however, the circulating neutrophils are mature. The absence of leukocyte precursors and increased leukocyte alkaline phosphatase (LAP) scores differentiates leukemoid reactions from chronic myelogenous leukemia (CML). A reversed differential indicates that there are more lymphocytes than neutrophils on a white blood cell differential count. Hypersegmentation of the neutrophils characterizes a right shift in myeloid maturation.

22. **The correct answer is C.** Red cell distribution width is a measure of anisocytosis, which is a variation of red blood cell size. Anisocytosis reports as part of a complete blood count (CBC). Normal ranges are 11 to 15%. Poikilocytosis refers to variation in the shape of red blood cells.

23. **The correct answer is C.** Peaked T waves, QRS widening, and biphasic QRS-T complexes on ECG indicate hyperkalemia. However, some patients with potassium levels of greater than 6 mEq/L may not demonstrate any ECG changes. Elevations in serum potassium are also a class effect of angiotensin-converting enzyme inhibitors. It is important to monitor potassium levels, especially in diabetic patients and those with impaired renal function. Patients who take NSAIDs concurrently are at increased risk for developing hyperkalemia due to decreased potassium excretion secondary to reduced aldosterone concentrations. Patients on potassium supplements, potassium-sparing diuretics, and salt substitutes (KCl) are also at increased risk. Symptoms/signs of hyperkalemia include arrhythmias, fatigue, paresthesias, muscle weakness, flaccid paralysis, abdominal distention, and diarrhea.

24. **The correct answer is D.** Transmission of *Giardia lamblia*, an intestinal protozoan, occurs via a fecal–oral route. Patients ingest the infected cysts and, when these become exposed to the acidic pH of the stomach, they transform into the motile pear-shaped trophozoite form. The trophozoite is easily recognizable by its four pairs of flagella and two symmetric nuclei with prominent karyosomes. The trophozoites encyst upon passage into the colon, and the passage of cysts in the feces completes the cycle. Infective eggs of *Ascaris lumbricoides* (roundworm) are resistant to environmental stressors. Upon ingestion, the larvae hatch in the small intestine, penetrate the wall of the small intestine, enter the portal circulation, and migrate into the lungs, where they can cause symptoms such as coughing and wheezing. The larvae ascend the bronchial tree, whereupon the patient coughs and expels them upward. At this point, the larvae are swallowed and then gain reentry into the intestines where final development into the adult worms occurs. Patient may present during this phase of infection with a variety of complaints ranging from, but not limited to, bowel obstruction, intussusception, volvulus, or expulsion of worms from body orifices. *Balantidium coli* is a large, ciliated protozoan that is easily recognizable in

both its cyst and trophozoite forms by its "sausage-shaped" macronucleus. Pigs are the most common reservoir for this organism. Although most infected individuals have no noticeable symptoms, they still may transmit the disease. Symptoms, if present, include diarrhea, abdominal pain, and hematochezia. *Dientamoeba fragilis* is unique among intestinal parasites in that it lacks a cyst form and infects humans via a fecal–oral route with ingestion of its nonflagellate trophozoite form. It has been proposed that coinfection with pinworm facilitates infection with this organism. It has a predilection for the proximal colon and cecum and causes a superficial localized irritation and inflammatory response of the colonic mucosa. The most common complaints are anorexia, abdominal pain, and intermittent mild diarrhea. The description of the stools is greenish-brown in color and ranging in consistency from watery to sticky.

25. **The correct answer is C.** The identification of multinucleated Reed-Sternberg cells on lymph node biopsy pathologically characterizes Hodgkin's lymphoma. Hodgkin's lymphoma demonstrates a bimodal age distribution, with one peak at ages 15 to 35 and another over the age of 55. Patients classically present with a painless enlarged lymph node, most commonly a cervical or supraclavicular node. Associated symptoms include fatigue, fever, night sweats, weight loss, and generalized pruritus and splenomegaly.

The Ann Arbor staging classification of Hodgkin's lymphoma is as follows:

Stage I: Involvement of a single lymph node region or single extralymphatic site

Stage II: Involvement of two or more lymph node regions on the same side of the diaphragm or one lymph node region and one contiguous extralymphatic site

Stage III: Involvement of lymph node regions on both sides of the diaphragm, which may include the spleen and/or limited contiguous extralymphatic organ or site

Stage IV: Disseminated involvement of one or more extralymphatic organs

Subclassifications of A and B refer to absence of constitutional symptoms or presence of constitutional symptoms, respectively.

26. **The correct answer is D.** The anion gap is an estimation of unmeasured anions (negatively charged molecules) in plasma and is calculated using the following formula:

$$\text{Anion Gap} = Na - (Cl + HCO_3)$$

The normal range is from 10 to 12. Students and practitioners alike created various mnemonics to identify causes of an increased anion gap. Two of the most frequently used ones are:

M: Methanol, metformin

U: Uremia

D: Diabetic ketoacidosis

P: Paraldehyde, propylene glycol

I: Infection, ischemia, isoniazid

L: Lactate

E: Ethylene glycol, ethanol

S: Salicylates, starvation

And

K: Ketones

I: Ingestion

L: Lactic acid (caused by infection or shock)

U: Uremia

27. **The correct answer is D.** Evidence of viral or aseptic meningitis on cerebral spinal fluid (CSF) analysis includes a normal or mildly elevated opening pressure, normal glucose, and a normal or slightly elevated protein concentration. The most characteristic feature of viral meningitis is lymphocyte pleocytosis, with counts less than 500 cells/µl. CSF findings in bacterial meningitis are increased opening pressures, increased protein of greater than 100 mg/ml, glucose of less than 50% of blood glucose, and a white cell predominance of polymorphonuclear cells.

28. **The correct answer is B.** Traditional treatment of venous thromboembolism, which includes deep vein thrombosis and pulmonary embolism, has been IV administration of heparin simultaneously with oral warfarin. Once the patient receives an initial bolus of IV heparin, then a continuous heparin drip follows. A partial thromboplastin time (PTT) should be drawn in 6 hours to assess initial response to therapy. Heparin is discontinued once the INR (international normalized ratio) values on warfarin attain a therapeutic level between 2 and 3 for 2 consecutive days. The patient then remains on oral anticoagulation therapy for an additional 6 months in the case of the first episode of deep vein thrombosis. Low-molecular-weight heparin, given subcutaneously, can also provide anticoagulation therapy. Its advantages include shorter hospital stays and no PTT monitoring.

29. **The correct answer is A.** The prothrombin time (PT) measures the time in seconds needed for clot formation in a plasma specimen upon the addition of tissue thromboplastin. It measures both the extrinsic pathway and the common pathway. The prothrombin time proves useful as a screening tool to assess bleeding tendencies, liver function, and vitamin K status. The PT also monitors warfarin therapy. The international normalized ratio (INR) reported as part of a PT standardizes results independent of the test methodology and reagents used. The desired therapeutic range for chronic atrial fibrillation is an INR of 2 to 3. In the absence of bleeding in this patient, it is appropriate to reduce the warfarin dose and recheck the PT/INR in 1 week. Holding the dose for 1 week could increase the patient's risk of a thrombotic event. Ingestion of leafy green vegetables high in vitamin K counteracts the effects of warfarin, resulting in shortened prothrombin times and decreased INR levels, therefore the practitioner should educate his or her patients accordingly. The partial thromboplastin time (PTT) measures the intrinsic and common pathways and monitors heparin therapy.

30. **The correct answer is D.** Alpha-fetoprotein is assessed on maternal blood (as part of a QUAD screen, which includes hCG, inhibin, and estriol) and amniotic fluid during pregnancy to evaluate for neural tube defects. It serves as a tumor marker for neuroblastoma, hepatocellular cancer, and nonseminomatis germ cell testicular cancers. Pure seminomas do not produce alpha-fetoprotein. The prostatic specific antigen (PSA), along with a digital rectal exam, are used to screen for prostate cancer in men over age 50. However, a recently released study states that men who are 75 years or older should not be screened for prostate cancer according to researchers from the U.S. Preventive Services Task Force (USPSTF). The authors state that for those with life expectancies of 10 or fewer years, there is a "small to none" incremental benefit and therefore the harm outweighs the benefit. These findings are in the *Annals of Internal Medicine* (see references at end of chapter). We advise the reader to investigate this important research for further elucidation. Increased PSA levels may be in benign conditions, such as prostatitis and benign prostatic hyperplasia, as well as following manipulative or disrupting procedures of the prostate gland.

31. **The correct answer is B.** Alpha-1 antitrypsin deficiency is an inherited disorder that causes a panacinar emphysema. Alpha-1 antitrypsin serves to protect the alveoli from antiproteases. Without this protection, the alveolar walls are destroyed by elastase, leading to emphysema. The manufacture of alpha-1 antitrypsin occurs in hepatocytes. Genetic

alterations in the structure of this molecule prevent its release from the hepatocytes, and ultimately results in liver damage. Liver disease manifests early as hepatitis or persistent neonatal jaundice and later as cirrhosis and hepatocellular cancer.

32. **The correct answer is A.** C-peptide or "connecting peptide" is a test used to assess the amount of endogenous insulin a patient produces. Beta cells of the pancreas produce proinsulin, which is composed of insulin and C-peptide. Measurement of the peptide is more accurate than measuring plasma insulin levels, because the liver extracts a significant portion of insulin from the portal vein before it reaches the peripheral circulation, depending on the patient's nutritional status. C-peptide matches up one-to-one to the amount of proinsulin produced. It quantifies the amount, if any, of residual beta cell function in type 1 diabetes and determines when injectable insulin is warranted in type 2 diabetes. Clinicians should monitor C-peptide levels in conjunction with insulin and glucagon levels in patients with hypoglycemia to identify the cause as well as to monitor response to treatment. In a patient who is currently on injectable insulin and experiences recurrent hypoglycemic episodes, a low C-peptide may indicate insulin abuse. In patients with polycystic ovary syndrome (PCOS), elevated C-peptide levels may reflect the degree of insulin resistance. Glycosylated hemoglobin measures overall glycemic control over the last 120 days.

33. **The correct answer is B.** The hepatitis B surface antigen (HBsAg) is the first serologic marker detected in a patient following exposure to hepatitis B virus. It corresponds closely to detectable HBV DNA and is generally positive at approximately 4 weeks after exposure. It wanes to nondetectable levels by 15 weeks following the appearance of symptoms. The hepatitis B e antigen (HBeAg) indicates acute hepatitis B and correlates with elevated virus titers and greater infectivity. Anti-Be denotes low levels of viral load, less infectivity, and reflects a good prognosis. Symptoms also present with an average of 12 weeks. IgM anti-HBc is detected at the onset of symptoms and progressively declines to nondetectable levels by approximately 6 to 8 months. It is the only marker positive during the "window" period. (Note that no test currently exists to measure HBcAg and IgG anti-HBc.) Total anti-HBc can last indefinitely and serves as a marker of past infection. After the disappearance of HBsAg and during the convalescent period, laboratory tests detect anti-HBs. Anti-HBs indicate recovery from disease and conferred immunity from reinfection. The persistence of HBsAg in the absence of anti-HBs indicates a carrier state. During the window period (after the disappearance of HBsAg and before the anti-HBs appears), the only serologic markers are IgM anti-HBc and total anti-HBc. The diagnosis of chronic hepatitis B is made when HBsAg and total anti-HBc are positive (two separate samples at least 6 months apart) or HBsAg and total anti-HBc are positive and IgM anti-HBc is negative from a single sample. For further information, the clinician is advised to review the CDC's tutorial at the following link: http://www.cdc.gov/hepatitis/Resources/Professionals/Training/Serology/training.htm#1.

34. **The correct answer is D.** Hyponatremia, defined as serum sodium levels less than 130 mEq/L, is the most common electrolyte imbalance found in hospitalized patients. It is more often due to a dilutional effect of water retention than to true sodium deficiency. In hospitalized patients, it generally relates to the infusion of hypotonic solutions.

35. **The correct answer is D.** Multiple myeloma is a malignancy of plasma cells and is characterized by overproduction of intact monoclonal immunoglobulins and Bence-Jones proteins, which are free immunoglobulin light chains. Symptoms include bone pain, anemia, and recurrent infection. Plasma cells infiltrate the bone marrow. Radiographic evidence includes osteoporosis and lytic lesions, especially in the axial skeleton. Serum protein electrophoresis demonstrates a monoclonal spike most frequently found in the beta or gamma globulin region. Peripheral smears of patients with multiple myeloma commonly demonstrate Rouleaux formation (from the French, "of rouleau," or "a roll"). The negatively charged globulins produced in multiple myeloma disrupt the exist-

ing electrical charge surrounding red blood cells, causing them to come within close proximity with their biconcave surfaces in opposition to each other, thereby forming groups that resemble stacks of coins. Rouleaux formation is not specific to multiple myeloma; it also occurs in infection and inflammatory disorders, diabetes, connective tissue disorders, and cancer.

36. **The correct answer is A.** The symptoms of diabetes insipidus (DI) result from the inability of the kidney to concentrate the urine due to either the lack of antidiuretic hormone (ADH, also known as vasopressin), as seen in central DI, or a defect in the kidneys' response to ADH, as seen in nephrogenic DI. Patients present with polydipsia and excretion of massive volumes of dilute urine. Head trauma may cause damage to the hypothalamus or pituitary gland and inhibit ADH production and release.

37. **The correct answer is A.** Hypermagnesemia can result from the administration of magnesium sulfate to preeclamptic and eclamptic patients. Symptoms are generally dose related and include flushing, nausea, loss of deep tendon reflexes, muscle weakness, flaccid paralysis, arrhythmias, hypotension, and coma. Treatment can include intravenous fluids, which serve to dilute extracellular magnesium, in combination with diuretics, which promote magnesium excretion. When magnesium levels are significantly elevated or when a patient is symptomatic, calcium gluconate is the appropriate treatment. Calcium directly counteracts the effects of magnesium.

38. **The correct answer is C.** Hereditary spherocytosis results from a genetic defect in erythrocyte membrane proteins, the most common being ankyrin. In the absence of these membrane-stabilizing proteins, red blood cells can no longer maintain their biconcave disk shape. They become spherical, and the spleen targets them for destruction. Heme degradation leads to increased bilirubin levels manifested clinically by jaundice. Treatment for this disorder is splenectomy, although this does not correct the inherent red blood cell membrane defect. The laboratory test that supports the diagnosis is osmotic fragility. Osmotic fragility measures red blood cell resistance to hemolysis when placed in increasingly hypotonic or dilute saline solutions. Spherocytes demonstrate increased osmotic fragility, which allows them to become easily lysed.

39. **The correct answer is B.** Schilling's test is performed to evaluate a patient with a determined vitamin B_{12} deficiency for pernicious anemia. The test has three stages. During the first stage, the patient ingests radiolabeled vitamin B_{12}, followed by an intramuscular injection of vitamin B_{12}. This serves to saturate the tissue binding sites to better facilitate urinary excretion of the radiolabeled vitamin B_{12}. Urine is then collected for 24 hours. A normal test is when the patient excretes at least 10% of the labeled vitamin B_{12}. If there is decreased excretion noted on the first stage testing, then there is a repeat of the first test along with administration of oral intrinsic factor. If excretion is normal after this second stage, then the patient has pernicious anemia. If excretion remains diminished, there can be a repeat of the test. The third stage incorporates administration of an antibiotic. A patient who has bacterial overgrowth in the small intestines, which competes for vitamin B_{12}, will have a normal labeled excretion after the third stage. If the patient fails to demonstrate normal excretion after the third stage, then the patient has the diagnosis of intestinal malabsorption.

40. **The correct answer is B.** A positive HLA-B27 gene is present in more than 90% of patients with ankylosing spondylitis. Antinuclear antigen (ANA) and rheumatoid factor (RF) are generally negative. An elevated C-reactive protein (CRP) is a general marker of inflammation and is not specific to ankylosing spondylitis.

REFERENCES

DeSai, S. P., and Isa-Pratt, S. (2002). *Clinician's guide to laboratory medicine: A practical approach*, 2nd ed. Lexi-Comp Inc., Cleveland, OH.

Hixson-Wallace, J. (2006). "Digoxin toxicity." *U.S. Pharmacist* 31(2): 28–36.

Kumar, N. (2007). "Nutritional neuropathies." *Neurologic Clinics* 25(1): 209–255.

Lee, M. (2004). *Basic skills in interpreting laboratory data*, 3rd ed. American Society of Health System Pharmacists, Bethesda, MD.

Lin, K., Lipsitz, R., Miller, T., and Janakiraman, S. (2008). "Benefits and harms of prostate-specific antigen: An evidence update for the U.S. Preventative Services Task Force." *Annals of Internal Medicine* 149: 185–199.

Pagano, K. D., and Pagano, T. J. (1998). *Mosby's manual of diagnostic and laboratory tests*. Mosby Inc., St. Louis.

Quiceno, G. A., and Cush, J. J. (2007). "Iatrogenic rheumatic syndromes in the elderly." *Rheumatic Disease Clinics of North America* 33(1): 123–134.

Vincent, E. C., and Goodwin, C. (2006). "What common substances can cause false positives on urine screens for drugs of abuse?" *The Journal of Family Practice* 55(10): 893–897.

Obstetrics and Gynecology

Rachel Catanzaro Ditoro, MSPAS, PA-C
Donna M. Agnew, MT (ASCP), MSPAS, PA-C

1. Approximately 5% of pregnant women screened for fetal neural tube defects will have falsely elevated serum alpha-fetoprotein (AFP) levels. Which of the following is *not* a common cause of false positive AFP levels?

    A. Inaccurate dating of gestational age
    B. Multiple gestation
    C. Fetal demise
    D. Chromosomal abnormalities

2. Which of the following is true with regard to chorionic villus sampling (CVS)?

    A. CVS is used in the second trimester to obtain villi for cytogenic testing.
    B. It is almost always performed transabdominally.
    C. It carries a lower miscarriage rate than amniocentesis.
    D. It is associated with distal limb defects.

3. Which of the following is *not* associated with the use of estrogen replacement therapy in postmenopausal women?

    A. Increased risk of stroke
    B. Decrease in low-density lipoprotein (LDL) cholesterol levels
    C. Increase in high-density lipoprotein (HDL) cholesterol levels
    D. Decrease in triglyceride levels

4. A G2P1001 female at 39 weeks gestation presents to the hospital with uterine contractions occurring every 5 minutes for the past hour and states that she "had her bloody show." You evaluate her and determine that she is 100% effaced and 6 cm dilated. This patient is in which of the following stages of labor?

    A. First stage, latent phase
    B. First stage, active phase
    C. Second stage
    D. Third stage

5. Which of the following does *not* increase a woman's risk for the development of breast cancer?

    A. Late menarche
    B. History of uterine cancer
    C. Late menopause
    D. Presence of genetic mutations in the *BRCA* genes

6. Which of the following is the most common presenting complaint for women with breast cancer?

    A. Breast mass
    B. Breast pain
    C. Nipple discharge
    D. Skin changes to the nipple and/or breast

7. A 24-year-old G2P0010 female presents to the office following a positive home pregnancy test. Based on her last menstrual period, she is 6 weeks pregnant. A pelvic ultrasound reveals no gestational sac nor intrauterine pregnancy and a 2.5-cm right tubal mass. The patient denies pelvic pain and vaginal bleeding. You decide to treat her with a single intramuscular dose of methotrexate. Which of the following would *not* be part of your treatment plan?

    A. Obtain day 1 β-hCG level.
    B. Give a second dose of methotrexate if β-hCG levels plateau.
    C. Obtain days 4 and 7 β-hCG levels.
    D. Perform dilatation and curettage.

8. Which of the following is the most common cause of secondary amenorrhea?

    A. Pregnancy
    B. Polycystic ovarian syndrome
    C. Anorexia nervosa
    D. Prolactinoma

9. A G1P0000 female at 30 weeks gestation presents to the emergency department with painless bright red vaginal bleeding for 30 minutes. Her uterus is nontender with palpation. Which of the following is the most likely diagnosis?

    A. Placenta previa
    B. Vasa previa
    C. Abruptio placentae
    D. Uterine rupture

10. A 30-year-old female presents complaining of unilateral, spontaneous serous discharge from her right nipple for 1 month. She has no significant past medical history, her periods are regular, and she takes no medication. Which of the following is the most likely cause for her discharge?

    A. Intraductal papilloma
    B. Intraductal carcinoma
    C. Prolactinoma
    D. Fibrocystic breast changes

11. Which of the following medications can be used safely in pregnancy to treat hypertension?

    A. labetalol
    B. enalapril
    C. hydrochlorothiazide
    D. magnesium sulfate

12. Which of the following signs is no longer a required criterion when making the diagnosis of preeclampsia?

    A. Hypertension
    B. Proteinuria
    C. Edema
    D. Seizures

13. An 18-year-old female presents complaining of vaginal discharge for the past 5 days. She describes the discharge as "somewhat itchy" and having a greenish color. She admits to having a new sexual partner. A wet mount of the discharge reveals flagellated cells. Which of the following medications should you prescribe in order to treat this patient?

    A. metronidazole 500 mg by mouth twice a day for 7 days
    B. One dose of fluconazole 150 mg by mouth
    C. doxycycline 100 mg by mouth twice a day for 7 days
    D. One dose of azithromycin 1 g by mouth

14. A 22-year-old G0P0 female presents complaining of severe lower abdominal and pelvic pain for 1 day. She admits to a fever of 101.5°F orally and "some" vaginal discharge for 2 days. She has an IUD in place and is sexually active with one partner for 6 months. She has no significant past medical history and takes no regular medications. Her last menstrual period was 7 days ago. Abdominal examination reveals moderate bilateral lower quadrant tenderness with palpation—the left side more so than the right side—active bowel sounds, and no rebound tenderness. Pelvic examination reveals a small amount of yellow discharge at the cervical os, moderate to severe tenderness with movement of the cervix and uterus, and palpation of the adnexa—the left side more so than the right side. The patient does not appear "toxic" and an in-office pregnancy test is negative. Which of the following would *not* be included in your treatment plan for this patient?

    A. Removal of the IUD.
    B. Give a single, intramuscular dose of ceftriaxone 250 mg, doxycycline 100 mg by mouth twice a day, plus metronidazole 500 mg by mouth twice a day for 14 days.
    C. Admit to the hospital for IV levofloxacin and doxycycline.
    D. ibuprofen 600 mg by mouth every 6 to 8 hours as needed for pain.

15. Which of the following is *not* a normal physiologic change seen in pregnancy?

    A. The presence of a diastolic ejection murmur secondary to increased cardiac output
    B. Increased glomerular filtration rate by approximately 50% over nonpregnant levels
    C. Respiratory tidal volume increases by approximately 40% over nonpregnant levels
    D. Plasma fibrinogen and Factor VIII levels nearly double

16. Rupture of membranes may be suspected when a patient reports having felt a "gush" of fluid from the vagina. Which of the following is *not* a test used to confirm this diagnosis?

    A. Pool test
    B. Nitrazine test
    C. Fern test
    D. Fetal fibronectin test

17. Which of the following is not a criterion when calculating the Bishop score to determine whether induction of labor will be required?

    A. Cervical consistency
    B. Cervical position
    C. Fetal station
    D. Fetal presentation

18. A 31-year-old African American female presents complaining of menorrhagia with periods lasting 10 days that she describes as "very heavy with clotting." She denies dysmenorrhea and dyspareunia. Her hemoglobin is 10 g/dl, and a pelvic ultrasound reveals a 4-cm submucosal leiomyoma. She states that she and her husband are trying to conceive. Which of the following is the most appropriate treatment plan for this patient?

    A. Uterine artery embolization
    B. Myomectomy
    C. Expectant management
    D. Begin a GnRH (gonadotropin-releasing hormone) agonist

19. A 57-year-old Caucasian female presents for her routine gynecologic exam. Her last period was 6 years ago. She denies any postmenopausal bleeding and takes no hormone replacement therapy (HRT). On physical examination, the vaginal mucosa is thin and atrophic. Bimanual exam reveals a small, freely mobile uterus, a nonpalpable right ovary, and a slightly palpable left ovary. She describes no discomfort with the pelvic exam. Which of the following is the most appropriate follow-up for this patient?

   A. See again in 1 year for her next routine exam.
   B. Repeat the bimanual exam in 3 to 6 months.
   C. Refer for exploratory laparoscopy.
   D. Begin HRT and follow-up in 6 months.

20. A 34-year-old Caucasian female presents complaining of pelvic pain that begins a few days before the onset of menses and lasts for the first 3 days into her period. She describes the pain as severe and says that it sometimes prevents her from going to work. She also admits to dyspareunia, especially just before her period, which is now interfering with her sexual relationship with her husband. Of the following, which is the most definitive means for diagnosing endometriosis in this patient?

   A. Pelvic ultrasound
   B. Pelvic CT scan
   C. Laparoscopy
   D. Pelvic MRI

21. Which of the following is considered the definitive treatment for endometriosis?

   A. Total hysterectomy and bilateral salpingo-oophrectomy
   B. Surgical ablation of endometrial implants
   C. Continuous administration of oral contraceptives
   D. Administration of a GnRH (gonadotropin-releasing hormone) agonist

22. A 27-year-old female presents for evaluation of a "sore" near her vagina for the past 2 days. On examination, you find a single round, red, firm 1-cm ulcer on her labia, shown below. The ulcer is not tender with palpation. A VDRL test is positive. The patient is allergic to penicillin. Which of the following medications would you prescribe in the treatment of this patient?

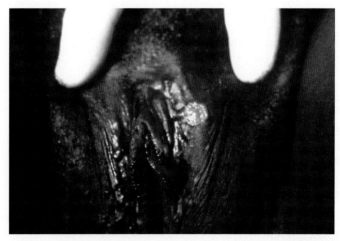

Courtesy of CDC

   A. doxycycline 100 mg by mouth twice a day for 2 weeks
   B. erythromycin 500 mg by mouth twice a day for 2 weeks
   C. acyclovir 400 mg by mouth three times a day for 2 weeks
   D. clindamycin 300 mg by mouth four times a day for 2 weeks

23. A 25-year-old nulliparous female presents for a routine gynecologic exam. Her periods are regular with a 32-day interval. She tells you that she and her husband would like to start a family. While counseling her about trying to become pregnant, you provide her with which of the following statements as advice?

    A. Ovulation occurs 14 days from the start of her period.

    B. Once ovulation has occurred, the egg is available for fertilization for 48 hours.

    C. If the egg remains unfertilized, her period will begin 14 days after ovulation has occurred.

    D. Healthy sperm will survive less than 24 hours inside the female body after ejaculation.

24. A 30-year-old female presents complaining of a painful "lump" in her vagina that has made it difficult for her to walk comfortably for the past 2 days. On physical examination, you palpate an exquisitely tender swelling, shown below. In order to treat and prevent recurrence of this vaginal swelling, which of the following would be the *least* appropriate course of treatment for this patient?

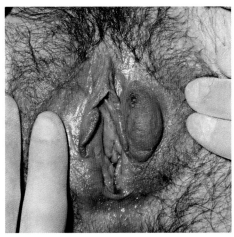

© Wellcome Trust Library/Custom Medical Stock Photo

    A. Incision and drainage, irrigation, insertion of a Word catheter

    B. Incision and drainage, marsupialization

    C. Incision and drainage, irrigation, antibiotics

    D. Incision and drainage, laser excision

25. Which of the following is the most appropriate course of treatment for the lesions shown below?

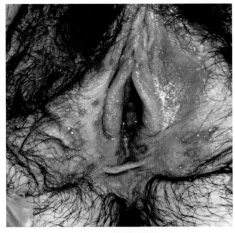

© Wellcome Trust Library/Custom Medical Stock Photo

A. benzathine penicillin G 2.4 million units intramuscularly, one dose
B. acyclovir 200 mg by mouth every 4 hours for 10 days
C. azithromycin 1 g by mouth, one dose
D. imiquimod 5% cream applied three times a week for 12 weeks

26. A 27-year-old female presents complaining of enlarged, painful "bumps" in her groin. She admits that these "bumps" have been present for the past 5 days and that she has also felt fatigued and "feverish." She states that a few weeks ago she noticed a small ulceration near the vaginal introitus, but it did not hurt and disappeared within a day or two. She admits to being sexually active and uses condoms "occasionally." Which of the following organisms is the cause of her condition?

A. *Chlamydia trachomatis*
B. *Treponema pallidum*
C. *Neisseria gonorrhoeae*
D. *Haemophilus ducreyi*

27. A 57-year-old postmenopausal female presents for a routine gynecologic exam. She admits to you that she has noticed some "changes" to her vagina over the past year. She states that the skin feels "tighter" and is sometimes "itchy." She also admits that sexual intercourse with her husband has become quite painful, and it is beginning to affect their relationship. Her last period was 5 years ago, and she denies any vaginal bleeding since that time. She also denies having any hot flashes or night sweats. Her past medical history is significant for well-controlled hypertension. Her only medication is hydrochlorothiazide 50 mg by mouth once a day. On physical examination, you note atrophic and thin vaginal mucosa and several hyperkeratotic, shiny white plaques, as shown below. Which of the following should be used to treat this patient?

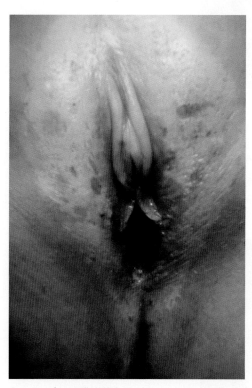

Courtesy of Joe Miller/CDC

A. clotrimazole cream 2%
B. estradiol vaginal cream 0.1%
C. clobetasol cream 0.05%
D. Oral hormone replacement therapy

28. A 60-year-old G3P3 African American postmenopausal female presents to your office requesting a bone mineral density (BMD) scan to test for osteoporosis. Her last period was 8 years ago, and she denies any vaginal bleeding since that time. She states she has a well-balanced diet, takes a daily multivitamin, consumes a small glass of red wine with dinner, and has smoked a half-pack of cigarettes for 25 years. She has no known family history of osteoporosis. She is 5′6″ tall and weighs 160 lbs. (BMI: 26). You agree to refer her for a BMD scan based on which of the following risk factors for osteoporosis?

A. Her history of cigarette smoking.
B. Her age—all women older than 60 years should have a BMD scan for osteoporosis.
C. You do not refer the patient for the BMD scan; she does not currently have enough risk factors to warrant it.
D. Her BMI is too high.

29. A 47-year-old G2P2 female presents for a routine gynecologic exam. While taking the patient's history, she hesitantly admits that she has recently been having a difficult time making it to the bathroom before "wetting herself." Based on the type of urinary incontinence this patient has described, which of the following therapies do you recommend?

A. Pessary
B. Surgery to restore the intra-abdominal position of the proximal urethra
C. Self-catheterization
D. An anticholinergic medication

30. Which of the following would *not* be in your differential diagnosis for galactorrhea?

A. Pituitary adenoma
B. Acromegaly
C. Hypothyroidism
D. Molar pregnancy

31. A 32-year-old G2P1001 Hispanic female who is 27 weeks pregnant has come to review the results of her glucose-tolerance test. The results are shown below. Based on these results, what is your advice to this patient?

Fasting = 100 mg/dl
1 hour = 195 mg/dl
2 hours = 170 mg/dl
3 hours = 140 mg/dl

A. She does not have gestational diabetes, but she should watch her diet and decrease her carbohydrate intake.
B. She has gestational diabetes and will be started on a short-acting insulin in combination with an intermediate-acting insulin in the morning and a short-acting insulin at dinner.
C. She has gestational diabetes and will be started on a 2,200 calorie/day diet with a decrease in her carbohydrate intake.
D. She does not have gestational diabetes and should continue her current diet.

32. A 31-year-old G2P2 female who is 3 weeks postpartum presents complaining of left breast swelling and tenderness for the past 24 hours. She states that she has been breastfeeding her newborn daughter since delivery without much difficulty prior to the onset of the breast swelling and discomfort. She has a temperature of 100.3°F oral. Physical exam reveals a focal area of erythema and tenderness on the affected breast (shown below) that is warmer in temperature that the rest of the breast. Which of the following would *not* be included in your treatment plan for this patient?

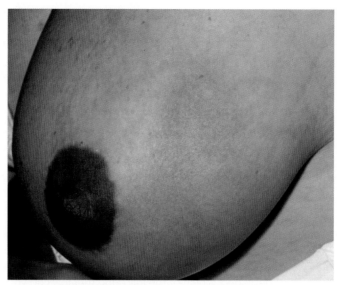

© SPL/Custom Medical Stock Photo

A. Continue breastfeeding
B. Warm compresses
C. Discontinue breastfeeding
D. dicloxacillin 250 mg by mouth four times a day for 7 days

33. Which of the following conditions is *not* associated with an elevated CA-125 level?

A. Endometriosis
B. Hepatic cirrhosis
C. Ovarian carcinoma
D. Hepatocellular carcinoma

34. A 45-year-old woman is concerned that she may be having "hot flashes." Her menses are less frequent and more erratic. Which of the following serum levels is the most accurate indicator of primary ovarian failure?

A. Prolactin >10 ng/ml
B. Androstenedione >600 ng/ml
C. Estradiol >30 pg/ml
D. Follicle-stimulating hormone >40 mIU/ml

35. Which of the following patients would be most at risk for endometrial carcinoma and therefore undergo a biopsy?

A. A 40-year-old nulliparous female with a history of breast cancer who is currently taking tamoxifen and now has irregular vaginal bleeding
B. A 50-year-old perimenopausal female with intermittent "spotting" for the past 6 months
C. A 32-year-old female with 2 months of abnormal bleeding after starting combined oral contraceptive pills
D. A 16-year-old female with irregular menses for 2 years

36. A 31-year-old G1P0 female who is 36 weeks pregnant presents for an obstetric checkup. She states that "the baby isn't moving as much as before." You refer her for a nonstress test to assess fetal movement. Which of the following results indicate normal fetal move-ment in a reactive nonstress test?

A. Two decelerations with fetal movements over 40 minutes
B. One acceleration with movement over 1 hour
C. Five decelerations with movements over 20 minutes
D. Two accelerations with movements over 20 minutes

37. A 21-year-old female presents with the complaint of "bumps near her vagina" for the past week. She admits to being sexually active with a new partner. On examination, you find multiple, nontender, rounded, pearly papular lesions (shown below). Which of the following is the most likely diagnosis?

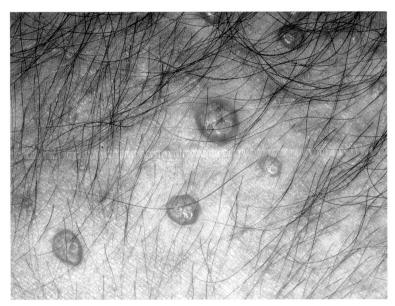

© Medical-on-Line/Alamy Images

   A. Molluscum contagiosum
   B. Condylomata latum
   C. Condylomata acuminata
   D. Herpes simplex

38. A 33-year-old female returns to the office to discuss the results of her abnormal Pap test. You explain to her that her Pap screening showed cervical changes consistent with moderate dysplasia (CIN II). Which of the following is the most appropriate next step for this patient?

   A. Dilation and curettage
   B. Colposcopy with directed biopsy
   C. Cone biopsy
   D. Repeat Pap smear in 6 months

39. An 18-year-old G1P0 female presents to the office complaining of vaginal bleeding following a positive home pregnancy test "about a month ago." She states that her periods are usually regular with a 30-day interval and that her last period was approximately 12 weeks ago. She admits that she has had severe nausea and vomiting and has had difficulty "keeping food down" for the past week. On physical examination, you see blood in the vaginal vault and her uterus can be palpated just below the umbilicus. No adnexal masses or tenderness can be palpated. You refer her for a pelvic ultrasound and a serum β-hCG level. Her β-hCG level is 240,000 mIU/ml, and her ultrasound reveals "multiple hypoechoic areas with no gestational sac or fetus present." Which of the following is the most likely diagnosis?

   A. Hydatidiform mole
   B. Threatened abortion
   C. Ectopic pregnancy
   D. Erythroblastosis fetalis

40. A diagnosis of adenomyosis would most likely be made in which of the following patients?

    A. A 21-year-old nulliparous female with dysmenorrhea and dyspareunia

    B. A 40-year-old multiparous female with menorrhagia, premenstrual pelvic pain, dysmenorrhea, and a symmetrically enlarged uterus

    C. A 38-year-old multiparous female with menorrhagia, no dysmenorrhea, and an irregular bulky uterus

    D. A 59-year-old nulliparous female with several recent episodes of vaginal bleeding whose last menstrual period was 7 years ago

41. You are at the delivery of a newborn baby boy, and are asked to obtain a 5-minute Apgar score for him. You assess the baby and determine that he is actively moving, his heart rate is 101 beats per minute, he is crying, and he is pink in color with somewhat pale extremities. Which of the following is the correct Apgar score?

    A. 7

    B. 8

    C. 9

    D. 10

42. A 34-year-old G2P1011 female presents with her fourth *Candida* vaginitis infection this year. Her past medical history is significant only for seasonal allergic rhinitis in the spring and fall for which she takes an over-the-counter antihistamine, as needed. She admits to being sexually active with a single male partner and denies any recent antibiotic use. Which of the following concurrent diseases should you consider in this patient given her history and presentation?

    A. Dermatitis

    B. Diabetes mellitus

    C. Polycystic ovarian syndrome

    D. Systemic lupus erythematosus

43. A 27-year-old G2P1001 female now 14 weeks pregnant presents complaining of "cramps" and "spotty" vaginal bleeding for the past 18 hours. Speculum exam shows blood in a closed cervical os. The uterus is nontender with palpation. Which of the following is the most likely diagnosis for this patient?

    A. Threatened abortion

    B. Inevitable abortion

    C. Complete abortion

    D. Incomplete abortion

44. Which of the following is *not* associated with polycystic ovarian syndrome?

    A. Hyperandrogenism

    B. Insulin resistance

    C. Infertility

    D. Metromenorrhagia

45. A 30-year-old female presents for her routine gynecologic exam. She is a G3P2012 with a history of two full-term vaginal deliveries without complications 5 years ago and 3 years ago, respectively. She has a history of one ectopic pregnancy, which was medically managed. She has used a combination of the rhythm method and condoms for contraception to date and asks you to recommend an alternative means of contraception. She admits to menses that are regular in cycle but heavy in flow and oftentimes associated with debilitating dysmenorrhea. She denies smoking, a history of migraines, liver disease, or coagulopathies. On physical examination, she has a BMI of 38 with no abnormal findings on breast or pelvic exams. Which of the following is the best form of contraception for this patient?

A. Copper IUD
B. Medroxyprogesterone acetate (DMPA) 150 mg every 3 months
C. Transdermal patch
D. Vaginal ring

46. Which of the following statements is true with regard to fetal hemoglobin?

A. It is transferred across the placenta.
B. It has a higher affinity for oxygen than adult hemoglobin.
C. It cannot transport oxygen.
D. It is completely replaced by adult hemoglobin within the first 4 weeks of life.

47. In a pregnant, untreated Rh-negative female, erythroblastosis fetalis would most likely occur in which of the following pregnancies?

A. Her first Rh-positive fetus
B. Her first Rh-negative fetus
C. Her second Rh-negative fetus
D. Her second Rh-positive fetus

48. A 66-year-old multiparous female presents to your office because she is concerned about some "light" vaginal bleeding that has happened twice in the past month. She admits to taking hormone replacement therapy for 10 years, but states she stopped taking it 10 years ago. She is treated for hypertension and hypercholesterolemia, which have been well controlled with medication and dietary changes for the past 20 years. Given her presenting complaint, you immediately begin evaluating this patient for which of the following conditions?

A. Ovarian cancer
B. Cervical cancer
C. Endometrial cancer
D. Breast cancer

49. Which of the following organisms produces a preformed toxin that causes toxic shock syndrome?

A. *Staphylococcus aureus*
B. *Chlamydia trachomatis*
C. *Streptococcus pyogenes*
D. *Staphylococcus epidermidis*

50. During labor, the fetal heart rate may show variability in the form of decelerations, which are described as early, late, or variable. Which of the following is the most likely cause of late decelerations?

A. Umbilical cord compression
B. Uteroplacental insufficiency
C. Head compression
D. Fetal movement

ANSWERS

1. **The correct answer is D.** Initial maternal serum alpha-fetoprotein (AFP) screening is performed at 15 to 20 weeks gestation and is useful in detecting nearly 85% of all open neural tube defects. Falsely elevated values may be due to other structural abnormalities, inaccurate gestational age dating, multiple gestation, or fetal demise. False positive levels should be repeated for accuracy and correlated with ultrasound examinations, amniotic fluid AFP, and acetylcholinesterase levels to secure diagnosis. Although low maternal AFP values are found with Down syndrome, chromosomal abnormalities and genetic diseases are better detected with amniocentesis and chorionic villus sampling.

2. **The correct answer is D.** Chorionic villus sampling (CVS) is performed in the first trimester, usually between 10 and 12 weeks gestation, allowing for earlier and safer pregnancy termination in the case of cytogenetic defects. It is more commonly performed transcervically than transabdominally. The transabdominal approach carries about the same miscarriage rate as amniocentesis, whereas the transcervical procedure incurs an increased risk of pregnancy loss over amniocentesis. Benefits include direct, rapid DNA and cytogenic testing, because cytotrophoblasts obtained from first-trimester placentas are more likely to be viable and in metaphase than amniotic cells. Negative aspects of CVS are that it does not diagnose neural tube defects and is associated with distal limb defects.

3. **The correct answer is D.** Oral estrogen replacement therapy for postmenopausal women can increase high-density lipoprotein (HDL) cholesterol and triglycerides and lower low-density lipoprotein (LDL) cholesterol. The World Health Initiative conducted a prospective randomized clinical trial to assess the health effects of estrogen alone and combined estrogen/progestin replacement. When cardiovascular risks exceeded benefits, the combined arm of the study was discontinued. The data revealed that combined hormonal therapy increased the risk of myocardial infarction, stroke, thromboembolic disease, and breast cancer and reduced the risk of colorectal cancer and hip fractures. The estrogen-only arm of the study was later halted because of increased risk of stroke. Signs and symptoms of menopause include hot flashes, vaginal atrophy, and sleep disturbances resulting from decreased production of estradiol-17β by ovarian follicles. Exogenous estrogen therapy may include estradiol-17β and its metabolites estrone and estriol alone or in combination with a synthetic progestin (as in the case of a patient with an intact uterus). Note that unopposed estrogen in a patient with an intact uterus can result in endometrial hyperplasia, placing the patient at increased risk for endometrial carcinoma. Alternative, nonhormonal therapies for menopausal symptoms include soy; black cohosh; selective serotonin reuptake inhibitors (SSRIs); dietary modifications, such as the avoidance of spicy foods, caffeine, and alcohol; and increased aerobic exercise.

4. **The correct answer is B.** The stages of labor are defined as follows:

- First stage: Time between the onset of labor and full cervical dilatation
- Second stage: Time between full cervical dilatation and delivery of the infant
- Third stage: Time between delivery of the infant and delivery of the placenta
- Fourth stage (as listed in some references): The immediate postpartum period, approximately 2 hours after the delivery of the placenta (this stage has the highest risk of maternal hemorrhage)

The first stage of labor is further divided into two phases: latent and active. The latent phase includes the initial indications of labor, such as passage of the mucus plug, cervical effacement, and irregular contractions, leading to slow, early cervical dilatation. Once a patient achieves 4 to 5 cm of dilatation, she enters the active phase. During the active phase, contractions become more frequent with longer, more intense peaks with shorter rest periods and cervical dilatation is accelerated. Mechanisms of labor, also referred to as *cardinal movements of labor*, describe fetal positioning through the birth canal during a vertex delivery. These movements facilitate navigation of the fetal head through the maternal bony pelvis and include the following:

- Engagement
- Flexion
- Descent
- Internal rotation
- Extension
- External rotation

5. **The correct answer is A.** In the United States, a woman's overall cumulative risk of developing breast cancer is one in eight. After gender, her greatest risk factor is advancing age. Other risk factors for the development of breast cancer reflect endogenous/exogenous estrogen exposure, such as early menarche (prior to age 12), nulliparity, late menopause (after age 50), and long-term estrogen replacement. Radiation exposure also places a patient at higher risk. Women with a history of uterine cancer are also at risk for the development of breast cancer, and vice versa. Gene mutation in BRCA genes increase a woman's risk of breast cancer.

6. **The correct answer is A.** In the majority of cases, women with breast cancer initially present with a self-discovered painless mass. Early masses tend to be mobile but develop indistinct borders and become adherent to supporting ligaments and underlying fascia as the cancer advances. Nipple discharge and *peau d'orange* skin changes are usually late findings and carry a poor prognosis. Fibrocystic breast changes (the most common form of benign breast disease) are associated with diffuse bilateral cyclic breast pain and engorgement. Fibroadenomas, another benign breast condition, typically occur in young women and are characterized by a firm, painless, mobile mass, usually measuring between 1 and 3 cm.

7. **The correct answer is D.** Ectopic pregnancy refers to the implantation of the fertilized ovum outside the uterine cavity. Medical management of a small, nonruptured ectopic pregnancy in an asymptomatic patient would include methotrexate therapy. A baseline β-hCG is obtained followed by repeat levels on days 4 and 7. A persistent rise or plateau of β-hCG levels would suggest methotrexate failure and would be managed by either a subsequent dose of methotrexate or surgical treatment. Dilatation and curettage is reserved for the evacuation of uterine products of conception. Ninety-five percent of ectopic gestations occur in the fallopian tubes, with the majority of these occurring in the ampulla. The primary risk factor for ectopic pregnancy is a history of salpingitis. Other risk factors include history of a previous ectopic pregnancy, maternal age over 35 years, multiparity (more than 3 pregnancies), and African American or Hispanic ethnicity. Symptoms include abdominal or pelvic pain resulting from a distended fallopian tube and/or peritoneal irritation caused by the presence of blood. Diagnosis is made by the failure of quantitative β-hCGs to double every 48 hours in conjunction with ultrasonography.

8. **The correct answer is A.** The most common cause of secondary amenorrhea (defined as the absence of menses for more than three cycles or 6 consecutive months in a previously menstruating woman) is pregnancy. Hypothalmic disorders, androgen disorders, and elevated prolactin levels caused by pituitary adenomas, psychogenic disorders (anorexia nervosa), and alterations of the genital outflow tract are other common causes of secondary amenorrhea. The most common *anatomic* cause of secondary amenorrhea is Asherman's syndrome, in which there is scarring of the endometrium.

9. **The correct answer is A.** Painless vaginal bleeding is the hallmark of placenta previa. Placenta previa typically presents as acute onset of painless, profuse, bright red vaginal bleeding after 28 weeks gestation. In placenta previa, the placenta is implanted low within the uterine segment, partially or completely obstructing the presenting fetal part. In vasa previa, the umbilical vessels cross the internal cervical os prior to the presenting part. This presents with sudden onset of vaginal bleeding with fetal tachycardia shortly after the rupture of membranes. An emergent cesarean section is then warranted to prevent fetal exsanguination. Abruptio placenta, the premature separation of a normally implanted placenta after 20 weeks gestation and prior to birth, is characterized by uterine or back pain and either a visible or concealed hemorrhage (when blood is trapped between the uterus and detached placenta). Uterine rupture will also result in painful vaginal bleeding.

10. **The correct answer is A.** Unilateral spontaneous serous or serosanguinous discharge from a single duct is usually caused by an intraductal papilloma and less frequently

by an intraductal carcinoma. Prolactin-producing adenomas produce a milky, bilateral breast discharge. Fibrocytic breast changes in premenopausal women produce spontaneous multiple-duct greenish-brown discharge, which may be unilateral or bilateral, and is most apparent just prior to the onset of menses. Oral contraception may cause a clear, serous, or milky discharge from single or multiple ducts that resolves upon discontinuation of the medication. Purulent discharge from a single breast may suggest a subareolar abscess.

11. **The correct answer is A.** Methyldopa is recommended by many obstetricians as the first-line antihypertensive medication in pregnancy. Labetolol is an alpha-1 adrenergic blocker and a nonselective β-adrenergic blocker that appears to be safe in pregnancy. It is not teratogenic and minimally crosses the placenta. Nifedipine, a calcium-channel blocker, is reported to be safe in pregnancy. However this was not studied as extensively as methyldopa and labetolol. ACE inhibitors are contraindicated in pregnancy, because they are associated with neonatal renal dysfunction. The use of diuretics such as HCTZ and furosemide throughout pregnancy is controversial.

12. **The correct answer is C.** The classic triad for preeclampsia includes hypertension, edema, and proteinuria. Risk factors for the development of preeclampsia include preexisting hypertension, renal disease, diabetes mellitus, multiple gestations, nulliparity, and a positive family history. Recent recommendations are to eliminate edema as a diagnostic criterion for preeclampsia, because it is frequently seen in normotensive pregnancies and is not always present in eclamptic patients. Edema seen in preeclamptic patients is generally persistent after resting supine and involves the upper extremity, face, and sacral area. Additional physical exam findings include hyperreflexia and liver tenderness secondary to hepatic capsular distention. Preeclampsia presenting in the first two semesters should raise suspicion for molar pregnancy or maternal lupus. Once there is an onset of seizures, the patient is eclamptic. The patient may be stabilized with magnesium sulfate, with close maternal and fetal monitoring. Definitive treatment is delivery of the fetus by either induction or cesarean delivery.

13. **The correct answer is A.** Trichomonas vaginitis is characterized by a profuse, frothy, greenish, foul-smelling discharge often accompanied by vaginal pruritis. Diagnosis is confirmed by direct visualization of motile unicellular flagellate protozoa on saline wet mount. FDA-approved treatment is metronidazole for all sexual partners. Bacterial vaginosis, an infection of anaerobic bacteria in combination with *Gardnerella vaginalis*, is characterized by a thin gray-white to yellow discharge that exhibits a musty odor. Mixing bacterial vaginosis vaginal secretions with 10% KOH causes the release of amines detected by a fishy odor, constituting a positive whiff test. Clue cells, which are epithelial cells stippled with bacteria, are visualized microscopically on KOH preparation. Treatment is with metronidazole or clindamycin. Candida vaginitis presents with vaginal pruritis and a thick, white, "cottage cheese" discharge. Diagnosis is confirmed by demonstrating hyphae and budding yeast on saline wet mount. Treatment includes topical imidazoles or oral fluconazole as a 150 mg single dose. Azithromycin and doxycycline are the treatment regimens for *Chlamydia trachomatis* infection, which is implicated in cervicitis and pelvic inflammatory disease.

14. **The correct answer is C.** This patient may be treated as an outpatient because she appears nontoxic with a temperature of <102.2°F (30°C) and is capable of taking oral medications. Treatment should also include removal of her IUD, broad-spectrum antibiotic therapy, analgesics, and bed rest, with close follow-up care. Centers for Disease Control recommendations for treatment of mild to moderately severe acute pelvic inflammatory disease (PID) include a single intramuscular dose of ceftriaxone 250 mg (or other parenteral third-generation cephalosporins; i.e., cefoxitin plus probenicid, ceftizoxime, cefotaxime) and doxycycline 100 mg by mouth twice a day for 14 days with or without

metronidazole 500 mg by mouth twice a day for 14 days. If the patient does not respond within 72 hours on oral therapy, the patient warrants reevaluation and perhaps parenteral therapy. New guidelines no longer favor fluoroquinolone antibiotics as first-line treatment of PID and gonococcal infections due to increasing resistance since 1999.

15. **The correct answer is A.** Physiologic changes seen in pregnancy include increased renal profusion reflected in an increased glomerular filtration rate, increased tidal volume and inspiratory capacity, and increased levels of circulating coagulation factors. Systolic murmurs may result from increased cardiac output and increased blood flow across the aortic and pulmonic valves. Diastolic murmurs are not an expected finding and require further evaluation. Other cardiac exam findings in pregnancy include a loud second heart sound split with inspiration and an S3 gallop in the third trimester. A mammary soufflé is a blowing, continuous, high-pitched functional cardiac murmur heard over the breast in late pregnancy and during lactation due to increased flow through the internal mammary artery.

16. **The correct answer is D.** Rupture of membranes is confirmed with sterile speculum examination looking for evidence of pooling (accumulation of amniotic fluid in the posterior fornix), a positive nitrazine test (amniotic fluid demonstrates an alkaline pH of 7.0 to 7.25, which turns nitrazine paper blue), and ferning (amniotic fluid air-dried on a glass slide forms a fernlike pattern of crystallization). A fetal fibronectin test serves as a predictor assay for preterm delivery in patients with preterm labor. A negative test has a greater predictive value for ruling out delivery within 2 weeks, whereas a positive test lacks sensitivity.

17. **The correct answer is D.** Fetal presentation is not included in the calculation of a Bishop score. Bishop scoring evaluates cervical and pelvic parameters prior to the elective induction of labor. Criteria include cervical consistency, positioning, dilatation, and effacement, as well as fetal station graded in relation to the ischial spines of the pelvis. Points (0, 1, 2, 3) are assigned based on the status of each of these criteria. Fetal presentation is determined by the fetal part that lies lowest in the birth canal and may be assessed with Leopold maneuvers. Leopold maneuvers are a series of four palpations of the fetus through the gravid abdominal wall. They determine fetal lie, presentation, and position. The four Leopold maneuvers are:

- Determine what occupies the fundus.
- Determine the location of small parts of the fetus.
- Identify descent of the presenting part.
- Identify the cephalic prominence.

18. **The correct answer is B.** Myomectomy is the treatment of choice for a symptomatic patient who wishes to preserve fertility. During the second and third trimesters of pregnancy leiomyomas increase rapidly in size, become vascularly deprived, and undergo degenerative changes that can cause an acute painful episode, possibly precipitating preterm labor. Complications of leiomyomas during labor include obstruction of the pelvic outlet and fetal malpresentation. Uterine artery embolization and pharmacologic inhibition of estrogen secretion with gonadotropin-releasing hormone agonist (GnRH) analogues are not recommended in patients who desire future childbearing. Expectant management may result in fibroid growth, inhibiting fertility.

19. **The correct answer is C.** In the postmenopausal patient, the ovaries are less responsive to the effects of gonadotropins. Follicular activity diminishes to essentially none within 3 years. Any palpable ovarian enlargement in a postmenopausal female warrants laparoscopic (surgical) evaluation for ovarian neoplasm. Nearly 25% of all ovarian tumors in postmenopausal women are found to be malignant.

20. **The correct answer is C.** Endometriosis is the implantation of functioning endometrial stroma and glands outside the uterine cavity. Multiple lesions are more common than single implants, with the ovary being the most frequently affected anatomic site. Endometriosis presents with the classic triad of dysmenorrhea, dyspareunia, and infertility, yet approximately 20% of women are asymptomatic. Although an exact cause is unknown, some theories include retrograde menstruation, coelomic metaplasia, and vascular lymphatic dissemination. Laparoscopy provides direct visualization of lesions and tissue biopsy for a definitive diagnosis. Lesions vary in gross appearance from red petechiae to darkly pigmented "powder burn" implants. Pelvic ultrasound, CT, and MRI cannot definitely make the diagnosis of endometriosis.

21. **The correct answer is A.** Hormonal therapy is directed against the stimulation and bleeding of the endometrial tissue and disease progression and includes oral contraceptives, progestins, danazol, and gonadotropin-releasing hormone. Danazol and the aromatase inhibitors serve to create a hypoestrogenic environment. NSAIDs provide mild relief of cyclic pelvic pain. Although surgical ablation alone also provides symptomatic relief, it carries a probable risk of reoccurrence. Definitive treatment is total abdominal hysterectomy with bilateral salpingo-oophorectomy with ablation and excision of residual lesions and secondary adhesions.

22. **The correct answer is A.** Syphilis is a chronic systemic illness caused by the spirochete *Treponema pallidum*. It is most often transmitted by sexual contact. It is called the "great masquerader" because of its wide variety of clinical presentations. After an incubation period of approximately 21 days from the time of exposure, the primary lesion appears at the site of inoculation. It begins as a small, painless papule that ulcerates into a chancre with firm, indurate borders. The chancre lasts about 2 to 6 weeks and then spontaneously resolves. The secondary stage then ensues, which is marked by fever, malaise, headache, lymphadenopathy, and a mucocutaneous rash. The rash is diffuse and includes the palms and soles, yet spares the face, with the exception of the perioral area. In warm, moist areas, papules coalesce to form condyloma lata, which are highly infectious, because they are loaded with spirochetes. These lesions also spontaneously resolve after a few weeks, and the infected individual then enters a latency stage. The third stage is characterized by neurologic and cardiac manifestations. The spirochete can be identified by darkfield microscopy, direct immunofluorescent techniques, silver stains, and PCR (polymerase chain reaction). Serologic testing is divided into nontreponemal tests (RPR, VDRL, USR, and TRUST) and the confirmatory treponemal tests (FTA-ABS, MHA-TP). Parenteral penicillin G is the drug of choice for all stages of syphilis. Doxycycline is an acceptable alternative treatment in patients who are allergic to penicillin.

23. **The correct answer is C.** The menstrual cycle is divided into the follicular (proliferative) and luteal (secretory) phases. Variation in menstrual cycle length is due to fluctuations in the proliferative phase of the uterine cycle, which can vary the time of ovulation. The secretory phase (time from ovulation to onset of menses, if the egg remains unfertilized) remains relatively constant at about 14 days. Therefore, if fertilization does not occur a woman should expect onset of menses 12 to 16 days after ovulation. After ovulation, the human ovum is only available for fertilization for up to 24 hours. Sperm are able to fertilize the ovum up to 48 hours after coitus. Although sperm may only last a few hours in the acidic environment of the vagina, they may remain for days within the cervical mucus. Human pregnancy normally lasts 40 weeks from the last normal menstrual period (LNMP). Mathematical calculation of the estimated date of delivery (EDD) is performed using Nägele's rule: LNMP – 3 months + 7 days (added to the first day of the LNMP).

24. **The correct answer is C.** Treatment of a Bartholin gland abscess includes incision and establishment of an opening to facilitate drainage. A Word catheter is a short catheter with an inflatable balloon tip. The balloon is inflated in the abscess cavity and is left in

place for a few weeks to promote epithelialization of the drainage tract. Marsupialization provides a larger incision to secure drainage. Excision of the cyst is recommended in recurrent cases and in the postmenopausal patient. Incision and drainage, irrigation, and antibiotic therapy alone result in recurrent infection.

25. **The correct answer is B.** Herpes simplex virus (HSV) is a DNA virus with two serotypes. Although most cases of genital herpes are caused by HSV-2, increasing numbers of cases are caused by HSV-1. Asymptomatic viral shedding can be a source of infection. Primary infection is accompanied by systemic symptoms such as fever, malaise, and inguinal adenopathy and is generally more severe than recurrent outbreaks. Dermatologic manifestations include prodromal localized burning at the site of inoculation followed by eruption of grouped vesicles that progress to painful ulcerations. Treatment of primary and recurrent infections, as well as daily suppressive therapy, includes antivirals, such as acyclovir, valacyclovir, and famciclovir. Benzathine penicillin G is used to treat syphilis. Azithromycin is used to treat genital infections caused by *Chlamydia trachomatis*. Imiquimod cream is employed in the treatment of genital warts due to human papillomavirus.

26. **The correct answer is A.** Lymphogranuloma venereum is a sexually transmitted disease caused by *Chlamydia trachomatis*. The first manifestation of infection is a painless vesicle that ulcerates and disappears in 2 to 3 days, often going unnoticed. Inguinal lymphadenopathy develops in 1 to 3 weeks following the initial lesion, progressing to bubo formation. Diagnosis can be made with culture, but serologic testing (complement-fixation tests) is more commonly employed, with LGV titers above 1:64 confirming diagnosis. Recommended treatment is azithromycin or doxycycline for 21 days.

27. **The correct answer is C.** Lichen sclerosis is a common benign chronic inflammatory dermatologic disorder that presents in the non-hair-bearing areas of the vulva, perineum, and perianal regions. The skin typically becomes thin and white with decreased elasticity. In time the epithelium becomes hyperkeratotic and atrophied. High-potency steroidal creams, such as clobetasol, are most effective in the symptomatic treatment of lichen sclerosis. The condition does not predispose the patient to the development of malignant lesions. Atrophic vaginitis may occur as a result of a lack of estrogen. It can cause dyspareunia secondary to vaginal dryness. In the absence of estrogen, the vaginal mucosa becomes thin, pale, and transparent, with loss of normal rugae. Symptoms of atrophic vaginitis respond to either topical or oral hormonal replacement. Clotrimazole is the treatment for *Candida* vaginitis.

28. **The correct answer is A.** Smoking is this patient's greatest risk factor for the development of osteoporosis. Osteoporosis is defined by the World Health Organization as a T-score of less than 2.5 on bone densitometry. A T-score of −1.0 to −2.5 denotes osteopenia, or low bone mass. Peak bone mass is achieved in the third decade of life. In postmenopausal patients, the amount of bone resorption by osteoclasts exceeds the amount of new bone formed by osteoblasts. Hormones, such as parathyroid hormone, that stimulates osteoclast resorption, and calcitonin, which inhibits osteoclast resorption, have active roles in blood calcium regulation. Risk factors for the development of osteoporosis include female gender, Caucasian race, advancing age, positive family history, hyperthyroidism, small stature, and cigarette smoking. Osteoporosis can result in increased fracture risk, with vertebral, hip, and wrist fractures occurring in order of frequency. Treatment includes calcium supplementation with a suggested dose of 1,200 to 1,500 mg of calcium per day for a postmenopausal female. Calcium supplements are best taken in three divided doses after meals to enhance absorption. Vitamin D is also prescribed at doses of 400 to 800 IU a day. Bisphosphanates are considered first-line antiresorptive therapy and are prescribed with stringent dosing instructions to prevent the development of esophagitis. Calcitonin and selective estrogen receptor modulators are treatment options in certain patients.

29. The correct answer is D. Urge incontinence, or overactive bladder, is suggested by urinary frequency accompanied by a strong sensation of impending urinary leakage. Conservative treatment includes behavioral modification, such as bladder training, timed voiding, and Kegel exercises. Because acetylcholine is the primary neurotransmitter involved in bladder contraction, pharmacologic treatment of overactive bladder includes agents that exert an anticholinergic effect. Pessaries are used to treat cystoceles. Self-catheterization is reserved for patients with a neurogenic bladder or postvoid residuals. Surgical correction is considered in cases of bladder prolapse.

30. The correct answer is D. Galactorrhea is lactation in the absence of nursing. Pituitary adenomas secrete prolactin and may also co-secrete growth hormone, leading to acromegaly. Patients with primary hypothyroidism often have an increase in thyroid-releasing hormone (TRH). TRH stimulates the release of prolactin from the pituitary gland and promotes the release of thyroid hormone from the thyroid gland. Molar pregnancy (hydatidiform mole) is a type of gestational trophoblastic disease; it can be complete or partial. A complete molar pregnancy develops when a sperm fertilizes an empty ovum, resulting only in placental development, which produces β-hCG. An incomplete or partial molar pregnancy occurs when two sperm fertilize a single ovum, causing an abnormal embryo and placenta. Galactorrhea is not a symptom of molar pregnancy.

31. The correct answer is C. Initial screening for gestational diabetes during pregnancy includes a 1-hour, 50-gram oral glucose load challenge between 24 and 28 weeks gestation. If the glucose level is greater than 130 mg/dl at 1 hour, then a 3-hour glucose-tolerance test is indicated using a 100-gram oral glucose load. The American Diabetes Association bases the diagnostic criteria for gestational diabetes on two abnormal results on the 3-hour, 100-gram oral glucose-tolerance test, with normal values as follows: fasting, 95 mg/dl; 1 hour, 180 mg/dl; 2 hour, 155 mg/dl; and 3 hour, 140 mg/dl. Appropriate treatment for this patient is carbohydrate restriction and a caloric intake of 1,800 to 2,400 kcal/day to improve glycemic control. Insulin therapy would be initiated only if the patient could not meet targeted goals with diet modification and exercise alone.

32. The correct answer is C. Mastitis, or cellulitis of the breast, occurs in the first few weeks to months in the postpartum period. Patients present with localized areas of breast erythema and pain. Causative organisms include *Staphylococcus*, *Streptococcus*, and *Escherichia coli*. The treatment of infectious mastitis includes antibiotics, analgesics, local heat, and breast support. Breastfeeding should be continued to promote breast emptying. Only if there is suspicion of an abscess should breastfeeding be discontinued.

33. The correct answer is D. Cancer antigen 125 (CA-125) is a tumor marker used to support the diagnosis of ovarian cancer, monitor response to treatment, and survey for reoccurrence. Elevated levels greater than 35 U/ml are seen in conditions that affect the peritoneum, such as cirrhosis, pancreatitis, endometriosis, pelvic inflammatory disease, and pregnancy. Elevated levels are not an indication of hepatocellular carcinoma. Alpha-fetoprotein is a tumor marker used to detect hepatomas; CA19-19 monitors hepatobiliary carcinomas. Carcinoembryonic antigen is elevated in patients with colorectal cancer, but it is not a good screening tool for this malignancy.

34. The correct answer is D. During menopause, levels of both FSH (follicle-stimulating hormone) and LH (luteinizing hormone) rise. FSH levels rise in response to decreasing estradiol secretion by the ovaries. FSH has a slower clearance from the bloodstream and therefore maintains higher levels than seen with LH.

35. The correct answer is A. A patient who is nulliparous with a previous history of breast cancer is most at risk for the development of endometrial carcinoma. Perimenopausal spotting, abnormal bleeding in the first few months after starting oral contraception, and irregular menstrual cycles in the first few years after menarche are normal findings in healthy females.

36. **The correct answer is D.** A reactive or reassuring nonstress test (NST) is defined as normal with two or more fetal heart accelerations with movements over 20 minutes. These accelerations should exceed 15 beats per minute above baseline and last at least 15 seconds. A reactive NST suggests that the fetus is not neurologically compromised or in an acidotic state.

37. **The correct answer is A.** These flesh-colored, dome-shaped, pearly, umbilicated lesions are most representative of molluscum contagiosum due to poxvirus. Condylomata latum are moist papules filled with spirochetes that appear during the second stage of syphilis. Condylomata acuminata (genital warts) appear as cauliflower-like lesions that generally coalesce. The lesions associated with herpes simplex infection are typically painful grouped vesicles.

38. **The correct answer is B.** Initial evaluation of cervical dysplasia would include colposcopy and biopsy of suspicious lesions. Dilation and curettage is of no value. Cone biopsy is performed to assess the degree of invasion if the initial biopsy proves positive. Repeating the Pap smear in 6 months is not a prudent option for an advancing CIN II lesion.

39. **The correct answer is A.** Hydatidiform mole represents an abnormal pregnancy in which the uterus is distended with grapelike vesicles in the absence of a fetus or gestational sac. Diagnosis is made by serial quantitative β-hCG levels and ultrasound. It should be suspected in any pregnancy that reports bleeding in the first half of the pregnancy, hyperemesis gravidarum, uterine size larger than expected for gestation age, and the onset of preeclampsia prior to 24 weeks gestation.

40. **The correct answer is B.** This is the classical presentation of adenomyosis. The patient presentation in answer A would raise suspicion for endometriosis. Answer C describes an irregular bulky uterus found with uterine fibroids. The patient profile in D would require further evaluation for endometrial cancer.

41. **The correct answer is C.** The Apgar score is a means of quantitatively evaluating a newborn's status after birth. Scores ranging from 0 to 2 are assigned based on the assessment of five categories that reflect the newborn's cardiorespiratory and neurologic condition. Total scores are obtained at 1 and 5 minutes after birth. The mnemonic APGAR (actually named by Virginia Apgar, MD [anesthesiologist and pediatrician] in 1952) stands for *a*ctivity (muscle tone), *p*ulse (heart rate), *g*rimace (reflex irritability), *a*ppearance (skin color), and *r*espiration (crying). Scoring criteria follow:

Heart rate: 0, absent; 1, slow (<100 bpm); 2, >100 bpm

Respirations: 0, absent; 1, slow, irregular; 2, good, crying

Muscle tone: 0, limp; 1, some flexion of extremities; 2, active motion

Reflex irritability: 0, nonresponsive to stimulus; 1, grimace; 2, cough or crying

Color: 0, blue, pale; 1, body pink with blue extremities; 2, completely pink

42. **The correct answer is B.** Diabetes mellitus predisposes a patient to recurrent *Candida* vaginitis. Women with diabetes have an increased glucose concentration in vaginal secretions and an alteration in the body's immune defenses.

43. **The correct answer is A.** *Threatened* abortion is defined as vaginal spotting or bleeding prior to the 20th completed week of gestation without cervical dilatation or passage of the products of conception. It may or may not be accompanied by uterine contractions. In an *inevitable* abortion the cervix is dilated and the membranes may have ruptured, but the products of conception have not passed. In a *complete* abortion, the fetus and placenta are expelled prior to the 20th completed week of gestation. Patients may have some residual spotting, but pain and heavy bleeding usually resolve. In an *incomplete* abortion, bleeding persists as only some, but not all, the products of conception pass

an open cervical os. Incomplete abortions generally occur between 6 and 14 weeks gestation. *Missed* abortion is fetal demise prior to 20 weeks without expulsion of the conceptus. Missed abortion may be treated with laminaria insertion, which serves to dilate the cervix, followed by an aspiration procedure. Misoprostol, a prostaglandin vaginal suppository, can also be used to promote labor and cervical ripening.

44. **The correct answer is D.** Polycystic ovarian syndrome (PCOS), or Stein-Leventhal syndrome, presents with hirsutism, truncal obesity, amenorrhea or oligomenorrhea, infertility, and insulin resistance. Polycystic ovaries appear in a classic "string of pearls" appearance on ultrasound. Lab findings in patients with PCOS are increased androgen levels, such as DHEAS, increased LH/FSH ratios, lipid abnormalities, and hyperglycemia.

45. **The correct answer is B.** Medroxyprogesterone injection is the preferred method of contraception for this patient because it does not increase her risk for arterial or venous disease. Although early studies revealed an average 5-pound yearly weight gain with depot medroxyprogesterone acetate (DMPA) after 1 year of use, recent randomized trials discount this associated weight gain. The copper IUD would not be wise in a patient with a history of ectopic pregnancy, because the rate of ectopic to intrauterine pregnancies is higher in patients with IUDs. The transdermal patch has decreased efficacy in patients over 90 kg due to diminished absorption. Vaginal rings need to be inserted high into the vagina, which may prove to be difficult for this patient to self-insert.

46. **The correct answer is B.** The umbilical cord contains two arteries and one vein. Oxygenated blood is carried to the fetus via the umbilical vein from the placenta. The major hemoglobin of the fetus from 8 weeks gestation to term is fetal hemoglobin, or hemoglobin F. Fetal hemoglobin is composed of four heme groups and four globin (two alpha and two gamma) chains. Fetal hemoglobin has a greater affinity for oxygen than adult hemoglobin. Hemoglobin F is essentially replaced by adult hemoglobin by 12 weeks after delivery.

47. **The correct answer is D.** Hemolytic disease of the newborn (erythroblastosis fetalis) may be caused by antibodies directed against any of the blood group antigens with anti-Rh_o(D) the most clinically significant. If a Rh_o(D)-negative woman carries a Rh_o(D)-positive fetus and fetal cells pass into the maternal circulation, then the mother could become sensitized and produce antibody to Rh_o(D) antigen. Fetal cells can enter the mother's circulation during the third trimester or during delivery. Other causes of fetomaternal bleeding can occur as a result of spontaneous or induced abortion, amniocentesis, ectopic pregnancy, or abruption placentae. Anti-Rh_o (D) usually causes no harm to the fetus during the first pregnancy. This antibody, once produced, remains in the maternal circulation and can cross the placenta and present a threat to Rh-positive fetuses in subsequent pregnancies. Rh_o(D) immune globulin provides passive immunity by coating and destroying the fetal cells, thus shielding them from the mother's immune system and preventing antibody production. As a routine precaution, a Rh_o(D)-negative mother will receive Rh_o(D) immune globulin at 28 weeks gestation, even if the antigen status of the fetus is unknown. Another vial is administered to the mother within 72 hours after delivery.

The Kleihauer-Betke test is used to estimate the amount of fetal cells in the maternal circulation. A blood sample is drawn from the mother, and the red blood cells undergo an acid elution. Fetal red blood cells are resistant to the acid and remain pink, whereas maternal red blood cells are susceptible to the acid and appear clear. This estimate can provide valuable information about the extent of the bleed and determine the amount of immune globulin required. One vial contains 300 mcg of Rh_o(D) immune globulin.

48. **The correct answer is C.** A postmenopausal female who experiences vaginal bleeding warrants evaluation for endometrial cancer, because this is the most common presenting symptom.

49. The correct answer is A. Toxic shock syndrome is caused by a preformed toxin produced by *Staphylococcus aureus*. Toxin production requires a neutral pH and an aerobic environment. Investigations by the Centers for Disease Control (CDC) correlated the syndrome with the use of superabsorbent tampon use. The clinical course is characterized by the acute onset of fever, hypotension, vomiting, watery diarrhea, headache, myalgias, and sore throat. It is accompanied by a diffuse, macular, erythematous rash over the face, trunk, and proximal extremities, eventually leading to desquamation of the entire skin, including palms and soles.

50. The correct answer is B. Late decelerations in the fetal heart rate suggest fetal hypoxemia secondary to uteroplacental insufficiency. Early decelerations are due to head compressions resulting from uterine contractions. Variable decelerations are usually related to cord compressions.

REFERENCES

Armstrong, C. (2007). ACS Recommendations on MRI and Mammography for Breast Cancer Screening. *American Family Physician*, 75(11): 1715–1716.

Beckman, C. R. B., Ling, F. W., Laube, D. W., Smith, R. P., Barzansky, B. M., and Herbert, W. N. P. (2006). *Obstetrics and gynecology*, 5th ed. Lippincott Williams & Wilkins, Philadelphia, PA.

Barton, J. R. (2008). Hypertension in pregnancy. *Annals of Emergency Medicine*, 51(3 Suppl): S16–S17.

Centers for Disease Control (CDC). (2007). Updated recommended treatment regimens for gonococcal infections and associated conditions—United States, April 2007. (Online). Available at www.cdc.gov/std/treatment/2006/updated-regimens.htm.

DeCherney, A. H., Nathan, L., Goodwin, T. M., and Laufer, N. (2007). *Current diagnosis and treatment obstetrics and gynecology*, 10th ed. McGraw-Hill Companies, New York.

Gass, M., and Dawson-Hughes, B. (2006). Preventing osteoporosis-related fractures: An overview. *American Journal of Medicine*, 119(4 Suppl 1): S3–S11.

Goldman, L., and Ausiello, D. (2008). *Cecil medicine*, 23rd ed. Saunders Elsevier, Philadelphia, PA.

Miltenburg, D. M., and Speights, V. O. (2008). Benign breast disease. *Obstetrics and Gynecology Clinicians of North America*, 35(2): 285–300.

Mukul, L. V., and Teal, S. B. (2007). Current management of ectopic pregnancy. *Obstetrics and Gynecology Clinicians of North America*, 34(3): 403–419.

Norton, M. E., Hopkins, L. M., Pena, S., Krantz, D., and Caughey, A. B. (2007). First-trimester combined screening: Experience with an instant results approach. *American Journal of Obstetrics and Gynecology*, 196(6): 606.e1–606.e5.

Sakornbut, E., Leeman, L., and Fontaine, P. (2007). Late pregnancy bleeding. *American Family Physician*, 75(8): 1199–1206.

Setji, T. L., and Brown, A. J. (2007). Polycystic ovary syndrome: Diagnosis and treatment. *American Journal of Medicine*, 120(2): 128–132.

Singletary, S. E. (2003). Rating the risk factors for breast cancer. *Annals of Surgery*, 237(4): 474–482.

Swea, A., Hacker, T. W., and Nuovo, J. (1999). Interpretation of electronic fetal heart rate during labor. *American Family Physician*, 59(9): 2487–2500.

Thorneycroft, I. H., Lindsay, R., and Pickar, J. H. (2007). Body composition during treatment with conjugated estrogens with and without medroxyprogesterone acetate: Analysis of the women's health, osteoporosis, progestin, estrogen (HOPE) trial. *American Journal of Obstetrics Gynecology*, 197: 137.e1–137.e7.

Wagner, L. K. (2004). Diagnosis and management of preeclampsia. *American Family Physician*, 70(12): 2317–2324.

Pediatrics

Keith Herzog, MD

1. The HIB vaccine is composed of which of the following?
    A. Inactivated organisms
    B. Live, attenuated virus
    C. A toxoid
    D. A protein–polysaccharide conjugate

2. Which of the following is an absolute contraindication to administering the DtaP vaccine?
    A. A child with an ear infection and fever of 101°F who otherwise appears to be well
    B. A history of inconsolable crying for 2 hours after a DtaP on a previous visit
    C. Allergic reaction to the vaccine on a previous dose
    D. A history of a cousin who had a bad reaction to the same vaccine

3. A 1-year-old child adopted from Russia comes to you for the first time. The adoptive parents are unable to provide the child's immunization records. Which of the following would be the most appropriate management of this child?
    A. Give as many (age-appropriate) vaccines as possible on the first visit.
    B. Defer vaccination until records are available.
    C. Defer vaccination if the child has symptoms of an upper respiratory tract infection.
    D. Send serum for antibody titers to assess immune status before giving any vaccines.

4. Which of the following are significant sources of ongoing pertussis transmission?
    A. Young infants who are unimmunized
    B. Adolescents and young adults
    C. Elderly patients
    D. Contaminated surfaces in the rooms of infected patients

5. A 3-year-old child presents with a chief complaint of sore throat. She also has a fever of 102°F, a runny nose, a hacking cough, and hoarseness. Several family members have similar symptoms. Which of the following is the most likely etiologic agent for her symptoms?
    A. Group A *Streptococcus*
    B. Epstein-Barr virus
    C. Adenovirus
    D. *Mycoplasma pneumoniae*

6. Which of the following is typically the most important clue to the diagnosis of otitis media?
    A. Red tympanic membrane
    B. Lack of sharp light reflex
    C. Impaired mobility of the tympanic membrane by insufflation
    D. Fever

Pediatrics

7. Which of the following would help differentiate sinusitis from an uncomplicated cold in children?
   A. Sinus transillumination
   B. Fever for 1 day
   C. Mucoid rhinorrhea
   D. Runny nose for longer than 10 days

8. A 2-year-old child presents with a 2-day history of temperature of 101°F, runny nose, and "noisy breathing." Examination reveals an alert child in mild respiratory distress with stridor when agitated. He is able to drink without difficulty. Which of the following is the most likely cause of this illness?
   A. Epiglottitis caused by *Haemophilus influenzae* type B
   B. Bacterial tracheitis caused by *Staphylococcus aureus*
   C. Viral laryngotracheobronchitis (croup) caused by parainfluenza
   D. Peritonsillar abscess caused by Group A *Streptococcus*

9. An 8-year-old boy presents with fever and sore throat for 3 days that has become much worse over the last 24 hours and is most severe on the left side. On examination, he is febrile, ill appearing, and drooling, but is not in respiratory distress. Which of the following is the most likely diagnosis?
   A. Croup (viral laryngotracheobronchitis)
   B. Peritonsillar abscess
   C. Epiglottitis
   D. Bacterial tracheitis

10. Which of the following is the most common cause of failure to thrive in an infant?
    A. Nutritional deprivation
    B. Cystic fibrosis
    C. Cerebral palsy
    D. Inflammatory bowel disease

11. Which of the following developmental milestones would you expect to see in a healthy 7-month-old infant?
    A. Feeds self
    B. Follows one step verbal commands
    C. Rolls from back to stomach
    D. Uses pincer grasp

12. Why should table (cow's) milk not be introduced into a child's diet until 12 months of age?
    A. Cow's milk contains too much fat for infants.
    B. Infants are frequently lactose intolerant.
    C. Cow's milk contains levels of vitamin D that are toxic to infants.
    D. Consumption of cow's milk can result in iron deficiency.

13. Which of the following should be the first step in evaluating a child with speech delay?
    A. Hearing evaluation
    B. Referral to a speech therapist
    C. Psychology referral
    D. Anticipatory guidance

311

14. Which of the following is the most common cause of jaundice appearing on day 2 or 3 of life?

   A. Physiologic jaundice
   B. Hemolytic disease of the newborn
   C. Biliary atresia
   D. Hepatitis

15. Which of the following is the most common cause of cardiac arrest in children?

   A. Myocardial infarction
   B. Poisoning
   C. Trauma to the chest
   D. Respiratory failure

16. Which of the following statements is FALSE regarding idiopathic scoliosis?

   A. It is more commonly diagnosed in adolescent females
   B. Thoracic dextroscoliosis is the most common type
   C. In curvatures of 30° or more, rib cage deformity may be evident
   D. Curvatures > 40° require corrective bracing

17. A previously well, afebrile 18-month-old child who presents with an abrupt onset of respiratory distress is most likely to have which of the following?

   A. Croup
   B. Epiglottitis
   C. Foreign-body aspiration
   D. Bacterial pneumonia

18. A febrile 2-year-old child with respiratory distress and diffuse crackles/rales most likely has which of the following?

   A. Tuberculosis
   B. Viral pneumonia
   C. Bacterial pneumonia
   D. *Mycoplasma pneumonia*

19. Which of the following is the most likely cause of chronic cough in a 10-year-old child?

   A. Tuberculosis
   B. Whooping cough
   C. Asthma
   D. Foreign-body obstruction

20. Which of the following is considered to be the most ominous finding in a patient with severe asthma?

   A. Persistent cough despite albuterol and steroid therapy
   B. A respiratory rate of 30 breaths per minute
   C. Both inspiratory and expiratory wheezing
   D. Altered mental status

21. The chest x-ray of a patient with bacterial pneumonia usually reveals which of the following?

   A. Diffuse bilateral patchy infiltrates
   B. Multiple lobes of one lung involved
   C. Single lobe total or partial consolidation
   D. Reticulonodular infiltrates

22. Which of the following is the most appropriate treatment for bronchitis in children?

    A. ampicillin
    B. Supportive care
    C. erythromycin
    D. corticosteroids

23. Which of the following physical examination findings is most helpful in differentiating Lyme disease from another bacterial infection of the knee?

    A. The size of the effusion is usually smaller in Lyme disease.
    B. Warmth of the joint is less frequent in Lyme disease.
    C. The degree of disability/limitation of range of motion is usually less in Lyme disease.
    D. Point tenderness is absent in Lyme disease.

24. A 4-year-old child presents with complaints of fever, medial knee pain, and a limp. However, the physical examination reveals full range of motion of the knee, with no effusion or bony tenderness. Which of the following is the most likely diagnosis?

    A. Osteomyelitis of the distal femur or proximal tibia
    B. Bacterial arthritis of the knee
    C. Toxic synovitis or bacterial arthritis of the hip
    D. An occult fracture of the distal femur or proximal tibia

25. A 7-year-old child falls off his bike and scrapes his knee but gets up and resumes biking. Three days after the accident he presents to the emergency department with a 36-hour history of a temperature of 102°F, a swollen knee, and markedly decreased range of motion. Which of the following would be the most appropriate first step in the management of this patient?

    A. Apply an ACE compression wrap, keep the leg elevated, and give ibuprofen.
    B. Obtain a complete blood count and blood culture and begin cephalexin.
    C. Obtain a Lyme titer and begin amoxicillin.
    D. Aspirate joint fluid for gram stain and culture as well as cell count.

26. Which of the following is the most common predisposing condition in children with a first urinary tract infection (UTI)?

    A. Close contact with another child with a UTI
    B. Poor perineal hygiene
    C. Structurally abnormal kidneys demonstrated on ultrasound
    D. Vesicoureteral reflux demonstrated on cystourethrogram

27. An 18-month-old child presents with a fever of 104°F for 6 days without localizing signs or symptoms except for poorly described abdominal pain. Examination reveals mild left side abdominal tenderness, but no rebound. Which of the following would be the most appropriate component of further evaluation?

    A. Obtain a rectal swab for routine stool culture.
    B. Consult the surgical service to rule out appendicitis.
    C. Obtain a catheterized urinalysis and urine culture.
    D. Order an abdominal obstruction series.

28. Which of the following would be the most reliable laboratory indicator of urinary tract infection?

    A. Urine dipstick for leukocyte esterase and nitrites
    B. Urine culture
    C. Urine gram stain
    D. Microscopic urinalysis

29. Which of the following organisms is the most common cause of community-acquired (vs. hospital-associated) urinary tract infections (UTIs) in the United States?

    A. *Enterococcus faecalis*
    B. *Pseudomonas aeruginosa*
    C. *Escherichia coli*
    D. *Staphylococcus aureus*

30. A 2-week-old infant presents to the emergency department with a 12-hour history of listlessness and poor feeding with no other localizing symptoms; specifically, she has had no upper respiratory symptoms or vomiting or diarrhea. On physical examination, she has a temperature of 103°F rectally, a heart rate of 200 beats per minute, and a respiratory rate of 60 breaths per minute. She has decreased tone and poor perfusion. The physical examination is otherwise unrevealing. Which of the following is the most likely underlying reason for this child's symptoms?

    A. Severe dehydration with hypovolemic shock
    B. Heart failure with cardiogenic shock
    C. Child abuse
    D. Sepsis

31. Which of the following is the proper sequence of events for emergency management of an infant with septic shock?

    A. Provide antibiotics, fluids, and oxygen and consider endotracheal intubation.
    B. Give oxygen, consider endotracheal intubation, obtain venous access for IV fluid support, obtain a blood culture, and provide antibiotics.
    C. Obtain a blood culture, a urine culture, and a spinal fluid sample; give antibiotics; and provide IV fluids.
    D. Obtain a CT scan of the head and a chest x-ray, supply oxygen, and give furosemide.

32. Which of the following is the most likely cause of bacterial sepsis in a neonate?

    A. Group B *Streptococcus*
    B. *Streptococcus pneumoniae*
    C. *Haemophilus influenzae*
    D. *Neisseria meningitidis*

33. Which of the following is a late sign of septic shock in an infant?

    A. Increased heart rate
    B. Decreased systolic blood pressure
    C. Increased respiratory rate
    D. Irritability or lethargy

34. Which of the following is the most common cause of meningitis in infants and children?

    A. Enterovirus
    B. *Streptococcus pneumoniae*
    C. Adenovirus
    D. *Neisseria meningitidis*

35. Which of the following cerebrospinal (CSF) findings would be most suggestive of viral (aseptic) meningitis?

    A. WBC of 1,400 with 90% polys, 3 RBC, protein 210, glucose 20
    B. WBC of 6 with 10% polys, 90% lymphocytes, RBC 42,000, protein 100, glucose 60
    C. WBC of 2 with 10% polys, 90% lymphocytes, 10 RBC, protein 23, glucose 74
    D. WBC of 390 with 30% polys, 70% lymphocytes, 20 RBC, protein 76, glucose 80

36. A 6 lb 10 oz full-term infant is born to a G1P1 female without pregnancy complications. The infant is discharged to home in good condition with a "normal" physical exam. At 4 weeks, the infant presents with a 1-week history of progressively worsening feeding, increased work of breathing, and poor color. On examination, the infant is afebrile but has increased heart rate and respiratory rate with increased work of breathing. A 5/6 harsh holosystolic murmur is now heard. This child most likely has which of the following congenital heart defects?

A. Small atrial septal defect
B. Large ventricular septal defect
C. Mitral valve prolapse
D. Transposition of the great vessels

37. Which of the following is the most significant sequelae of Kawasaki disease?

A. Renal dysfunction
B. Coronary artery aneurysms
C. Hepatitis
D. Adenopathy

38. Which of the following typically signifies a pathologic heart murmur in an infant?

A. It has a vibratory quality.
B. It is 2/6 in intensity.
C. It is holosystolic.
D. It is best heard in the back and both axillae.

39. In a child presenting with syncope, which of the following historic findings would be *most* indicative of cardiac problems?

A. Past history of a murmur
B. Family history of a grandmother who died at age 87 of a heart attack
C. Syncope when standing up quickly
D. Syncope with exercise

40. Which of the following findings in a child should raise concern about coarctation of the aorta?

A. Pulsus paradoxus
B. Widened pulse pressure
C. A 2/6 murmur at the left sternal border
D. O_2 saturation (pulse oximetry) markedly higher in the upper extremity than the lower extremity

41. A 12-year-old child with cystic fibrosis with very few hospitalizations presents with 2 weeks of increasing exercise intolerance, cough, and low-grade fever. Which of the following is the most likely explanation for these symptoms?

A. Pneumonia due to *Moraxella catarrhalis*
B. Cardiac failure due to pulmonary hypertension
C. Bronchopneumonia due to *Pseudomonas aeruginosa*
C. Malabsorption, leading to hypoalbuminemia and secondary pulmonary edema

42. An 18-month-old child with sickle-cell disease (hemoglobin S) presents with 3 days of a runny nose and a temperature of 101.5°F. Which of the following is the best management approach for this patient?

A. Treat with cold and cough preparation and follow-up in the morning.
B. Perform appropriate cultures and begin empiric intravenous antibiotics in the hospital.
C. Prescribe amoxicillin and follow-up first thing in the morning.
D. Prescribe around-the-clock acetaminophen and ibuprofen (alternating) to manage the fever.

43. A 3-year-old child presents with a 3- to 4-week history of poorly localized pain in the upper and lower extremities and back along with a low-grade temperature (maximum of 101°F). Physical examination reveals a temperature of 100.4°F; a pulse of 150 beats per minute, regular; and a respiration of 30 breaths per minute. The child appears tired and pale, and further examination reveals lymphadenopathy and hepatosplenomegaly. Which of the following would be the most appropriate initial evaluation in this patient?

   A. A bone scan to evaluate for osteomyelitis
   B. A complete blood count and bone marrow aspirate to rule out leukemia
   C. A CT of the abdomen to evaluate the hepatosplenomegaly
   D. Liver-associated enzymes to assess for hepatitis

44. A 6-month-old child presents with 12 hours of colicky abdominal pain and vomiting that has recently become bilious; there is no fever or diarrhea. Which of the following is the most appropriate initial presumptive assessment?

   A. Viral gastroenteritis
   B. Intestinal obstruction
   C. Urinary tract infection
   D. *Salmonella typhii* infection

45. Which of the following is the most common identifiable cause of gastroenteritis in childhood?

   A. *Salmonella*
   B. Enterovirus
   C. Rotavirus
   D. *Campylobacter*

46. A 5-week-old infant presents with 2 days of vomiting that has increased over the last 24 hours. The vomit is not bilious or bloody. On physical examination, the abdomen is full, but soft. Mucous membranes are tacky. Electrolytes reveal a hypochloremic, hypokalemic metabolic alkalosis. X-ray results are shown below. Which of the following is the most likely diagnosis?

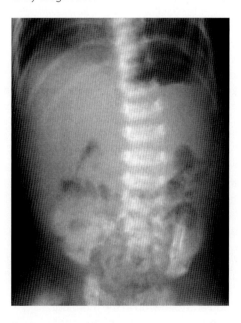

   A. Intussusception
   B. Urinary tract infection
   C. Pyloric stenosis
   D. Incarcerated inguinal hernia

47. A 9-year-old girl presents with 36 hours of abdominal pain that began in the mid-abdomen and now has migrated to the right side. She has had vomiting after the onset of pain, and the most recent episode is bilious. She now has a temperature of 101°F. She prefers to lie motionless, and her abdomen is tender on the right side with rebound tenderness. Which of the following is the most likely diagnosis?

A. Intussusception
B. Urinary tract infection
C. Appendicitis
D. Pelvic inflammatory disease

ANSWERS

1. **The correct answer is D.** Vaccines are made in several ways, and their overall safety and effectiveness depend on how a particular vaccine is made and what it contains. Vaccines are made in four ways: (1) *Killed vaccines* contain killed bacteria or inactivated viruses; (2) *live, attenuated vaccines* contain bacteria or viruses that have been altered; (3) *toxoid vaccines* contain toxins (or poisons) produced by the organism that are then rendered harmless; and (4) *component vaccines* contain parts of the bacteria or viruses. The HIB vaccine is a component vaccine composed of a protein–polysaccharide conjugate. Other examples of component vaccines include the hepatitis A and B (Hep A and B) vaccines and the *pneumoccocal* conjugate vaccine. Viruses are inactivated with chemicals such as formaldehyde. Examples of inactivated (killed) vaccines include the polio vaccine (IPV) and the influenza vaccine. Live, attenuated vaccines usually are created from the naturally occurring pathogen itself. Viruses are weakened (or attenuated) from viruses whose virulence has deteriorated from multiple passages of cell culture. Examples of live, attenuated vaccines include the measles vaccine, the mumps vaccine, and the rubella (German measles) vaccine, which are all found in the MMR vaccine. Other examples of live, attenuated vaccines include the oral polio (OPV) and varicella (chickenpox) vaccines. Toxoid vaccines are made by treating toxins (or poisons) produced by bacteria with heat or chemicals, such as formalin, to destroy their ability to cause illness. Toxoid vaccines include the diphtheria toxoid vaccine, and the tetanus toxoid vaccine, each of which may be given alone or as part of DTP, DTaP, or dT vaccines.

2. **The correct answer is C.** An allergic reaction to any vaccination is an absolute contraindication for continuation of the series for obvious reasons. Other contraindications for administration of the DtaP vaccine include Guillian-Barré syndrome or other neurologic disorders. A reaction in a second-degree relative is not a contraindication, nor is a history of crying. In a child with a fever who otherwise appears well, the clinician should use his or her best judgment. The practitioner should consider carefully the benefits and risks of this vaccine in these circumstances. If the risks are believed to outweigh the benefits, withhold the vaccination; if the benefits are believed to outweigh the risks (e.g., during an outbreak or foreign travel), give the vaccine.

3. **The correct answer is A.** As many age-appropriate vaccines should be given on the first visit as possible. Those vaccines that follow schedules should then be followed as per recommendations. The other choices present a problem in that the child will still not be protected against the various illnesses vaccinations are supposed to prevent. The catch-up immunization schedule is shown in the following figure.

Recommended Immunization Schedule for Persons Aged 0–6 Years—UNITED STATES • 2008

For those who fall behind or start late, see the catch-up schedule

Vaccine ▼ Age ▶	Birth	1 month	2 months	4 months	6 months	12 months	15 months	18 months	19–23 months	2–3 years	4–6 years
Hepatitis B [1]	HepB	HepB		see footnote 1		HepB					
Rotavirus [2]			Rota	Rota	Rota						
Diphtheria, Tetanus, Pertussis [3]			DTaP	DTaP	DTaP	see footnote 3	DTaP				DTaP
Haemophilus influenzae type b [4]			Hib	Hib	Hib	Hib					
Pneumococcal [5]			PCV	PCV	PCV	PCV				PPV	
Inactivated Poliovirus [6]			IPV	IPV		IPV					IPV
Influenza [6]						Influenza (Yearly)					
Measles, Mumps, Rubella [7]						MMR					MMR
Varicella [8]						Varicella					Varicella
Hepatitis A [9]						HepA (2 doses)				HepA Series	
Meningococcal [10]										MCV4	

Range of recommended ages

Certain high-risk groups

This schedule indicates the recommended ages for routine administration of currently licensed childhood vaccines, as of December 1, 2007, for children aged 0 through 6 years. Additional information is available at www.cdc.gov/vaccines/recs/schedules. Any dose not administered at the recommended age should be administered at any subsequent visit, when indicated and feasible. Additional vaccines may be licensed and recommended during the year. Licensed combination vaccines may be used whenever any components of the combination are indicated and other components of the vaccine are not contraindicated and if approved by the Food and Drug Administration for that dose of the series. Providers should consult the respective Advisory Committee on Immunization Practices statement for detailed recommendations, including for high-risk conditions: http://www.cdc.gov/vaccines/pubs/ACIP-list.htm. Clinically significant adverse events that follow immunization should be reported to the Vaccine Adverse Event Reporting System (VAERS). Guidance about how to obtain and complete a VAERS form is available at www.vaers.hhs.gov or by telephone, 800-822-7967.

4. **The correct answer is B.** According to the Centers for Disease Control (CDC), the rate of endemic pertussis in this age group is extraordinarily high (some states report 150 to 200 cases per 1,000), and as such represent a significant source of transmission. Elderly patients and young unimmunized infants do not have significant rates of pertussis. Contaminated surfaces have negligible transmission rates of this disease.

5. **The correct answer is C.** Over 51 serotypes of adenoviruses produce a variety of clinical syndromes. Adenoviral infections are usually self-limited and are frequently found among infants, children, and military recruits. This child has symptoms of the common cold, which is primarily the manifestation with which most of us are familiar. This is characterized by rhinitis, malaise, and pharyngitis, with or without fever (seen frequently in non–*Streptococcal* exudative pharyngitis). The Epstein-Barr virus causes infectious mononucleosis; it frequently manifests as malaise, fever, pharyngitis, lymphadenopathy, and splenomegaly. *Mycoplasma pneumoniae* is usually seen in an older population, such as college students or others living in close quarters with many other people. Symptoms do not usually include rhinorrhea or hoarseness.

6. **The correct answer is C.** Hallmarks of this diagnosis are otalgia, often in conjunction with an upper respiratory infection; erythema of the tympanic membrane; and hypomobility of the membrane to insufflation. Often, one or more symptoms are not present; however, the buildup of fluid behind the membrane will reduce the mobility to insufflations, thus alerting the practitioner to the diagnosis. Loss of the light reflex may or may not be indicative of otitis media; it might just be absent due to an allergic condition or other fluid buildup. Fever, although a frequent finding in otitis media, is nonspecific and could be due to other causes.

7. **The correct answer is D.** The common cold is usually self-limited, frequently lasting less than a week. Symptoms that last for more than 1 week (and less than 4 weeks) are hallmarks of diagnosis. Diminished sinus transillumination (less transillumination in fluid versus air) may be due to a transient adenovirus or allergic response. The same holds true for fever or mucoid rhinorrhea.

8. **The correct answer is C.** The term *croup* does not refer to a single illness, but rather a group of conditions involving inflammation of the upper airway that leads to a cough that sounds like a bark, particularly when a child is crying. The caregiver might also describe noisy breathing. Similar symptoms may occasionally be caused by bacteria or an

318

allergic reaction, although most cases of croup are caused by viruses, most commonly parainfluenza virus. Other cases may involve adenoviruses, influenza, respiratory syncytial viruses, and measles. Most children with viral croup are between the ages of 3 months and 5 years. Symptoms are most severe in children younger than 3 years of age. Croup may be accompanied by fast or difficult breathing and sometimes a grunting noise or wheezing while breathing. The patient may have cold symptoms such as rhinorrhea for a few days and may also have fever. As the upper airway (the lining of the windpipe and the voice box) becomes progressively inflamed and swollen, the child may become hoarse, with a harsh, barking cough. If the upper airway becomes swollen to the point where it is partially blocked off, it becomes even more difficult for a child to breathe, especially if agitated. This happens with severe croup. The viruses may cause inflammation further down the airway, including the bronchi and the lungs. Patients with epiglottitis typically have narrowed airways and present with drooling and marked dysphagia. Patients with bacterial tracheitis resemble croup patients; however, the symptoms may be intermediate between those of epiglottitis and croup. The presentation is either acute or subacute. Patients may have high fevers, a toxic appearance, stridor, respiratory distress, and high white blood cell counts. Cough is frequent, and this patient does not have one. In the subacute presentation, children experience several days of viral croup-like symptoms and either do not respond to standard treatment or clinically worsen. The prodrome is usually an upper respiratory infection, followed by progression to higher fever, cough, inspiratory stridor, and a variable degree of respiratory distress. Patients with peritonsillar abscess typically present with severe sore throat pain, trismus, odynophagia, and medial deviation of the soft palate, along with a muffled voice (the "hot potato" voice). The practitioner should also note the uvula typically deviates *away* from the abscess.

9. **The correct answer is B.** Patients with peritonsillar abscess typically present with severe sore throat pain, trismus, odynophagia, and medial deviation of the soft palate, along with a muffled voice (the "hot potato" voice). Following treatment, peritonsillar cellulitis either resolves or develops into a peritonsillar abscess. Existence of an abscess is confirmed by needle aspiration. The literature supports treatments ranging from needle aspiration, incision and drainage, to tonsillectomy. Complications, such as extension into adjacent structures, are possible if it is left untreated or treated improperly. The term *croup* does not refer to a single illness, but rather a group of conditions involving inflammation of the upper airway that leads to a cough that sounds like a bark, particularly when a child is crying. The caregiver might also describe noisy breathing. Similar symptoms may occasionally be caused by bacteria or an allergic reaction, although most cases of croup are caused by viruses, most commonly the parainfluenza viruses. Other cases may involve adenoviruses, influenza, respiratory syncytial viruses, and measles. Most children with viral croup are between the ages of 3 months and 5 years. Symptoms are most severe in children younger than 3 years of age. Croup may be accompanied by fast or difficult breathing and sometimes a grunting noise or wheezing while breathing. The patient may have cold symptoms such as rhinorrhea for a few days and may also have fever. As the upper airway (the lining of the windpipe and the voice box) becomes progressively inflamed and swollen, the child may become hoarse, with a harsh, barking cough. If the upper airway becomes swollen to the point where it is partially blocked off, it becomes even more difficult for a child to breathe especially if agitated. This happens with severe croup. The viruses may cause inflammation further down the airway, including the bronchi and the lungs. Patients with epiglottitis typically have narrowed airways and present with drooling and marked dysphagia. Patients with bacterial tracheitis resemble croup patients; however, symptoms may be intermediate between those of epiglottitis and croup. The presentation is either acute or subacute. Patients may have high fevers, a toxic appearance, stridor, respiratory distress, and high white blood cell counts. Cough is frequent, and this patient does not have one. In the subacute presentation, children experience several days of viral crouplike symptoms and either do not respond to standard treatment or clinically worsen. The prodrome is usually an upper

respiratory infection, followed by progression to higher fever, cough, inspiratory stridor, and a variable degree of respiratory distress.

10. **The correct answer is A.** The most common cause of failure to thrive is nutritional deprivation. Without adequate nutrition, humans have difficulty surviving. In fact, in cases of failure to thrive clinicians are urged to examine all the contributing factors, including possible child maltreatment. Cystic fibrosis is the most common chronic lung disease of young adults. Cerebral palsy is a nonprogressive neurologic disorder that involves motor damage. Most cases develop in utero (75%), with 5% of cases occurring during childbirth and approximately 15% during childhood. It is the second most expensive developmental disability to manage during a lifetime. Inflammatory bowel disease is primarily a disease of adults.

11. **The correct answer is C.** A 6- to 8-month-old child is expected to roll from back to stomach. The other answers are developmental milestones expected to occur later in the child's life.

12. **The correct answer is D.** Infants who rely on a diet of cow's milk are at high risk of anemia during the first years of life, because cow's milk is low in iron (about 2.6 mg Fe per 1,000 kcal). The recommended daily iron consumption for children between the ages of 6 months and 5 years is 10 mg, which corresponds to diets with iron densities of 11.7 mg, 7.7 mg, and 5.6 mg for children aged 6 to 11 months, 12 to 35 months, and 36 to 60 months, respectively. In addition to being poor in iron, cow's milk does not contain heme iron, the form that is best absorbed by the body. Research has also found that cow's milk has the potential to inhibit the absorption of both heme and nonheme iron present in other foods consumed by the child. The high fat content is not a problem, especially when you consider the high fat content of breast milk. Infants usually are not lactose intolerant. In fact, lactase enzyme levels are highest in infants. The levels of vitamin D in table milk are not generally toxic to infants.

13. **The correct answer is A.** Obviously, an evaluation of a child's hearing is paramount in determining the reasons for speech delay. Frequently, speech delay is a result of partial or full deafness. Referral to a speech therapist or psychologist without ascertaining the pathologic causes (if any) is premature. Anticipatory guidance is also premature in the absence of an accurate diagnosis.

14. **The correct answer is A.** Jaundice is a common condition among newborns and requires medical attention. The yellow coloration of the skin and sclera in newborns with jaundice is the result of accumulation of unconjugated bilirubin. In most infants, unconjugated hyperbilirubinemia reflects a normal transitional phenomenon. However, because unconjugated bilirubin is neurotoxic and can cause death in newborns and lifelong neurologic sequelae in infants who survive, the presence of neonatal jaundice frequently results in diagnostic evaluation. Neonatal physiologic jaundice results from simultaneous occurrence of elevated bilirubin production due to increased breakdown of fetal erythrocytes and a low hepatic excretory capacity. This is caused by low concentrations of the binding protein ligand in the hepatocytes and the low activity of glucuronyl transferase, the enzyme responsible for binding bilirubin to glucuronic acid, thus making bilirubin water soluble (conjugation). Hemolytic disease of the newborn, erythroblastosis fetalis, occurs in one of two situations. The first is where there is blood type incompatibility between mother and fetus. This usually occurs when an Rh negative mother has an Rh positive child (inherited from an Rh positive father). This frequently occurs in the mother's second or third pregnancy. The second situation is ABO incompatibility. ABO incompatibility disease usually limits to those fetuses with A or B antigens whose mothers have type O blood. Usually, one-third of these babies show evidence of the mother's antibodies in their bloodstream, but only a small percentage develop symptoms of ABO incompatibility disease. Hemolytic disease of the newborn is three times more likely

among Caucasian than African Americans. Biliary atresia occurs due to obliteration or discontinuity of the extrahepatic biliary system, resulting in obstruction of bile flow. It is the most common surgically treatable cause of cholestasis encountered during the newborn period; however, it is not the most common cause of neonatal jaundice. The more common neonatal type is characterized by a progressive inflammatory lesion, which suggests a role for infectious and/or toxic agents causing bile duct obliteration. However, no single etiologic feature of this problem has been identified. The overall incidence in the United States is 1 per 10,000 to 15,000 live births. Hepatitis, particularly hepatitis C, can be transmitted from an infected mother to the newborn, but it is not the most common form of neonatal jaundice.

15. **The correct answer is D.** Far and away, respiratory failure secondary to foreign-body aspiration or organic causes is the primary cause of cardiac arrest in children. Poisoning runs a distant second, followed by chest trauma, and, rarely, if ever, myocardial infarctions.

16. **The correct answer is D.** Curvatures greater than 40° prove resistant to bracing and may require spinal fusion. Answers A, B, and C are all true statements.

17. **The correct answer is C.** In healthy children, especially in this age group, an abrupt onset of respiratory distress is usually due to foreign-body aspiration. The literature notes that approximately 75% of children from infancy to 6 years of age with respiratory distress have a foreign-body obstruction. The most common causes do not include croup, epiglottitis, or pneumonia, although all of these are potential precursors of respiratory distress.

18. **The correct answer is B.** Viruses are the most common cause of pneumonia in children. Diffuse crackles rather than discrete or specific lobar rales tilt the diagnosis in the direction of a viral origin. Bacterial pneumonia typically is discrete or well rounded, affecting one or more lobes. *Mycoplasma pneumonia* is a subset of bacterial pneumonia and presents much the same way, albeit usually with less respiratory distress. Tuberculosis is common among the homeless, immunocompromised individuals, and individuals from foreign countries where the disease is prevalent. This condition presents with classic signs of pneumonia, including tachypnea, nasal flaring, grunting, dullness to percussion, egophony, decreased breath sounds, and crackles. However, a febrile 2-year-old child presenting as described in the question most likely has viral pneumonia.

19. **The correct answer is C.** Cough is the most common reason patients seek medical attention for respiratory complaints. Acute coughs can mean a host of various conditions, but chronic cough in children is most likely the result of undiagnosed asthma. The second most common cause of cough in children is nasal and/or sinus disease or other upper respiratory conditions. A foreign body can cause recurrent unilateral pneumonia or acute respiratory distress. Tuberculosis, which presents with cough, is not the most likely cause.

20. **The correct answer is D.** All of the choices may indicate serious complications; indeed, inspiratory and expiratory wheezing may be indicative of status asthmaticus. However, altered mental status indicates significant hypoxia and impending catastrophe.

21. **The correct answer is C.** Viruses are the most common cause of pneumonia in children. Diffuse crackles rather than discrete or specific lobar rales tilt the diagnosis in the direction of a viral cause. Bacterial pneumonia typically is discrete or well rounded, affecting one or more lobes. This presents radiographically with partial or complete consolidation. Bacterial pneumonia can progress to multiple lobes; however, the most common radiographic presentation is typically in a single lobe. Diffuse patchy infiltrates can be present in several conditions, ranging from tuberculosis to other chronic lung diseases. Reticulonodular infiltrates are usually present in fibrotic lung diseases, including, but not limited to, asbestosis.

22. **The correct answer is B.** In children, acute bronchitis usually lasts 1 to 2 weeks and is self-limited. Treatment is usually limited to supportive care such as a vaporizer or humidifier or supportive medications for cough or fever. Antibiotics are not indicated due to the probable viral and self-limited nature of the disease. Steroids similarly should not be given, because the risk/benefit ratio is too high and they are not typically useful.

23. **The correct answer is C.** Patients with bacterial effusions of the knee typically have larger effusions, which cause decreased ROM and more disability. The other statements are incorrect.

24. **The correct answer is C.** With any orthopedic presentation, the clinician should examine the joints proximal and distal to the area in question. When the examination is essentially unremarkable for the joint in question, then other areas should be examined. Usually, it is the proximal area that will have the problem. Toxic synovitis and bacterial arthritis are more likely in this patient due to the fever. When patients, especially overweight adolescents, present only with pain and a limp, the clinician should look for signs of aseptic necrosis. Osteomyelitis may present with fever, but typically physical findings are present to support such a diagnosis. Patients with septic arthritis of the knee present in the same fashion. An occult fracture of the distal femur or proximal tibia can be ruled out with the appropriate radiographs, and although pain may radiate into the hip, it is unlikely that the patient will present with fever or absence of physical signs in the area in question.

25. **The correct answer is D.** Judging from the patient's history, this patient likely has cellulitis and a bacterial effusion in the knee. The essential diagnostic test is aspiration and culture. Aspiration of fat globules floating in the effusion may also reveal an occult fracture. An ACE wrap and elevation with ibuprofen for pain without knowing the culture of the effusion is inappropriate and could prove dangerous to the child. The history does not support obtaining a Lyme titer. A complete blood count should be obtained. The aspirate will probably contain *Staphylococcus* species, but a confirmatory aspirate would make the prescribing of the cephalosporin more appropriate.

26. **The correct answer is D.** Abnormalities such as a vesicoureteral reflux and hydronephrosis are common, with vesicoureteral reflux being the most common congenital abnormality. Close contact with another infected child is extremely unlikely to cause a urinary tract infection (UTI). Poor perineal hygiene may lead to a UTI if bacteria are transmitted when wiping after voiding; however, this is also unlikely.

27. **The correct answer is C.** Urinary tract infections (UTIs) are the most common nosocomial infection in the United States and are very common among nonhospitalized patients. Based on the choices provided in the question, a UTI is the most likely cause. The patient has mild left-sided tenderness without rebound, thus the absence of peritoneal signs tends to put appendicitis low on the differential list. Few rectal abnormalities in a child could cause the symptoms as listed. An abdominal obstruction series is inappropriate, because the history does not support a diagnosis of intestinal obstruction.

28. **The correct answer is B.** Culture and sensitivity is the most reliable indicator of a urinary tract infection (UTI). The other tests are primary tests that will point the clinician toward a diagnosis, but not confirm it.

29. **The correct answer is C.** Urinary tract infections (UTIs) are the most common nosocomial infection in the United States. *Escherichia coli* is the most common pathogen in these cases.

30. **The correct answer is D.** This child is clearly septic, as demonstrated by her vital signs (including the very high fever). Nothing in the patient's presentation (especially the physical examination) indicate dehydration with hypovolemia. Although a 2-week-old infant

may have heart failure secondary to a congenital disorder, the physical examination does not bear this out. No clear signs or symptoms of child maltreatment are present.

31. **The correct answer is B.** Elements of all the choices would be correct in the resuscitation of an infant in septic shock. However, the clinician is advised to recall the ABCs of resuscitation—*a*irway, *b*reathing, and *c*irculation. Septic shock patients are typically hypoxemic and require supportive oxygen therapy (usually 100%). To support the airway, endotracheal intubation must be considered. Venous access for IV fluids and necessary medication administration is paramount. Blood cultures should be obtained to identify the pathogen(s) causing the sepsis, and appropriate antibiotic administration should follow. A CT scan of the head may be appropriate if the diagnosis supports a neurologic cause; however, this is not delineated in the question.

32. **The correct answer is A.** Septic shock is the most common cause of shock seen by internists in the United States. At present, *Streptococcus agalactiae* (Group B *Streptococcus*) is the most likely cause of bacterial sepsis in a neonate. This has changed from a few years ago, when *Haemophilus influenzae* was the most common cause. The widespread vaccination of children with the HiB vaccine has dramatically reduced this number. *Streptococcus pneumoniae* and *Neisseria sp.* are common, but not the most common.

33. **The correct answer is B.** Tachycardia, tachypnea, and irritability or lethargy are typically initial presenting signs of septic shock in infants. A decreased systolic blood pressure is an ominous late sign.

34. **The correct answer is A.** Viruses are the most common cause of meningitis in infants and children, with enteroviruses being the most prevalent. *Streptococcus pneumoniae* and *Neisseria meningitidis* are common bacterial causes; however, most cases of meningitis are of viral origin.

35. **The correct answer is D.** Viral (aseptic) meningitis usually produces a spinal fluid that is clear to cloudy with normal glucose and increased protein. The opening pressure can be normal to increased with a predominance of lymphocytes.

36. **The correct answer is B.** Ventricular septal defect is the most common congenital heart defect in children. Coarctation of the aorta is the most common cyanotic congenital defect. The symptoms for all of the listed abnormalities present with varying degrees of difficulty; however, in this patient, the severity of the symptoms increases the likelihood that this is a ventricular septal defect.

37. **The correct answer is B.** Kawasaki disease was initially described in 1967 by Tomisaku Kawasaki. It is also known as mucocutaneous lymph node syndrome and is present primarily in children younger than 5 years of age; however, it is occasionally seen in adults. The disease typically presents with fever of at least 5 days duration and four of the following five physical signs:

    1. Extremity changes including erythema, edema, and desquamation/induration. The child may refuse to bear weight as a result. Desquamation of the fingers and toes begins in the periungual region, is usually observed 1–2 weeks after the onset of fever, and may involve the palms and soles (75% of patients). The hand/feet induration is also known as Beau's lines.
    2. Bilateral bulbar conjunctivitis not typically associated with exudates (85% of patients).
    3. Nonvesicular, generalized polymorphous rash. The rash may be limited to the groin or lower extremities (80% of patients).
    4. Unilateral cervical lymphadenopathy typically greater than 1.5 cm and unilateral. This finding is more common in Asia. Occurrence is approximately 40%.
    5. Lip and oral cavity changes, which may include strawberry tongue (with prominent papillae), dry/fissured or swollen lips, or pharyngeal erythema (90% of patients).

In 25% of untreated patients, arteritis of the coronary vessels may occur, which can lead to myocardial infarction and/or arterial aneurysm. Adenopathy is not a major sequelae of the disease. Patients do not typically present with renal dysfunction or hepatitis.

38. **The correct answer is C.** In infants, pathologic murmurs include all diastolic murmurs; all holosystolic, late systolic, or continuous murmurs; loud murmurs >3/6; and those with associated cardiac abnormalities. The other parameters listed are not always or usually pathologic.

39. **The correct answer is D.** Syncope with increased cardiac demand is most worrisome. As the myocardial oxygen demand increases in these children, the heart is unable to maintain the oxygen levels needed to maintain cerebral function. A past history of a murmur may or may not have pathologic implications, and it rarely does in the case of innocent murmurs. A positive family history of coronary disease is notable in that the child should be aware of the increased risk for cardiac problems later in life, but it is not worrisome at this time. Syncope while standing up quickly may be benign and just a positional hypotension or it may be indicative of a significant problem. However, syncope with exercise is most troublesome.

40. **The correct answer is D.** The usual presentation of coarctation of the aorta is systemic hypertension. Patients present with an associated bicuspid aortic valve and absent or weak femoral pulses. Systolic pressures are also higher in the upper extremities compared to the lower extremities, which would lead to higher pulse oximetry in the upper versus the lower extremities. Cardiac catheterization can provide definitive gradient information across the lesion. A pulsus paradoxus and a widened pulse pressure are present in aortic aneurysms. A II/VI murmur can be caused by several conditions and is nonspecific in this case.

41. **The correct answer is C.** Cystic fibrosis is the most common severe respiratory chronic disorder in young adults and the most common fatal hereditary disorder of Caucasians in the United States. Cystic fibrosis is caused by abnormalities in the apical membranes of the cystic cells' chloride channel that result in altered chloride transport. This causes the production of abnormal mucus that eventually obstructs glands and ducts. Pneumonia typically occurs in these patients due to *Pseudomonas aeruginosa*. Clinicians are cautioned to watch for resistant strains in patients with chronic episodes of *Pseudomonas*. Lung transplantation is currently the only definitive treatment for advanced cystic fibrosis.

42. **The correct answer is B.** Sickle-cell disease is an autosomal recessive disorder in which abnormal hemoglobin leads to chronic hemolytic anemia, resulting in several clinical problems. Acute painful episodes may be due to vasoocclusion and can be provoked by infection, dehydration, and hypoxia. If a patient presents with fever, such as in this question, the clinician must assume infection and admit the patient for diagnostic cultures and appropriate antimicrobial treatment. Due to the range of infections that may be present, blind treatment with amoxicillin would be inappropriate. Supportive treatment, as described in answers A and D, is ill-advised in this situation.

43. **The correct answer is B.** The child's symptoms are worrisome and point strongly to leukemia (most commonly ALL) as a potential cause. Most of the symptoms of acute leukemia are due to replacement of normal bone marrow elements by malignant cells. The infection is usually due to neutropenia. Patients generally appear pale and have purpura and petechiae. Fever is common, and patients typically present with enlargement of the liver, spleen, and lymph nodes. The complete blood count will ascertain the presence of neutropenia, and the bone marrow analysis will confirm the diagnosis. A CT of the abdomen will only indicate whether hepatosplenomegaly is present; it will not determine the cause. This patient has no specific findings of osteomyelitis, and there is no indication hepatitis should be considered.

44. **The correct answer is B.** Intestinal obstruction typically presents with crampy abdominal pain that is progressive. Vomiting frequently occurs and is typically bilious. Although there may be an initial passage of stool or diarrhea, in most cases this ceases. Viral gastroenteritis is the most common cause of abdominal pain in children; however, the pain is typically self-limited and is usually not described as progressive. Urinary tract infections would not typically present in this fashion. *Salmonella* poisoning generally presents with pain, fever, and diarrhea.

45. **The correct answer is C.** Viral gastroenteritis is the most common cause of abdominal pain in children. Rotaviruses are the most common viral cause. The Norwalk virus, adenovirus, and enterovirus are also frequent causes of gastroenteritis. The most common bacterial agents include *Escherichia coli*, *Yersinia sp.*, *Campylobacter sp.*, *Salmonella sp.*, and *Shigella sp.*

46. **The correct answer is C.** Pyloric stenosis, or infantile hypertrophic pyloric stenosis (IHPS), is the most common cause of intestinal obstruction in infancy. Pyloric stenosis occurs secondary to hypertrophy and hyperplasia of the muscular layers of the pylorus, causing a functional gastric outlet obstruction. The usual age of onset is 3 weeks of age; however, this can range from those aged 3 to 12 weeks. Classically, the infant will have nonbilious vomiting or regurgitation, which may become projectile (up to 70%), after which the infant is still hungry. Emesis may be intermittent or occur after each feeding. The infant may begin to show signs of dehydration and malnutrition, such as poor weight gain, weight loss, decreased urinary output, lethargy, and shock. The infant may develop jaundice, which usually resolves upon correction of the disease. The classic signs of IHPS are becoming less common. The mean age of presentation is getting significantly younger, and infants are not developing the physical signs or electrolyte abnormalities they were 20 years ago. Additionally, the availability of diagnostic imaging is allowing clinicians to make this diagnosis before other clinical manifestations appear. Intussusception occurs when one portion of the bowel slides into the next, much like the pieces of a telescope. It is the most common cause of intestinal obstruction in children between the ages of 3 months and 6 years and most often occurs in children between 5 and 10 months of age (80% occur before a child is 24 months old). Children with an intussusception have intense abdominal pain, which often begins so suddenly that it causes loud, anguished crying and makes the child draw the knees up to the chest. The pain is usually intermittent, but recurs and becomes stronger. Other common symptoms include abdominal swelling or distention; passing stools mixed with blood and mucus, known as "currant jelly" stool; bilious vomiting; lethargy; grunting; and shallow respirations. Urinary tract infections may cause pain, but not the symptoms as described. An incarcerated inguinal hernia can cause vomiting and inguinal pain, but it does not usually cause an electrolyte disturbance.

47. **The correct answer is C.** Appendicitis is the most common surgical condition in children who present with abdominal pain. Lymphoid tissue or a fecalith obstructs the appendiceal lumen, the appendix becomes distended, and ischemia and necrosis may develop. Patients with appendicitis classically present with visceral, vague, poorly localized, periumbilical pain. Within 6 to 48 hours, the pain becomes parietal as the overlying peritoneum becomes inflamed; the pain then becomes well localized and constant in the right iliac fossa. Intussusception occurs when one portion of the bowel slides into the next, much like the pieces of a telescope. It is the most common cause of intestinal obstruction in children between the ages of 3 months and 6 years and most often occurs in children between 5 and 10 months of age (80% occur before a child is 24 months old). Children with an intussusception have intense abdominal pain, which often begins so suddenly that it causes loud, anguished crying and makes the child draw the knees up to the chest. The pain is usually intermittent, but recurs and becomes stronger. Other common symptoms include abdominal swelling or distention; passing stools mixed with

blood and mucus, known as "currant jelly" stool; bilious vomiting; lethargy; grunting; and shallow respirations. A urinary tract infection is unlikely given the peritoneal signs, and pelvic inflammatory disease is rarely, if ever, seen in a 9-year-old child.

REFERENCES

Behrman, R. E., Kliegman, R. M., and Jenson, H. B. (2008). *Nelson textbook of pediatrics*, 17th ed. Elsevier Publishing, Philadelphia, PA.

Centers for Disease Control (CDC). (2004). Guide to contraindications to vaccinations. (Online). Available at www.cdc.gov/vaccines/recs/vac-admin/contraindications.htm. Accessed August 21, 2007.

Frizzell, R. A., Rechkemmer, G., and Shoemaker, R. L. (1986). "Altered regulation of airway epithelial cell chloride channels in cystic fibrosis." *Science* 233(4763): 558–560.

Long, S. S., Pickering, L. K., and Prober, C. G. (eds.). (2003). *Principles and practice of pediatric infectious diseases*, 2nd ed. Elsevier Publishing, Philadelphia, PA.

Zitelli, B. J., and Davis H. W. (eds.). (2002). *Atlas of pediatric physical diagnosis*. Mosby Publishing, St. Louis, MO.

General Urology

Irvin H. Hirsch, MD
Mark L. Pe, MD
Eleanor Davis, PA-C

1. Which of the following is *not* a risk factor for prostate cancer?
   A. Family history of prostate cancer
   B. Racial background
   C. History of benign prostatic hypertrophy
   D. Older age

2. Which of the following does *not* elevate serum prostate-specific antigen (PSA)?
   A. Adenocarcinoma of the prostate
   B. Benign prostatic hyperplasia
   C. Prostatitis
   D. Surgical ablation of prostate tissue

3. Which of the following is the American Cancer Society's current recommendation for prostate cancer screening in men?
   A. Health care providers should offer the option of an annual prostate-specific antigen (PSA) test and a digital rectal examination in men 50 years and older who are at average risk of developing prostate cancer.
   B. Health care providers should offer the option of an annual PSA in men 50 years and older who are at average risk of developing prostate cancer.
   C. Health care providers should offer the option of a biannual PSA and digital rectal examination in men 50 years and older who are at average risk of developing prostate cancer.
   D. Health care providers should offer the option of an annual PSA in men 60 years and older who are at average risk of developing prostate cancer.

4. Which of the following are the most common sites of prostate cancer metastasis?
   A. Lymph nodes, bone, and testicles
   B. Kidney, lymph nodes, and bone
   C. Lymph nodes, bone, and lung
   D. Bone, liver, and brain

5. Which of the following is the most common type of prostate cancer?
   A. Small cell carcinoma
   B. Adenocarcinoma
   C. Squamous cell carcinoma
   D. Transitional cell carcinoma

6. Which of the following is *not* a common cause of community-acquired urinary tract infections (UTIs)?

    A. *Escherichia coli*
    B. *Klebsiella pneumoniae*
    C. *Serratia marcescens*
    D. *Proteus vulgaris*

7. Which of the following microscopic findings is considered to be the minimum criteria for significant hematuria?

    A. Greater than 20 red blood cells per high power field
    B. Greater than 5 red blood cells per high power field
    C. Greater than 12 red blood cells per high power field
    D. Greater than 3 red blood cells per high power field

8. Which of the following is the most common site of metastasis of prostate carcinoma?

    A. Breast
    B. Liver
    C. Lung
    D. Bone

9. Which of the following is most consistent with the finding of a positive Prehn's sign?

    A. Testicular cancer
    B. Epididymitis
    C. Testicular torsion
    D. Varicocele

10. Which of the following is the proper description of a grade III cystocele?

    A. Descent of the organ toward the introitus
    B. Descent of the organ outside of the introitus with straining
    C. Descent of the organ outside of the level of the introitus without straining
    D. None of the above

11. von Hippel Lindau syndrome is associated with which of the following genitourinary malignancies?

    A. Penile squamous cell carcinoma
    B. Testicular seminoma
    C. Renal cell carcinoma
    D. Prostatic adenocarcinoma

12. Which of the following is the most appropriate imaging for a patient presenting with pain, a flank mass, and gross hematuria?

    A. CT scan of the abdomen without contrast
    B. MRI of abdomen and pelvis
    C. Renal ultrasound
    D. CT urogram

13. An 8-year-old child presents with complaints of sudden onset of testicular pain. A positive "blue dot sign" is found on physical examination. Which of the following is the most likely diagnosis?

    A. Testicular cancer
    B. Torsed appendix testis
    C. Epididymitis
    D. Varicocele

14. Which of the following is *not* a risk factor for carcinoma of the bladder?

    A. History of tobacco use

    B. Occupational exposure to aromatic amines

    C. History of recurrent urinary tract infections

    D. History of cystitis from chronic indwelling catheters

15. Which of the following is *not* a contraindication for the use of sildenafil?

    A. Concomitant nitrate use

    B. Documented retinopathy

    C. Concomitant alpha blocker use

    D. Patients prone to priapism

16. Which of the following is *not* typically a risk factor for erectile dysfunction?

    A. Hypercholesterolemia

    B. Smoking

    C. Hyperthyroidism

    D. Diabetes mellitus

17. A 55-year-old male presents complaining of progressively worsening nocturia and weak urinary stream. A digital rectal examination reveals a large 45-g, nontender, nonboggy prostate, without any nodularity. He is found to have a postvoid residual of 85 ml. His prostate-specific antigen (PSA) is 1.2 ng/ml, and his urinalysis is unremarkable. Which of the following is the most appropriate medical treatment for this patient?

    A. Anticholinergic alone (e.g., oxybutinin)

    B. 5α-reductase inhibitor (e.g., finasteride) and α-blocker (e.g., tamsulosin)

    C. 5α-reductase inhibitor alone (e.g., finasteride)

    D. Dietary modification and recheck in 2 months

18. Which of the following is the most common etiology of organic erectile dysfunction?

    A. Vascular disease

    B. Medications

    C. Surgical procedures

    D. Endocrine disorders

19. A 60-year-old male with a 40-pack-year history of tobacco use presents with a 3-week history of gross, painless hematuria. After obtaining a history and a physical, which of the following would *not* be included in his workup?

    A. CT urogram

    B. Urinalysis, urine culture, and cytology

    C. Cystoscopy

    D. Immediate operative intervention

20. A 40-year-old female presents complaining of severe, intermittent, left-side flank pain that radiates to her groin, along with episodes of nausea and vomiting. You suspect that she is passing a kidney stone. Which of the following would be the imaging study of choice to confirm your diagnosis?

    A. Abdominal x-ray of kidneys, ureters, and bladder (KUB)

    B. Renal ultrasound

    C. Noncontrast CT of the abdomen and pelvis

    D. MRI of the abdomen and pelvis

21. A 45-year-old male presents complaining of a 3-day history of fever and chills, dysuria, urinary frequency, and urinary urgency. Urinalysis is positive for nitrites, leukocyte esterase, and 20 white blood cells per high-power field. Digital rectal examination reveals a tender, boggy prostate. Which of the following is the most likely diagnosis?

   A. Renal colic with an infected stone
   B. Acute pyelonephritis
   C. Acute bacterial prostatitis
   D. Cystitis

22. A 27-year-old male comes to the office with a new onset of left scrotal swelling. The swelling is constant and is not associated with straining. Physical examination reveals a nontender, but enlarged, hard, nodular testicle. Which of the following is the most likely diagnosis?

   A. Indirect inguinal hernia
   B. Testicular cancer
   C. Hydrocele
   D. Orchitis

23. A 45-year-old female with no significant medical history presents with intermittent right-sided flank pain. She denies any fevers, chills, or urinary symptoms. Workup reveals a 5-mm mid-ureteral stone. Which of the following is the most appropriate next step?

   A. Ureteroscopy and laser lithotripsy of stone
   B. ESWL (extracorporeal shockwave lithotripsy)
   C. PCNL (percutaneous nephrolithotomy)
   D. Hydration, pain management, and observation

24. A 62-year-old male presents for his annual physical examination. A digital rectal examination performed in the office revealed a small prostatic nodule on the right. One month ago his serum prostate-specific antigen (PSA) was 5.1 ng/ml. Which of the following is the most appropriate next step?

   A. Follow-up in 6 months for a repeat physical examination and repeat PSA
   B. Referral to a urologist for prostate biopsy
   C. A trial of fluoroquinolone antibiotics and repeat physical examination and PSA in 6 weeks
   D. Start an alpha blocker (e.g., tamsulosin) for treatment of benign prostatic hypertrophy (BPH)

25. Which of the following is *not* an appropriate treatment for clinically localized prostate cancer?

   A. Radical prostatectomy
   B. Brachytherapy or external beam radiation
   C. Active surveillance
   D. Radical ipslateral prostatectomy

26. A 63-year-old male presents for an annual physical examination. He has been taking tamsulosin and finasteride for treatment of benign prostatic hyperplasia (BPH) for 3 years. A digital rectal examination performed in the office was normal. His annual prostate-specific antigen (PSA) is 2.7 ng/ml. His PSA prior to that was 2.0 ng/ml. Which of the following is the most appropriate next step?

   A. Refer patient to a urologist for prostate biopsy.
   B. Follow-up in 1 year for annual digital rectal examination and PSA
   C. Start fluoroquinolone antibiotic and repeat PSA in 6 weeks.
   D. Follow-up in 6 months with digital rectal examination and PSA.

27. A 54-year-old male initially presents with gross painless hematuria. He is found to have low-grade, nonmuscular invasive bladder cancer. Which of the following is the most appropriate treatment option?

A. Intravesical immunotherapy with Bacillus Calmette-Guerin (BCG)
B. Systemic chemotherapy with gemcitabine and cisplatinum
C. Radical cystectomy
D. Radiation therapy

28. Which of the following is the most common histologic type of bladder cancer?

A. Adenocarcinoma
B. Squamous cell carcinoma
C. Transitional cell carcinoma
D. Small cell carcinoma

29. Which of the following is the most common type of kidney stone?

A. Magnesium ammonium phosphate
B. Calcium oxalate
C. Uric acid
D. Cystine

30. A healthy 30-year-old female presents to your office with a 3-day history of urinary frequency, urgency, and dysuria. Urinalysis is positive for leukocyte esterase and 15 white blood cells per high-power field. Which of the following is the most likely diagnosis?

A. Bladder stone
B. Transitional cell cancer of the bladder
C. Vaginitis
D. Uncomplicated bacterial cystitis

31. Prostate cancer most commonly occurs in which area of the prostate?

A. Peripheral zone
B. Transition zone
C. Central zone
D. Anterior zone

32. Which of the following is how most renal masses are discovered?

A. Episode of hematuria
B. Flank pain
C. Incidental finding on imaging study
D. Flank mass

33. Which of the following is the most common pathogen for community-acquired, noncomplicated urinary tract infections?

A. *Klebsiella oxytoca*
B. *Escherichia coli*
C. *Enterococcus faecalis*
D. *Staphylococcus saprophyticus*

34. The erectile dysfunction medications sildenafil, tadalafil, and vardenafil belong to which of the following drug classes?

A. Nitric oxide synthase inhibitors
B. Guanylate cyclase inhibitors
C. Alpha 1-receptor inhibitors
D. Phosphodiesterase-5 inhibitors

35. Which of the following neurotransmitters is responsible for the initiation of erections?

    A. Acetylcholine
    B. Nitric oxide
    C. Norepinephrine
    D. Dopamine

36. Which of the following is an absolute contraindication for taking a phosphodiesterase-5 inhibitor?

    A. Nitrates or nitric oxide
    B. Alpha blockers
    C. A history of myocardial infarction within the past 3 years
    D. All of the above

37. A 57-year-old male presents complaining of increased urinary frequency, urinary urgency, nocturia three to four times a night, and weak stream. A uroflow was taken, which showed a urinary stream of 12 ml/sec. His urinalysis was normal. The patient's postvoid residual was 175 ml. A digital rectal examination reveals a symmetric, 60-g prostate. You diagnose the patient with benign prostatic hypertrophy (BPH). Which of the following would be the most appropriate next step in management of this patient?

    A. Initiate treatment with an alpha blocker (e.g., tamsulosin).
    B. Recommend surgical intervention [e.g., transurethral resection of the prostate (TURP)].
    C. Initiate treatment with an anticholinergic medication (e.g., oxybutinin).
    D. Initiate treatment with saw palmetto.

38. A 62-year-old male presents complaining of worsening urinary frequency, urgency, and weak stream. He tells you that he voids every 30 minutes to 1 hour and that he wakes up three to four times a night to void. He feels that he does not completely empty his bladder after voiding. He has been on tamsulosin and finasteride for 2 years, but he feels as though his symptoms are progressing. Over the past year, he has been diagnosed with three urinary tract infections and was seen in the emergency room for an episode of urinary retention. Which of the following would be the most appropriate recommendation?

    A. Change tamsulosin to alfuzosin.
    B. Change finasteride to dutasteride.
    C. Refer the patient to a urologist for a transurethral resection of the prostate (TURP).
    D. Place an indwelling Foley catheter.

39. A 57-year-old male is seen in your clinic for an annual physical examination. He has a history of benign prostatic hypertrophy (BPH), for which you prescribed him tamsulosin 2 years prior. He states that his stream has gotten weaker and that he is still waking up two to three times a night to void. He says that he is voiding every hour, which he is unhappy about. Which of the following is the most appropriate next step?

    A. Start saw palmetto.
    B. Start 5α-reductase inhibitor (e.g., finasteride).
    C. Refer the patient to a urologist for a transurethral resection of the prostate (TURP).
    D. Change tamsulosin to alfuzosin.

ANSWERS

  1. The correct answer is C. Benign prostatic hypertrophy (BPH) is not a known risk factor for prostate cancer. However, family history, age, and ethnicity have all been found to affect prostate cancer risk. Age is the most important risk factor for the development of many cancers, including prostate cancer. Most diagnoses of prostate cancer are made in men older than age 65. The incidence of prostate cancer is higher in African American men than in Caucasian men. It has been found that having a father or brother with prostate cancer significantly increases one's risk of developing this disease.

2. **The correct answer is D.** Prostate-specific antigen (PSA) is a protein produced by prostatic epithelial cells and periurethral glands. Serum PSA elevation is a result of disrupted prostatic architecture. Elevation of PSA may be seen in benign prostatic hypertrophy (BPH) or prostatic malignancy. Infection of the prostate may also produce transient serum elevations of PSA. Surgical ablation of the prostate tissue for BPH or prostate cancer will reduce PSA levels.

3. **The correct answer is A.** The American Cancer Society recommends that health care professionals offer men 50 years or older who are at average risk of developing prostate cancer the options of an annual prostate-specific antigen (PSA) test and digital rectal examination for early detection of prostate cancer. Screening should start between ages 40 to 45 in African American men or men with a family history of prostate cancer.

4. **The correct answer is C.** The most common sites of metastasis, in decreasing order of occurrence, are pelvic lymph nodes, bone, and lung.

5. **The correct answer is B.** More than 95% percent of prostate cancers are adenocarcinomas.

6. **The correct answer is C.** *Escherichia coli* is responsible for the majority (85%) of community-acquired urinary tract infections (UTIs). Other gram-negative enterobacteriaceae, gram-positive *Enterococcus faecalis,* and *Staphylococcus saprophyticus* are responsible for the remainder of most community-acquired infections.

7. **The correct answer is D.** A finding of greater than three red blood cells per high power microscopic field is significant microscopic hematuria.

8. **The correct answer is D.** Prostate cancer most commonly metastasizes to the bone.

9. **The correct answer B.** Alleviation of pain with scrotal elevation is a positive Prehn's sign. This is often found during evaluation of patients suffering from epididymitis. Testicular cancer may present as a firm, painless mass or as scrotal heaviness, enlargement, or discomfort. Testicular torsion is characterized by the acute onset of testicular pain in the absence of voiding symptoms. Torsion most typically occurs in the young teen, and on examination the affected testis generally lies superiorly to the contralateral testis. A varicocele represents an engorgement and dilatation of the internal spermatic veins. It is usually asymptomatic and diminishes in size with the patient supine. It frequently occurs on the left side, because the left spermatic vein empties into the left renal vein, whereas the right spermatic vein empties directly into the inferior vena cava.

10. **The correct answer B.** A grade III cystocele is described as the descent of the bladder outside of the introitus with straining.

11. **The correct answer is C.** von Hippel Lindau disease is an autosomal dominant condition manifested by cerebellar hemangioblastomas; retinal angiomas; cysts of the pancreas, kidney, and epididymis; epididymal cystadenoma; pheochromocytoma; and clear cell renal carcinoma. It is not associated with any of the other choices.

12. **The correct answer is D.** This patient's presentation is suspicious for renal mass. The most appropriate imaging would be a CT urogram, which is a CT of the abdomen and pelvis with IV contrast, without contrast, and with delayed excretion of contrast images. Any lesion that enhances upon administration of contrast is suspicious for renal cell carcinoma. None of the other choices is appropriate in this situation.

13. **The correct answer is B.** The "blue dot sign" is when a small tender lump at the upper pole of the testicle appears to be blue because the skin is kept fastened over the mass. This is found with a torsed appendix testis.

14. **The correct answer is C.** Smoking, occupational exposure to chemicals, chronic indwelling catheters, and pelvic irradiation all increase one's risk of bladder cancer. Urinary tract infections have not been shown to affect a patient's risk for bladder cancer.

15. **The correct answer is C.** Contraindications to sildenafil include nitrate use, retinopathy, and priapism. Although many clinicians do not recommend taking sildenafil within 4 hours of taking an alpha blocker, use of alpha blockers is not an absolute contraindication.

16. **The correct answer is C.** There are numerous risk factors for erectile dysfunction (ED). Many of these can be reduced with lifestyle modifications. Risk factors for the development of ED include cardiovascular diseases, smoking history, hypercholesterolemia, pelvic surgery, medications, depression, multiple sclerosis, Parkinson's disease, and lumbar disc disease. Hyperthyroidism is not a risk factor for ED.

17. **The correct answer is B.** Common medications for the treatment of benign prostatic hypertrophy (BPH) include 5α-reductase inhibitors and alpha blockers. Although the patient may benefit from finasteride, it may take up to 6 months for improvement of bladder outlet obstructive symptoms. Starting the patient on an alpha blocker in combination with a 5α-reductase inhibitor will allow him to see an improvement in less than 1 week. Anticholinergics would not alleviate, and could actually worsen, this patient's symptoms.

18. **The correct answer is A.** The most common cause of erectile dysfunction is organic. The most common etiology of organic erectile dysfunction is vascular disease.

19. **The correct answer is D.** This patient's history and presentation are concerning for urologic malignancy. His extensive smoking history puts him especially at risk for bladder cancer; however, hematuria may occur anywhere along the urinary tract. The proper workup for hematuria is upper tract (kidneys and ureters) evaluation in the form of a CT urogram or intravenous pyelogram (*IVP*), lower tract evaluation (bladder and urethra) through cystoscopy, and evaluation of urine for infection (urinalysis and urine culture) or presence of malignant cells (cytology). Although he may indeed have bladder carcinoma and require surgical intervention, it is not absolute. Other treatment(s) may be utilized instead of operative intervention. Choices A through C will ascertain the diagnosis and allow the clinician to plan appropriately.

20. **The correct answer is C.** Noncontrast CT of the abdomen and pelvis is the study of choice for assessing the presence of stones in the urinary tract. It is highly sensitive and specific, it can be performed in a fairly expeditious manner, and it provides an accurate anatomic representation of the location of the calculus. A radiograph of the kidney, ureter, and bladder (KUB) may detect the presence of stones; however, radiolucent calculi, such as uric acid calculi, will be missed. Ultrasound accuracy frequently depends on the technician, and stones in the mid- to distal ureter may be missed. Magnetic reasonance imaging (MRI) is an expensive and time-consuming imaging modality; it should not be used as first-line imaging of urinary calculi.

21. **The correct answer is C.** This constellation of findings most likely represents acute bacterial prostatitis. Prostatitis is the most common urologic diagnosis in men younger than age 50. The etiology is ascending colonization of the urinary tract, leading to infection of the prostate. Patients typically experience fevers, chills, and malaise, along with urinary symptoms such as dysuria, frequency, and urgency. Perineal pain may be present as well. Treatment typically consists of long-term course (at least 4 weeks) of antibiotics. Fluoroquinolones are the antibiotics of choice; however, trimethoprim-sulfamethoxazole

may be used as well. Patients presenting with high fevers and signs of sepsis should be admitted to the hospital for IV antibiotics, hydration, and careful observation.

22. **The correct answer is B.** Testicular cancer is the most common solid tumor in men ages of 20 to 34. Typical presentation is a firm nodule or painless swelling of one testicle; however, 10% may present with signs of metastatic disease: shortness of breath, anorexia, nausea, vomiting, back pain, or bone pain. Approximately 90% of testicular tumors are germ cell tumors, either seminoma or nonseminoma. The most common risk factor for testicular cancer is a history of cryptorchidism. Initial workup includes a scrotal ultrasound, serum tumor markers [lactate dehydrogenase (LDH), alpha fetoprotein (AFP), and human choriogonadotropin (HCG)], CHEM 7, liver function tests, and a chest x-ray.

23. **The correct answer is D.** Approximately 90% of stones less than or equal to 5 mm will spontaneously pass within 40 days. For this patient, a trial of passage is warranted. The patient should receive analgesia in the form of narcotics or NSAIDs. She should be encouraged to drink plenty of fluids and strain her urine for stones. She should follow-up in 1 month with a repeat imaging study to assess the progression of the stone.

24. **The correct answer is B.** This patient has an abnormal digital rectal examination and a high serum prostate-specific antigen (PSA), two indications for prostate biopsy. The American Cancer Society and American Urological Association recommend prostate cancer screening to begin at age 50 for men with a life expectancy of at least 10 years and at age 40 for men with an increased risk of prostate cancer (family history or African American men). Screening consists of an annual PSA and digital rectal examination. Indications for prostate biopsy are: abnormal digital rectal examination, elevated PSA, or a significant increase in PSA compared to prior tests (PSA velocity ≥0.75 ng/ml).

25. **The correct answer is D.** Opinions differ; there is no obvious "right" answer for the treatment of clinically localized prostate cancer. Discussing treatment options is an involved process that must be tailored to the patient's needs. Each modality has advantages and disadvantages. Studies have shown similar recurrence-free survival rates for low-risk prostate cancer patients who undergo either surgery or radiation; however, both treatment modalities can adversely affect quality of life. Some physicians recommend active surveillance or even hormonal therapy based on the patient's comorbidities. Education should be multidisciplinary; patients need to be counseled on the risks and benefits of each treatment option, on how each treatment will affect his quality of life, and on how it will affect his lifetime goals.

26. **The correct answer is A.** The patient should be referred to a urologist for a prostate biopsy. The patient has been taking finasteride for 3 years. Finasteride is a 5α-reductase inhibitor that subsequently lowers serum and intraprostatic dihydrotestosterone (DHT) levels. 5α-reductase converts testosterone to dihydrotestosterone (DHT), the major androgen in the prostate. This facilitates benign stromal growth of the prostate. Finasteride lowers DHT levels and shrinks the prostate gland. Prostate volume regression is maximal at 6 months. In addition, finasteride reduces prostate-serum antigen (PSA) levels by approximately 50%. This patient's PSA is 2.7 ng on finasteride; his actual PSA is 5.4 ng/ml, which is elevated.

27. **The most appropriate answer is A.** This patient should be treated with Bacillus Calmette-Guerin (BCG). BCG is an attenuated, live bacillus vaccine generated from *Mycobacterium bovis*. Instillation of BCG into the bladder reduces the recurrence and progression of non-muscle invasive bladder cancer. BCG stimulates an immune response that helps destroy tumor cells. It is initially given in the outpatient setting once a week for 6 weeks (total of six doses). Complications include cystitis, dysuria, hematuria, malaise, fever, and sepsis. To prevent complications, do not instill if the patient has grossly bloody urine or has a urinary tract infection.

28. The correct answer is C. Transitional cell carcinoma (TCC) is the most common type of bladder cancer. The bladder, ureters, and renal pelvis are lined by transitional cell epithelium. Because these surfaces are constantly exposed to urine, TCC can occur anywhere along the urinary tract.

29. The correct answer is B. Kidney stones are most commonly composed of calcium oxalate. The most common cause of formation of these stones is dehydration. Magnesium ammonium phosphate stones are associated with urinary tract infections. Uric acid stones are associated with high uric acid levels in the urine. These stones are radiolucent and can occur in patients with gout, myeloproliferative disorders, chronic diarrhea, or who are undergoing chemotherapy. Cystine stones occur in patients with cystinuria, an inherited autosomal recessive disorder. These patients have impaired transport of the amino acids cystine, ornithine, lysine, and arginine (COLA).

30. The correct answer is D. This patient has an acute uncomplicated bacterial cystitis, An uncomplicated UTI is defined as an infection of a urinary tract that does not have any structural or functional abnormalities. The treatment is a 3-day course of antibiotics, usually trimethoprim-sulbactam, nitrofurantoin, or a fluoroquinolone.

31. The correct answer is A. The majority (70%) of prostate cancers are found in the peripheral zone. Benign prostatic hyperplasia (BPH), however, occurs predominantly in the transition zone.

32. The correct answer is C. With the increased use of abdominal CT scans, ultrasounds, and MRIs for a variety of medical reasons, the majority of renal masses are now detected incidentally. Most renal masses are asymptomatic, although patients may experience flank pain, hematuria, or a palpable flank mass. It is estimated that over 50% of renal cell carcinomas are discovered incidentally.

33. The correct answer is B. *Escherichia coli* is the most common urinary pathogen for both community-acquired (85%) and nosocomial (50%) urinary tract infections (UTIs). The most common route of infection is through fecal flora ascending into the bladder from the perineal area. Treatment for uncomplicated UTIs is a 3-day course of trimethoprim-sulfamethoxazole, nitrofurantoin, or a fluoroquinolone antibiotic.

34. The correct answer is D. Sildenafil, tadalafil, and vardenafil are the most common medications used to treat erectile dysfunction (ED). They belong to a drug class called phosphodiesterase type 5 (PDE5) inhibitors. They facilitate an erection by inhibiting the degradation of cGMP by PDE5 in the arterial smooth muscle cells of the penis. This allows for decreased intracellular calcium, causing smooth muscle relaxation of the cavernosal arteries, which leads to increased blood flow and subsequent erection. The 2005 American Urological Association guidelines recommend PDE5 inhibitors as first-line therapy for treatment of ED, unless contraindicated.

35. The correct answer is B. Nitric oxide is released from parasympathetic nerve cells, initiating a cascade of events that result in erection. Nitric oxide binds to guanylate cyclase on arterial smooth muscle cells located in the cavernosa of the penis. Guanylate cyclase then forms cGMP from GTP. cGMP leads to decreased intracellular calcium, causing smooth muscle relaxation of the cavernosal arteries, which leads to increased blood flow and subsequent erection.

36. The correct answer is A. Phosphodiesterase type 5 (PDE5) inhibitors are absolutely contraindicated in patients taking nitrates or nitric oxide. The PDE5 inhibitors could potentiate the effect of nitric oxide in the patient, which could cause life-threatening hypotension. Patients taking alpha blockers can take PDE5 inhibitors; however, they should be warned to watch for dizziness and hypotension. Some physicians recommend taking the alpha blocker and the PDE5 inhibitor 4 hours apart from one another. A PDE5 inhibitor is questionable if a patient has a history of severe cardiovascular disease or a recent history (past 6 months) of a cardiovascular event, such as a stroke, myocardial infarction, or arrhythmia. In these cases, a consultation with a cardiologist should be considered.

37. **The correct answer is A.** Alpha blockers are the first-line treatment option for management of benign prostatic hypertrophy (BPH). As part of the aging process, many men will experience benign enlargement of the prostate, which may subsequently cause symptoms of urinary obstruction. These symptoms are called *lower urinary tract symptoms*, or LUTS. LUTS include urinary frequency, nocturia, urinary urgency, incomplete emptying, weak urinary stream, postvoid dribbling, and difficulty initiating stream. In men, the prostate and the bladder neck are abundant in alpha-1A receptors. Alpha blockers such as tamsulosin are specific for these receptors; they subsequently relax the smooth muscle in the prostate and bladder neck, allowing for an improved urinary stream and a decrease in LUTS. This particular patient presents with LUTS. Measurement of his urinary stream reveals decreased flow (flow less than 15 ml/sec is suggestive of obstruction). In addition, the patient has an elevated postvoid residual (normal men should retain little to no urine after voiding), and examination reveals an enlarged prostate (normal prostate volume is 20 g). The next course of action would be to start him on an alpha-1A blocker.

38. **The correct answer is C.** This patient presents with signs and symptoms of urinary obstruction from benign prostatic hypertrophy (BPH). His symptoms have worsened despite medical management with tamsulosin and finasteride. High postvoid residuals and urinary stasis have led to urinary tract infections (UTIs) and an episode of retention. These findings provide a compelling argument for surgical intervention. Changing medications within the same drug class will not help, because studies have shown similar efficacy of each drug within its respective class. Strong indications for surgery are recurrent UTIs, recurrent or persistent urinary retention, bladder stones, renal insufficiency secondary to BPH, and substantial bother from symptoms. These patients have usually failed medical management with alpha blockers and 5α-reductase inhibitors. The gold standard urologic intervention is transurethral resection of the prostate, or TURP.

39. **The correct answer is B.** This patient is complaining of worsening obstructive voiding symptoms from benign prostatic hypertrophy (BPH) despite taking an alpha blocker (tamsulosin). The next step would be to add a 5α-reductase inhibitor such as finasteride. Studies have shown that both alpha blockers and 5α-reductase inhibitors can individually prevent BPH progression, but the combination provides a synergistic effect, preventing progression better than each medication alone.

REFERENCES

Abeloff, M. D., Armitage, J. O., Neiderhuber, J. E., Kastan, M. B., and McKenna, W. G. (2004). *Clinical oncology*, 3rd ed. Churchill-Livingstone, Philadelphia, PA.

American Cancer Society. ACS cancer detection guidelines: Cancer-related checkup. (Online). Available at www.cancer.org/docroot/PED/content/PED_2_3X_ACS_Cancer_Detection_Guidlines_36.asp?sitearea=PED. Accessed May 22, 2007.

Bostwick, D., Crawford, E., Higano, C., et al. (2005). *American Cancer Society's complete guide to prostate cancer*. American Cancer Society Health Promotions, Atlanta, GA.

Brunicardi, F. C., Andersen, D. K., Billiar, T. R., Dunn, D. L., Hunter, J. G., Matthews, J. B., Pollock, R. E., and Schwartz, S. I. (2006). *Schwartz's principles of surgery*, 8th ed. McGraw-Hill Publishers, New York.

Gomella, L. G. (2000). *The 5-minute urology consult*. Philadelphia, Lippincott Williams and Wilkins, Philadelphia, PA.

Graham, S. D., Jr., Glenn, J. F., and Keane, T. E. (1998). *Glenn's urologic surgery*, 6th ed. Lippincott Williams and Wilkins, Philadelphia, PA.

Kumar, V., Abbas, A. L., and Fausto, N. (2005). *Robbins and Cotran: Pathologic basis of disease*, 7th ed. Elsevier-Saunders, Philadelphia, PA.

Townsend, C. M., and Mattox, K. L. (2004). *Sabiston textbook of surgery*, 17th ed. Elsevier-Saunders, Philadelphia, PA.

Wein, A. J., Kavoussi, L. R., Novick, A. C., Partin, A. W., and Peters, C. A. (2007). *Campbell-Walsh urology*, 9th ed. Saunders, Philadelphia, PA.

Wieder, J. A. (2005). *Pocket guide to urology*, 2nd ed. Griffith Publishing, Boise, ID.

Renal Medicine

Barry Korn, DO, DPM, DAAPM

1. Which of the following is *not* a risk factor for chronic kidney disease?

   A. Diabetes mellitus
   B. Hypertension
   C. "Honeymooner's cystitis"
   D. Urinary obstruction

2. Which of the following is *false* concerning the glomerular filtration rate (GFR)?

   A. GFR is an indication of functioning kidney mass.
   B. It is an important consideration for the dosing of certain medications.
   C. Creatinine clearance as measured by a 24-hour urine collection usually underestimates the GFR.
   D. Patients with the same creatinine levels may have different estimated GFRs.

3. Proteinuria may be decreased and the progression of chronic kidney disease slowed by the utilization of which of the following?

   A. Calcium-channel blockers
   B. Angiotensin-converting enzyme inhibitors
   C. Beta blockers
   D. Alpha blockers

4. Which of the following urine sediment findings would you most commonly see in patients with glomerulonephritis?

   A. Red blood cell casts
   B. White blood cell casts
   C. Eosinophils
   D. Granular casts

5. Which of the following is *not* true of renal artery stenosis?

   A. The majority of cases are due to atherosclerosis.
   B. Prevalence decreases with age.
   C. Prevalence increases with diabetes.
   D. Refractory hypertension may never develop, therefore many cases would remain undetected.

6. A 60-year-old obese male presents with flank pain, hematuria, and a palpable abdominal mass. He has fatigue and anemia. Which of the following is the most likely diagnosis?

   A. Renal cell carcinoma
   B. Bladder cancer
   C. Nephrothiasis
   D. Cystitis

7. Which of the following is *not* usually a complication of polycystic renal disease?

   A. Aortic aneurysms
   B. Crohn's disease
   C. Intracerebral aneurysms
   D. Recurrent urinary tract infections

8. Which of the following is the most common form of glomerulonephritis worldwide?

   A. Poststreptococcal glomerulonephritis
   B. IgA nephropathy
   C. Rapidly progressive glomerulonephritis
   D. Tubulointerstitial nephritis

9. Which of the following is *not* characteristic of the nephritic syndrome?

   A. Absence of protein
   B. Hypoalbuminemia
   C. Edema
   D. Hyperlipidemia

10. A 46-year-old male presents with a sudden onset of excruciating right flank pain. The pain occurs in "waves" and refers into the right lower abdomen and groin. The pain is now radiating to the tip of the penis. In which of the following conditions do these symptoms most commonly occur?

   A. Appendicitis
   B. Cholecystitis
   C. Diverticulitis
   D. Ureteral stone

11. Which of the following laboratory tests must a clinician order before performing an intravenous pyelogram (IVP)?

   A. Alkaline phosphatase
   B. Serum creatinine
   C. Aspartate aminotransferase (AST)
   D. Alanine transaminase (ALT)

12. Which of the following is *false* regarding hemolytic-uremic syndrome?

   A. The cause is *Escherichia coli* O157:H7.
   B. It is the least common cause of acute renal failure in children.
   C. Testing reveals microangiopathic anemia.
   D. Testing reveals thrombotic thrombocytopenia.

13. Which of the following best defines oliguria?

   A. <800 ml of urine per day
   B. <700 ml of urine per day
   C. <600 ml of urine per day
   D. <500 ml of urine per day

14. Which of the following typically is not a cause of prerenal failure?

   A. NSAIDs
   B. Diuretics
   C. Hypovolemic shock
   D. Prostatic hypertrophy

15. Which of the following is *not* usually associated with urinary tract infection (UTI)?

   A. Dysuria
   B. Negative leukocyte esterase
   C. Positive nitrites
   D. White blood cells in urine

16. Which of the following is *not* a risk factor for complicated pyelonephritis?

    A. Age greater than 60 years
    B. Polycystic kidney disease
    C. Female sex
    D. Corticosteroid use

17. Which of the following is *not* a preoperative risk for patients with chronic kidney disease?

    A. Hypokalemia
    B. Hypertension
    C. Hypoglycemia
    D. Anemia

18. Which of the following is *not* a common cause of chronic kidney disease?

    A. Diabetes mellitus
    B. Hypotension
    C. Ischemia
    D. Toxins

19. To predict the glomerular filtration rate (GFR) in patients with chronic kidney disease, which of the following information is not a requirement for the Cockcroft-Gault equation?

    A. Age
    B. Weight in pounds
    C. Serum creatinine
    D. Sex

20. Which of the following is *not* usually a cause of sterile pyuria?

    A. Tuberculosis
    B. Bladder tumors
    C. Sedentary lifestyle
    D. Corticosteroids

21. A 4-year-old girl presents with an abdominal mass, gross hematuria, and fever. Abdominal CT scan defines the mass to be of renal origin. Which of the following is the most likely cause of the mass?

    A. Wilms' tumor
    B. Polycystic kidney disease
    C. Hydronephrosis
    D. Renal calculi

22. Which of the following is the leading cause of acute nephritic syndrome?

    A. Urinary tract infection
    B. Drug reaction
    C. Ischemia
    D. Poststreptococcal glomerulonephritis

23. Which of the following is the definitive test for diagnosis of acute interstitial nephritis?

    A. Urinalysis
    B. CT scan
    C. BUN/creatinine
    D. Renal biopsy

24. Which of the following is *not* a contraindication for renal biopsy?

    A. Acute renal failure
    B. Bleeding diathesis
    C. Solitary kidney
    D. Sepsis

25. Which of the following is *not* a functional role primarily attributed to the kidney?

    A. Erythropoiesis
    B. Renin secretion
    C. Sodium regulation
    D. Urobilinogen excretion

ANSWERS

1. **The correct answer is C.** "Honeymooner's cystitis" represents an ascending urinary tract infection (UTI) typically caused by minor trauma during sexual intercourse. The name "honeymooner's cystitis" resulted from the increased incidence of cystitis among new brides. Recurrent UTIs are a risk factor for chronic kidney disease, as are the other choices. The one or few instances of cystitis among "honeymooners" is not a recurrent UTI, and therefore not a cause of chronic kidney disease.

2. **The correct answer is C.** The glomerular filtration rate (GFR) is a useful measure of over-all renal function. It measures the amount of plasma ultrafiltered across the glomerular capillaries, which correlates with the ability of the kidneys to filter various substances. A 24-hour urine creatinine clearance estimation is remarkably accurate. An incomplete or a prolonged collection is a common source of error; a complete collection is usually accurate.

3. **The correct answer is B.** Angiotensin-converting enzyme (ACE) inhibitors are antihy-pertensive agents that act by inhibiting the conversion of angiotensin I into angiotensin II (a powerful vasoconstrictor), thus helping to reduce blood pressure. ACE inhibitors may decrease proteinuria by reducing glomerular selectivity, slowing the progression of chronic kidney disease. Other factors, such as a general reduction in blood pressure and sodium excretion, can also reduce proteinuria. High sodium intake reduces the an-tiproteinuric effects of ACE inhibitors, so this would make sense. The other medications would not have this effect. Alpha-blockers aid in reducing outflow obstruction.

4. **The correct answer is A.** Dipstick and microscopic evaluation will reveal evidence of hematuria, moderate proteinuria and red cell casts, and white cells. Red cell casts are specific for glomerulonephritis.

5. **The correct answer is B.** The prevalence of renal artery stenosis *increases* with age. All the other choices are correct.

6. **The correct answer is A.** Renal cell carcinoma typically presents with flank pain and hematuria along with a palpable mass in approximately one-third of cases. The triad of flank pain, hematuria, and a mass is usually a sign of advanced disease. Bladder cancer does not generally present with a palpable abdominal mass (usually pelvic) and does not usually present with flank pain. Nephroliths (kidney stones) present with flank pain and hematuria, but not a palpable abdominal mass. Cystitis may present with hema-turia and flank pain, but no palpable mass. Typically, cystitis presents with suprapubic pressure or pain.

7. **The correct answer is B.** Colonic diverticuli is a complication of polycystic renal disease, but Crohn's disease usually is not. All of the other conditions are potential complications of polycystic kidney disease.

8. **The correct answer is B.** IgA nephropathy, also known as Berger's disease, the most common form of glomerulonephritis, presents with deposition of IgA in the glomerular

mesangium. An episode of gross hematuria is the most common presenting complaint. This is frequently associated with an upper respiratory infection.

9. **The correct answer is A.** Although the proteinuria may be mild or moderate, it is still present, especially if the glomerulonephritis worsens. All of the other answers are present during the nephritic syndrome.

10. **The correct answer is D.** This is an obvious presentation of nephrolithiasis. It is probably located in a mid to lower arc of the ureter, as witnessed by the radiation of pain into the penis. Appendicitis typically presents with periumbilical pain radiating to the right lower quadrant along with anorexia and/or nausea and vomiting. Cholecystitis may present with right upper quadrant pain, often in conjunction with a fatty meal intake. Diverticulitis presents with a left lower quadrant pain.

11. **The correct answer is B.** The practitioner must determine the serum creatinine level. There is a relative contraindication to order the IVP in patients at increased risk for acute renal failure, which includes patients with a serum creatinine greater than 2 mg/dl. Other imaging modalities, such as CT and MRI replaced the intravenous pyelogram (IVP), once the standard imaging procedure for evaluation of the urinary tract.

12. **The correct answer is B.** Hemolytic-uremic syndrome (HUS) occurs most commonly in children. Fortunately, the mortality rate is generally low (approximately 5%). All of the other signs/symptoms listed occur with HUS.

13. **The correct answer is D.** Oliguria is <500 ml of urine a day. Some texts list oliguria as <400 ml of urine a day.

14. **The correct answer is D.** Prerenal failure occurs as a result of a variety of conditions; however, prostatic hypertrophy is not usually one of them. Prostatic hypertrophy may result in urinary flow obstruction leading to postrenal failure.

15. **The correct answer is B.** Urinary tract infections are associated with a positive leukocyte esterase in urine samples. Nitrites may be positive in infections involving gram negative organisms.

16. **The correct answer is C.** All of the answers are risk factors for complicated pyelonephritis except female sex. Complicated pyelonephritis occurs more commonly in the male sex.

17. **The correct answer is A.** All of the listed answers are preoperative risk factors for patients with kidney disease except for hypokalemia. Hyperkalemia is a preoperative risk factor for patients with kidney disease. Current estimates indicate preoperative hyperkalemia to be as high as 19 to 38% in patients with chronic or end-stage renal disease. This statistic is significant as research through the years attributes hyperkalemia to cardiac arrhythmia. Indeed, cardiovascular disease is the most common cause of death in patients with renal disease, however, recent unpublished data finds no correlation between arrhythmia and hyperkalemia in this patient population. We urge the clinician to follow future research closely. Although no recommendations exist for safe preoperative potassium values, one study believes practitioners should avoid general anesthesia in chronic kidney disease patients with serum potassium levels above 5.5 mEq per L (5.5 mmol per L). Intravenous administration of an insulin-dextrose combination or bicarbonate, and polystyrene binding resins or dialysis can remove excess stores of potassium, thus temporarily improving hyperkalemia. Of course, dialysis is the treatment of last resort.

18. **The correct answer is B.** All are contributing factors except for hypotension. Hypertension usually "contributes" to chronic kidney disease through several factors, although the clinician should understand that this is a case of reciprocal causation. In other words, does the hypertension cause chronic kidney disease or does chronic kidney disease cause hypertension? The answer is both. Typical "causes" of chronic kidney disease (or the reverse) from hypertension include increased sympathetic activity, chronic renal transplant dysfunction, extracellular volume expansion, renin-angiotensin aldosterone stimulation, renovascular disease, or perhaps preexisting cases of essential hypertension.

19. **The correct answer is B.** All of the parameters listed are necessary to calculate creatinine clearance, except the weight should be in kilograms, not pounds.

20. **The correct answer is C.** All of the answers listed can cause sterile pyuria except for a sedentary lifestyle. Exercise can cause sterile pyuria. Heavy exercise (especially in long-distance runners) could cause microtrauma to the urinary vasculature, thus causing hematuria. Classically, this condition occurs as a result of tuberculosis.

21. **The correct answer is A.** Wilms' tumor (nephroblastoma) is a rare kidney cancer that affects children. It is the fifth most common pediatric malignancy and the most common renal tumor in children. The tumor may arise in three clinical settings, the study of which resulted in the discovery of the genetic abnormalities that lead to the disease. The settings for Wilms' tumor are (1) sporadic, (2) in association with genetic syndromes, and (3) familial. Although researchers slowly determined some of the molecular biology of Wilms' tumor, the exact cellular mechanisms involved in the etiology of the tumor remain under investigation.

22. **The correct answer is D.** All conditions listed in the question may cause nephritic syndrome; however the leading cause is poststreptococcal glomerulonephritis.

23. **The correct answer is D.** A biopsy is the definitive modality to diagnose this condition. The other modalities may or may not assist in the diagnosis, but there is no substitute for tissue samples and pathologic analysis.

24. **The correct answer is A.** All of the choices listed are contraindications for invasive renal biopsy except for acute renal failure, which may indeed be the reason for the biopsy in the first place.

25. **The correct answer is D.** The human kidneys (approximately 250 g total weight), with approximately 2 million nephrons, receive the highest blood flow per gram of organ weight in the body, amounting to approximately 1 liter/min of renal blood flow (RBF). The kidney generates a glomerular filtrate of 100 ml/min, of which almost 99% reabsorbs along the nephrons, and approximately 1% excretes as urine. The kidney performs high, nonselective filtration and almost complete reabsorption of the filtrate through highly ordered and regulated tubular reabsorption and secretion. The principal function of the kidney is to maintain homeostasis of our extracellular fluid (ECF)—despite wide variations of daily fluid and electrolyte intake. Indeed, this remarkable function of high filtration and high reabsorption is exactly what permits great flexibility in daily fluid and electrolyte intake with daily water intake varying from 0 to 30 liters/day. The kidneys also function in maintenance of acid-base balance. Urobilinogen is one of the substances excreted in the 1% of urine. Erythropoiesis, renin secretion, and regulation of sodium are primary functional roles of the kidney.

REFERENCES

Fauci, A. S., Braunwald, E., Kasper, D. L., Hauser, S. L., Longo, D. L., Jameson, J. L., and Loscalzo, J. (2008). *Harrison's textbook of internal medicine*, 17th ed. McGraw-Hill Medical Publishing, New York.

Goldman, L., and Ausiello, D. (2008). *Cecil medicine*, 23rd ed. Saunders Elsevier, Philadelphia, PA.

Krishnan, M. (2002). "Preoperative care of patients with kidney disease." *American Family Physician* 66(8): 1471–1476.

Kurokawa, K. (1998). "Tubuloglomerular feedback: Its physiological and pathophysiological significance." *Kidney International* 54(S71–S74): 1523–1755.

McPhee, S. J., Papadakis, M. A., and Tierney, L. M. (2007). *Current medical diagnosis and treatment*. McGraw-Hill Medical Publishers, New York.

21

Emergency Medicine

Michael Lucca, MD, FACEP, FAAEM
Henry D. Unger, MD, FACEP

1. A 12-year-old boy was playing in his backyard when he suddenly collapsed. Neighbors found him gasping for air and with a swollen face. The paramedics arrive and find him to be unconscious. Physical examination reveals marked facial swelling, stridor, and a generalized erythematous, maculopapular rash, as shown below. His vital signs are as follows: blood pressure, 80/50 mmHg, left arm, supine; pulse, 130 beats per minute and weak; respiratory rate, 26 breaths per minute and labored; and a temperature of 98.6°F. Which of the following is the most likely cause for this patient's symptoms?

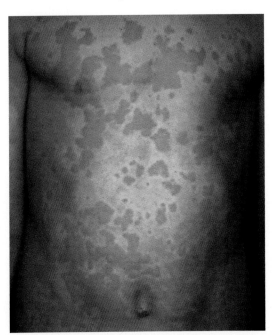

    A. Nonlethal hypersensitivity response
    B. Toxic shock
    C. Anaphylactic shock
    D. Acute myocardial infarction

2. A 24-year-old man presents with a single stab wound just to the left of his sternum. He arrives at the hospital with a blood pressure of 80/60 mmHg, right arm, supine; pulse of 140 beats per minute and thready; and a respiratory rate of 26 breaths per minute. His skin is cool and clammy, and he is incoherent. Physical examination reveals clear, bilateral bronchovesicular breath sounds, no tracheal deviation, muffled heart sounds, and distended neck veins. Furthermore, you note that the patient's peripheral pulses

diminish dramatically with inspiration. Which of the following is the most likely etiology for this patient's symptoms?

A. Hypovolemic shock
B. Cardiogenic shock
C. Tension pneumothorax
D. Cardiac tamponade

3. A 52-year-old female presents to the emergency department complaining of intermittent fever over the past few weeks. It occurs at night and is associated with shaking chills and sweats. She has a headache and myalgias, but no other symptoms. She tells you she was "fine" when she came back from India 2 months ago. Which of the following etiologic agents is most consistent with this presentation?

A. Hepatitis A
B. Hepatitis B
C. *Salmonella* sp.
D. *Plasmodium* sp.

4. Which of the following is the most common cause of chronic persistent traveler's diarrhea?

A. *Escherichia coli*
B. *Salmonella enteriditis*
C. *Shigella sonnei*
D. *Giardia lamblia*

5. A 24-year-old man presents to the emergency department with numbness and tingling of his arms and shoulder pain. He has just returned from a vacation in the tropics where he was scuba diving. He dove that morning and flew home that afternoon. Which of the following is the most appropriate management for this patient?

A. NSAIDs
B. Narcotics
C. Skeletal muscle relaxants
D. Transfer to a hyperbaric chamber

6. Which of the following is the hallmark of acute mountain sickness?

A. Headache
B. Nausea/vomiting
C. Dizziness
D. Fatigue

7. A 52-year-old female was on vacation and dove into a freshwater lake. Her head struck something in the water, causing her to lose consciousness. She was rescued by bystanders, one of whom was a physician assistant. She is nonresponsive and apneic. She has a faint pulse. Which of the following is the most appropriate first step in the management of this patient?

A. Begin rescue breathing.
B. Start chest compressions.
C. Hyperextend her neck to open her airway.
D. Clear her airway of secretions and maintain C-spine control.

8. Which aspect of a patient's history most likely predicts injuries sustained in a traumatic event?

A. AMPLE history
B. Mechanism of injury
C. Past medical history
D. Social history and past drug use

9. Which type of intravenous line is the most useful in children younger than age of 5 with signs of shock and no peripheral IV access?

   A. Femoral line
   B. Subclavian line
   C. Peripherally inserted central catheter (PICC) line
   D. Intraosseous line

10. Which of the following is *not* a common sign of shock?

    A. Confusion
    B. Agitation
    C. Tachycardia
    D. Hypertension

11. Which type of local anesthetic should *not* be used on digits, the penis, or the tip of the nose?

    A. 2% lidocaine without epinephrine
    B. Bupivicaine without epinephrine
    C. 1% lidocaine with epinephrine
    D. Procaine without epinephrine

12. Which of the following is the most effective technique to minimize infection in repair for nonfacial or scalp wounds in the emergency department?

    A. Prophylactic oral antibiotics
    B. Topical antibiotics
    C. High-pressure wound irrigation
    D. Sterile dressings

13. Which of the following organisms is most commonly associated with cat bites?

    A. *Pasteurella multocida*
    B. *Staphylococcus aureus*
    C. *Eikenella corrodens*
    D. *Clostridium perfringens*

14. Which of the following is true of rabies in the United States?

    A. Dogs are the most common vector for rabies.
    B. Squirrel bites have a high incidence of rabies.
    C. Bat exposure without a documented bite warrants rabies prophylaxis.
    D. Monkeys do not carry rabies.

15. Which of the following is *false* concerning hypothermia?

    A. Hyperglycemia is common.
    B. Tachycardia is the initial rhythm in hypothermia.
    C. Osborn J waves may be seen on the electrocardiogram in hypothermic patients.
    D. Hypothermia occurs when the core body temperature is below 32°C (89.6°F).

16. Which of the following does *not* cause an anion gap metabolic acidosis?

    A. Diabetic ketoacidosis
    B. Diarrhea
    C. Methanol
    D. Ethylene glycol

17. Which of the following does *not* characterize anticholinergic toxicity?

    A. Cool, moist skin
    B. Urinary retention
    C. Elevated temperature
    D. Confusion
    E. Tachycardia

18. Shingles is the reactivation later in life of which of the following viruses?

    A. Herpes simplex I
    B. Rubeola
    C. Parvovirus
    D. Varicella zoster

19. Which of the following is the most common cause of uncomplicated urinary tract infection (UTI)?

    A. *Pseudomonas aeruginosa*
    B. *Proteus mirabilis*
    C. *Klebsiella pneumoniae*
    D. *Escherichia coli*

20. The following radiograph demonstrates a fracture of the most commonly fractured carpal bone. Which of the following is this bone?

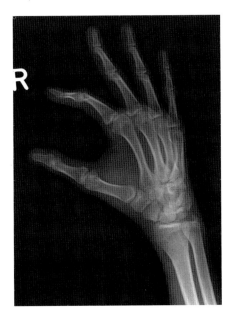

    A. Lunate
    B. Triquitrium
    C. Scaphoid
    D. Capitate

21. Which of the following is the most commonly dislocated major joint in the body?

    A. Elbow
    B. Knee
    C. Ankle
    D. Shoulder

22. Which of the following is *not* a characteristic of compartment syndrome?

    A. Pain
    B. Hyperesthesia
    C. Absent pulses
    D. Compartment pressures above 40 mmHg

23. A 35-year-old female presents to the emergency department complaining of abdominal pain, nausea, and vomiting over the past 12 hours. On examination, she is ill appearing. Vital signs reveal a mild tachycardia without fever. She is tender to palpation in the epigastric and right upper quadrant regions. Regarding initial evaluation and treatment, which of the following tests can be eliminated?

    A. Urine β-hCG
    B. An abdominal CT scan
    C. Amylase and lipase
    D. Ultrasound of the right upper quadrant

24. A 65-year-old male presents to the emergency department complaining of severe chest pain associated with ptosis and miosis of the right eye. Which of the following is the most likely diagnosis?

    A. Infarct in the distribution of the left middle cerebral artery
    B. Aortic dissection
    C. Unstable angina
    D. Pulmonary embolism

25. In which of the following situations would treatment with hyperbaric oxygen best be indicated?

    A. Patient suffering from smoke inhalation with carbon monoxide level of 15 ppm
    B. Patient with hypoxia following a near drowning (freshwater)
    C. Diabetic patient with a new ulcer on the dorsum of the right foot
    D. Patient with numbness and weakness of both lower extremities 2 hours after scuba diving

26. A 4-year-old child is brought to the emergency department because of an abrupt onset of coughing and choking. On arrival at the emergency department, the symptoms have resolved and the patient is comfortable. A radiograph of the chest and abdomen reveals the presence of a coin in the stomach. Which of the following is the most appropriate treatment?

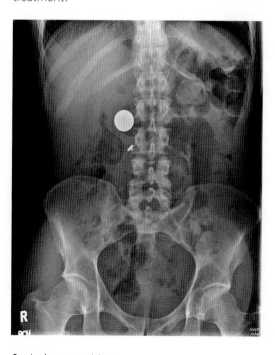

    A. Induce vomiting.
    B. Attempt to retrieve the coin by performing an endoscopy.
    C. Attempt to retrieve the coin with a nasogastric tube.
    D. Educate the parents regarding home safety and discharge the patient.

27. A 35-year-old male presents to the emergency department complaining of retrosternal burning chest pain that is worse with swallowing. It is slightly better when sitting upright. The pain has been constant over the past 2 days. The electrocardiogram reveals diffuse ST elevations and PR segment depressions. Which of the following is the most appropriate therapy?

A. Thrombolytics
B. NSAIDs
C. Urgent transfer to the cardiac catheterization lab
D. Beta blockers

28. A 25-year-old female with a history of an anxiety disorder presents to the emergency department. She tells you that her heart is racing and her breathing feels "short." She thinks it may be due to lack of sleep, because she just returned from a long vacation yesterday and was too uncomfortable on the 8-hour plane ride to sleep. She has run out of her lorazepam and is requesting a refill. Her only other medication is oral contraceptives. The electrocardiogram reveals sinus tachycardia with no acute changes. Which of the following is the most appropriate next step in the management of this patient?

A. Obtain a contrast CT scan of the chest.
B. Provide the patient with a dose of lorazepam, a prescription, and a referral to her psychologist.
C. Order a D-dimer.
D. Test her thyroid-stimulating hormone (TSH) level.

29. A 50-year-old patient presents to the emergency department with left-sided weakness. His CT scan shows no evidence of cerebral hemorrhage. Which of the following would *not* be a contraindication to the use of thrombolytic therapy in this patient?

A. Dementia
B. Prior history of intracranial bleeding
C. Patient awakened with symptoms 2 hours ago
D. Poorly controlled hypertension

30. A healthy appearing 55-year-old patient presents with left lower quadrant pain, a minimally elevated white blood cell count, and a CT scan (shown below) that reveals pericolonic inflammatory changes and a thickened colonic wall. Which of the following would *not* be appropriate treatment for this patient?

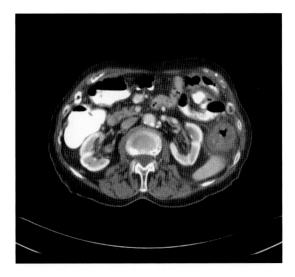

A. Surgery
B. IV fluids and nothing by mouth
C. Placement of a nasogastric tube
D. Metronidazole and a quinolone antibiotic

31. A patient presents with generalized abdominal pain, anorexia, and pain upon rectal examination. The WBC count is within the lab's normal limits. Which of the following statements is the most likely diagnosis?

 A. Appendicitis
 B. Bacteremia
 C. Diverticulitis
 D. Ascending cholangitis

32. Which of the following tests would *not* be indicated in the acute treatment of a 20-year-old female with abnormal vaginal bleeding, shoulder pain, and tachycardia?

 A. Cervical cultures
 B. β-hCG and pelvic ultrasound
 C. Tilt test
 D. Type and cross

33. Which of the following typically is *inappropriate* in the treatment of a patient with bleeding esophageal varices?

 A. Packed red blood cells
 B. Vasopressin
 C. Epinephrine
 D. Football helmet

34. A 20-year-old male presents with drooping of the right side of his face. He is unable to wrinkle his forehead, and when he attempts to close his eyes the right eye rolls backwards. He has detected a change in his ability to taste foods, and he winces when you speak because your voice seems loud. The remainder of his examination is benign. Which of the following is *incorrect* regarding this patient's condition?

 A. The condition is associated with Lyme disease.
 B. A CT scan of the brain is indicated to confirm diagnosis.
 C. Oral prednisone should be administered along with an antiviral agent.
 D. Herpes simplex virus has been associated with this condition.

35. A 50-year-old diabetic patient presents with crushing chest pain, a normal electrocardiogram, and an initial negative set of cardiac serum markers. Which of the following statements is true regarding this patient?

 A. The patient is at low risk for a myocardial infarction.
 B. Unstable angina is a likely diagnosis.
 C. Coronary artery disease is not present.
 D. The negative predictive value of the first set of negative enzymes is high.

36. A patient is brought to the emergency department following an intentional overdose of acetaminophen. Which of the following is true of regarding this patient?

 A. Oral acetylcysteine is easily tolerated.
 B. Gastric lavage is a first-line approach if the patient presents within 4 hours of ingestion.
 C. A metabolic acidosis and a respiratory alkalosis are seen with significant ingestions.
 D. Activated charcoal hemoperfusion is an important part of the management strategy.

37. A 42-year-old male patient presents to the emergency department with an intensely pruritic rash on both hands and arms following exposure to "poison ivy" 3 days ago while working in his garden. The lesions, which are shown below, are erythematous, edematous, and contain vesicles draining clear fluid. In some areas, a well-defined linear distribution is noted. Which of the following is *not* true concerning this patient's condition?

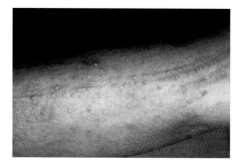

A. Treatment includes oral steroids for at least 2 weeks.
B. The rash is contagious if another person contacts the draining fluid.
C. Use of a dose pack of steroids may exacerbate the condition.
D. Cleansing the skin with copious amounts of water up to 20 minutes following the exposure to the toxin can prevent development of the rash.

38. A 60-year-old obese male presents to the emergency department following an abrupt onset of severe back pain. He is hypertensive and diaphoretic. His abdominal examination is benign. His urinalysis reveals three to four red blood cells per high-power field. The patient's clinician has called ahead and asked that you treat him for his kidney stone. Which of the following is the most appropriate diagnostic study to obtain for this patient?

A. Abdominal flat film
B. Electrocardiogram
C. Renal ultrasound
D. CT abdomen and pelvis

39. A 70-year-old patient with a history of chronic obstructive pulmonary disease (COPD) is being evaluated for possible pneumonia. She is placed on 4 liters of oxygen via nasal cannula, because her pulse oximetry registers in the low 80s. Your examination of the patient reveals that she is somnolent and confused. The triage note states that she was awake and alert at the time of arrival. Which of the following statements is most likely to be true?

A. She will be tachypneic when you examine her.
B. Her blood gas will reveal a marked decrease in her carbon dioxide.
C. Her serum bicarbonate will be elevated.
D. Providing more oxygen will improve her mental status.

40. A renal dialysis patient is brought into the emergency department in cardiac arrest. She is intubated, and CPR is initiated. She is in ventricular fibrillation. Despite repeated shocks, you are unable to convert her rhythm. Which of the following is the most urgent task to perform?

A. Obtain an arterial blood gas to assess her pH.
B. Administer sodium bicarbonate, calcium gluconate, insulin, and dextrose.
C. Perform synchronous cardioversion.
D. Look for "U" waves on her electrocardiogram.

41. A victim of a 20-foot fall from a ladder is brought to the emergency department by paramedics. His blood pressure is 80/50 mmHg, right arm, supine; his pulse is 56 beats per minute and regular; his respiratory rate is 24 breaths per minute and regular; and his temperature is 95°F. He is awake, alert, and speaking clearly. His hypotensive blood pressure is most likely the result of which of the following?

A. Spinal shock
B. Hypovolemic shock
C. Cardiogenic shock
D. Cardiac tamponade

42. A patient seeks emergency care for loss of sensation in his toes after hiking through subzero temperatures while wearing constrictive boots. He states his toes feel like "wood." His toes are shown below. Which of the following statements is *not* true concerning this patient?

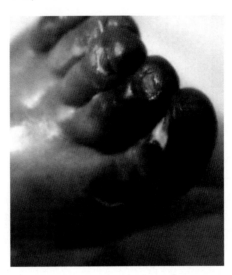

   A. The extremities should be rewarmed slowly in a water bath at 30°C.
   B. Hemorrhagic bullae should be left intact.
   C. Tetanus prophylaxis should be provided.
   D. Administer narcotic medication, because warming causes excessive pain.

43. An elderly patient presents to the emergency department complaining of severe abdominal pain. On examination, her abdomen is found to be soft with minimal tenderness. Despite the paucity of findings on physical examination, she is extremely uncomfortable, and her abdominal pain has her writhing on the table. She has heme-positive stools and an irregular heartbeat. Which of the following is likely to be true?

   A. An arterial blood gas will reveal a metabolic acidosis.
   B. Her obstruction series will reveal air fluid levels.
   C. She has a low pain threshold.
   D. This condition has a low mortality rate.

44. A 54-year-old male with a long history of alcohol abuse presents to the emergency department with nausea and vomiting following a night of heavy drinking. He states he has been vomiting for "much of the night." Although his emesis was initially limited to gastric contents, it has now become blood tinged. He is mildly tachycardic, and his epigastric region is tender to palpation. Which of the following is *least* likely to be present?

   A. Elevated lipase
   B. Elevated liver enzymes
   C. Profound anemia
   D. BUN/creatinine ratio <10

45. A type I diabetic patient is found unresponsive at home. He has been ill with vomiting for several days and has been unable to eat or take his normal medications. On arrival at the emergency department his blood pressure is 70/50 mmHg, left arm, supine, and his heart rate is 140 beats per minute. Which of the following is the most appropriate initial therapy?

   A. Bolus of normal saline
   B. Insulin therapy
   C. Antibiotics
   D. Beta blockade

46. During the month of July, a construction worker is brought to the emergency department because he has become confused and lethargic while working outside on the roof of a building. Which of the following statements is *incorrect* with regard to his diagnosis?

A. Core temperatures can exceed 105°F.
B. Rhabdomyolisis can lead to renal failure.
C. Disseminated intravascular coagulation (DIC) may be present.
D. Altered mental status is an unusual finding.

ANSWERS

1. The correct answer is C. Anaphylaxis is essentially a severe hypersensitivity reaction to an allergen, which may include environmental or pharmacologic causes or a response to envenomation. It affects multiple systems and usually involves hypotension and/or airway compromise. It is typically characterized by laryngeal edema, bronchospasm, and respiratory distress, which may progress to vascular collapse and shock. Patients in anaphylaxis or preanaphylaxis may exhibit intense pruritus and urticaria or angio-edema. Current clinical thought is that anaphylaxis refers to both IgE-mediated and non-IgE-mediated reactions. Mild allergic reactions may progress to a severe systemic response, anaphylaxis, and death; however, answer A is incorrect due to the severity of symptoms described. Toxic shock syndrome results from infection with *Staphylococcus aureus* or *Streptococcus pyogenes* and usually presents with fever, pain, and a generalized maculopapular or petechial rash that desquamates. Symptoms may progress to hypotension, shock, and death, but it does not present so acutely as in this scenario. Although myocardial infarction may ultimately result in or present with hypotension and shock, the history, signs, and symptoms of this patient do not warrant its consideration as the diagnosis.

2. The correct answer is D. The classic presentation of cardiac tamponade is Beck's triad: decreased systemic pressure, muffled or absent heart sounds, and distended neck veins (from a raised central venous pressure). Pulsus paradoxus (>10 mmHg decline in systolic pressure at the end of inspiration) and dyspnea further increase the likelihood of the diagnosis of cardiac tamponade. Tamponade occurs when fluid or blood accumulates between the pericardium and heart. If the heart is surrounded or filled with pericardial fluid, then the physical compression means that there is less blood in the ventricle available for ejection to the lungs or body. This is principally a problem where patients have sustained penetrating and/or blunt trauma to the sternum or in close proximity to the sternum. In this case, the patient suffered a knife wound that probably perforated the heart wall, which caused an accumulation of blood between the pericardium and the heart, ultimately compressing the heart. All of the answer choices provided may present with tachypnea, tachycardia, and hypotension. The clinician must look to the etiology of the symptoms. Answer A is incorrect because hypovolemic shock results from a loss of volume and may present with the symptoms as described, with the exception of increased venous pressure (distended neck veins). B is incorrect because cardiogenic shock (especially with left-sided heart failure) increases fluid in the lungs, which can overwhelm the capacity of the pulmonary lymphatics, causing interstitial and eventually alveolar edema. This patient did not have adventitious sounds, so it is unlikely that the etiology of his symptoms is cardiogenic shock. The end result of his tamponade may result in cardiogenic shock, however. The patient is obviously in shock, and one would expect to see tracheal deviation with a tension pneumothorax that leads to shock, therefore making C an incorrect answer.

3. The correct answer is D. Malaria is most common in the tropical regions of Africa, New Guinea, Haiti, Central America, and the Indian subcontinent. The classic presentation of malaria is fever spikes, chills, and rigors occurring at regular intervals. The fever is irregular at first. Furthermore, this patient traveled to a malaria endemic area. Answers A and B are incorrect because hepatitis usually presents with flulike symptoms, such as malaise, fatigue, nausea, vomiting, anorexia, and right upper quadrant pain or discomfort. The patient may also present with jaundice. C is not the answer because *Salmonella* usually presents with nausea, vomiting, and diarrhea within 6 to 48 hours following ingestion of contaminated food or water sources.

4. **The correct answer is D.** Although *Escherichia coli* is usually responsible for causing acute episodes of traveler's diarrhea (with enterotoxigenic *E. coli* [ETEC] being the most frequently isolated pathogen), chronic cases are more likely due to a protozoan infection. Chronic persistent traveler's diarrhea is most likely caused by *Giardia lamblia*.

5. **The correct answer is D.** The patient is exhibiting signs of decompression sickness (DCS). The appropriate treatment for decompression sickness is a hyperbaric oxygen chamber. The patient was at increased risk because he flew home after diving, which is not recommended following deep sea diving. Patients are at increased risk for air embolism and/or the bends following diving, and flight on the same day of a dive increases the risk. NSAIDs, narcotics, and muscle relaxants would not treat the cause of the pain and are thus incorrect.

6. **The correct Answer is A.** Headache is the hallmark of acute mountain sickness (AMS). AMS is defined as the presence of headache in an unacclimatized person who arrives at greater than 2,500 m (8,000 ft). In addition to headache, the patient with AMS may experience nausea or vomiting, dizziness, fatigue, shortness of breath with exertion, increased urination, and frequent night awakenings with sleep. Acetazolamide, a carbonic anhydrase inhibitor, is sometimes prescribed as a prophylactic. It increases urinary bicarbonate secretion, which results in an acidic blood pH, which, in turn, stimulates ventilation. This serves to accelerate acclimatization.

7. **The correct answer is D.** Following the tenets of ABC (airway, breathing, circulation), the airway must be opened before beginning rescue breathing or chest compressions. This patient probably has suffered a potential C-spine fracture. In trauma, airway management must be combined with C-spine control.

8. **The correct answer is B.** The mechanism of injury frequently gives clues as to the physical aspects of the injury and thus what injury has most likely been sustained. Answer A is incorrect. AMPLE refers to: *a*ge and *a*llergies; available *m*edications; *p*ast medical history; *l*ast meal; and *e*vents leading to current condition. The AMPLE history is not necessarily predictive of the type of injury. C is incorrect for the reasons mentioned with the AMPLE history. Social history and past drug use are not predictive of injuries sustained in an event.

9. **The correct answer is D.** Pediatric resuscitation courses now stress the use of interosseous lines for vascular access during resuscitation. A, B, and C are incorrect due to the difficulty and time required to obtain vascular access. Approximately one-quarter of pediatric resuscitation cases require 10 minutes or more for access, and this number is higher in children younger than 2 years of age.

10. **The correct answer is D.** Answers A, B, and C are all signs of shock, although the heart rate may be normal in the early stages of shock and bradycardic in later, more fulminant stages. The patient is rarely hypertensive in shock, because shock lends itself to vascular compromise and poor perfusion.

11. **The correct answer is C.** Epinephrine causes vasospasm, which can cause the affected area to become hypoxic. This may ultimately lead to necrosis of the area. The other choices are all acceptable local anesthetics.

Emergency Medicine

12. **The correct answer is C.** High-pressure wound irrigation is an effective method to remove bacteria and/or other contaminants within the wound. High-pressure irrigation has not proven to be effective in highly vascular wounds, such as the scalp or face, when there is no difference in the rate of infection or cosmetic appearance. A, B, and D are incorrect. In some studies, groups taking prophylactic antibiotics have shown to have higher rates of infection than controls. The literature is mixed in this regard. Topical antibiotics have shown mixed results as well in the healing rates of noninfected wounds.

13. **The correct answer is A.** This organism is prevalent in feline oral cavities and is the most commonly isolated organism in cat bites. Cat bites are treated with amoxicillin/clavulanic acid to cover for this organism. *Eikenella corrodens* is the organism most commonly found in human bite wounds. *Staphylococcus aureus* can cause a variety of wound infections not specific to cat bites. *Clostridium perfringens* is implicated in gas gangrene.

14. **The correct answer is C.** Since 1980, bats infected with rabies are the most common cause of human exposure in the United States. Answer A is incorrect because dogs are the most common vector in the rest of the world, but not the United States. Rodents, domestic ferrets, lagomorphs (rabbits and hares), dogs, and cats are not usually carriers of rabies in the United States. Monkeys have been known to carry rabies, especially where monkey populations are prevalent.

15. **The correct answer is D.** Hypothermia is diagnosed when the core body temperature is at or below 35°C (95°F). All of the other choices are incorrect, because hypothermia, accidental or otherwise, may present with one of the signs or symptoms listed in the choices.

16. **The correct answer is B.** The mnemonic MUDPILES is used to describe the causes of anion gap metabolic acidosis: *m*ethanol, *u*remia, *d*iabetic ketoacidosis, *p*araldehyde, *p*henformin (or metformin); *i*ron, *i*soniazid; *l*actic acidosis (cyanide, H_2S, CO, MetHb), *e*thylene glycol, *s*alicylates. Diarrhea is not a cause of anion gap metabolic acidosis. Diarrhea may cause a metabolic acidosis, albeit with a normal anion gap.

17. **The correct answer is A.** Signs and symptoms are best remembered as described in *Tintinalli's Emergency Medicine*: "Dry as a bone (dry skin, especially the axillae); red as a beet (flushed from vasodilation); hot as Hades (warm, perhaps febrile); blind as a bat (dilated pupils, visual hallucinations); mad as a hatter (dramatic delirium and visual hallucinations); and stuffed as a pipe (absent or hypoactive bowel sounds and decreased gastric motility along with a palpable bladder due to urinary retention)." Cool, moist skin is not seen in anticholinergic toxicity.

18. **The correct answer is D.** Shingles is the most common manifestation of varicella zoster viral infection in immunocompromised patients. It is cause by the herpes zoster virus. The other viruses do not cause the condition. Herpes simplex I causes cold sores (herpes labialis).

19. **The correct answer is D.** *Escherichia coli* causes >95% of all cases urinary tract infections. Answers A, B, and C are more commonly isolated from patients with other types of infections or conditions.

20. **The correct answer is C.** The scaphoid bone is the most commonly fractured carpal bone, especially in children, who comprise >88% of all broken scaphoid bones. A, B, and D are incorrect.

21. **The correct answer is D.** The shoulder is the most commonly dislocated major joint in the body. Shoulder injuries in athletes account for approximately 13% of all joint injuries, with shoulder dislocations accounting for approximately 50% of all dislocations.

22. **The correct answer is C.** Compartment syndromes are serious emergency complications that should be considered in any fracture within an enclosed osseofacial space where there is pain and paresthesias. Historically, compartment syndromes exhibited the "five Ps:" pain, pallor, pulselessness, paresthesia, and paralysis. This is no longer the case. In a conscious, oriented patient, the hallmark finding is pain that is disproportionate to the injury or physical findings. Pain on passive stretching of the muscle groups is also an important physical finding. Skin color, capillary refill, and distal pulses are considered to be unreliable indicators, because the pressure necessary to produce compartment syndrome is well below arterial pressure. Diminished pulses suggest ancillary pathologic conditions responsible for reduced arterial flow.

23. **The correct answer is B.** Approximately 7 to 10% of patients with abdominal pain have life-threatening conditions, even without hemodynamic instability. Answer A is incorrect, because pregnancy should be ruled out in all patients of childbearing age. C is incorrect, because this patient does not meet the typical diagnostic criteria for pancreatic conditions, and therefore an amylase and lipase profile is unlikely to be of use. An ultrasound of the right upper quadrant has rapidly become the diagnostic test of choice due to its relative ease and noncomplicating nature. Emergency department transabdominal or transvaginal ultrasound can help to identify intrauterine pregnancies; abdominal aortic aneurysms; intraperitoneal fluid, such as pus; hemorrhage; and intestinal contents. Helical CT has rapidly become the diagnostic test of choice in nonobstetric abdominal pain, but for initial evaluation ultrasound is the most appropriate test.

24. **The correct answer is B.** This is a relatively rare presentation of aortic dissection wherein the patient has Horner's syndrome (ptosis and miosis, facial flushing, and anhidrosis on one side) along with chest pain. Other rarely encountered clinical manifestations of aortic dissection include upper airway obstruction or hoarseness, hemoptysis, or dysphagia. A variety of conditions can mimic aortic dissection; however, the presence of the chest pain in a 65-year-old male along with the miosis and ptosis strongly points to aortic dissection. The other choices are part of a differential diagnosis in a patient with chest pain; however, they can be ruled out based on this information.

25. **The correct answer is D.** The patient probably has decompression sickness and, as such, requires hyperbaric oxygen therapy (HBOT). The use of HBOT in decompression sickness is widely accepted. HBOT has been described as useful in other cases such as clostridial and other necrotizing soft-tissue infections; certain problem wounds; delayed or late radiation injury to soft tissue and bone; and, in some of the literature, carbon monoxide inhalation. However, the use of HBOT in the case of carbon monoxide inhalation is controversial. Several authors will not call for future randomized control trials, underscoring the controversy surrounding this treatment. As always, the clinician is advised to remain current with prevailing evidence. When faced with a question in which one answer *may* be acceptable, the test-taker is advised to go with the choice that is incontrovertibly the correct choice to make—in this case, D.

26. **The correct answer is D.** This child swallowed a small, blunt object, and it has not lodged or obstructed in any fashion. Therefore, no treatment is necessary other than reassurance and education. A true foreign body is classified according to its physical characteristics (e.g., small, medium, or large; blunt or sharp; long or pointed). Plain films of the appropriate area (neck, chest, and abdomen) are necessary to localize the foreign body. Any foreign body in the esophagus should be removed. Most small, blunt objects beyond the esophagus will pass uneventfully.

27. **The correct answer is B.** This patient has pericarditis, as evidenced by the history, pain pattern, and the electrocardiogram. The other interventions are all appropriate in a patient with suspected or confirmed myocardial infarction.

28. The correct answer is A. Although this patient has a past history of anxiety disorder treated with lorazepam, the clinician should not ignore the shortness of breath and tachycardia that followed an 8-hour airplane trip. Also, anxiety can cause tachycardia, so the pulmonary embolism must first be ruled out; therefore, at this particular time, a referral to her psychologist is inappropriate. This patient is at high-risk for pulmonary embolism, and it must be ruled out before proceeding with any other course of action. C is incorrect; D-dimer should be used, but is not specific for making the diagnosis, rather more useful in excluding the diagnosis. Choice D, obtaining thyroid-stimulating hormone (TSH) levels, is an appropriate test to investigate hyperthyroidism, which can cause tachycardia, but the pulmonary embolism must first be ruled out.

29. The correct answer is C. Contraindications to fibrinolytic therapy are classified as absolute and relative. Answers A and D are incorrect because they are both relative contraindications to therapy. B is an absolute contraindication to therapy. Ideally, treatment should begin in less than 3 hours from time of symptom onset.

30. The correct answer is A. This patient has signs and symptoms consistent with diverticulitis, although the patient has not progressed to a more serious condition. Treatment of diverticulitis includes bowel rest, gastric decompression, IV fluids, and antibiotics, such as listed in choice D. Surgery would not be appropriate treatment for this patient at this time. Complications of acute diverticulitis, such as abscess formation or significant bowel perforation, would be indications of surgery.

31. The correct answer is A. Up to 20% of patients with acute appendicitis have a normal white blood cell count. Also, these patients frequently present with pain upon rectal examination due to irritation of the peritoneal cavity during the colonic manipulation. B is incorrect; as a general rule, the higher the white blood cell count, the greater the likelihood of bacteremia. C is incorrect; diverticulitis is usually accompanied with an elevated white cell count and left lower quadrant pain. D is incorrect; ascending cholangitis has a high mortality rate, and it will almost always manifest with an elevated white blood cell count.

32. The correct answer is A. This patient has a clinical picture consistent with an ectopic pregnancy. A is not a correct choice for diagnostic testing at this time. Cultures may ultimately play a role in determining if this patient has a sexually transmitted infection (STI), but plays no role in the acute treatment of an ectopic pregnancy. β-hCG will confirm if the patient is in a gravid state; the tilt test will determine volume loss; pelvic ultrasound will identify the presence or absence of an intrauterine pregnancy; and type and cross will prepare the patient for a blood transfusion in the case of a ruptured ectopic pregnancy, as indicated by the tachycardia.

33. The correct answer is C. Epinephrine is not an appropriate treatment for bleeding esophageal varices. Answers A, B, and D are all appropriate treatments for actively bleeding esophageal varices. The use of a football helmet is appropriate and refers to the use of a Sengstaken-Blakemore tube, which is placed in the stomach and esophagus and held in place by a helmet.

34. The correct answer is B. This patient has Bell's palsy. Answers A, C, and D are all correct. A CT scan would be unnecessary in such a case as clear-cut as this one.

35. The correct answer is B. Answer A is incorrect; ruling out a myocardial infarction requires two to three sets of enzymes. Answer D is incorrect; the negative predictive value of one set of enzymes is approximately 50% (flip of a coin). Normal electrocardiograms and negative enzymes do not rule out the presence of coronary artery disease (a stress test and/or catheterization would be necessary for that), and with this patient's complaint and risk factors, the presence of disease is likely to be high. It is important to remember, however, that negative enzymes and a normal electrocardiogram never rule out angina as the source of chest pain.

36. **The correct answer is B.** Acetaminophen overdose presents with several difficulties, with up to 20% of patients suffering profound liver failure. Answer A is incorrect; Acetylcysteine is a pungent sulfur-smelling compound usually tolerated with great difficulty. Lavage is seldom used for decontamination of the stomach in cases of overdose after 4 hours have passed. This patient presents within the accepted therapeutic window. Aspiration is a risk, and the airway should be protected if lavage is attempted. Answer C is incorrect; a mixed acid-base disturbance is seen with aspirin (not acetaminophen), and if an ingestion is suspected charcoal hemoperfusion has no established role in treatment.

37. **The correct answer is B.** Answer A is not the answer and therefore a true statement. Poison ivy (*Toxicodendron* dermatitis) requires a prolonged course of steroid therapy. Answer C is incorrect; short treatments with steroid dose packs can result in a recrudescence of the lesions. Once the toxin (urushiol) contacts the skin for longer than 20 minutes, there is little that can be done to avoid the outbreak. Therefore, it is important to wash the area within 20 minutes of exposure, thus answer D is incorrect. After the resin is removed, the lesions are no longer contagious. Therefore, no one can be contaminated by the serous drainage from the vesicles days later.

38. **The correct answer is D.** An aortic dissection must be ruled out in a hypertensive male patient in his 60s who presents with an abrupt onset of pain. Answers A, B, and C are all incorrect. A flat film of the abdomen and an electrocardiogram will provide little useful information in identifying this entity. A renal ultrasound would be helpful in determining the presence of a hydronephrosis, but the most appropriate test to identify an aortic pathology (which is the most dangerous among the differential diagnoses) is a CT. A CT is also useful because it can identify other causes of pain, including the renal colic the patient's clinician says he has in the first place. The presence of a few red blood cells should not lead the examiner to believe that the diagnosis must be renal.

39. **The correct answer is C.** This patient is suffering from hypercarbia (CO_2 retention), resulting from a high FiO_2 (inspired oxygen). This will suppress her respiratory drive, resulting in CO_2 elevation of and development of acidosis. Because the patient has chronic obstructive pulmonary disease (COPD), her chronic CO_2 elevation results in a compensatory increase in bicarbonate. Providing additional oxygen will probably further suppress her drive to breathe and exacerbate her clinical condition.

40. **The correct answer is B.** This patient is likely hyperkalemic, and these medications will drive her potassium intracellularly. Synchronized cardioversion will not be effective in the presence of fibrillation. Although you do want to obtain an arterial blood gas to assess her pH, as well as other indices, it will not solve this patient's problem therefore it is not the most urgent task. Identifying U waves on an electrocardiogram may satisfy an intellectual quest, but it is not what should be done.

41. **The correct answer is A.** The mechanism of injury, combined with hypotension and bradycardia, is a classic presentation of spinal shock. Answers B, C, and D are incorrect, because nothing indicates any of the other types of shock.

42. **The correct answer is A.** In cases of frostbite, all wet, constricting clothing should be removed and rapid, not slow, rewarming should occur in a warm water bath of 40–42°C (104–107.6°F). This will maximize the speed of rewarming without the danger of burns. The clinician should avoid refreezing, because this can cause a great deal of damage. Intact blisters should be left alone. Pain medications should be given, because rewarming is painful. Updating tetanus is also important.

43. **The correct answer is A.** Early findings include metabolic acidosis secondary to tissue ischemia. Mesenteric ischemia occurs when the blood supply to the mesentery is compromised for any reason. Answer B is incorrect because air/fluid levels are routinely seen in intestinal obstruction, and this is not an obstruction. Answer D is incorrect because of the high mortality rate in patients with risk factors such as atrial fibrillation. Pain that is out of proportion to physical findings is common and is the hallmark of this condition. Whether this patient has a low pain threshold is immaterial to the presentation at hand.

44. **The correct answer is D.** This patient has a long history of alcohol abuse, which could precipitate pancreatitis and, as such, an elevated serum lipase. Forceful and repeated vomiting may cause a Mallory-Weiss tear. This could cause small amounts of blood in the vomitus. However, the blood loss is unlikely to be severe, and therefore the prospect of a profound anemia is unlikely. From repeated emesis he is likely to be dehydrated, thus his BUN/creatinine ratio would be greater than 20. His liver enzymes most likely would be elevated due to his history of alcohol abuse.

45. **The correct answer is A.** This patient is likely to be in diabetic ketoacidosis and, as such, hypovolemic. Therefore, the initial therapy should include rapid hydration. Insulin can be given *after* fluid resuscitation is initiated. Antibiotics may be necessary if an infectious etiology is present; however, they are not part of initial therapy. D is absolutely incorrect because beta blockade should never be used to slow the heart rate in the face of hypovolemia.

46. **The correct answer is D.** Multisystem organ failure is common in severe cases, and core temperatures can reach 105° to 106°F. Altered mental status is seen in all cases of heat stroke.

REFERENCES

American Heart Association. (2005). *Guidelines for cardiopulmonary resuscitation and emergency cardiac care*. American Heart Association, Dallas, TX.

Auerbach, P. S. (2001). *Wilderness medicine*, 4th ed. Mosby Publishers, St. Louis.

Brunicardi, F. C., Andersen, D. K., Billiar, T. R., Dunn, D. L., Hunter, J. G., Matthews, J. B., Pollock, R. E., and Schwartz, S. I. (2006). *Schwartz's principles of surgery*, 8th ed. McGraw-Hill Publishers, New York.

Centers for Disease Control and Prevention. (2006). Travelers' diarrhea. (Online). Available at www.cdc.gov/ncidod/dbmd/diseaseinfo/travelersdiarrhea_g.htm.

Chudnofsky, C. R., Custalow, C. B., and Dronen, S. C. (2004). *Clinical procedures in emergency medicine*, 4th ed. Saunders Publishing, Philadelphia, PA.

Cohen, J., and Powderly, W. G. (2004). *Infectious diseases*, 2nd ed. Mosby–Elsevier, Philadelphia, PA.

Cummings, C. W., Flint, P. W., Haughey, B. H., Robbins, K. T., Thomas, R., Lederer, F. L., Harker, L. A., Richardson, M. A., and Schuller, D. E. (2005). *Otolaryngology head and neck surgery*, 4th ed. Mosby Publishers, Philadelphia, PA.

DeLee, J. C., Drez, D., and Miller, M. D. (2003). *DeLee and Drez's orthopaedic sports medicine*, 2nd ed. Saunders Publishing, Philadelphia, PA.

Feldman, M., Freidman, L. S., and Brandt, L. J. (2006). *Sleisenger and Fortran's gastrointestinal and liver diseases*, 8th ed. Saunders Publishing, Philadelphia, PA.

Ferri, F. F., Cooper, E., and McClure, M. (2007). *Practical guide to the care of the medical patient*, 7th ed. Mosby-Elsevier, Philadelphia, PA.

Hazinski, M. F., ed. (2002). *Textbook of pediatric advanced life support*. American Heart Association, Dallas, TX.

Kasper, D. L., Braunwald, E., Fauci, A. S., Hauser, S. L., Longo, D. L., Jameson, J. L., and Isselbacher, K. J., eds. (2005). *Harrison's principles of internal medicine*, 16th ed. The McGraw-Hill Companies, New York.

Marx, J. A. (2006). *Rosen's emergency medicine: Concepts and clinical practice*, 6th ed. Mosby-Elsevier, Philadelphia, PA.

Rakel, R. E., and Bope, E. T. (2007). *Conn's current therapy*, 59th ed. Saunders Publishing, Philadelphia, PA.

Roberts, J. R., Hedges, J. R., Chanmugam, A. S., Mandell, G. L., Bennett, J. E., and Dolin, R. (2005). *Principles and practice of infectious diseases*, 6th ed. Churchill-Livingstone, Elsevier, Philadelphia, PA.

Tintinalli, J. E., Kelen, G. D., Stapczynski, J. S., Ma, O. J., and Cline, D. M. (2004). *Tintinalli's emergency medicine*. McGraw-Hill Publishers, New York.

Townsend, C. M., and Mattox, K. L. (2004). *Sabiston textbook of surgery*, 17th ed. Saunders Publishing, Elsevier, Philadelphia, PA.

Zipes, D. P., Libby, P., Bonow, R. O., and Braunwald, E. (2005). *Braunwald's heart disease: A textbook of cardiovascular medicine*, 7th ed. Elsevier Saunders Publishing, Philadelphia, PA.

Endocrinology

Renee E. Amori, MD
Richard D. Siegel, MD

1. A 29-year-old man presents to the emergency department after a syncopal episode. He regained consciousness in transport and is able to report that for the last 6 to 7 months he has experienced fatigue, weight loss, and dizziness. He appears ill, and his skin pigment is darker than you would expect. His supine blood pressure is 110/65 mmHg, and his heart rate is 96 beats per minute. He is unable to sit upright without experiencing symptoms of orthostasis. His labs are significant for hyperkalemia and hyponatremia. Which of the following laboratory results would you would expect with this condition?

   A. High serum cortisol, high adrenocorticotropic hormone (ACTH)
   B. High serum cortisol, low ACTH
   C. Low serum cortisol, high ACTH
   D. Low serum cortisol, low ACTH

2. Which of the following corticosteroids does *not* interfere with the serum cortisol assay?

   A. Prednisone
   B. Hydrocortisone
   C. Prednisolone
   D. Dexamethasone

3. Which of the following is *not* associated with hyperkalemia?

   A. Chronic renal insufficiency
   B. Secondary adrenal insufficiency from exogenous glucocorticoid use
   C. ACE-inhibitor therapy
   D. Primary adrenal insufficiency from autoimmune adrenalitis

4. Which of the following hormones is *not* secreted from the adrenal cortex?

   A. Aldosterone
   B. Epinephrine
   C. Cortisol
   D. Testosterone

5. A 56-year-old female presents for an annual physical examination. She has been feeling fatigued, but has not noticed any increased thirst or urination. She is 63 inches tall and weighs 183 pounds (BMI 32.4). You order some routine laboratory data. Her nonfasting blood glucose level is 174 mg/dl. Which of the following is the next best step?

   A. Nothing additional is required.
   B. Check a fasting-glucose level.
   C. Check a hemoglobin A_1C.
   D. Prescribe metformin 500 mg once daily.

6. An 18-year-old male presents to the local emergency department with nausea, vomiting, and abdominal pain. His blood pressure is 110/60 mmHg, and he is awake but visibly uncomfortable. His abdomen is soft, nontender, and without masses. His renal function and urine output are within normal limits. He states, "I've never experienced anything like this before in my life." His laboratory values are shown below. Which of the following should *not* be included in his orders?

Glucose 560 mg/dL	Urine+ for glucose, ketones
Potassium 3.6 mEq/L	Serum ketones are positive
CO_2 11 mEq/L	ABG with a pH 7.15
Anion gap 16	Amylase, lipase are both normal

   A. Order intravenous fluids.
   B. Order potassium chloride.
   C. Start an infusion of bicarbonate.
   D. Order IV insulin at 0.1 units/kg/hr.

7. A 35-year-old man sees you to establish primary care. He was diagnosed with type 1 diabetes mellitus at the age of 12. He has been taking insulin glargine and insulin lispro for the past 2 years, but no other medications. He checks his blood glucose "when he remembers" and has not had routine blood work for "a few years." On examination, his blood pressure is 146/70 mmHg. You order routine blood and urine tests. He returns for follow-up 4 weeks later. His hemoglobin A_1C is 8.8%, and his urine microalbumin/creatinine ratio is 250 ug/mg Cr. On this visit, his blood pressure is 140/90 mmHg, and he reports that his wife "made" him check his blood pressure at the local pharmacy. At that time the reading was 138/85 mmHg. With regards to his blood pressure, which of the following is the most appropriate recommendation?

   A. Do nothing.
   B. Begin hydrochlorothiazide.
   C. Begin metoprolol.
   D. Begin lisinopril.

8. A 31-year-old woman has had type 1 diabetes since the age of 9. In the past 2 years, she has had excellent glycemic control with a hemoglobin A_1C <7% using her continuous subcutaneous insulin infusions. Prior to this, she had suboptimal control, with her A_1C ranging from 8 to 10%. She has recently had a dilated eye exam and was noted to have mild retinopathy. Which of the following should you tell her regarding these findings?

   A. She should not have children.
   B. This condition will not progress.
   C. She should have an eye exam every 2 years.
   D. Strict glycemic control will decrease the risk of progression.

9. A 55-year-old man was recently hospitalized for chest pain. He was diagnosed with diabetes mellitus. A hemoglobin A_1C drawn during hospitalization which was 8.2%. His creatinine is 1.2 mg/dl. He is 67 inches tall and weighs 267 pounds (BMI 41.8). His father had "borderline diabetes" and his aunt was "taking the needle" for her "sugar." You refer him to a nutritionist and diabetes educator, counsel him on exercise and weight loss, and give him a glucometer to self-monitor his fingerstick blood glucose values. You see him 3 months later for a follow-up visit. His diet has improved, but he has not lost weight. His A_1C remains at 8.1%. Which of the following is the next best step in the management of his diabetes mellitus?

   A. Give him 3 more months to lose weight.
   B. Begin glipizide.
   C. Begin metformin.
   D. Begin pioglitazone.

10. A 78-year-old female is brought to the emergency department after falling at home. She is a frail woman, with a history of type 2 diabetes mellitus, for which she takes glyburide 10 mg daily, metformin, and pioglitazone. In the emergency department, her fingerstick blood glucose is 56 mg/dl. Her creatinine has increased to 1.5/mg/dl (1 year ago). Which of the following is the most appropriate management for this patient?

    A. Stop the glyburide.
    B. Stop the glyburide and metformin.
    C. Stop all oral agents and begin insulin.
    D. Make no changes.

11. Which of the following is *not* an adverse effect associated with pioglitazone monotherapy?

    A. Weight gain
    B. Hypoglycemia
    C. Increased incidence of congestive heart failure
    D. Lower extremity edema

12. Which of the following screening tests is *not* recommended for evaluating microvascular complications of diabetes mellitus?

    A. Yearly barium swallow study for gastroparesis
    B. Yearly urine microalbumin/creatinine ratio for nephropathy
    C. Yearly foot exam with monofilament testing for peripheral neuropathy
    D. Yearly dilated retinal exam for retinopathy

13. According to the Adult Treatment Program III (ATP III), the low-density lipoprotein (LDL) goal for a patient considered to be "moderate risk" is which of the following?

    A. <70 mg/dl
    B. <100 mg/dl
    C. <130 mg/dl
    D. <160 mg/dl

14. Which of the following class of medications is the most effective at decreasing low-density lipoprotein (LDL) cholesterol?

    A. Bile acid resins
    B. Fibric acids
    C. HMG CoA reductase inhibitors (statins)
    D. Nicotinic acid (niacin)

15. Which class of medication is the most effective at increasing high-density lipoprotein (HDL) cholesterol?

    A. Bile acid resins
    B. Fibric acids
    C. HMG CoA reductase inhibitors (statins)
    D. Nicotinic acid (niacin)

16. Which of the following is considered a coronary artery disease risk equivalent?

    A. Hypothyroidism
    B. Postmenopausal status
    C. Diabetes mellitus
    D. Elevated cardiospecific C-reactive protein

17. Which of the following does *not* decrease triglyceride levels?

    A. Bile acid resins
    B. Fibric acids
    C. Fish oil
    D. Nicotinic acid (niacin)

18. A 39-year-old woman presents to your office with fatigue and weight gain. She is concerned about her thyroid function. Her history is significant for menorrhagia, which has improved using an oral contraceptive agent. Her mother has been diagnosed with hypothyroidism. Her neck exam is noncontributory, with no palpable thyroid abnormality. You agree that thyroid hormone levels are indicated, and the results are as follows:

Thyroid-stimulating hormone (TSH) = 1.47/µU/ml

Total thyroxine = 12.9/ng/dl

Total triiodothyronine = 280/ng/dl

Free T4: 1.5 ng/dl

Which of the following is the most appropriate next step?

A. A thyroid ultrasound
B. An iodine-123 uptake and scan
C. Antithyroid peroxidase antibodies
D. No additional testing is indicated.

19. A 45-year-old man presents with neck pain. An MRI of the neck was ordered to evaluate his complaint. In addition to his degenerative joint disease, multiple thyroid nodules were noted. He denies other complaints. A dedicated thyroid ultrasound was ordered. The report describes a heterogeneous thyroid with three hypoechoic nodules in the right lobe, the largest measuring 1.5 × 0.9 × 0.9 cm and one hypoechoic nodule in the left lobe measuring 0.6 × 0.7 × 0.7 cm. Which of the following would be the most appropriate step in the management of this patient?

A. No additional testing is indicated.
B. A thyroid uptake and scan
C. Test for thyroid-stimulating hormone (TSH)
D. Ultrasound-guided, fine-needle aspiration of the dominant nodule

20. A 22-year-old female presents with weight loss, palpitations, and tremor. She is 3 months postpartum, and her normal menstrual cycle has not resumed. She has lost some weight, despite an increased appetite. Her exam is significant for a nontender thyroid that is normal in size and texture. Her heart rate is 96 beats per minute. Her skin is warm and dry, with palmar erythema. Labs reveal a thyroid-stimulating hormone (TSH) of <0.001/µU/ml and a free T4 of 2.6/ng/dl. She is breastfeeding. You order an iodine-123 uptake and scan, which shows diffuse uptake in the thyroid. Which of the following is the best initial management for this patient at this time?

A. No treatment is indicated.
B. Ablation with radioactive iodine-131.
C. Perform a total thyroidectomy.
D. Begin antithyroid medications (propylthiouracil or methimazole).

21. A 57-year-old woman presents to the local emergency department with confusion. Her family reports that she was well until 3 days ago, when she began to cough. Today, in addition to the cough, she had a rapid heartbeat and did not recognize her children. She is now lethargic and febrile, with a temperature of 101°F. Her heart rate is 126 beats per minute, and her respiratory rate is 24 breaths per minute. A goiter is visible in her neck, and her lung exam is significant for rhonchi. Which of the following would not be consistent with a diagnosis of thyroid storm?

A. Her fever
B. Her heart rate
C. Her mental status change
D. Her respiratory rate

22. An 84-year-old female with a history of hypercholesterolemia, stroke (s/p left carotid endarterectomy), and hypertension presents for a routine office visit. She complains of fatigue. Routine lab work shows that her thyroid-stimulating hormone (TSH) is 12/μU/ml. Which of the following is the best initial management?

    A. Begin levothyroxine 0.025 mg daily.
    B. Begin levothyroxine 0.025 mg daily and repeat TSH in 4 to 6 weeks.
    C. Begin levothyroxine 0.025 mg daily and repeat TSH in 1 year.
    D. Begin levothyroxine based on 1.6 mcg/kg ideal body weight.

23. A 44-year-old female presents with fatigue, weight gain, and dry skin. Her thyroid exam is unremarkable. Her family history is significant for a sister with hypothyroidism. The patient's thyroid-stimulating hormone (TSH) is 12/μU/ml. Which of the following tests is indicated?

    A. No additional testing is indicated.
    B. Thyroid uptake and scan
    C. Free T4
    D. Thyroid ultrasound

24. Which of the following is *not* appropriate management for patients with low bone mass?

    A. 1,500 mg of calcium and 800 IU of vitamin D daily
    B. Smoking cessation
    C. Weight-bearing exercise
    D. Low-protein diet

25. A 67-year-old woman presents with back pain. She has not fallen or suffered an injury. Six months ago, she had a dual-energy x-ray absorptiometry (DXA) with a spine T score of −1.3 and a femoral neck T score of −1.9. She is not on any medications for metabolic bone disease. Plain films of her back are shown below. Which of the following is the most appropriate treatment option for this patient?

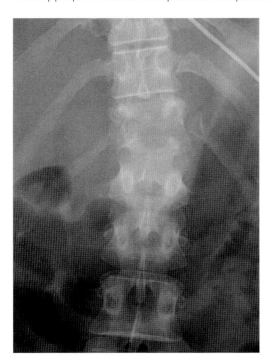

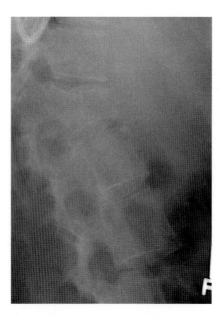

A. No treatment is indicated.
B. Begin oral alendronate.
C. Begin calcitonin nasal spray.
D. Begin raloxifene.

26. A 48-year-old man has had three episodes of nephrolithiasis in the past 2 years. Which of the following lab patterns would you expect if he had primary hyperparathyroidism?

    A. Elevated parathyroid hormone (PTH), elevated serum calcium
    B. Elevated PTH, low serum calcium
    C. Low PTH, elevated serum calcium
    D. Low PTH, low serum calcium

27. A patient has a serum calcium of 8.0 mg/dl and an albumin of 2.0 g/dl. In light of these findings, which of the following is the corrected calcium?

    A. 9.0 mg/dl
    B. 9.6 mg/dl
    C. 10.2 mg/dl
    D. 10.8 mg/dl

28. Which of the following antihypertensive medications typically increases serum calcium levels?

    A. Hydrochlorothiazide (HCTZ)
    B. Atenolol
    C. Lisinopril
    D. Amlodipine

29. Which of the following is *not* part of the diagnostic criteria for polycystic ovarian syndrome?

    A. Clinical or biochemical evidence of increased androgens
    B. Oligomenorrhea
    C. Exclusion of other causes of signs/symptoms
    D. An elevated luteinizing hormone (LH)/follicle-stimulating hormone (FSH) ratio

30. Women with polycystic ovarian syndrome are at increased risk of developing which of the following?

    A. Hyperthyroidism
    B. Type 2 diabetes
    C. Rheumatoid arthritis
    D. Ulcerative colitis

31. Which of the following is *not* usually seen after menopause?

    A. Decreased bone mass, especially in the spine
    B. Lower high-density lipoprotein (HDL) cholesterol
    C. Lower levels of circulating estrogens
    D. Higher levels of testosterone

32. A 24-year-old woman presents with amenorrhea for the past 4 months. Which of the following is the most appropriate first test(s) to order?

    A. Prolactin
    B. Thyroid-stimulating hormone (TSH)
    C. Follicle-stimulating hormone (FSH) and luteinizing hormone (LH)
    D. β-hCG

33. Which of the following medications have *not* been associated with gynecomastia?

    A. Spironolactone
    B. Cimetidine
    C. Phenytoin
    D. NSAIDs

34. Six months ago a 47-year-old patient had a resection of a nonsecreting pituitary adenoma that was impinging on his optic chiasm. His postoperative course has essentially been uncomplicated, and he has not required thyroid or adrenal supplementation. He does report fatigue, decreased erectile function, and decreased facial hair growth. His early morning serum total testosterone is 85 ng/dl, his follicle-stimulating hormone (FSH) is 3.1 IU/L, and his luteinizing hormone (LH) is 2.1 IU/L. You discuss androgen replacement therapy with him, and he agrees on a trial of transdermal testosterone. Which of the following would typically *not* be necessary to monitor 3 months after beginning this androgen therapy?

    A. Liver function tests
    B. Prostate-specific antigen
    C. Morning testosterone
    D. Gonadotropin-releasing hormone (GnRH)

35. A 44-year-old man was involved in a motor vehicle accident. A CT scan of the head shows a pituitary adenoma. An MRI of the pituitary with gadolinium confirms the presence of a pituitary macroadenoma, with extension to the suprasellar region and impingement on the optic chiasm. Your biochemical workup leads you to suspect a nonsecretory pituitary adenoma. He undergoes transphenoidal surgery for decompression of the optic chiasm. Which of the following is this patient at risk of developing?

    A. Secondary hypogonadism
    B. Secondary hyperadrenalism
    C. Secondary hyperthyroidism
    D. Secondary hypotension

36. A 33-year-old woman presents with amenorrhea for 6 months, galactorrhea, and breast tenderness. A pregnancy test is negative, and her serum prolactin is 123 ng/ml. An MRI of the pituitary with gadolinium demonstrates a 0.8-cm enhancing lesion within the sella turcica. Which of the following is the treatment of choice for this condition?

    A. Dopamine agonist therapy (cabergoline or bromocriptine)
    B. Trans-sphenoidal surgery
    C. Radiation therapy
    D. Craniotomy

37. A 42-year-old woman presents with fatigue, weight gain for 3 years, and proximal muscle weakness. She takes medications for hypertension. She has plethora, acne, and central adiposity on examination. Which of the following would *not* be an appropriate screening test for this patient?

    A. 24-hour urine for free cortisol
    B. 11 P.M. salivary cortisol
    C. 1 mg dexamethasone-suppression test
    D. Morning serum cortisol

38. Which of the following conditions is *not* usually associated with hyponatremia?

    A. Severe hypertriglyceridemia
    B. Hypothyroidism
    C. Adrenal insufficiency
    D. Nausea and vomiting

39. A 17-year-old female presents with headaches. An MRI is ordered. It demonstrates a symmetrically enlarged pituitary gland that has no enhancing lesions after gadolinium. The pituitary stalk is midline; the superior portion of the gland has a convex appearance. The patient has no significant past medical history. She has had normal pubertal development; her menses are regular. Which of the following is most consistent with this scenario?

    A. Nonsecreting pituitary adenoma
    B. Rathke's cleft cyst
    C. Craniopharnygioma
    D. Normal pubertal development

ANSWERS

1. **The correct answer is C.** This patient has primary adrenal insufficiency. The patient presents with orthostatic hypotension, weight loss, and fatigue, which are consistent with primary adrenal insufficiency. Low serum cortisol and elevated adrenocorticotropic hormone (ACTH) is the expected pattern. ACTH stimulates cortisol release from the adrenal glands, and cortisol provides feedback to the pituitary to regulate ACTH. Answer A may be seen in Cushing's syndrome (ACTH-secreting pituitary adenoma causing hypercortisolemia). Answer B is seen with Cushing's syndrome (hypercortisolemia from an adrenal adenoma). Answer D is secondary adrenal insufficiency, such as seen after a pituitary surgery.

2. **The correct answer is D.** Dexamethasone does not interfere with the serum cortisol assay. All of the other corticosteroids listed interfere with the serum cortisol assay, making this the appropriate choice when you want an accurate result with this assay.

3. **The correct answer is B.** Secondary adrenal insufficiency is not typically associated with a potassium imbalance. Secondary adrenal insufficiency from any cause, though most often from adrenal suppression from chronic glucocorticoid use or pituitary surgery, generally causes suppression of cortisol, but not mineralocorticoid, production.

4. **The correct answer is B.** The clinician should recognize which hormones originate from the adrenal cortex and adrenal medulla. Aldosterone and cortisol are both found in the cortex. Androstenedione, epinephrine, norepinephrine, and dopamine are all generated by the adrenal medulla. Testosterone is synthesized in the testes.

5. **The correct answer is B.** The patient's age (>45) and BMI (>25) put her at risk for developing type 2 diabetes mellitus. The simplest screening test is a fasting blood glucose value. For nonpregnant adults, a diagnosis of diabetes mellitus is made when: (1) the fasting glucose is >126 mg/dl; (2) a 75-g oral glucose tolerance test yields a blood glucose of >200 mg/dl; or (3) a "casual" glucose is >200 mg/dl with the classic symptoms of polyuria, polydipsia, and weight loss. Answer A is incorrect, because additional testing is indicated. Answer B is incorrect, because hemoglobin A_1C is not included in the diagnostic criteria for diabetes mellitus. Answer D is incorrect, because a specific diagnosis should be established prior to treatment.

6. **The correct answer is C.** This patient has diabetic ketoacidosis. He needs aggressive fluid repletion and intravenous insulin. Even though the serum potassium is normal, his body is depleted of potassium. The intravenous insulin will cause potassium to move from the extracellular compartment to the intracellular compartment, thus potassium repletion is indicated when the potassium is <4.0 mEq. The insulin infusion should be initiated and continued until the anion gap is corrected and the serum ketones have been cleared from the blood. However, despite the severe acidemia, a bicarbonate infusion is not indicated if the pH is >7.0.

7. **The correct answer is D.** The patient has type 1 diabetes mellitus with microalbuminuria. His blood pressure goal should be <130/80 mmHg. Clearly, answer A is incorrect. Although hydrochlorothiazide (HCTZ) and metoprolol are excellent agents for blood pressure control, an ACE inhibitor is the first-line agent in a patient with type 1 diabetes mellitus and presence of microalbuminuria or hypertension without microalbuminuria. Ample data show that inhibition of the renin–angiotensin–aldosterone system using ACE inhibitors in patients with type 1 diabetes mellitus and angiotensin receptor blockers (ARBs) in type 2 diabetes mellitus delay progression of renal disease.

8. **The correct answer is D.** Diabetic retinopathy is a common microvascular complication of both type 1 and type 2 diabetes mellitus. The progression of retinopathy is directly related to glycemic control, as shown by the Diabetes Control and Complications Trial (DCCT) and the United Kingdom Prospective Diabetes Study (UKPDS). When hemoglobin A_1C is <7%, microvascular complications are minimized. Generally, patients with diabetes should have a dilated eye exam once per year. Women who have diabetes mellitus should not be discouraged from conceiving but should receive preconception counseling that emphasizes the need to have strict glycemic control for at least a year prior to pregnancy. Pregnant women with diabetes may have a worsening of existing retinopathy that must be followed closely by ophthalmology during each trimester.

9. **The correct answer is C.** Although all of the choices are reasonable, ample evidence supports the use of metformin as the first-line agent in type 2 diabetes mellitus. Metformin improves the dysfunctional hepatic gluconeogenesis that occurs in type 2 diabetes. Unlike the other agents listed, metformin is not associated with weight gain. Metformin can decrease hemoglobin A_1C by 1 to 2%. The most common adverse events are gastrointestinal discomfort and diarrhea. However, in patients with impaired renal function metformin clearance can be altered and lead to lactic acidosis. Its use should be avoided in patients with renal impairment, in men with creatinine >1.5, and in women with a creatinine >1.4. Regardless of sex, a glomerular filtration rate of <60 is also reason to discontinue metformin, despite creatinine levels. Care should also be taken when using metformin in patients with hepatic impairment.

10. **The correct answer is B.** Sulfonylureas promote insulin secretion by binding to the sulfonylurea receptors on the beta cells, causing secretory granules to release preformed insulin. One known adverse event with this class of antidiabetes medications is the risk for hypoglycemia. Insulin secretion is promoted even when the patient is fasting. Both sulfonylureas and insulin are cleared by the kidney, thus care should be taken when using this class of agents in the elderly as well as in those with renal impairment or irregular eating patterns. Glyburide is metabolized into active fragments, thus hypoglycemia related to this medication can be severe and prolonged. Given the clinical scenario, it is best to stop the glyburide and metformin.

11. **The correct answer is B.** Pioglitzaone is an insulin-sensitizing agent that binds to the PPAR-gamma receptor. It is not associated with hypoglycemia when used in monotherapy, but is well known to cause weight gain and lower extremity edema. Although evidence suggests that pioglitazone may have beneficial effects on the cardiovascular system, there is an increased frequency of congestive heart failure exacerbations.

12. **The correct answer is A.** Microvascular complications of diabetes are well documented and are minimized when hemoglobin A_1C is maintained at 6.5 to 7%. It is recommended that a dilated eye exam, a urine microalbumin test, and a foot examination be done on at least a yearly basis. In addition, routine vaccinations and dental exams should be encouraged. Although gastroparesis is a common complication of diabetes mellitus, at present, an accurate screening method, or even definitive diagnostic tests, are not available for this complication.

13. **The correct answer is C.** The updated ATP III classification has low, moderate, moderately high, and high risk stratifications, and the low-density lipoprotein (LDL) goals vary accordingly. Patients with cardiovascular disease or disease equivalents (such as diabetes) are considered high risk and should have an LDL goal of <100 mg/dl. In very high risk patients, some consider an LDL <70 mg/dl to be a reasonable goal. A low-risk patient (0 to 1 risk factors for cardiovascular disease) should have an LDL <160 mg/dl. A moderate risk patient has 2 or more risk factors and a 10-year cardiovascular disease <10% based on Framingham risk assessment and should have an LDL goal of <130 mg/dl.

14. **The correct answer is C.** All of the agents can decrease low-density lipoprotein (LDL) modestly, but HMG-CoA reductase inhibitors are the most effective at decreasing LDL cholesterol.

15. **The correct answer is D.** Few medications increase high-density lipoprotein (HDL) cholesterol. Diet, exercise, and estrogens help increase HDL cholesterol, but of the agents listed niacin increases HDL cholesterol the most. Fibric acid derivatives are the second most effective.

16. **The correct answer is C.** Although elevated C-reactive protein and postmenopausal status may influence coronary artery disease (CAD) risk stratification, of the options listed only diabetes mellitus is considered a CAD risk equivalent. Hypothyroidism can be associated with abnormal cholesterol panels, and patients with hyperlipidemia should be screened for hypothyroidism with a thyroid-stimulating hormone (TSH).

17. **The correct answer is A.** Fish oil supplements and fibric acid derivatives are very effective at decreasing triglyceride levels. Nicotinic acid can also decrease triglycerides, but bile acid resins do not. Bile acid resins may actually increase triglyceride levels.

18. **The correct answer is D.** The third-generation thyroid-stimulating hormone (TSH) is the most sensitive test of thyroid hormone levels. TSH may be elevated or decreased when other parameters are normal. Total T4 and total T3 levels represent hormone levels bound to thyroid-binding globulin (TBG), and conditions where TBG is elevated

can also increase total T4 and total T3 levels. This patient's estrogen-containing oral contraceptive pills are causing an increase in circulating TBG with a measured increase in total T4 and total T3. This pattern also occurs during pregnancy. Other medications that can affect TBG include antiepileptics and tamoxifen. However, the TSH is normal, thus she is biochemically euthyroid. Without a palpable abnormality on examination, a thyroid ultrasound is not indicated. An iodine uptake and scan would be considered if the TSH was low, but that is not indicated here. Although many practitioners may check anti-thyroid-peroxidase (TPO) antibodies, this is not indicated, because the patient is biochemically euthyroid. If the antibodies had been checked and were positive, she would be at risk for developing autoimmune thyroid disease in the future and should have a TSH screening once a year.

19. **The correct answer is C.** It is estimated that 50% of the population has a thyroid nodule, 90% of these being benign adenoma. Only 4 to 7% of nodules are actually palpable on exam. Often they are discovered as this nodule was; that is, incidentally when evaluating other structures within the neck. Answer A is incorrect, because thyroid hormone levels should be evaluated. A thyroid uptake and scan is only indicated in the presence of low thyroid-stimulating hormone (TSH), indicating hyperthyroidism. An ultrasound-guided fine-needle aspiration is reasonable based on the size of the nodule, but the patient should be proven to be biochemically euthyroid prior to undergoing this procedure.

20. **The correct answer is D.** The patient's labs and scan are consistent with autoimmune hyperthyroidism (Graves' disease). The absence of the textbook diffuse, symmetrically enlarged thyroid is not an uncommon finding. Surgery, radioactive iodine ablation (RIA), and antithyroid drugs (ATDs) are all reasonable approaches for treatment of Graves' disease. However, in the United States surgery is the third-line treatment option and is usually reserved for patients who cannot tolerate other treatment options. In the United States, treatment with RIA or ATDs is largely a matter of patient choice. Ablation with RIA has a very high likelihood of postablation hypothyroidism requiring thyroid hormone replacement. ATDs are useful and induce remission in approximately 50% of patients after 1 to 2 years of use. However, although rare, ATDs can cause agranulocytosis and hepatic damage, thus liver function tests and complete blood counts should be monitored during treatment. Patients should also be instructed to contact their practitioner if they develop a severe sore throat and very high fever (suggestive of agranulocytosis). The ATDs available in the United States are propylthiouracil and methimazole. Although RIA is not contraindicated in this case, the patient would have to express her breast milk and discard it for several weeks to prevent her infant from ingesting any of the radioactive iodine. Most patients and practitioners would probably elect to begin with an ATD, at least until the patient has completed breastfeeding, because both are considered safe in breastfeeding mothers. Using ATDs does not preclude the use of radioactive iodine, although iodine treatment failures are more common following propylthiouracil treatment than following methimazole use.

21. **The correct answer is D.** Tachypnea is not necessary for the diagnosis of thyroid storm. Thyroid storm is a form of decompensated hyperthyroidism. Often there is a precipitating event, such as infection. Tachycardia, hyperpyrexia, and mental status change in the presence of biochemical hyperthyroidism are required for the diagnosis. Thyroid storm presents a risk for high-output cardiac failure. Beta blockers, antithyroid medications, and glucocorticoids are indicated for treatment of thyroid storm.

22. **The correct answer is B.** This patient has hypothyroidism and hypercholesterolemia and requires treatment. However, given that the patient is elderly, you should begin low-dose levothyroxine therapy and repeat a thyroid-stimulating hormone (TSH) test in 4 to 6 weeks with further dose adjustments. In a younger patient, one without coronary artery disease (CAD) or CAD risk equivalents, you can consider full thyroid hormone

replacement at a dose of 1.6 mcg/kg ideal body weight. In an older patient, graded titration is generally still recommended, and some would advocate using 12.5 mcg daily as the initial dose.

23. **The correct answer is A.** You know the diagnosis. No additional testing is required. This patient has signs and symptoms of hypothyroidism and an elevated thyroid-stimulating hormone (TSH). No additional imaging is indicated if the thyroid exam is normal. A 123-iodine uptake and scan is not necessary in this case.

24. **The correct answer is D.** The clinician should recognize the importance of lifestyle changes for osteoporosis. There are modifiable and nonmodifiable risk factors for metabolic bone disease. Nonmodifiable risk factors include age, family history of osteoporosis, personal history of fragility fracture, and postmenopausal state. Modifiable risk factors include calcium and vitamin D intake, tobacco use, alcohol use, and exercise. Other risk factors include corticosteroid use and increased risk for falls. A low-protein diet has no role in the treatment of osteoporosis.

25. **The correct answer is B.** The World Health Organization (WHO) defines osteopenia as a T score on bone densitometry of −1 to −2.5; osteoporosis as a T score of −2.5 or less; and severe osteoporosis as a T score of −2.5 with fragility fractures. The presence of a fragility fracture increases the risk of future fractures. This patient has decreased bone density with a fragility fracture, thus treatment for osteoporosis is clearly indicated. Adequate calcium and vitamin D supplementation is essential to therapy. Oral bisphosphonates are the first-line treatment, and alendronate confers a fracture-risk reduction at both the spine and hip. These are available in once-weekly preparations and are associated with acid reflux and esophageal erosion. Patients should be instructed to take the alendronate on an empty stomach, with 8 oz of water, remain upright for 1 hour after taking the dose, and wait 1 hour before eating. Intravenous bisphosphonates are indicated only if oral bisphosphonates are not tolerated. Calcitonin was used prior to the development of the bisphosphonates, but has been replaced with more effective medications. Raloxifene is very useful for patients with low bone density at the spine, but has not shown the same at the hip and is generally not a first-line agent.

26. **The correct answer is A.** Primary hyperparathyroidism presents with a high parathyroid hormone (PTH) level and high calcium. High PTH and low calcium is consistent with vitamin D deficiency. A low PTH and high calcium causes concern for humoral hypercalcemia. A low PTH and low calcium is seen with hypoparathyroidism. When hypoparathyroidism occurs, it is most often following a thyroidectomy or parathyroidectomy. However, congenital hypoparathyroidism can present in childhood.

27. **The correct answer is B.** Serum calcium levels need to be evaluated in the context of the patient's albumin levels. Low albumin levels can falsely lower the serum calcium. You should correct the serum calcium as follows: Ca + 0.8 × (4.0 − serum albumin). In this case, the corrected calcium is as followings: 8 + 0.8 × (4 − 2) = 9.6 mg/dl.

28. **The correct answer is A.** Hydrochlorothiazide (HCTZ) is associated with hypercalcemia. All of the other antihypertensives typically do not raise calcium levels. In patients with calcium metabolism difficulties (e.g., patients with parathyroid problems) and hypertension, HCTZ should not be the drug of choice.

29. **The correct answer is D.** The elevated LH:FSH ratio is not included in the Rotterdam criteria. A 2003 consensus conference recognized that polycystic ovary syndrome (PCOS) can be diagnosed when, in the absence of other causes for signs and symptoms, a patient demonstrates two of the following: oligo- or anovulation, clinical or biochemical signs of hyperandrogenism, or polycystic ovaries demonstrated on transvaginal ultrasound. The LH:FSH ratio is no longer considered reliable for diagnosis.

30. **The correct answer is B.** Women with polycystic ovary syndrome (PCOS) are more likely to develop obesity. However, PCOS is associated with metabolic abnormalities, regardless of BMI, and these patients are at increased risk of developing type 2 diabetes.

31. **The correct answer is D.** The change in the ratio of estrogen to testosterone is due to the decrease in estrogen levels; the amount of testosterone produced does not change. Bone density in the spine does decrease (particularly in the first 5 years following menopause), and the decrease in circulating estrogens impacts the high-density lipoprotein (HDL) cholesterol level.

32. **The correct answer is D.** Pregnancy must always be ruled out first in a female with amenorrhea. The other tests may be indicated based on history and physical exam.

33. **The correct answer is D.** Numerous medications have been associated with gynecomastia. All of the medications listed, including androgens, have been associated with gynecomastia, excluding NSAIDs. Others include, but are not limited to, metoclopromide, narcotics, phenytoin, tricyclic antidepressants, ACE inhibitors, protease inhibitors, and haloperidol.

34. **The correct answer is D.** This patient is a candidate for androgen replacement therapy. Following pituitary surgery, hypogonadism is among the earliest anterior pituitary deficiencies noted. Injectable and transdermal preparations are available; however, transdermal preparations are generally favored. All of the answers listed should be checked at baseline, including a digital rectal examination, and at 3 months after therapy. If normal, then the blood counts and prostate-specific antigen (PSA) test and a digital rectal examination can be performed yearly thereafter. It is not necessary to check gonadotropin-releasing hormone (GnRH), because it is released from the hypothalamus, not the pituitary.

35. **The correct answer is A.** Generally, everyone who undergoes pituitary surgery is at risk for developing anterior and posterior pituitary deficiencies. The hormones of the anterior pituitary include follicle-stimulating hormone (FSH), luteinizing hormone (LH), thyroid-stimulating hormone (TSH), adrenocorticotropic hormone (ACTH), and growth hormone (GH). The hormones of the posterior pituitary include vasopressin (ADH) and oxytocin. In the immediate postoperative period, vasopressin deficiency and adrenal insufficiency are the primary concerns. After surgery, thyroid hormone function and adrenal function are initially tested. However, patients will need to be monitored for hypogonadism as well.

36. **The correct answer is A.** This patient has a prolactinoma. These prolactin-secreting pituitary adenomas usually respond very well to medical therapy with dopamine agonists (DA), such as cabergoline or bromocriptine, and even macroadenomas have been shown to decrease in size with DA treatment. Surgery is generally only used when medications cannot be tolerated, and it is associated with recurrence of hyperprolactinemia. Radiation or gamma-knife therapy is not commonly used.

37. **The correct answer is D.** The clinician should suspect Cushing's syndrome in this patient. The signs and symptoms of elevated cortisol levels are very nonspecific; fortunately, hypercortisolemia is not common. However, many practitioners mistakenly use a serum cortisol as a screening test. Cortisol levels, in general, are unreliable as a screening test. A 24-hour urinary-free cortisol (UFC) or late-night salivary cortisol (LNSC) is the most common and most useful screening test. The overnight dexamethasone suppression test, where the 1-mg dose is taken by the patient at 10 P.M. and a fasting cortisol is drawn between 8 and 9 A.M. the following morning, is often used in conjunction with the UFC and LNSC for screening. Screening for hypercortisolemia can be difficult, because it can be affected by medications, medical comorbidities (such as depression, dementia,

chronic renal insufficiency, or obstructive sleep apnea), changes in diurnal rhythms (when a patient changes shifts at work frequently), and alcoholism.

38. **The correct answer is A.** Severe hypertriglyceridemia, hyperglycemia, and hyperproteinemia are associated with pseudohyponatremia. This phenomenon is a laboratory abnormality where increased solute levels in the blood interfere with the sodium assay. Hypothyroidism and adrenal insufficiency cause hypothyroidism from decreased free-water clearance. In addition, primary adrenal insufficiency with alterations in the renin–angiotensin–aldosterone system can also lead to hyponatremia. Nausea and vomiting are very strong stimulants of antidiuretic hormone (ADH) release, causing resorption of free water from the kidney.

39. **The correct answer is D.** This patient has headaches, but no evidence of a pituitary adenoma on MRI. During normal pubertal development and pregnancy, the pituitary can appear symmetrically enlarged. It is reasonable to confirm that the patient's anterior pituitary is functioning properly, but this is most likely a normal physiologic enlargement of the pituitary gland.

REFERENCES

American Association of Clinical Endocrinologists (AACE) and Associazione Medici Endocrinologi (AME) Task Force on Thyroid Nodules. (2006). "AACE/AME medical guidelines for clinical practice for the diagnosis and management of thyroid nodules." *Endocrine Practice*, 12(1): 63–102.

Adrogue, H. A., and Madias, N. E. (2000). "Hyponatremia." *New England Journal of Medicine*, 342(21): 1581–1589.

American Diabetes Association. (2008). "Standards of medical care for diabetes mellitus." *Diabetes Care*, 31(S1): S12–S54.

Androgen Deficiency Syndromes in Men Guideline Task Force. (2006). "Testosterone therapy in adult men with androgen deficiency syndromes." *Journal of Clinical Endocrinology & Metabolism*, 91(6): 1995–2010.

Braunstein, G. D. (2007). "Gynecomastia." *New England Journal of Medicine*, 357: 1229–1237.

Casanueva, F. F., Molitch, M. E., Schlechte, J. A., Abs, R., Bonert, V., Bronstein, M. D., Brue, T., Cappabianca, P., Colao, A., Fahlbusch, R., Fideleff, H., Hadani, M., Kelly, P., Kleinberg, D., Laws, E., Marek, J., Scanlon, M., Sobrinho, L. G., Wass, J. A., and Giustina, A. (2006). "Guidelines of the Pituitary Society for the diagnosis and management of prolactinomas." *Clinical Endocrinology*, 65(4): 265–273.

Chanson, P., Daujat, F., Young, J., Bellucci, A., Kujas, M., Doyon, D., and Schaison G. (2001). "Normal pituitary hypertrophy as a frequent cause of pituitary incidentaloma: A follow-up study." *Journal of Clinical Endocrinology & Metabolism*, 86(7): 3009–3015.

Cooper, D. S. (2005). "Antithyroid drugs." *New England Journal of Medicine*, 352(9): 905–917.

Dufour, D. R. (2007). "Laboratory tests of thyroid function: Uses and limitations." *Endocrinology Metabolism Clinics of North America*, 36(3): 579–594.

Hirsch, I. (2005). "Insulin analogues." *New England Journal of Medicine*, 352(2): 174–183.

Hueston, W. J. (2001). "Treatment of hypothyroidism." *American Family Physician*, 64(10): 1717–1724.

Johanson, K. (1999). "Efficacy of metformin in the treatment of NIDDM: A meta-analysis." *Diabetes Care*, 22: 33–37.

Kitabchi, A. E., Umpierrez, G. E., Murphy, M. B., Barrett, E. J., Kreisberg, R. A., Malone, J. I., and Wall, B. M. (2001). "Management of hyperglycemic crisis in patients with diabetes." *Diabetes Care*, 24(1): 151–161.

Master-Hunter, T., and Heiman, D. L. (2006). "Amenorrhea: Evaluation and treatment." *American Family Physician*, 73(8): 1374–1382.

Mauck, K. F., and Clarke, B. L. (2006). "Diagnosis, screening, prevention, and treatment of osteoporosis." *Mayo Clinic Proceedings*, 81(5): 662–672.

National Cholesterol Education Program. Detection, evaluation, and treatment of high blood cholesterol in adults (ATP III). (Online). Available at www.nhlbi.nih.gov/guidelines/cholesterol/atp3xsum.pdf.

Nayak, B., and Hodak, S. P. (2007). "Hyperthyroidism." *Endocrinology & Metabolism Clinics of North America*, 36(3): 617–657.

Nayak, B., and Burman, K. (2006). "Thyrotoxicosis and thyroid storm." *Endocrinology & Metabolism Clinics of North America*, 35(4): 663–686.

Nieman, L. K., and Ilias, I. (2005). "Evaluation and treatment of Cushing's syndrome." *American Journal of Medicine*, 118(12): 1340–1346.

Nelson, H. D. (2008). "Menopause." *Lancet*, 371(9614): 760–770.

Rotterdam ESHRE/ASRM-sponsored PCOS Consensus Workshop Group. (2004). "Revised 2003 consensus on diagnostic criteria and long-term health risks related to polycystic ovary syndrome (PCOS)." *Human Reproduction*, 19(1): 41–47.

Vance, M. L. (1994). "Hypopituitarism." *New England Journal of Medicine*, 330(23): 1651–1662.

Hematology/Oncology

Dale Bryansmith, MD
Donna M. Agnew, MT (ASCP), MSPAS, PA-C

1. Which of the following is *not* included in the classic triad of findings seen in primary polycythemia vera?

   A. Elevated red blood cell mass
   B. Increased erythropoietin levels
   C. Normal arterial oxygen saturations
   D. Splenomegaly

2. A 38-year-old male who complains of increasing fatigue is found to have a macrocytic anemia. Which of the following symptoms would best support a vitamin B_{12} deficiency as the etiology of this megaloblastic anemia?

   A. Angular cheilitis
   B. Glossitis
   C. Diarrhea
   D. Paresthesias

3. Which of the following is *not* included in the treatment of hemochromatosis?

   A. Chelation therapy
   B. Dietary modification
   C. Phlebotomy
   D. Vitamin C supplementation

4. What red blood cell morphology would most likely be seen in the peripheral blood smear of a patient with a mechanical heart valve?

   A. Elliptocytes
   B. Schistocytes
   C. Spherocytes
   D. Target cells

5. Which of the following medications is most likely to cause pancytopenia and an aplastic bone marrow?

   A. Ceftriaxone
   B. Chloramphenicol
   C. Streptomycin
   D. Tetracycline

6. Which red blood cell inclusions are seen in patients with G6PD (glucose-6-phosphate dehydrogenase) deficiency and represent precipitated, denatured hemoglobin (as shown on the supravital stained smear shown below)?

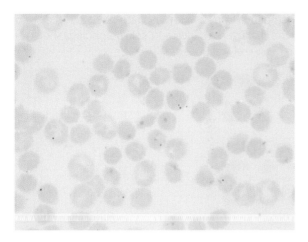

A. Döhle bodies
B. Heinz bodies
C. Howell-Jolly bodies
D. Pappenheimer bodies

7. A 53-year-old male welder presents complaining of intermittent, colicky, diffuse abdominal pain and constipation for the past 2 months. He denies dyspepsia, nausea, vomiting, early satiety, fever, weight loss, cold intolerance, hematochezia, or melena. He had no abnormal findings on colonoscopy 9 months ago. He is found to be anemic, with a hemoglobin of 10.5 g/dl and a mean corpuscular volume (MCV) of 80. His reticulocyte count is 2.6%. His white blood cell and platelet counts are normal. His peripheral blood smear is shown below. Based on his history and laboratory findings, what would be the most appropriate next step in the evaluation of this patient?

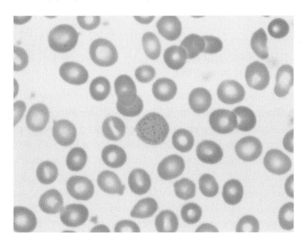

A. Barium imaging study
B. Hemoglobin electrophoresis
C. Thyroid function tests
D. Heavy metal levels

8. A 51-year-old male has suffered recurrent upper respiratory infections in the past year and progressively worsening fatigue the past 6 months. He describes an upper abdominal "fullness" without any associated gastrointestinal complaints. Initial laboratory testing reveals pancytopenia. On physical examination, you note significant pallor and hepatosplenomegaly. An attempt at a bone marrow aspirate resulted in a dry tap, and bone marrow biopsy reveals the characteristic "fried egg" cell morphology shown below. Which of the following is the most likely diagnosis?

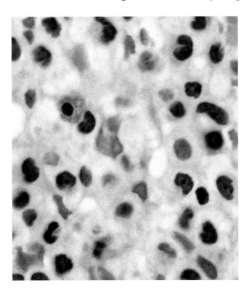

A. Aplastic anemia
B. Hairy cell leukemia
C. Non-Hodgkin's lymphoma
D. Paroxysmal nocturnal hemoglobinuria

9. Which of the following tests best confirms that a patient is in a vaso-occlusive sickle-cell crisis?

A. Elevated hemoglobin F levels
B. Positive metabisulfite (deoxygenation) test
C. Presence of sickle cells on peripheral smear
D. Presence of SS on hemoglobin electrophoresis

10. A 25-year-old graduate student presents complaining of a nonpruritic rash over her lower extremities for the past week. She admits to easy bruising, gingival bleeding with flossing, and an episode of significant epistaxis this morning. She reports no other symptoms except for an upper respiratory infection 3 to 4 weeks ago that spontaneously resolved with over-the-counter cold preparations. On physical examination, there are numerous petechiae on the lower extremity but no hepatosplenomegaly or lymphadenopathy. Her complete blood count reveals a platelet count of 7,000/mm^3, with otherwise normal parameters. Prothrombin time (PT), partial thromboplastin time (PTT), and thrombin time (TT) are normal, with negative ASO titer, HIV screening, and β-hCG. Which of the following is the most likely diagnosis?

A. Hemophilia A
B. Henoch-Schönlein purpura
C. Idiopathic thrombocytopenia purpura
D. von Willebrand's disease

11. Which of the following disorders does *not* show a predominance of white blood cells, as depicted below?

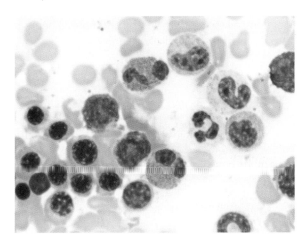

   A. Connective tissue disease
   B. Dermatologic allergic conditions
   C. Inflammatory bowel disease
   D. Parasitic infections

12. Which of the following is the pathognomonic finding for acute myelogenous leukemia (shown below)?

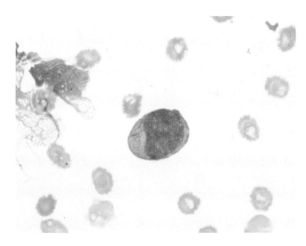

   A. Auer rod
   B. Pelger-Huet cell
   C. Plasma cell
   D. Reed-Sternberg cell

13. A 69-year-old retired carpenter presents complaining of progressively worsening thoracic back and rib pain that is exacerbated with movement. Radiographic findings reveal diffuse "punched out" lytic bone lesions. Based on the patient's history and radiographic findings, you order additional blood work and a bone marrow aspiration and biopsy. Which of the following is *not* a significant criterion for the specific diagnosis of multiple myeloma in this patient?

   A. A monoclonal serum protein >3.5 g
   B. Hypercalcemia >12 mg/dl
   C. Marrow plasmocytosis >30%
   D. Radiographic evidence of osteolytic bone lesions

14. Evaluation of a 73-year-old Italian female with a past medical history of cirrhosis, chronic obstructive pulmonary disease (COPD), and osteoarthritis reveals the following laboratory values: hemoglobin, 9.0 g/dl; decreased serum iron and total iron-binding capacity (TIBC); increased ferritin; normal RDW (red cell distribution width); and normal hemoglobin electrophoresis. Which of the following is the most likely diagnosis?

    A. Anemia of chronic disease
    B. β-thalassemia
    C. Iron deficiency anemia
    D. Sideroblastic anemia

15. You recently diagnose a patient with rheumatoid arthritis and wish to initiate pharmacologic treatment. With which of the following medications are you required to prescribe supplemental folic acid to prevent the development of a macrocytic anemia?

    A. Etanercept
    B. Methotrexate
    C. Placquenil
    D. Sulfasalazine

16. You initiate iron supplementation on a 51-year-old female who has iron deficiency anemia secondary to dysfunctional uterine bleeding from fibroids. Which of the following tests would be an initial positive indicator of her bone marrow's response to treatment?

    A. Increased hemoglobin
    B. Increased mean corpuscular volume (MCV)
    C. Increased ferritin
    D. Increased reticulocyte count

17. Which of the following is the most common inherited disorder of hemostasis?

    A. Factor V Leidin deficiency
    B. Hemophilia
    C. Protein C deficiency
    D. von Willebrand's disease

18. Which of the following best describes the cause of sickle-cell anemia?

    A. A single DNA base change that encodes for the substitution of valine for glutamine during β-globin chain synthesis
    B. A genetic defect that results in a reduced rate of synthesis of one of the globin chains
    C. The substitution of two γ chains for β chains in the hemoglobin molecule
    D. Weak covalent bonds between the heme and globin portions of the molecule, which facilitates sickling

19. Which of the following is the major factor in the regulation of erythropoiesis?

    A. Erythropoietin levels
    B. Pulmonary capillary pCO_2
    C. Renal blood flow
    D. Tissue oxygen tension

20. What is the mechanism of action of hydroxyurea in the treatment of sickle-cell disease?

    A. It increases erythropoietin levels.
    B. It prevents the deoxygenation of blood.
    C. It stimulates the production of hemoglobin F.
    D. It stimulates the immune system to fight infections.

21. A 42-year-old African American female presents with a recent onset of fatigue, dyspnea, and dark urine. On physical examination, she is jaundiced and tachycardic. Laboratory results reveal the following:

White blood cell: 10,000/mm^3

Hemoglobin: 7.2 g/dl

Mean corpuscular volume (MCV): 103

Platelets: 378,000/mm^3

Reticulocyte count: 21%

Aspartate aminotransferase (AST): 41 U/l

Alanine aminotransferase (ALT): 63 U/l

Total bilirubin: 16.2 mg/dl

Direct bilirubin: 4.1 mg/dl

BUN: 16 mg/dl

Creatinine: 1.1 mg/dl

Which of the following tests would be most helpful in determining the exact cause of her anemia?

A. Serum B$_{12}$ and folate levels
B. Direct Coombs'
C. Haptoglobin
D. Hemoglobin electrophoresis

22. Which of the following most commonly initiates a workup for prostatic cancer?

A. Elevated serum screening prostate-specific antigen (PSA) levels
B. A palpable nodule detected on digital rectal examination
C. Obstructive voiding symptoms
D. Metastatic bone disease

23. Which of the following statements is *false* regarding ovarian cancer?

A. It is a surgically staged disease.
B. Most patients are diagnosed with late-stage (III or IV) disease.
C. CA-125 is diagnostic.
D. Early symptoms are vague and nonspecific.

24. The presence of the Philadelphia chromosome confirms the diagnosis of which of the following leukemias?

A. Acute lymphocytic leukemia
B. Acute myelogenous leukemia
C. Chronic lymphocytic leukemia
D. Chronic myelogenous leukemia

25. Which of the following patients is *least* at risk for the development of a macrocytic anemia?

A. A 41-year-old morbidly obese female who has undergone gastric bypass surgery
B. A 28-year-old female who is a strict vegan
C. A 38-year-old male with a history of Crohn's disease
D. A 30-year-old male with a history of juvenile arthritis

26. Which of the following family histories would *not* place a patient at increased risk for colon carcinoma?

A. Diverticular disease
B. Familial adenomatous polyposis
C. Inflammatory bowel disease
D. Peutz-Jeghers syndrome

27. Which of the following anemias would most likely be depicted by the peripheral blood smear shown below?

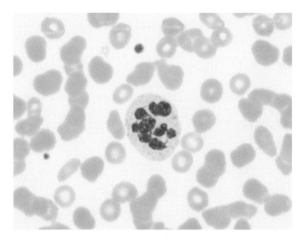

A. Hereditary spherocytosis
B. Iron deficiency anemia
C. Pernicious anemia
D. Thalassemia

28. A 5-year-old child presents to your office complaining of a persistent cough and fever of 2 weeks' duration. He notes associated pain across his ribs, which his mother attributed to strain caused by coughing. This morning he experienced a slight nosebleed. On physical examination, you note pallor, axillary adenopathy, hepatospenomegaly, and diffuse tenderness over the ribs bilaterally. The initial laboratory results are as follows: hemoglobin, 9.8 g/dl; platelets, 98,000/mm^3; white blood cells, 31,000/mm^3; aspartate aminotransferase (AST), 118 U/l; alanine aminotransferase (ALT), 200 U/l; bilirubin, 0.6 mg/dl; BUN, 10 mg/dl, and normal prothrombin time (PT) and partial thromboplastin time (PTT). A peripheral smear is shown below. Which of the following is the most likely diagnosis?

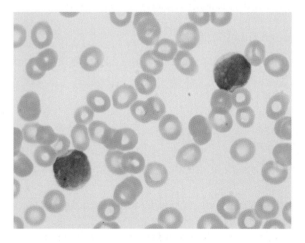

A. Acute myelogenous leukemia
B. Acute lymphoblastic leukemia
C. Infectious mononucleosis
D. Hodgkin's disease

29. Which symptom is *not* typically associated with severe iron deficiency anemia?

    A. Cheilosis

    B. Dysphagia

    C. Nail clubbing

    D. Pica

30. A 37-year-old woman is concerned about a breast lump she discovered during self-examination. On physical examination, a 3-cm mass is palpated deep in the upper outer aspect of her left breast at the 1 o'clock position. There is no dimpling, skin changes, nipple inversion, or galactorrhea. The axillary and supraclavicular nodes are nonpalpable. Mammogram and ultrasound are negative. Which of the following is the most appropriate next step in the management of this patient?

    A. Repeat the mammogram in 6 months.

    B. Refer the patient for a surgical biopsy.

    C. Obtain an MRI of the left breast.

    D. Reassure the patient because the tests were negative.

31. What radiographic ultrasound finding is most suggestive of a benign etiology in a patient found to have an adnexal mass?

    A. Ascites

    B. Calcifications

    C. Multiple septations

    D. Solid mass

32. Which of the following primary cancers is matched incorrectly with its most common site of initial metastasis?

    A. Colon, liver

    B. Prostate, bone

    C. Lung, brain

    D. Breast, ovaries

33. Which of the following is *false* regarding chronic lymphocytic leukemia (CLL)?

    A. It usually presents in patients older than age 50, with a higher incidence in males.

    B. Symptoms may include fatigue (especially after exercise), painless lymphadenopathy, weight loss, and night sweats.

    C. A valuable diagnostic test, in addition to bone marrow aspirate and biopsy, is blood-flow cytometry.

    D. Initiating chemotherapy in the early stages of the disease, even if the patient is asymptomatic, has been proven to reduce mortality.

34. Which type of anemia is best represented by cells identified by Prussian blue staining?

    A. Hereditary spherocytosis

    B. Iron deficiency anemia

    C. Sideroblastic anemia

    D. Thalassemia

35. A 2-day postpartum woman has become hypotensive and is in respiratory distress. She delivered a healthy 7 lb., 3 oz. male at 37 weeks' gestation via a cesarean delivery secondary to preterm premature rupture of membranes (PPROM). Her catheter urine reveals gross blood, and she is oozing blood from her intravenous site. Which of the following tests would *not* confirm disseminated intravascular coagulation in this patient?

    A. Increased prothrombin time (PT) and partial thromboplastin time (PTT)

    B. Increased fibrinogen

    C. Positive D-dimer

    D. Thrombocytopenia

36. Which of the following coagulation factors is *not* synthesized in the liver?

    A. Fibrinogen
    B. Factor II
    C. Factor VIII
    D. Factor X

37. Which statement is *false* regarding Hodgkin's lymphoma?

    A. It has a poorer prognosis than non-Hodgkin's lymphoma.
    B. The most common site for lymphadenopathy is the cervical area.
    C. Asymptomatic lymphadenopathy may be present.
    D. The etiology of Hodgkin's disease is unknown.

38. Which of the following represent the greatest risk for the development of breast cancer?

    A. A woman who began menarche after the age of 15
    B. A woman who breastfed all three of her children
    C. A woman who has a family history of breast cancer in a first-degree relative
    D. A woman who is Native American

39. The peripheral smear of a patient with β-thalassemia characteristically shows which of the following red blood cell morphologies?

    A. Basophilic stippling
    B. Spherocytes
    C. Microcytic hypochromic red blood cells
    D. Target cells

40. A 58-year-old male is hospitalized for treatment of a pulmonary embolism. He has a past medical history of hypertension, which is well controlled with an angiotensin II receptor blocker (ARB)–hydrochlorothiazide (HCTV) combination antihypertensive. After 4 days in the hospital, the patient has developed thrombocytopenia. Which of the following is the most likely cause of thrombocytopenia in this patient?

    A. ARB
    B. HCTZ
    C. Heparin
    D. Warfarin

ANSWERS

1. **The correct answer is B.** Primary polycythemia vera is a myeloproliferative disorder that classically presents with symptoms of headache, epitaxis, dizziness/vertigo, splenomegaly and generalized pruritus after bathing. Although it involves proliferation of all three hematopoietic cell lines, there is a predominant elevation in red blood cell mass irrespective of erythropoietin production. *Serum levels of erythropoietin are generally low to normal.* Red blood cells function properly and maintain normal arterial oxygen saturation levels. Bone marrow appears hypercellular with absent iron stores. The most significant complication of polycythemia vera is thrombosis due to blood hyperviscosity and platelet dysfunction. The treatment of choice is phlebotomy, which reduces red blood cell mass and hyperviscosity. Other treatment options include antihistamines (symptomatic relief of pruritus); myelosuppressive therapy (hydroxyurea); allopurinol (if indicated, to reduce serum uric acid); low-dose aspirin (antiplatelet effect and symptomatic relief of microvascular symptoms, such as headache); and, in some cases, splenectomy. Alkylating agents should be avoided, as they can stimulate leukocyte production and may precipitate the conversion to an acute leukemia.

2. **The correct answer is D.** Neurologic symptoms are the hallmark of vitamin B_{12} deficiency. Demyelination results in paresthesias, muscle weakness, and ataxia. Mental status changes can range from forgetfulness or irritability to overt psychosis. Angular cheilitis is generally seen in iron deficiency anemia, which is a microcytic anemia. Both vitamin B_{12} and folate deficiencies affect the mucosal epithelium of the gastrointestinal tract and may cause symptoms of glossitis and diarrhea.

3. **The correct answer is D.** Primary hemochromatosis is an autosomal recessive disorder that results in accumulation and deposition of iron as hemosiderin. Signs and symptoms include bronze discoloration of the skin, arthralgias, cardiac arrhythmias and cardiomyopathies, loss of libido, hepatomegaly, and glucose intolerance. Liver biopsy has been the gold standard for diagnosis, but genetic testing for the *HFE C282Y* mutation may also provide a reliable diagnosis. Liver biopsy provides valuable information regarding the extent of liver damage and is of prognostic value. Treatment options include chelation therapy with deferoxamine and phlebotomies to deplete both serum iron and iron stores. Avoidance of foods that are rich in iron, such as red meat and raw shellfish, is also recommended. Vitamin C enhances iron absorption from the gut and should be avoided in patients with hemochromatosis.

4. **The correct answer is B.** The shearing forces of a mechanical heart valve may fragment the red blood cells, causing them to appear as schistocytes on peripheral smear (shown below). Fragmented red blood cells may also be seen in patients with disseminated intravascular coagulation. Elliptocytes (ovalocytes) result from bipolar aggregation of hemoglobin in the red blood cells, which causes the cells to elongate. They are seen in hereditary elliptocytosis, thalassemia, and sickle-cell anemia. A spherocyte is a round red blood cell that lacks an area of central pallor due to being "packed" with hemoglobin, as indicated by an increased mean cell hemoglobin concentration (MCHC). Spherocytes demonstrate increased osmotic fragility and are seen in hereditary spherocytosis and in immune hemolytic anemia. Target cells (codocytes) demonstrate a central area and peripheral rim of hemoglobin separated by a pale concentric zone. They can be indicative of hemoglobinopathies, liver disease, or iron deficiency anemia.

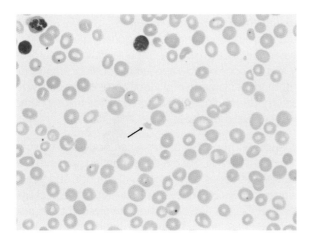

5. **The correct answer is B.** An adverse effect of chloramphenicol is bone marrow suppression and aplastic anemia. Ceftriaxone can cause gallbladder sludging. Streptomycin has ototoxic side effects. Tetracycline is responsible for teeth-staining in young children.

6. **The correct answer is B.** Heinz bodies are red blood cell inclusions of denatured hemoglobin. Visualization of Heinz bodies requires supravital stains, because they are not seen with Wright's stain. Döhle bodies are pale-blue stained areas seen within the cytoplasm of neutrophils and are representative of residual RNA. They are seen in bacterial

infections when the production of granulocytes is expedited. Howell-Jolly bodies are red blood cell inclusions of DNA remnants; they can be viewed with both Wright's and supravital stains. They are commonly seen in hemolytic anemias and in postsplenectomy patients. Pappenheimer bodies are small, blue iron granules that usually appear in clusters near the periphery of the red blood cell. They are seen in sideroblastic anemia and postsplenectomy patients. They may be seen on Wright's stain, but are confirmed with Prussian blue stain.

7. **The correct answer is D.** As a welder, this patient is at risk for chronic exposure to heavy metals, especially lead. Lead is found in many industrial materials, such as paint, solders, pottery, plumbing, and storage batteries (in 1978, the use of lead in household paints was restricted by the Consumer Product Safety Commission). Symptoms of heavy metal poisoning via inhalation or ingestion include constipation, colicky abdominal pain, headache, mood liability, and decreased cognition. Peripheral neuropathies may also occur, the most common being a weakness in the extensor muscles of the hand, resulting in a wrist drop. Lead toxicity in children has been correlated with learning disabilities. Lead toxicity may cause bluish lines known as Burton's lines along the gingiva. Peripheral blood smears often reveal microcytic, hypochromic red blood cells containing coarse basophilic stippling. Treatment includes chelating agents, such as EDTA (ethylenediaminetetraacetic acid) and succimer (DSMA).

8. **The correct answer is B.** Hairy cell leukemia is a cancer of mature B lymphocytes. It is comparable to a slow-growing form of chronic lymphoid leukemia. These abnormal B lymphocytes have fine peripheral projections that give them their characteristic name. Although an exact etiology has not been determined, proposed causes include exposure to agricultural insecticides, radiation, and even sawdust. There is male predominance, with a male to female ratio of 5:1. The median age at diagnosis is 52 years. Pancytopenia is characteristic of the disease, which predisposes patients to fatigue; recurrent infections, especially to atypical organisms; and bleeding tendencies. Splenomegaly is a hallmark physical exam finding, whereas peripheral lymphadenopathy is seen in less than 10% of patients. Circulating cells on peripheral smear are TRAP (tartrate-resistant acid phosphatase) positive. A significant decrease in circulating monocytes is unique to hairy cell leukemia. Infiltration of cells within the bone marrow usually results in dry taps. On core biopsy, these cells have a central nucleus surrounded by abundant cytoplasm, giving a "fried egg" appearance. In aplastic anemia, there is pancytopenia without hepatosplenomegaly or lymphadenopathy, and the bone marrow appears hypocellular. Non-Hodgkin's lymphoma presents with a nontender, enlarged lymph node and is diagnosed by lymph node biopsy. Paroxysmal nocturnal hemoglobinuria is noted by the triad of hemolytic anemia, pancytopenia, and large vessel thrombosis.

9. **The correct answer is C.** A vaso-occlusive crisis occurs when sickle cells occlude the microcirculation, leading to organ ischemia. Such a crisis manifests as severe, acute painful episodes and may include the bones, joints, soft tissues, lungs, abdomen, and internal organs, such as the liver, spleen, or kidneys. Skin ulcerations, especially over the bony prominences, can occur. Central nervous system involvement can result in seizures, transient ischemic attacks (TIAs), or even coma. Elevations in hemoglobin F, a positive metabisulfite (deoxygenation) test, and the demonstration of hemoglobin SS on electrophoresis support the diagnosis of sickle-cell disease, but are not necessarily indicative of vaso-occlusive crises. Sickle cells seen on peripheral smear support the diagnosis of an acute crisis.

10. **The correct answer is C.** This is the textbook presentation of acquired idiopathic thrombocytopenia purpura (aITP, formerly known as ITP). Acquired idiopathic thrombocytopenic purpura (aITP) is an autoimmune condition in which IgG antibody is produced against platelets, marking them for destruction by splenic macrophages. Labora-

tory studies reveal an isolated thrombocytopenia. Patients are usually young females who report no systemic complaints and have no evidence of splenomegaly on exam. Splenectomy is an effective treatment for ITP because it eliminates both the source of antibody production and platelet destruction. Hemophilia A is an X-linked, recessive disorder (seen primarily in males) that results in a deficiency in functional coagulation factor VIII. Bleeding can vary in severity, from episodes involving major trauma or surgery to spontaneous hemarthroses. Laboratory findings with hemophilia are a prolonged partial thromboplastin time (PTT) with a normal prothrombin time (PT), platelet counts, bleeding times, and thrombin times. Henoch-Schölein purpura (HSP) is a vasculitis caused by the deposition of IgA, complement component 3 (C3), and immune complexes in arterioles, capillaries, and venules. It is often seen in children. It is also described as being preceded by a recent upper respiratory infection. In addition to the palpable purpura, patients experience abdominal pain, edema, gastrointestinal bleeding, and hematuria. Antistreptolysin O titers are elevated in approximately 20 to 50% of patients with HSP. In von Willebrand's disease, there is a defective or deficient von Willebrand factor, which is a glycoprotein that is synthesized by megakaryocytes and endothial cells and plays a role in platelet adhesion. Platelet counts and morphology would be expected to be normal, with the exception of type 2B, which may have intermittent thrombocytopenia. Bleeding times are generally prolonged in von Willebrand's disease.

11. **The correct answer is C.** On Wright's stain, the cytoplasmic granules of the eosinophil stain a characteristic red-orange color due to an arginine-rich protein contained within. Eosinophils normally constitute 1 to 3% of the total leukocyte differential count. Eosinophilia is defined as >500 eosinophils per microliter of blood and is encountered in allergic reactions (asthma, eczema, hay fever), connective tissue disease (rheumatoid arthritis), parasitic or helminthic infections, and in some malignancies (Hodgkin's disease, chronic myelogenous leukemia, and mycosis fungoides). Inflammatory bowel disease is not marked by eosinophilia, but rather an activation and increased secretion of inflammatory cytokines.

12. **The correct answer is A.** The hallmark of acute myelogenous leukemia is the presence of more than 30% leukemic blasts in the peripheral blood (French-American-British [FAB] classification) or bone marrow and the presence of Auer rods. Auer rods are elongated azurphilic cytoplasmic inclusions that represent fused lysosomal granules. They are not always present in acute myelogenous leukemia (AML), and they are sometimes seen in some myeloproliferative disorders. When present, they distinguish between myelogenous and lymphoid leukemias and are pathognomonic for AML. Pelger-Huët anomaly is a benign, inherited dominant disorder of granulocyte maturation. It is characterized by "spectacle-shaped," bilobed nuclei. It is clinically relevant to distinguish Pelger-Huët cells from band forms representative of a left shift. Mature plasma cells are seen in chronic lymphoid leukemia. Reed-Sternberg cells are bilobed ("owl's eyes") or multinucleated giant cells; they are essential to the diagnosis of Hodgkin's lymphoma.

13. **The correct answer is B.** The following comprise a definitive diagnosis of multiple myeloma: a minimum of 10% of the bone marrow is composed of plasma cells; radiographic lytic, "punched-out" bone lesions; and monoclonal immunoglobulins demonstrated in the blood or urine. Hypercalcemia can be a manifestation of the disease, but it is not a required finding for the diagnosis and it is not specific to multiple myeloma. Multiple myeloma involves the malignant proliferation of plasma cells, a form of B lymphocytes responsible for the production of antibodies (humoral immunity). Plasma cells are unique in that they manufacture only one type of immunoglobulin, and thus are referred to as being monoclonal. Characteristic monoclonal spikes appear on serum electrophoresis. IgG is the most common spike, followed by IgA. Antibodies are comprised of Fc (heavy) and Fab (light) chains. If cleaved, the Fab portion, or light chain, may be found in the urine and is referred to as the Bence Jones protein.

14. **The correct answer is A.** This laboratory profile clearly depicts anemia of chronic disease resulting from the effects of chronic inflammation. Inflammatory cytokines cause the liver to produce increased amounts of hepicidin. Hepicidin is responsible for inhibiting iron absorption and suppressing the release of iron from iron stores. Iron delivery to the bone marrow is reduced in spite of normal or increased iron stores. An additional proposed mechanism includes the upregulation of leukocyte production in the face of inflammation, shifting the myeloid-to-erythroid ratio. In iron deficiency anemia, there are decreased iron and ferritin stores, increased total iron-binding capacity (TIBC) and red blood cell distribution width (RDW), and normal hemoglobin electrophoresis. β-thalassemia would demonstrate an increased hemoglobin A2 level on hemoglobin electrophoresis. Sideroblastic anemia would likely reveal increased iron, ferritin, and RDW, with a normal TIBC and hemoglobin electrophoresis pattern.

15. **The correct answer is B.** Methotrexate is the disease-modifying antirheumatic drug (DMARD) of choice for the initial treatment of rheumatoid arthritis. Methotrexate acts by inhibiting the metabolism of folic acid. It competitively and reversibly inhibits the enzyme dihydrofolate reductase, which converts folic acid to the more active form, tetrahydrofolate.

16. **The correct answer is D.** Reticulocyte counts generally increase 4 to 7 days after initiation of therapy, with restoration of the hemoglobin to a normal range within 2 months. Replenishment of ferritin stores may take several months to a year.

17. **The correct answer is D.** von Willebrand's disease is the most common congenital disorder of hemostasis. It is an autosomal dominant disorder that reflects either a quantitative (type I and III) or a qualitative (IIA, IIB) deficiency in von Willebrand factor. von Willebrand factor facilitates platelet adhesion and serves as the plasma carrier protein for antihemophilic factor (Factor VIII). Patients with von Willebrand's disease experience gingival bleeding, epistaxis, easy bruising, menorrhagia, and postpartum bleeds. Laboratory findings include prolonged bleeding times, normal platelet counts and morphology, and decreased von Willebrand's factor antigen or ristocetin cofactor. Patients are recommended to avoid aspirin and NSAIDs. DDAVP (desmopressin acetate) releases stored von Willebrand factor from endothelial cells and is used prior to minor procedures. Significant acute bleeding episodes are treated with von Willebrand factor replacement, cryoprecipitate, or platelet transfusions, depending on the severity of the bleed.

18. **The correct answer is A.** Sickle-cell disease results from a single base change that encodes for a valine substitution for glutamine in the sixth position of the β-globin chain, leading to the formation of defective hemoglobin known as hemoglobin S.

19. **The correct answer is D.** Tissue hypoxia is the primary stimulus to erythropoiesis, exerting its effect directly on the kidney to release erythropoietin. Hypoxia caused by residing at high altitudes, chronic cardiopulmonary disease, and sleep apnea result in a polycythemia.

20. **The correct answer is C.** Hydroxyurea is used in the treatment of chronic myelogenous leukemia, acute myelogenous leukemia, polycythemia vera, and psoriasis. In the management of sickle-cell disease, the drug is used to induce the production of hemoglobin F, which is composed of two γ chains instead of the defective β chains of hemoglobin S. Hemoglobin F also has higher affinity for oxygen. Fetal hemoglobin is the predominant hemoglobin prior to birth. The replacement of fetal hemoglobin by hemoglobin A initially occurs during the third trimester of pregnancy. By increasing hemoglobin F concentrations, hydroxyurea is used to prevent, not treat, vaso-occlusive crises.

21. **The correct answer is B.** The definitive test for the diagnosis of an autoimmune hemolytic anemia is the direct Coomb's, or antiglobulin, test. Coomb's reagent is rabbit IgM

antibody produced against human IgG or complement. In an autoimmune anemia, the patient's red blood cells are coated with IgG antibody. Mixing the patient's red blood cells with Coomb's reagent "bridges the gap" between the red blood cells (counteracting the normal opposing negative charges) and results in agglutination. Although the mean corpuscular volume (MCV) is elevated, vitamin B_{12} or folate deficiency would not account for the abnormal liver function tests or markedly elevated reticulocyte count. Haptoglobin is a plasma protein that binds free hemoglobin when released from red blood cells. It serves as an indicator of hemolysis but is not specific in testing for an autoimmune cause of the destruction. Hemoglobin electrophoresis is used to identify thalassemia and sickle-cell anemia.

22. **The correct answer is A.** Prostate cancer is diagnosed in more that 60% of cases because of elevated screening prostate-specific antigen (PSA) levels, because most patients are asymptomatic at the time of diagnosis. Approximately 85% of prostate cancers are located posteriorly, which is the only portion of the prostate gland palpable on digital rectal examination. Any focal nodules or areas of induration require further evaluation with a prostate biopsy. It is much less common for prostate cancer to be diagnosed because of a presenting symptom of voiding symptoms or pelvic or bone pain secondary to metastatic disease.

23. **The correct answer is C.** After endometrial cancer, ovarian cancer is the most common gynecologic malignancy. Ovarian cancer often presents insidiously with nonspecific gastrointestinal complaints, such as early satiety or change in bowel habits. It is associated with diets high in saturated fats. Multiparity and anovulatory cycles appear to be protective factors. The prognosis is much better with early detection; however, because of the lack of symptoms, the disease usually is confirmed in the later stages. Pelvic ultrasound plays an important role in the evaluation of adnexal masses. Cancer antigen-125 (CA-125) is not a reliable screening tool for ovarian cancer; it is better used to monitor treatment response. Cancer antigen-125 may be increased in other conditions that can cause peritoneal inflammation, such as pancreatic, gastric, colon, and endometrial cancers. Surgery is the cornerstone of staging and treatment of ovarian cancer.

24. **The correct answer is D.** Philadelphia chromosome is a chromosomal abnormality in which the long arms of chromosomes 9 and 22 are translocated. It is found in approximately 95% of cases of chronic myelogenous leukemia (CML). The presence of the Philadelphia chromosome alone is not sufficient evidence of the diagnosis of CML, because it has also been found in some cases of acute lymphoblastic leukemia and acute myelogenous leukemia. Chronic myelogenous leukemia is characterized by a leukocytosis and a left shift of the myelogenous series, with more mature forms predominating and less than 5% blasts present on peripheral blood smear.

25. **The correct answer is D.** Cyanocobalamin, vitamin B_{12}, is found primarily in foods that come from animals, such as fish, meat, poultry, eggs, milk, and milk products. It is for this reason that strict vegans need to supplement their diets with vitamin B_{12}. B_{12} attaches to gastric intrinsic factor and is absorbed by the terminal ileum of the small intestines. Because the most common site of involvement in Crohn's disease is the terminal ileum, malabsorption can occur. Patients who undergo gastric bypass surgery for treatment of severe obesity may encounter nutritional deficiencies in iron, calcium, vitamins D and B_{12}, and folate. Rheumatoid arthritis is more apt to cause anemia of chronic disease; it is not directly associated with the development of macrocytic anemia.

26. **The correct answer is A.** Colon cancer is the second leading cause of death due to malignancy in the United States. Risk factors for the development of colon cancer include African American ethnicity, a family history of colon cancer or adenomatous polyps, a diet rich in fats and red meats, and inflammatory bowel disease. Colonoscopy is the diagnostic test of choice, because it affords biopsy of a suspicious lesion to confirm

malignancy. If the colonoscopy does not reach the cecum (less than 5% of cases) or if there is an obstructing lesion, a barium enema or "virtual colonoscopy" (CT colonography) becomes an alternative diagnostic modality. Tumor-node-metastasis (TNM) cancer staging is used more frequently than the previously used Duke staging. Family history for diverticulosis does not place a patient at increased risk for colon cancer. Diverticulosis refers to small herniations, or "outpouchings," of the intestinal or colonic mucosa. Peutz-Jeghers syndrome is an inherited autosomal dominant disorder characterized by mucocutaneous, hyperpigmented macules and hamartomatous intestinal polyps. Patients with Peutz-Jeghers syndrome are at risk for bleeding, intussusceptions, and bowel obstructions. These patients also are at increased risk of developing certain types of cancers, especially gastrointestinal cancers.

27. **The correct answer is C.** Hypersegmented neutrophils and macrocytic ovalocytes strongly suggest a megaloblastic anemia. The peripheral smear of patients with hereditary spherocytosis demonstrates anisocytosis and the presence of dense, uniform spherocytes that lack an area of central pallor. Both iron deficiency anemia and thalassemia demonstrate microcytic, hypochromic red blood cells. There is a greater degree of anisocytosis and poikilocytosis in thalassemia than in iron deficiency anemia. Target cells are also seen on smears of patients with thalassemia.

28. **The correct answer is B.** Acute lymphoblastic leukemia (ALL) is the most common leukemia of childhood, constituting 80% of all cases. Peak incidence is 3 to 7 years of age. In ALL there is proliferation of the lymphoid precursors, leading to a hypercellular bone marrow with greater than 20% lymphoblasts. Patients may experience bleeding episodes secondary to the thrombocytopenia and infections due to the neutropenia. Fatigue, gingival hyperplasia and bleeding, bone pain, and lymphadenopathy are common presenting symptoms. Treatment of children with ALL is divided into three chemotherapy stages: induction, consolidation, and maintenance. The duration of treatment regimens for most children with ALL is 2 to 3 years. Although only 20 to 30% of adults are cured with standard chemotherapy treatments, the cure rate in children can reach 80 to 95%.

29. **The correct answer is C.** Symptoms of severe iron deficiency anemia include mucosal and skin changes such as atrophic glossitis and cheilosis. Some patients will admit to pica, which is an unusual food craving for ice, dirt, or starch, which actually proves the patient is deficient in iron. Brittleness or spooning of the nails, known as koilonychias, can also occur. Clubbing of the nails is generally indicative of chronic hypoxia and is seen more commonly in patients with chronic pulmonary disorders. Dysphagia can occur as a result of esophageal web formation, as seen in Plummer-Vinson syndrome, a long-standing iron deficiency condition. Once an occult blood loss has been excluded or inadequate intake or cause of malabsorption identified, iron supplementation should be initiated. Ferrous sulfate 325 mg by mouth three times a day with meals is usually recommended. An acidic environment is required for the release of ferric iron from food sources, an important fact to consider in patients concurrently taking proton-pump inhibitors. Calcium also decreases the bioavailability of iron. Ascorbic acid has been found to promote absorption of ferric and ferrous iron. Parenteral iron is reserved for those patients intolerant to oral iron or who are refractory to trial of oral therapy. Transfusion with packed red blood cells may be indicated for those patients who demonstrate a continued blood loss or who are hemodynamically unstable.

30. **The correct answer is B.** Patients with a palpable or suspicious mass should undergo biopsy, regardless of mammography, ultrasound, or MRI findings. In the United States, a woman's overall lifetime risk of developing breast cancer is one in eight. Risk factors are a positive family history, especially a first-degree relative with a history of breast cancer, or *BRCA-1* and *BRCA-2* genetic mutations. Others include early menarche, nulliparity, first full-term pregnancy after age 35, and late menopause. The sensitivity of mammography

depends on a variety of factors, such as breast density, which is reflective of the patient's age, and tumor size and location. MRI testing of patients at high risk of developing breast cancer, such as patients with a family history and those with a genetic predisposition, is becoming widely accepted as a useful screening modality. However, no radiologic test should substitute for biopsy.

31. **The correct answer is B.** Calcifications on an ovarian mass are relatively benign. Compare this with calcifications in the lung or breast where their presence is more ominous. A solid mass is typically indicative of an advanced malignancy, as is the presence of ascites, a protein-rich fluid that occurs in response to malignancy of inflammation. These are both ominous signs. Sonographic findings, such as septations, are also typically indicative of malignancy.

32. **The correct answer is D.** Breast cancer typically metastasizes to the brain, lung, and bone, which should not be surprising considering the location. Metastasis to the ovaries, although possible, is unlikely. The colon, prostate, and lung all metastasize as noted in the question—again, consider the anatomic location of each area.

33. **The correct answer is D.** Patients in the early stage of disease who are stable may initially be monitored, because chemotherapy has not been proven advantageous in these patients. Treatment options for chronic lymphocytic leukemia include corticosteroids, monoclonal antibody therapy, and splenectomy.

34. **The correct answer is C.** Prussian blue staining is used to identify ringed sideroblasts, which represent iron deposits within the mitochondria surrounding the nucleus of the red blood cell. Sideroblastic anemia results from the inability of heme to incorporate into the protoporphyrin ring during hemoglobin synthesis. Iron accumulates and is deposited within the red blood cells. It can be an inherited or acquired disorder. Some drugs, such as isoniazid and ethanol, can induce such an anemia. Laboratory findings demonstrate increased serum iron, transferrin saturation, and ferritin levels, with a decreased total iron-binding capacity. Hematocrit levels are generally in the 20 to 30% range. In some cases, treatment with moderate to high doses of vitamin B_6 not only improve hemoglobin levels, but reverse the anemia.

35. **The correct answer is B.** Disseminated intravascular coagulation (DIC) may occur as a result of a myriad of conditions, such as septicemia, trauma, tissue necrosis, obstetric complications, vascular disorders, and cancer. Laboratory findings classically include low or depleted fibrinogen levels, thrombocytopenia, positive D-dimer, and prolonged prothrombin times. The partial thromboplastin time (PTT) results are variable and may or may not be prolonged in DIC.

36. **The correct answer is C.** All of the factors listed are synthesized in the liver except for Factor VIII. Factor VIII is synthesized by platelets and the endothelium.

37. **The correct answer is A.** Non-Hodgkin's lymphoma has a poorer prognosis than Hodgkin's disease. The etiology is unknown; however, the Epstein-Barr virus (EBV) has been implicated in some of the literature. In up to 80% of patients, asymptomatic lymphadenopathy above the diaphragm may be present. The most common site for lymphadenopathy occurs (in order of occurrence) in the cervical and axillary areas and, less commonly, the inguinal area. Splenomegaly or hepatomegaly may also be present. As you would expect, patients with HIV have a higher incidence of non-Hodgkin's lymphoma than the non-HIV population. The typical patient presents with symptoms in large part consisting of nonintentional weight loss, night sweats, and fever.

38. **The correct answer is C.** Caucasian women have a slightly higher risk of developing breast cancer than African American women. Those with the lowest risk include Asian, Hispanic, and Native American women. Early menarche imparts a greater risk of

developing breast carcinoma than later menarche, and multiparity and breastfeeding actually reduce the risk of developing breast cancer. Two of the greatest risks for developing and dying from breast carcinoma are breast cancer in a first-degree relative and a personal history of breast cancer.

39. **The correct answer is D.** The classic finding in β-thalassemia is the presence of target cells. These cells can be described as a peripheral rim of hemoglobin with a small amount in the center and a cleared area between the two, thus giving the appearance of a target (shown below). Basophilic stippling can be seen in α- or β-thalassemia, but it is not as common, and certainly not the classic finding. Basophilic stippling is also found in heavy metal poisoning. Microcytic, hypochromic red blood cells are typically found in iron deficiency anemia. Spherocytes are usually found in hereditary spherocytosis.

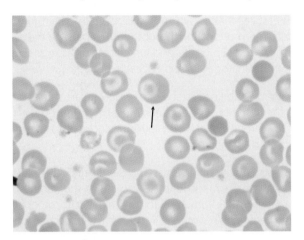

40. **The correct answer is C.** Heparin-induced thrombocytopenia (HIT) is a common drug-induced cause of low platelet counts. It occurs secondary to a reaction of IgG autoantibodies with platelet factor 4 in combination with heparin. There is a lower risk of HIT with low-molecular-weight heparin than unfractionated heparin. Hydrochlorothiazide has also been implicated in the cause of thrombocytopenia, but not as frequently as heparin. Warfarin affects vitamin K synthesis. The antidote, in fact, for warfarin overdose is vitamin K. The vitamin K coagulation factors are Factors II, VII, IX, and X. Angiotensin II receptor blockers (ARBs) do not affect platelets. The most common side effect of an ARB would be hyperkalemia.

REFERENCES

Bartella, L., Smith, C. S., Dershaw, D. D., and Lieberman, L. (2007). "Imaging breast cancer." *Radiologic Clinics of North American*, 45(1): 45–67.

deVos, S. (2006). "Historical overview and current state of art in diagnosis and treatment of Hodgkin's and Non-Hodgkin's lymphoma." *PET Clin*, 1(3): 203–217.

Fauci, A. S., Braunwald, E., Kasper, D. L., Hauser, S. L., Longo, D. L., Jameson, J. L., and Loscalzo, J. (2008). *Harrison's textbook of internal medicine*, 17th ed. McGraw-Hill Medical Publishing, New York.

Goldman, L., and Ausiello, D. (2008). *Cecil medicine*, 23rd ed. Saunders Elsevier, Philadelphia, PA.

Heeney, M. M., and Ware, R. E. (2008). "Hydroxyurea for children with sickle cell disease." *Pediatric Clinics of North America*, 55(2): 483–501.

Killip, S., Bennett, J. M., and Chambers, M. D. (2007). "Iron deficiency anemia." *American Family Physician*, 75(5): 671–678.

Lee, G. R., Bithell, T. C., Foerster, J., Athens, J. W., and Lukens, J. N. (1993). *Wintrobe's clinical hematology*, Volumes 1 and 2, 9th ed. Lea & Febiger, Malvern, PA.

Levi, M. (2005). "Disseminated intravascular coagulation: What's new?" *Critical Care Clinics*, 21(3): 449–467.

Robertson, J., Lillicrap, D., and James, P. D. (2008). "von Willibrand Disease." *Pediatric Clinics of North American*, 55(2): 377–392.

Tierney, Jr., L. M., McPhee, S. J., Papadakis, M. A. (2008). *Current medical diagnosis and treatment.* McGraw-Hill Companies, New York.

CHAPTER

24

Surgery

Jennifer Arnold, MHS, PA-C
Richard L. Commaille, PA-C

1. A 2-year-old child presents with sudden onset of cramping and abdominal pain. His evaluation is consistent with a bowel obstruction. He also passed a small amount of "currant jelly" blood per rectum. You palpate an elongated mass in the right upper quadrant of the abdomen. Operative intervention revealed the following photograph to be the mass you palpated (see below). Which of the following is the most common pathologic lead point for this condition?

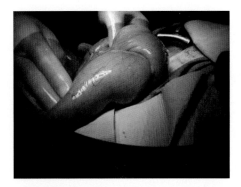

   A. Carcinoid
   B. Meckel's diverticulum
   C. Rectal polyps
   D. Adenocarcinoma

2. A 60-year-old male smoker presents to your office with intermittent dysphagia, halitosis, and excessive salivation. You obtain the radiograph shown below. Which of the following is the most likely cause for this patient's condition?

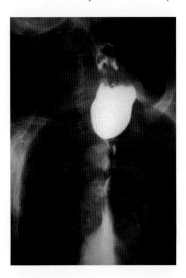

A. Plummer-Vinson syndrome
B. Schatzki rings
C. Zenker's diverticulum
D. Achalasia

3. A 45-year-old male presents to the emergency department after a night of heavy drinking punctuated by several episodes of vomiting with an acute upper gastrointestinal bleed. Of note in the patient's history is hepatitis C and cirrhosis. Which of the following is the most likely cause of the patient's upper gastrointestinal bleed?

A. Boerhaave's syndrome
B. Barrett's esophagitis
C. Mallory-Weiss tear
D. Peptic ulcer

4. Which of the following is the most common location for the appendix?

A. Retrocecal
B. Medial to McBurney's point
C. Lateral to McBurney's point
D. Preileal

5. Appendicitis is most common in which of the following age groups?

A. 7 to 11 years
B. 15 to 25 years
C. 35 to 45 years
D. Older than 50 years

6. Which of the following best defines diverticulum?

A. Local inflammation of a bowel outpouching
B. Luminal obstruction of a bowel outpouching
C. The existence of diverticula without inflammation
D. Perforation of the colon

7. Which of the following is the most common location for diverticular disease?

A. Sigmoid colon
B. Descending colon
C. Ascending colon
D. Transverse colon

8. In which of the following circumstances would you *not* expect to see abnormal calcifications on an abdominal flat plate?

A. Cholelithiasis
B. Crohn's disease
C. Ureterolithiasis
D. Phleboliths

9. Complications following a splenectomy may be immediate or delayed. Which of the following represents a complication that may occur years later?

A. Dumping syndrome
B. Postoperative hemorrhage
C. Overwhelming postsplenectomy sepsis
D. Subphrenic abscess

10. Which of the following is *not* a usual precipitating factor for acalculous cholecystitis?

A. Prolonged fasting
B. Sepsis
C. Dehydration
D. Aerobic activity

11. Primary sclerosing cholangitis is associated with which of the following diseases?

    A. Chagas disease

    B. Ulcerative colitis

    C. Typhlitis

    D. Schistosomiasis

12. Incarceration of abdominal contents into a hernia sac is most common with which of the following hernias?

    A. Parastomal hernia

    B. Paraesophageal hernia

    C. Direct hernia

    D. Femoral hernia

13. A 60-year-old male presents complaining of localized pain to the left of the umbilicus near the edge of the rectus muscle. You are unable to palpate a mass, but you suspect this pain may represent a hernia. Which of the following types of hernias is most likely in this location?

    A. Epigastric

    B. Grynfeltt's

    C. Richter's

    D. Spigelian

14. Which of the following is the best imaging technique to diagnose the hernia in the scenario described in Question 13?

    A. CT scan

    B. Abdominal x-ray

    C. Hepatobiliary iminodiacetic acid (HIDA) scan

    D. Laparoscopy

15. Which of the following is *not* usually associated with angiodysplasia occurring in the ascending colon?

    A. End-stage renal disease

    B. von Willebrand's disease

    C. Aortic stenosis

    D. Pancreatic cancer

16. Which of the following is the hallmark of an acute lower gastrointestinal bleed?

    A. Melena

    B. Hemoptysis

    C. Hematochezia

    D. Diverticulosis

17. Procidentia must be differentiated from prolapsed incarcerated internal hemorrhoids. Which of the following would confirm the diagnosis of procidentia?

    A. The mucosa may have a rose-like appearance.

    B. The mucosa has concentric folds.

    C. There may be extreme pain.

    D. The rectum is always reducible.

18. Which of the following is the most common life-threatening complication of portal hypertension?

    A. Sepsis

    B. Hepatorenal syndrome

    C. Bleeding from esophageal varices

    D. Portal vein thrombosis

19. Which of the following is the most common cause of chronic cholecystitis?

   A. Cholelithiasis
   B. Chronic pancreatitis
   C. Chronic alcohol abuse
   D. Primary sclerosing cholangitis

20. A patient presents with pneumobilia and small-bowel obstruction. Which of the following are the most common sites of obstruction, secondary to gallstones?

   A. Duodenum and transverse colon
   B. Ileum and sigmoid colon
   C. Jejunum and ascending colon
   D. Cecum and descending colon

21. The use of balloon tamponade to control bleeding from esophageal varices is as effective as pharmacologic intervention in stabilizing hemodynamically compromised patients. Which of the following would *not* be considered definitive treatment of esophageal variceal bleeding?

   A. Transjugular intrahepatic portosystemic shunt placement
   B. Endoscopic variceal sclerosis
   C. Esophageal transection
   D. Repeated lavage with ice water

22. Extramammary Paget's disease, which is commonly found in the perianal area, is a rare form of adenocarcinoma arising from which of the following?

   A. Endocrine glands
   B. Exocrine glands
   C. Apocrine glands
   D. Crypts of Mortgagni

23. Which of the following is the most common primary bone malignancy found in teenagers and young adults?

   A. Osteogenic sarcoma
   B. Chondrosarcomas
   C. Fibrosarcomas
   D. Malignant fibrous histiocytomas

24. During an elective thyroidectomy, the superior laryngeal nerve may be injured. This would result in development of which of the following?

   A. Dysphagia
   B. Hoarseness
   C. Precision in pitch
   D. Airway compromise

25. A 57-year-old female presents complaining of bloody discharge from her left breast. This is most consistent with which of the following?

   A. Galactocele
   B. Carcinoma
   C. Papilloma
   D. Mastitis

26. Senescent breast hypertrophy may occur in males older than age 50 and may be associated with which of the following medications?

   A. Atenolol
   B. Digoxin
   C. Clindamycin
   D. Albuterol

27. Ischemic orchitis following an inguinal hernia repair usually occurs at which of the following points?

    A. 2 to 5 days postoperative

    B. Immediately postoperative

    C. Within 24 hours of surgery

    D. 1 week postoperative

28. A 24-year-old female presents to the emergency department with right lower quadrant pain and a positive β-hCG. Ultrasound confirms an intrauterine pregnancy. Surgery for suspected appendicitis should be delayed during which of the following?

    A. First trimester

    B. Second trimester

    C. Third trimester

    D. No delay is necessary.

29. Which of the following is the best procedure for diagnosing the site of an upper gastrointestinal bleed in a patient with portal hypertension?

    A. Ultrasound

    B. CT scan

    C. Upper gastrointestinal series

    D. Endoscopy

30. Which of the following is a contraindication to performing a laparoscopic cholecystectomy?

    A. Morbid obesity

    B. Liver cirrhosis

    C. Previous upper abdominal surgery

    D. Uncontrolled coagulopathy

31. Which of the following is the most common cause of esophageal perforation?

    A. Iatrogenic

    B. Trauma

    C. Foreign bodies

    D. Vomiting

32. Which of the following is the most common sign of malignant carcinoid syndrome?

    A. Diarrhea

    B. Right heart valvular disease

    C. Cutaneous flushing

    D. Asthma

33. Which of the following is *not* a characteristic finding associated with anal fissures?

    A. Sentinel tag

    B. Pain on defecation

    C. Bleeding

    D. Lesions at 9 and 3 o'clock

34. Ulcerative colitis usually presents with which of the following?

    A. Anal fissures and fistulas

    B. Abscesses

    C. Pain and constipation

    D. Bloody diarrhea

35. A male patient presents with intractable peptic ulcer disease and persistent diarrhea. Which of the following is the most likely cause of his problem?

A. Ulcerative colitis

B. Zollinger-Ellison syndrome

C. Ischemic enterocolitis

D. Gastric outlet obstruction

36. Severe pancreatitis may be associated with left flank discoloration secondary to bleeding. This discoloration is described as which of the following?

A. Cullen's sign

B. Grey Turner's sign

C. Sentinel loop sign

D. Cutoff sign

37. A 72-year-old male was brought to the emergency department by his family. The patient complains of weight loss and periumbilical pain that occurs approximately 30 minutes after eating. He notes that the pain resolves after several hours but repeats after each meal. He has no history of peptic ulcer disease. Which of the following is the most likely cause for this patient's pain?

A. Acute mesenteric occlusion

B. Venous congestion

C. Mesenteric angina

D. Mesenteric thrombosis

38. A 22-year-old white male presents to the emergency department with fever and pain in the midline buttock region. On examination, you find an abscess in the postsacral intergluteal fold, as shown below. This condition is most consistent with which of the following?

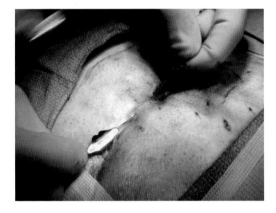

A. Perianal abscess

B. Pilonidal cyst

C. Fistula-in-ano

D. Hidradenitis suppurativa

39. A 55-year-old female is diagnosed with breast cancer. She elects to have a modified radical mastectomy rather than a lumpectomy. Which of the following nerves should *not* be at risk for injury during the surgical dissection?

A. Phrenic nerve

B. Long thoracic nerve

C. Thoracodorsal nerve

D. Intercostal brachial cutaneous nerve

40. A 35-year-old female presents with a thyroid lesion in the left lobe less than 1 cm in size. In her youth, she had neck irradiation. The diagnosis of papillary carcinoma is confirmed with US-guided biopsy. Which of the following would be the appropriate surgical treatment?

    A. Near-total thyroidectomy
    B. Total thyroidectomy
    C. Left lobectomy and isthmectomy
    D. Chemotherapy

41. Which of the following is the most common location for colorectal cancer in men?

    A. Transverse colon
    B. Ascending colon
    C. Sigmoid colon
    D. Rectum

42. Which of the following statements is true of pancreatic pseudocysts?

    A. Pancreatic pseudocysts represent most cases of acute pancreatitis.
    B. The physical examination is usually unremarkable.
    C. An abdominal CT scan is the diagnostic study of choice.
    D. Pancreatic pseudocysts should always be drained.

43. In most patients, which of the following coronary arteries wraps the apex of the heart and anastamoses with the posterior descending artery?

    A. Right coronary artery
    B. Left circumflex artery
    C. Left anterior descending artery
    D. Diagonal artery

44. A 68-year-old male is admitted to the hospital with chest pain on exertion. The pain is mid-sternal, and he describes it as "sharp and burning." The electrocardiogram showed nonspecific ST changes. A cardiac catheterization revealed an ejection fraction of 65%, a 70% stenosed diagonal lesion, an 80% stenosed circumflex lesion, and a 90% stenosed lesion in the posterior descending artery. Which of the following is the most appropriate next step?

    A. Begin IV nitroglycerin and heparin.
    B. Place an intra-aortic balloon pump.
    C. Perform an echocardiogram for heart function.
    D. Perform an emergent coronary artery bypass graft.

45. Which of the following are the dilated pockets of the aortic root between the cusps and aortic wall from which the coronary arteries arise?

    A. Chordae tendoneae
    B. Sinuses of valsalva
    C. Fibrous skeleton
    D. Papillary muscles

46. Which of the following conduits for coronary artery bypass grafting surgery has the best long-term patency rate?

    A. Lesser saphenous vein
    B. Greater saphenous vein
    C. Internal mammary artery
    D. Radial artery

47. Which of the following is the most common site of a type A aortic dissection?

    A. Descending aorta distal to the left subclavian artery
    B. Ascending aorta 1 to 2 cm above the aortic sinus
    C. Ascending aorta just above the origin of left subclavian
    D. Area between the left carotid and left subclavian artery

48. A 68-year-old woman with a history of hypercholesterolemia, hypertension, and a 20-pack-year smoking history presents with angina, two syncopal episodes, and some shortness of breath with pedal edema. Her electrocardiogram revealed left ventricular hypertrophy, but no ST changes or Q waves. An echocardiogram revealed an aortic valve area <1.0 cm^2 and a left ventricular ejection fraction of 45%. Which of the following is the most appropriate next step for this patient?

A. Surgery for aortic valve repair
B. Surgery for aortic valve replacement
C. Cardiac catheterization to evaluate the coronary arteries
D. Percutaneous balloon valvotomy

49. Which of the following is *not* an absolute indication for surgery for native mitral valve infective endocarditis?

A. Severe regurgitation causing heart failure
B. Abscess of the valve annulus
C. Vegetation on the mitral leaflets <1 cm in size
D. Fungal or gram-negative infections

50. A 35-year-old male with a history of Marfan syndrome and a positive family history of aortic dissection is being followed by you for his ascending aortic aneurysm. When the aneurysm reaches which of the following sizes would you recommend that he have elective surgical repair?

A. 3 cm
B. 4 cm
C. 5 cm
D. 6 cm

51. A 60-year-old male was a belted driver in a head-on collision. He was brought to the emergency department via ambulance. He is complaining of head, neck, shoulder, chest, and back pain. His vitals on arrival are as follows: blood pressure, 90/68 mmHg; pulse, 118 beats per minute, regular; respiration, 20 breaths per minute, labored; and a temperature of 99.5°F. The results of his emergent CT axial scan are shown below. Which of the following is the most likely diagnosis?

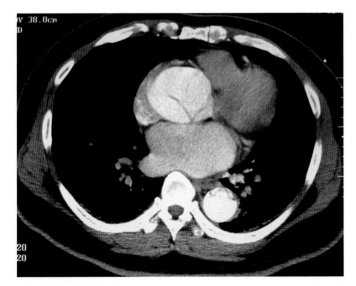

A. Lacerated liver
B. Type A dissection
C. Lacerated spleen
D. Pneumothorax

52. In a diabetic patient undergoing a coronary artery bypass graft (CABG), which of the following significantly increases the risk of sternal wound complications?

   A. Grafting the right internal mammary artery to the left anterior descending artery
   B. Excessive traction on the hemisternum with the Rultract
   C. Performing a full sternotomy
   D. The use of bilateral internal mammary arteries as conduit grafts

53. Prior to harvesting the radial artery for use as a conduit graft for a coronary artery bypass graft, which of the following must be performed to test for patency?

   A. CT scan
   B. Arteriogram of the radial and ulnar arteries
   C. Intraoperative Allen's test with the use of a pulse oximeter
   D. Preoperative Allen's test without the use of a pulse oximeter

54. Which of the following is the most appropriate medication for infusion into a patient during radial artery harvest to reduce arterial spasm?

   A. Nicardipine HCL
   B. Heparin
   C. Dobutamine
   D. Amiodarone

ANSWERS

1. The correct answer is B. Meckel's diverticulum is the most prevalent congenital anomaly of the gastrointestinal tract, affecting males more than females by a ratio of 3:2. This is considered a true diverticuli, because the walls contain all the layers normally found in the small intestine (see below). Intussusception is the most common cause of intestinal obstruction in the infant, and this child presents with the most common signs/symptoms of the condition. Meckel's diverticulum obstruction is rarely reduced by air or contrast media (compared to the success of this procedure in patients with intussusception), and thus the pathologic lead point is usually identified when operative intervention is performed.

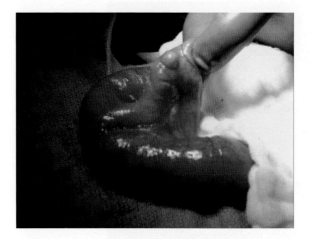

2. The correct answer is C. Zenker's diverticulum is a motility disorder of the pharyngo-esophageal segment of the intestine. For years, it was the most common recognized sign of pharyngoesophageal dysfunction and was originally "discovered" in 1769. Zenker's diverticula tend to enlarge progressively with time due to the decreased compliance of the skeletal portion of the cervical esophagus that occurs with aging. The patient presents with dysphagia, which is usually associated with spontaneous regurgitation of undigested material (leading to halitosis) that often interrupts eating or drinking. This can be severe enough to cause weight loss or aspiration. The diagnosis is made with a barium swallow. Endoscopy is not only difficult, but dangerous due to the attendant risk of perforation. Achalasia also presents with regurgitation and dysphagia, but the barium swallow demonstrates the lesion to be a narrowing of the distal esophagus (bird's beak sign). Schatzki rings are narrow bands of tissue at the distal end of the esophagus, and dysphagia is also common with this condition. Plummer-Vinson syndrome is characterized by dysphagia associated with atrophic oral mucosa, chronic anemia, and spoon-shaped fingers with brittle nail beds. This condition characteristically occurs in edentulous middle-aged women. Plummer-Vinson syndrome is also known as sidero-blastic dysphagia.

3. **The correct answer is C.** Mallory-Weiss tears are responsible for approximately 10% of all cases of acute upper gastrointestinal hemorrhage. It is most often a longitudinal tear in the gastric mucosa near the esophagogastric junction. It usually follows bouts of forceful retching. Boerhaave's syndrome is the actual rupture of the distal esophagus. It can also be caused by vomiting. However, Boerhaave's syndrome requires the presence of food in the rupture, whereas a Mallory-Weiss tear does not. It is thought that patients with a history of liver dysfunction have increased vasculature in the esophagus, and thus may have an increased risk for rupture and bleed. Barrett's esophagitis is due to reflux of gastric/duodenal contents into the esophagus. These patients present with symptoms of GERD (gastroesophageal reflux disease), such as pyrosis, thrash, or substernal discomfort. Peptic ulcer disease bleeding can present either acutely and dramatically or chronically and insidiously. However, in this case the history of chronic alcoholism, liver disease, and repeated vomiting lends one to the diagnosis of a Mallory-Weiss tear.

4. **The correct answer is A.** The appendix is located retrocecally in approximately 16% of patients.

5. **The correct answer is B.** Appendicitis (shown below) is one of the most common surgical emergencies presenting in the United States, accounting for approximately 200,000 appendectomies each year. It is most common in the 15-to-25 age group.

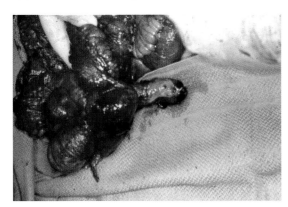

6. **The correct answer is D.** Although the suffix -itis commonly means "inflammation," it actually occurs later in the progression of the disease, not initially. There is a discrete perforation of the diverticulum itself, leading to a localized inflammation of the colonic wall or associated tissues. This may progress to complications such as fissures or abscesses. As a general rule, the original perforation seals itself, which usually isolates any paracolic infection from the lumen of the colon.

7. **The correct answer is A.** Diverticular disease is primarily a Western disease resulting from high consumption of processed food. It presents in the sigmoid colon in over one-half of patients. It presents in the descending colon in about 40% of patients, with

the entire colon accounting for the other 5 to 10% of patients. An acute diverticulitis is shown below.

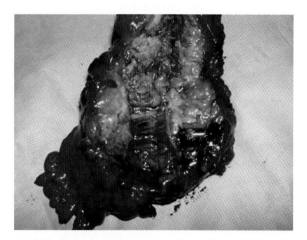

8. **The correct answer is B.** Crohn's disease presents radiographically with a thickened bowel wall with stricture ("string" sign) or fissuring, a cobblestone pattern, or the presence of skip lesions. Abnormal calcifications are not usually seen. In all of the answer options, calcifications are seen, and may even be pathognomonic of the condition.

9. **The correct answer is C.** Complications of splenectomy are relatively rare. The most common complications, which occur relatively soon postoperatively, are atelectasis, postoperative hemorrhage, and pancreatitis. Postsplenectomy, patients are susceptible to bacteremia due to decreased clearance of bacteria from the blood and decreased levels of IgM circulating in the blood. Most infections following splenectomy occur within 1 year following surgery; however, more than half occur more than 5 years postoperatively. The most common pathogens are encapsulated organisms such as *Streptococcus pneumoniae*, *Haemophilus influenzae*, and *Neisseria meningitidis*. Dumping syndrome is usually related to operations that impair the stomach's ability to regulate its rate of emptying. Splenectomy rarely interferes with emptying, and the signs/symptoms of dumping syndrome would appear earlier.

10. **The correct answer is D.** Acalculous cholecystitis—cholecystitis occurring in the absence of cholelithiasis—occurs in approximately one-fifth of cases of acute cholecystitis. Causes include cystic duct obstruction from other processes. It is most common in patients hospitalized with some other process—particularly in trauma victims. Aerobic physical activity is not a precipitating factor.

11. **The correct answer is B.** Extracolonic manifestations of ulcerative colitis are numerous, and there is no absolute relationship between severity of the colitis and the extracolonic manifestation. These manifestations include skin and mucous membrane lesions, such as aphthous stomatitis or erythema nodosum; uveitis; arthralgias and arthritis; and other hepatobiliary complications, such as cirrhosis, pericholangitis, sclerosing cholangitis, gallstones, and pancreatic insufficiency. Pericarditis and malnutrition are other extracolonic manifestations. Schistosomiasis is the second most common tropical disease in the world. There is no documented relationship between primary sclerosing cholangitis and schistosomiasis. The clinician should note that sclerosing cholangitis may require liver transplantation.

12. **The correct answer is D.** Femoral hernias are more likely to become incarcerated or strangulated due to their narrow anatomical neck. Parastomal and paraesophageal hernias are less likely to have abdominal contents within them due to their anatomic

locations. Direct hernias are a result of developed weakness of the transversalis fascia in Hesselbach's area. In general, direct hernias produce fewer symptoms than indirect inguinal hernias and are less likely to become incarcerated or strangulated.

13. **The correct answer is D.** A spigelian hernia is an acquired ventral hernia that occurs where the sheaths of the lateral abdominal muscles form the lateral rectus sheath. Patients usually present with pain localized to the hernia site aggravated by increased intra-abdominal pressure. Over time, the pain will become dull and diffuse, which muddles the picture. Epigastric hernias usually present as protrusions above the level of the umbilicus through the linea alba. They are more common in men between the ages of 20 and 50. In a Richter's hernia, it is usually on only one side of the intestinal wall, and it usually strangulates. This strangulation does not always result in intestinal obstruction. Grynfeltt's hernia, or lumbar hernia, refers to several hernias (congenital, spontaneous, and traumatic) that occur through the anatomic location known as Grynfeltt's triangle, which is an inverted triangle bounded by the 12th rib, the internal oblique abdominal muscle, and the sacrospinalis muscle, and then covered by the latissimus dorsi muscle.

14. **The correct answer is A.** Diagnosis of a spigelian hernia is difficult because it may not be palpable. These hernias may lay beneath the external oblique muscle. Both ultrasound and CT scans can help make the diagnosis. The other imaging modalities would be of little use, excepting laparoscopy, which is much too invasive to simply make the diagnosis.

15. **The correct answer is D.** Angiodysplasia is an acquired condition consisting of a focal submucosal vascular ectasia that frequently bleeds. It most often affects the elderly (older than 60 years of age). Most of these lesions are located in the cecum and proximal ascending colon, although some patients, especially younger patients, may present with lesions in the small bowel. All of the conditions listed have been associated with this condition, with the exception of pancreatic carcinoma.

16. **The correct answer is C.** Hematochezia is the passage of liquid blood or clots of varying color (maroon to bright red). The brighter the color, the more vigorous and acute the bleeding. It is the hallmark of an acute lower gastrointestinal bleed. Melena is the passage of black, tarry stools; it usually indicates a bleed that has allowed the blood to be partially digested, which negates the acute lower gastrointestinal characteristic. Hemoptysis is the coughing of blood, and the abnormal condition of diverticuli in the colon would not be a hallmark of an acute bleed. Hematemesis is the vomiting of blood.

17. **The correct answer is B.** Procidentia is a condition in which the rectum literally turns inside out. The etiology of this condition is controversial. Proposed causes include weak musculature of the pelvic floor and anal canal or herniation of the cul-de-sac. Procidentia occurs naturally with bowel movements in some larger mammals, but not in humans. The presence of concentric rings would confirm this diagnosis.

18. **The correct answer is C.** Due to the increase in portal pressures (i.e., portal hypertension), all attendant vascular structures that feed into the system must accommodate the pressure. The varicose veins of the esophagus are especially prone to this dilation. With any further increase in pressure, they may rupture and bleed, presenting a life-threatening complication. The other conditions, although possible complications, do not afford the immediate and most common life-threatening complication of esophageal variceal bleeding.

19. **The correct answer is A.** An ongoing or recurrent inflammation of the gallbladder results in chronic cholecystitis. The most common cause of this is cholelithiasis for the obvious reason that calculi can block the bile ducts and cause inflammation—and subsequent cholecystitis. The other conditions may cause acute and/or chronic cholecystitis, but they are not the most common causes.

20. **The correct answer is B.** A patient presenting with pneumobilia and a small-bowel obstruction should first be considered to have a gallstone ileus. The most common sites are the ileum and sigmoid colon.

21. **The correct answer is D.** The first three choices are all obviously more long-term and significant treatments. Ice-water lavage is temporary, at best, and certainly not definitive.

22. **The correct answer is C.** Paget's disease is a rare intraepithelial adenocarcinoma that occurs primarily in women who are in their 60s and 70s. It arises from the intraepidermal portion of the apocrine glands. It presents primarily as severe, intractable pruritus with an erythematous, eczematoid rash. If biopsy confirms the disease, a workup for a coexistent gastrointestinal carcinoma should be performed; such carcinomas are found in up to one-half of patients with Paget's disease.

23. **The correct answer is A.** Osteogenic sarcoma, also known as osteosarcoma, is the most common primary malignant tumor of the bone, affecting 0.25 cases per 100,000/year, or approximately 400 cases per year in persons less than 20 years of age. Most tumors arise in the distal femoral metaphysis, proximal tibial metaphysis, proximal humeral metaphysis, pelvis, or proximal femur. Most cases are adolescents, with a male to female ratio of 3:2.

24. **The correct answer is C.** Voice dysfunction after thyroidectomy may be caused by damage to the laryngeal nerves or lesions to strap muscles with laryngotracheal movement impairment. Injury to an external branch of the superior laryngeal nerve usually results in changes in voice pitch.

25. **The correct answer is C.** A papilloma is a tumor of variable size presenting in the epithelium of the duct network of the breast. Papilloma typically presents with serosanguinous or bloody discharge. Carcinoma rarely presents with discharge. Mastitis presents with inflammation and may have a purulent discharge, if any. Galactoceles are tumors within the milk-producing glands of the breast, and any discharge would be of a milk-like nature.

26. **The correct answer is B.** Medications with estrogen or estrogen-like compounds may cause gynecomastia. These drugs include digitalis, estrogens, anabolic steroids, and marijuana. Medications that inhibit testosterone production may have the same effect (cimetidine, ketoconazole, phenytoin, spironolactone, diazepam, and antineoplastic agents). The other medications listed do not have an effect upon the male breast.

27. **The correct answer is A.** Ischemic orchitis results in a painful swollen testis and can have devastating results. It occurs as a result of interruption of blood flow to the testicles and typically occurs 2 to 5 days after surgery.

28. **The correct answer is D.** Acute appendicitis can occur at any time during pregnancy, but it is statistically more prevalent during the first two trimesters. This diagnosis can prove more difficult due to the displacement of the appendix as the pregnancy continues. This diagnosis requires prompt surgical intervention. Delay can be deadly. The clinician should note that the risk of premature labor is 10 to 15%.

29. **The correct answer is D.** Once the patient is stabilized, location of the site of the bleed is best diagnosed with endoscopy. It should be performed with 24 hours of admission. The diagnostic yield is generally 80% or better.

30. **The correct answer is D.** Cholecystectomy is the most common gastrointestinal operation performed in the United States. Generally, slightly more than one-half of cases of cholecystitis resolve with antibiotics and supportive care, thus there are two schools of thought regarding the need for surgical intervention. Once the decision to surgically

intervene is made, laparoscopic intervention clearly has fewer complications; however, it can only be performed in approximately 50% of patients. As with any surgical intervention, bleeding is a concern, and due to the nature of laparoscopic cholecystectomy, it is especially a concern. Therefore, a patient with an uncontrolled coagulopathy poses an unacceptable risk for this procedure.

31. **The correct answer is A.** Perforation of the esophagus is a true medical emergency. It most commonly occurs as an untoward result of diagnostic or therapeutic procedures. Spontaneous perforation, also known as Boerhaave's perforation, is responsible for approximately 15% of cases. Foreign bodies and trauma result in approximately one-quarter of cases. Coughing, retching, and/or vomiting do increase intraesophageal pressure, which, by itself, would pose an increased risk for rupture, but because esophageal or extragastric pressure remains almost equal to intragastric pressure, stretching of the wall is minimal. Furthermore, in cadaver studies, stretching of the esophageal wall usually leads to a Mallory-Weiss tear, which causes bleeding rather than a rupture.

32. **The correct answer is C.** Malignant carcinoid syndrome is the constellation of symptoms typically exhibited by patients with metastases from carcinoid tumors. These tumors usually secrete excessive amounts of serotonin. The flushing is usually caused by the secretion of the tumoral hormone. Diarrhea is also common as a result of this, but facial flushing remains the most predominant manifestation.

33. **The correct answer is D.** Anal fissures typically present with a sentinel tag, pain with defecation, and bleeding due to the tearing. Lesions are usually found posteriorly in 90% of cases and anteriorly in 10% of cases. Lesions in both areas present in less than 1% of cases.

34. **The correct answer is D.** The classic presentation of ulcerative colitis is bloody diarrhea, lower abdominal cramps, and fecal urgency. Crohn's disease presents insidiously with intermittent bouts of low-grade fever, diarrhea, and right lower abdominal pain. The terminal ileum is the most frequent site of involvement of Crohn's disease.

35. **The correct answer is B.** Zollinger-Ellison syndrome presents as described in the question. These ulcers are usually less responsive to conventional therapy than other ulcers and typically are severe and unrelenting. Most ulcers are located in the proximal duodenum, although gastric and more distal ulceration occurs as well. Diarrhea is a frequent symptom and may occur in the absence of ulceration. Ulcerative colitis usually presents with bloody diarrhea. Ischemic enterocolitis presents with mild abdominal pain initially followed by the passage of bright-red blood from the rectum. Gastric outlet obstruction frequently presents as vomiting.

36. **The correct answer is B.** Grey Turner's sign presents in 1 to 2% of patients as a bluish discoloration in the flank as a result of hemorrhagic pancreatitis with dissection of blood into this area. Cullen's sign is when the blood dissects into the periumbilical area. Sentinel loop sign is a play on the isolated dilation of a segment of gut consisting of the jejunum, transverse colon, or duodenum adjacent to the pancreas. The cutoff sign refers to gas distention of the right colon that stops abruptly in the mid or left transverse colon. Both the sentinel loop and the colon cutoff signs are relatively nonspecific signs in pancreatitis.

37. **The correct answer is C.** Mesenteric vascular disease is not a single presenting entity but rather a constellation of symptoms resulting in a syndrome that can present as a complete occlusion of mesenteric arteries; thrombosis of mesenteric veins (portal); extraluminal obstruction of the arteries by aneurysms, fibrous bands, or tumors; aneurysms of splanchnic arteries; or trauma to the area. Acute mesenteric occlusion typically presents with pain that is out of proportion to the findings. Venous congestion and thrombosis

would present this way as well. Mesenteric angina is the most likely choice here due to the intermittent and anginal way in which the patient presents with pain. The likelihood of pain increases as oxygen demand rises (as is the case following a meal).

38. **The correct answer is B.** Pilonidal cysts or abscesses most commonly present in white males between the ages of 15 and 40. These patients are generally hirsute, heavy, and perspire heavily. The cysts are typically located on the midline or slightly lateral of midline near the coccyx or sacrum. It is an acquired infection of the natal cleft hair follicles, which subsequently rupture and cause pilonidal abscesses. These abscesses cause hair to be pulled into them, thus irritating the area further. Diagnosis is made upon physical examination. If Crohn's disease is suspected, then a more vigorous workup is recommended. Hidradenitis suppurativa is a skin infection of the axillae or groin consisting of multiple abscesses of the apocrine sweat glands. Fistula-in-ano are abscesses that have formed a communication between the anus and the perianal skin. Perianal abscesses are classified according to the area in which they develop.

39. **The correct answer is A.** The phrenic nerves lie along the lateral mediastinum and run from the thoracic inlet to the diaphragm. They travel through the upper chest, medial to the mediastinal pleura and the apex of the right or left lung. The right phrenic nerve lies lateral to the right brachiocephalic vein and the superior vena cava. The left phrenic nerve travels along the lateral aspect of the transverse arch of the aorta. The two nerves subsequently pass anterior to their respective pulmonary hila and then inferiorly in a broad vertical plane along the margin of the heart between the fibrous pericardium and the mediastinal pleura. A mastectomy, regardless of the approach, should not interfere with the phrenic nerves. All of the other three answer options are in the path of a mastectomy and, as such, should be identified during the procedure.

40. **The correct answer is C.** Papillary adenocarcinomas of the thyroid account for most of the cases of thyroid carcinoma. They usually appear at a young age and are slow-growing. The treatment of differentiated thyroid carcinoma is operative excision. The appropriate operation for this patient is a total lobectomy with isthmectomy. Subtotal or partial lobectomy is contraindicated because the recurrence of tumor is greater and survival would be shorter. Because this patient has undergone irradiation and has had a recurrence, it is not recommended that she undergo chemotherapy. Total thyroidectomy is an acceptable operation for patients with papillary adenocarcinomas. In much of the literature, however, there is concern of more risk to the recurrent laryngeal nerve and the parathyroid gland. Some studies have found a higher risk of recurrence in patients who had a total thyroidectomy. Furthermore, due to the patient's age and the risks of damage, left lobectomy and isthmectomy is the best choice.

41. **The correct answer is D.** The most common location for colon carcinoma is the rectum in men and the right colon in women.

42. **The correct answer is C.** Pancreatic pseudocysts are localized collections of fluid with high concentrations of pancreatic enzymes. They can occur as a complication of pancreatitis. They lack a true epithelial lining like congenital cysts or cystic neoplasms, hence the name *pseudocysts*. The diagnostic study of choice is the abdominal CT scan. Drainage of these cysts is next to impossible and should not be attempted unless there is infection. Pancreatic pseudocysts develop in around 2% of cases, and the physical presence of a mass is usually the first clinical manifestation.

43. **The correct answer is C.** The left anterior descending (interventricular) coronary artery continues from the bifurcation of the left main stem, coursing anteriorly and inferiorly in the anterior interventricular groove to the apex of the heart. The diagonals run along the anterolateral wall of the left ventricle. The left circumflex arises from the left main

at a right angle to the anterior interventricular branch and courses the atrioventricular groove and terminates near the outer margin of the left ventricle. The right coronary artery runs from the aorta anteriorly and laterally descending in the right atrioventricular groove and carving posteriorly at the acute margin of the right ventricle.

44. **The correct answer is A.** The patient has three vessels with >60% stenosis and is symptomatic. The patient needs a coronary artery bypass graft, but not emergently. He is stable and there is no mention of ischemia to the heart.

45. **The correct answer is B.** The sinuses of valsalva are the dilation of the aortic wall behind each of the cusps of the aortic valve as described in the question. There are generally three aortic sinuses: the left, the right, and the posterior. The left aortic sinus gives rise to the left coronary artery, and the right aortic sinus gives rise to the right coronary artery. Usually no vessels arise from the posterior aortic sinus, which is therefore known as the *noncoronary* sinus. Each aortic sinus also can be referred to as the sinus of Valsalva, the sinus of Morgagni, or Petit's sinus. Chordae tendinae are tendons that link the atrioventricular valves to the papillary muscles. The papillary muscles provide tension that prevents the valves from prolapsing into the atria during the high pressure gradient that forces the valves open.

46. **The correct answer is C.** The left internal thoracic artery (left internal mammary artery) anastomosed end to side to the left anterior descending artery has a 10-year patency of over 90% and reports of continued patency 15, 20, 25, and 30 years postoperative. The patency rates of a radial artery graft off the aorta are approximately 80% at 5 years. Early graft failure occurs during the first year in approximately 20 to 25% of all venous conduits.

47. **The correct answer is B.** This is the most common site of a type A dissection.

48. **The correct answer is C.** Although the patient does need an aortic valve replacement, based on her past medical history she should have a cardiac catherization to evaluate her coronary arteries in order to determine if she needs a coronary artery bypass graft as well.

49. **The correct answer is C.** The vegetation on the mitral leaflets must be mobile and >1 cm in size to be an absolute indication for surgery.

50. **The correct answer is C.** Patients with Marfan syndrome and a positive family history of dissection should have this elective procedure when the aneurysm reaches 5 cm or grows at a rate >1.0 cm per year.

51. **The correct answer is B.** CT arteriogram shows a type A dissection. The axial image shows a dissection flap in the mid ascending aorta. This patient needs emergent surgical treatment.

52. **The correct answer is D.** Taking down both internal mammary arteries decreases the blood flow to the sternum, which is already an area that has poor blood flow. This increases the likelihood of a sternal wound infection in any patient, but especially in a diabetic patient.

53. **The correct answer is C.** An intraoperative Allen's test is the best answer. Preoperatively, you would obtain a radial artery study showing mapping of the radial arteries and flow through them. A CT scan and arteriogram are not indicated.

54. **The correct answer is A.** While harvesting the radial artery, the patient must be on a calcium-channel blocker or nitroglycerin to decrease the spasm of the artery.

REFERENCES

Doherty, G. M. (2006). *Current surgical diagnosis and treatment*, 12th ed. McGraw-Hill Medical Publishing, New York.

Schwartz, S. (1999). *Principles of surgery*, 17th ed. McGraw-Hill Medical Publishing, New York.

Townsend, C. M. (2008). *Sabiston textbook of surgery*, 18th ed. Elsevier Publishing, Philadelphia, PA.

Mental Health and Illness

Mary Puckett, PhD, PA-C

1. An 83-year-old woman is brought to the office by her daughter, who says that she was well until earlier today, but has increasingly been "talking out of her head" over the past few hours. The patient's only medical history is hypertension, for which she takes lisinopril. The daughter counted her mother's pills and verified that the patient has neither under- nor overdosed. Vital signs, including oxygen saturation, and the physical examination are unremarkable. The neurologic exam is negative, with the exception that the patient often switches topics in her speech and is not oriented to the situation. Which of the following would be the best first test to order in terms of yield and cost-effectiveness?

   A. Urinalysis with culture
   B. CT of the head
   C. Chest x-ray
   D. Thyroid function test

2. A 51-year-old man with hypertension, dyslipidemia, depression, and history of tobacco use presents complaining of restlessness. He appears agitated and anxious. On review of his history, you note that his wife died 6 months ago and since that time he has required the addition of amlodipine to the hydrochlorothiazide for control of his hypertension. You also note that he has increased his tobacco use from half a pack to a pack and a half daily and has begun fluoxetine for depression. His only other medications are simvastatin and baby aspirin. Which of the following is the most likely cause of his agitation?

   A. amlodipine
   B. Tobacco
   C. fluoxetine
   D. simvastatin

3. In a patient on long-term lithium maintenance, which of the following tests should be monitored intermittently in addition to his lithium level?

   A. Ultrasound of the gallbladder
   B. Chest x-ray
   C. Thyroid stimulating hormone
   D. Serum lipids

4. In rapid-cycling bipolar disorder, the patient may go from manic to depressed within which of the following periods of time?

   A. 1 day
   B. 1 week
   C. 1 month
   D. 3 months

5. Which of the following is required for a diagnosis of attention-deficit hyperactivity disorder (ADHD)?

   A. The problem must be present in more than one setting (e.g., both home and school).
   B. The problem must have its onset prior to adulthood (age 18).
   C. The patient must not have coexisting depression.
   D. The patient must be observed for at least 6 months for the diagnosis to be made.

6. In a patient taking valproic acid for mood stabilization, it is most important to monitor which of the following, especially in the first 6 months?

   A. Parathyroid hormone (PTH) level
   B. Liver function
   C. Weight gain
   D. Amylase and lipase

7. Patient adherence to a medication regimen is most likely to be affected by which of the following?

   A. The patient's personality characteristics
   B. The patient's socioeconomic status
   C. The patient's relationship with the practitioner
   D. Dosing schedule or frequency

8. A significant symptom of early dementia is a decrease in executive functioning. In this context, *executive functioning* refers to which of the following abilities?

   A. Ability to direct the activities of others
   B. Ability to plan or organize one's own activities
   C. Ability to recall recent events
   D. Ability to recall remote events

9. Which of the following medications/drugs is most likely to cause a period of amnesia in some users?

   A. Alcohol
   B. Tobacco
   C. Venlafaxine
   D. Amitriptyline

10. Which if the following patients would be considered at greatest risk for *successful* suicide?

   A. A 30-year-old man whose wife recently left him
   B. A 70-year-old widower
   C. A 20-year-old woman recently diagnosed with HIV
   D. A 40-year-old woman who recently lost her job

11. Which of the following conditions *most* elevates a woman's risk of being the victim of domestic violence?

   A. Being unemployed
   B. Having more than four children
   C. Alcoholism
   D. A BMI >30

12. A 70-year-old man with osteoarthritis but no other medical diagnoses admits to hearing the voice of his wife, who died 3 weeks ago, when he is alone at night. He does not seem disturbed by this. Which of the following is the most appropriate course of action at this point?

   A. Order an MRI of the head.

   B. Order CT of the head, with and without contrast.

   C. Assume this is a normal part of bereavement if no additional symptoms occur.

   D. Prescribe a low dose of an antidepressant to see if these symptoms resolve.

13. A 47-year-old man is brought to the emergency department by his wife, who says, "I thought he just had a bad cold, but I'm afraid it's that bird flu." He has had a sore throat, cough, and congestion for a week and has been taking acetaminophen and an over-the-counter cough suppressant/expectorant for the past 2 days. This morning, he awoke with a fever (102°F), sweating, "the shakes," and "talking out of his head." When this didn't improve in an hour with additional acetaminophen and cough medicine, his wife brought him to the emergency department. He has a history of hypertension, obesity, and depression. His prescription medications include hydrochlorothiazide, lisinopril, and fluoxetine. Assuming other causes have been ruled out, what medication interaction would you suspect as the cause of his symptoms?

   A. Acetaminophen and dextromethorphan

   B. Acetaminophen and lisinopril

   C. Lisinopril and dextromethorphan

   D. Fluoxetine and dextromethorphan

14. If a patient's chart indicates that she is "oriented × 3," this means that she can correctly identify which three aspects of her situation?

   A. Person, place, and time

   B. Person, place, and age

   C. Person, time, and recent events (today only)

   D. Place, time, and age

15. A 33-year-old man complains that he "can't sleep." Further questioning reveals that his problem is not an inability to fall asleep, but rather a recent history of waking 2 hours before his usual time for arising and then lying in bed worrying. He then starts the day exhausted. However, he usually feels somewhat better as the day goes on, falling asleep without difficulty at bedtime. He asks for "that pill that keeps you asleep all night" that he has seen advertised. Before considering his request for a prescription, the clinician should first evaluate for symptoms of which of the following?

   A. Multiple sclerosis

   B. Depression

   C. Traumatic brain injury

   D. Mania

16. When a patient expresses a wish to quit smoking tobacco, the best evidence-based advice would be to do which of the following?

   A. Go "cold turkey"

   B. Consider a behavioral intervention for smoking cessation

   C. Consider medication to help with smoking cessation

   D. Consider a behavioral intervention plus medication

17. In the treatment of generalized anxiety disorder (GAD), _____ are most often used for acute management, but _____ may be a better choice for long-term treatment.

   A. Benzodiazepines, antidepressants

   B. Antidepressants, benzodiazepines

   C. Benzodiazepines, antipsychotics

   D. Beta blockers, antidepressants

18. Which of the following is typically *not* part of the diagnostic criteria for factitious disorder?

   A. The patient intentionally feigns signs or symptoms of a disease or injury.
   B. The factitious disease may be either physical or psychologic.
   C. The patient is motivated to assume the sick role.
   D. The patient gains something external for being sick (e.g., disability payments).

19. In a young patient with a major depressive disorder, the clinician should be alert for which of the following second diagnoses?

   A. Anxiety
   B. Bulimia
   C. Confusion
   D. Dissociative disorder

20. A 27-year-old male presents to a family practice clinic and, during his initial interview with the clinician, makes it clear that he is a well-known author of several books and is also an expert at golf, having turned down an offer to be the golf pro at the local country club. His only medical complaint is his prematurely receding hairline, for which he is sure medical science has a "cure." On subsequent office visits, he is arrogant and demanding with the office staff, complaining loudly if others are taken back for their appointments before him and telling the receptionist that he is a busy man who cannot afford to wait. On one occasion when he is asked to reschedule his appointment because his clinician is out with the flu, he complains that "she probably just wanted a day off." He displays no symptoms of anxiety or depression and continues to have no medical complaints except those related to his appearance. Which of the following psychiatric diagnoses would be most appropriate for this patient?

   A. Depersonalization disorder
   B. Dysthymia
   C. Passive-aggressive personality
   D. Narcissistic personality disorder

21. A 43-year-old woman complains of depression for the past 6 months. She has tried behavioral therapy with little benefit, though her therapist tells you the patient follows all instructions faithfully. On review of her medications, which of the following is the most likely cause of her depression?

   A. Sumatriptan taken as needed for migraines
   B. Lisinopril taken daily for hypertension
   C. St. John's wort, which she is taking to self-treat for depression
   D. Estrogen–progestin, which she takes for birth control

22. A 23-year-old man is brought by ambulance to the emergency department after having been a passenger in a motor vehicle accident. Although the presenting complaint is leg pain from a suspected fracture, the EMTs noted that the patient is agitated, paranoid, and not entirely rational. On physical examination, the patient is found to have scabbed lesions covering much of his arms, some of them infected. His teeth are in very poor repair with obviously poor oral hygiene. In addition to poor grooming and hygiene, the man is very thin and has an ammonia-like body odor. Although his altered mental status and recent motor vehicle accident warrant a head scan, you should also suspect which of the following?

   A. Methamphetamine abuse
   B. Marijuana use
   C. Generalized anxiety disorder
   D. Hysterical personality disorder

23. Fibromyalgia is currently classified as which of the following?

   A. A psychiatric disorder
   B. An orthopedic disorder
   C. A rheumatologic disorder
   D. A neurologic disorder

24. Which of the following is a negative symptom of psychosis?

   A. Hearing voices
   B. Thought broadcasting
   C. Clang associations
   D. Failure to attend to personal hygiene

25. Which of the following statements is true regarding delirium?

   A. There is no identifiable cause
   B. A likely cause usually can be identified.
   C. Antipsychotic medications rarely relieve the symptoms.
   D. These patients typically become violent.

26. Bulimia is typically associated with which of the following?

   A. Normal weight
   B. Morbid obesity
   C. Subnormal weight
   D. Dangerously subnormal weight

27. A patient who abruptly discontinues an antidepressant medication taken for several months may experience an antidepressant discontinuation syndrome, consisting of which of the following?

   A. Severe reactive depression
   B. Severe anxiety
   C. Hypersomnia, sinus congestion, and rash
   D. Nausea, insomnia, and headache

28. A 24-year-old female patient admits on questioning that her multiple bruises, which are in various stages of healing, were inflicted by her husband. She tells you that he has struck her multiple times during their 2-year marriage. However, she politely declines information about available resources, stating that her husband recently apologized and told her he is "trying to do better" and she wants to give him a chance to "reform on his own." Which of the following best describes this situation?

   A. People do change, and the patient and husband will do best working out their problems on their own.
   B. A cycle of apology and reform, followed by recurrent violence, is common in abusive relationships.
   C. The patient certainly can decline a referral, but the laws in every state require you to report spousal abuse.
   D. The patient needs to obtain a weapon to protect herself.

29. An adult patient with Down syndrome should be screened at regular office visits for several disorders that are more common in that population, including which of the following?

   A. Anorexia nervosa
   B. Rubella
   C. Cardiac valve dysfunction
   D. Rosacea

30. When dealing with a demanding patient who does not follow through with treatment recommendations, which of the following phrases could the clinician best use to improve communication?

    A. "You don't seem to have been able to do what I recommended."
    B. "What I understand you to say is that _____. Is that what you mean?"
    C. "To be honest, you make me feel inadequate."
    D. "Perhaps you should see a specialist about this."

31. Which of the following is not a common symptom of posttraumatic stress disorder (PTSD)?

    A. Hyperarousal
    B. Intrusive thoughts
    C. Alcohol abuse
    D. Self-mutilation

32. A 27-year-old woman complains of dyspepsia, occasional nausea, and frequent headaches for the past 5 years. Her symptoms have been worsening over the past 6 months. A gastrointestinal workup did not show significant findings, and thyroid function and other lab results are within normal limits. She has labile blood pressure, with readings in the office varying from the normal range to 162/88 mmHg when she is "upset." Tachycardia is observed concurrently with increased blood pressure. She consistently denies unusual stresses in her life, although she admits to feeling "nervous" a good bit of the time. Having ruled out the usual medical causes, which of the following is the most likely diagnosis?

    A. Obsessive-compulsive disorder
    B. Phobic disorder
    C. Panic disorder
    D. Generalized anxiety disorder

33. A 37-year-old woman presents as a new patient, explaining that she has seen many physicians without relief from her chronic back pain, which limits her daily activities. As part of your initial assessment, it is most important to evaluate which of the following?

    A. To assess what extent the pain is real
    B. Determine whether the patient receives disability payments related to the pain
    C. Ask whether the patient is married or single
    D. How many topical analgesic creams the patient uses

34. Most erectile dysfunction is due to which of the following?

    A. Psychologic factors
    B. Physiologic factors
    C. Social factors
    D. Cultural factors

35. A 23-year-old single man complains that he has trouble getting along with others at work. On further questioning, he is found to be introverted and withdrawn. He avoids contact with others as much as possible and does well enough at work so long as his only task is to write computer programs. However, he is failing in his new assignment to work with a team to develop a larger project. This seems to be due to his inability to make eye contact or to speak more than a few words at a time because he is "shy." He has never had close friends and does not date. He does enjoy his hobbies, which include stamp collecting, and he does not seem depressed. He does not have a thought disorder. This clinical picture is most representative of which of the following?

    A. Schizophrenia
    B. Bipolar disorder
    C. Antisocial personality
    D. Schizoid personality

36. A 32-year-old woman is admitted to the hospital because of a 3-month history of epigastric pain, nausea, and vomiting, with a weight loss of about 40 pounds. She states that she has no history of medical problems, with the exception of a hospitalization about 10 years ago for depression. She is 5'4" tall and states that she weighed 180 pounds about 3 years ago when she decided to lose weight. She successfully lost about 55 pounds with prudent diet and exercise and had maintained a weight of 125 pounds until 3 months ago, when she developed nausea and vomiting that have resulted in further weight loss to her current weight of 85 pounds. She denies depression, but is very concerned about the weight loss and wants to know what is wrong. She feels she is too thin and is worried about developing osteoporosis, for which being thin places her at increased risk. After the initial history and physical by the hospitalist, a consult should *first* be obtained from which of the following?

A. Psychiatry for possible anorexia
B. Psychiatry for possible bulimia
C. Gastroenterology
D. Oncology

37. A 21-year-old male college student is brought to the emergency department from a nearby university because he has developed a number of odd behaviors over the past 2 weeks. The nurse from student health who has brought him in states that he has quit attending classes, quit bathing, and stays in his room, refusing to come out. His roommate is afraid of him because he "talks out of his head," complaining that he is being sent threatening messages through the local radio station. After a thorough physical evaluation reveals no evidence of disease, which of the following psychiatric diagnoses should be considered?

A. Schizophrenia
B. Generalized anxiety disorder
C. Obsessive-compulsive personality disorder
D. Antisocial personality disorder

38. In which of the following situations is a 57-year-old male considered to have a problem with alcohol abuse?

A. He has more than 10 drinks per week.
B. He consumes "straight" alcohol (e.g., vodka with no mixer).
C. He has recently been arrested for driving under the influence of alcohol.
D. He has one drink per day, but it is before 3:00 P.M.

39. Which of the following habits is most likely to contribute to a diagnosis of depression in a 43-year-old man whose only prior medical diagnosis is a wrist fracture 6 months ago?

A. Consumption of about twice the recommended level of table salt in foods
B. Consumption of 8 to 10 servings of high-sugar foods daily
C. Failure to consume more than one to two servings of fruits and vegetables daily
D. Consumption of about six alcoholic drinks most days

40. In evaluating the effectiveness of antidepressant medication in a particular patient, it is important to consider the adequacy of which of the following?

A. Dose for patient body weight and rest periods of about 3 days a month
B. Dose and duration of treatment and adequate adherence to treatment
C. Rest periods during which medication is not taken
D. Vitamin intake to support recovery from depression

41. Why are monoamine oxidase inhibitors (MAOIs) usually the last choice among antidepressant medications?

A. They have potentially dangerous interactions with common foods.
B. They are very expensive.
C. They are difficult to obtain in the United States.
D. They are FDA approved for rheumatoid arthritis, but not for depression.

42. A 54-year-old man with chronic schizophrenia, seizure disorder, and cardiovascular disease is observed to smack his lips often and to make chewing motions much of the time, although there is nothing in his mouth. These symptoms are most likely a side effect of long-term use of which of the following?

    A. Paroxetine (a selective serotonin reuptake inhibitor)
    B. Lorazepam (a benzodiazepine)
    C. Phenytoin (an anticonvulsant)
    D. Risperdal (an atypical antipsychotic)

43. A 23-year-old man is brought to the emergency department by his wife because he has been sleeping only about 2 to 3 hours a night for the past 3 weeks. He has gradually become more active and sleeping less. In addition to his usual job as a financial advisor, he now spends most of his off-hours on his computer, trading stocks in markets around the world and day-trading in the U.S. market. He has made and lost large sums of money in the past 3 weeks, and has, in addition, purchased a vacation home in the Bahamas and made plans to fly there on weekends with his wife. When interviewed, he is very pleasant and upbeat, but declines to acknowledge the potentially harmful aspects of his behavior. His only medical history is of "pretty serious" depression about a year ago from which he has gradually recovered without treatment. Physical examination, mental status examination, routine laboratory tests, and drug screens are noncontributory. Which of the following should be first in the differential diagnosis?

    A. Psychosis
    B. Major depression
    C. Mania
    D. Posttraumatic stress disorder

44. A 35-year-old woman presents with the complaint that she has "felt bad" since switching to an "all natural, organic" diet a week ago. She complains of nausea, headache, and "not feeling right." She has no history of medical problems, but decided to "shape up" after reading a book on health. Dietary history reveals that she was consuming a typical Western diet prior to the change, including cereal with milk, coffee, and juice for breakfast; a sandwich and soft drink for lunch; and a restaurant meal with iced tea for dinner. Her snacks consisted of crackers and other typical snack foods, often with a cola drink. Since "reforming," she has whole grain cereal with soy milk for breakfast along with some fruit, a salad with whole grain crackers for lunch, and a meal of whole grains and vegetables for dinner. Her snacks consist of a fruit-and-nut mix from her local health food store. Her only liquids are soy milk and spring water. She takes no supplements, nor did she prior to her "reform." Which of the following is the likely source of her symptoms of nausea, headache, and general malaise?

    A. Allergy to soy
    B. Caffeine withdrawal
    C. Withdrawal from artificial colors and flavors in the typical Western diet
    D. Psychologic reaction to her radical change in diet

45. A 41-year-old male is sent to you for a disability evaluation. He states that the stress of his job has "gotten to him" and he "needs to be on disability." He frankly explains that he has plans to open a restaurant, which a disability income would allow him to do. He complains of headache and backache, but has no findings to support this after a thorough workup. In addition, he complains of pain on palpation directly over the spinous processes at every level of his spine, but denies pain on palpation of the paraspinous muscles. Which of the following is the most likely diagnosis?

    A. Fibromyalgia
    B. Somatoform disorder
    C. Factitious disorder
    D. Malingering

46. A low dose of a tricyclic antidepressant (TCA), such as amitriptyline, is commonly used to help patients sleep. Especially in geriatric patients, which type of side effect should be monitored in this off-label use of TCAs?

   A. Anticholinergic effects
   B. Hypertension
   C. Increased risk for gout
   D. Tardive dyskinesia

47. Which of the following classes of psychotropic medication is most often appropriate and effective as part of therapy for chronic pain?

   A. Antidepressants
   B. Benzodiazepines
   C. Antipsychotics
   D. Atypical antipsychotics

48. A patient with depression asks about psychotherapy. Based on the literature, you can tell him that there are two types of psychotherapy with demonstrated effectiveness in managing depression. Which of the following are these two types?

   A. Psychoanalysis and behavior therapy
   B. Behavior therapy and Gestalt therapy
   C. Cognitive behavior therapy and psychoanalysis
   D. Cognitive behavior therapy and interpersonal therapy

ANSWERS

1. **The correct answer is A.** Urinary tract infection is a relatively common cause of delirium in older individuals who may not have dysuria, fever, or other symptoms of infection. A head CT would be reasonable as an emergency evaluation in a person with hypertension, but this patient has no neurologic signs other than delirium, thus this would not be a cost-effective or high-yield first test. Chest x-ray is not indicated, because the patient has no respiratory signs or symptoms. Thyroid dysfunction typically causes symptoms of anxiety or depression rather than delirium.

2. **The correct answer is C.** Akathisia is a common side effect not only of antipsychotic medications, but also of selective serotonin reuptake inhibitors (SSRIs), including fluoxetine. Tobacco more often subjectively calms rather than agitates patients, so the increased tobacco use may be a result of his agitation but is probably not the cause. Amlodipine can cause palpitations and lightheadedness due to hypotension and should be considered, but restlessness would not typically be a part of this reaction. Simvastatin may cause dizziness and fatigue, but not agitation. Baby aspirin is an unlikely cause of restlessness and anxiety.

3. **The correct answer is C.** Lithium is the most commonly used mood stabilizer, but many patients on chronic lithium maintenance eventually develop hypothyroidism. Lithium does not typically affect the gallbladder, lungs, or lipids.

4. **The correct answer is D.** Rapid-cycling bipolar disorder, as reported in the literature, may occur in bipolar I or II disorders. The patient may have cycles as frequently as four times a year (every 3 months). Patients with classic bipolar disorder (now called bipolar I disorder) go through a complete cycle between mania and depression over a period of approximately a year, although there is considerable individual variation. Patients with bipolar II disorder cycle over a similar period of time, but cycle between hypomania and depression. Patients with cyclothymic disorder cycle over a similar period of time, but between hypomania and dysthymia. Note that it is common for patients to speak of

individuals with unstable mood, who change from happy or hyperactive to sad or irritable as frequently as daily or weekly as "bipolar." However, such individuals do not qualify for a diagnosis of bipolar disorder on the basis of these short-term mood swings. Another psychiatric diagnosis may or may not be appropriate for such individuals.

5. **The correct answer is A.** For a diagnosis of attention-deficit hyperactivity disorder (ADHD), symptoms must have their onset before age 7 and must occur in more than one setting. It is fairly common for teachers or parents to complain that a child is "hyper," when in fact the problem is with the environment rather than the child. Children may appear hyperactive because of poor environmental structure, boredom, or inability to meet the demands of a situation for other reasons. Inadequate parenting and poor individual educational programming are common causes of inattentiveness or bothersome behavior in children. Children may be seen as troublesome in school, at home, or in the community. A careful and comprehensive evaluation of the child in more than one environment must be undertaken for diagnosis. It would be wise to involve a school psychologist or social worker, a social services worker, or a social worker or psychologist from the community before making a diagnosis. It is possible for an individual with ADHD to have coexisting depression or other psychiatric disorder, and depression in individuals with ADHD becomes more common as they reach adolescence. However, for the diagnosis of ADHD, the hyperactivity and/or inattentiveness must *not* be due to another condition, such as pervasive developmental disorder, medication side effects, or a psychosis.

6. **The correct answer is B.** Valproic acid is commonly used as a mood stabilizer, and levels should be monitored and the dose adjusted accordingly. It causes a number of common side effects, including sedation, tremor, and gastrointestinal symptoms. However, the most important thing to monitor in the first 6 months is liver function, because fatal hepatotoxicity is a potential side effect of valproic acid and is most common in the first 6 months of use. Drug levels should be monitored periodically as well, and patients should be warned about the symptoms of valproic acid toxicity, which include confusion, coma, and cardiac arrest. Because of the potentially troubling side effects, even at therapeutic levels patients should fully understand the risks and benefits before beginning valproic acid.

7. **The correct answer is D.** Adherence to medication regimens is affected by a number of factors, most of them related to the medication and the medical setting rather than to personality characteristics. A simpler medication schedule (e.g., one medication rather than two, one dose a day rather than two or three) and a positive relationship with clinic staff improve medication adherence. Although it is certainly true that patients must have their basic needs for food, shelter, and security met before they can concern themselves with less immediate problems (e.g., the long-term effects of diabetes or hypertension), many patients whose basic needs are met and who have adequate income to afford medication still fail to take medication as prescribed. It is advisable to prescribe as few medications as possible and to make dosing as simple as possible. In addition, having someone in the clinic take the time to clearly explain to the patient the reason for the medication and the likely risks and benefits builds a relationship with the patient, which improves the chance of adherence. Some side effects, such as frequent urination, do decrease adherence, but they may be better tolerated if they are expected and explained in advance. Commonsense strategies to help patients remember medication are helpful. These may include putting an evening medication beside the toothbrush, use of pillboxes that have a container for each day of the week, and noting the date on the calendar when a monthly or weekly medication is due. It is also important to help patients avoid running out of medication, and the pharmacy may place a notice in the bag with the last refill of a medication to assist with this. Patients may need to note on the calendar when they need to call the pharmacy for refills, and clinicians probably

should schedule follow-up appointments in such a way that prescriptions are renewed in a timely fashion.

8. **The correct answer is B.** The diagnosis of dementia requires a relatively gradual onset of memory deficit coupled with at least one other cognitive deficit, such as disorientation to time, place, person, or situation; difficulty with language, motor tasks, or visual recognition of common objects; impaired attention; or impaired executive functioning. Executive functioning refers to the ability to consider appropriate alternatives and organize them so as to plan and carry out relatively complex activities effectively. It is important to know the patient's baseline ability in executive functioning, because some individuals may have lacked good executive functioning ability prior to the onset of dementia. In addition, it is important to rule out delirium before arriving at a diagnosis of dementia.

9. **The correct answer is A.** Alcohol abuse is one of the most common causes of amnesia. However, a patient experiencing amnesia often will fail to report it unless asked directly about "losing time" or "forgetting" what happened in the hours following alcohol use. The alcoholic, consistent with the tendency to minimize symptoms of this disorder, often accepts such blackouts as "normal." Although its use generally leads to addiction, tobacco use is not known to cause blackouts. Venlafaxine may cause increases in blood pressure and heart rate, dizziness, and drowsiness, but it does not cause amnesia. Amitriptyline is sometimes used to promote sleep, especially in geriatric patients, but it does not cause amnesia.

10. **The correct answer is B.** The following factors increase the risk of suicide: a first-degree relative who committed suicide, age older than 45 in men and 55 in women, unmarried status, higher socioeconomic class, and a feeling of hopelessness. Men are more often successful in their suicide attempts than women. Although any of the persons described in the answers may be suicidal, the 70-year-old man is in the highest-risk age range and is unmarried as well as male. Other risk factors for suicide include being a gay or lesbian youth, recent initiation of antidepressant medication, certain professions (including physician), and easy access to a means of suicide. A common method for the assessment of suicide risk with an individual patient is to ask about suicidal thought, access to means, and suicidal intent. For example, "Have you thought about suicide?" "Do you have a plan?" "Would you follow through with that plan?" Many, if not most, individuals have thought about suicide, but most lack a well-defined plan, and even fewer say they would carry out the plan.

11. **The correct answer is C.** Many victims of domestic violence, as well as many perpetrators, abuse alcohol. Unemployment and multiple children certainly may increase the stress in a home, and stress may increase the risk of many maladaptive behaviors, but alcoholism is more commonly associated with being the victim of abuse than is stress. In addition, stress from a variety of causes is ubiquitous. Socioeconomic status and increased BMI may be associated with stereotypes of domestic violence, but they are not reliable predictors.

12. **The correct answer is C.** In an otherwise healthy individual, hearing or even seeing a lost love one is considered a normal part of bereavement. An MRI of the head is useful to rule out metastatic disease, but this patient has no evidence of either cancer or neurologic dysfunction. Likewise, a CT of the head is useful for assessing potential intracranial bleed, but this patient has no other symptoms. The clinician should be alert for the possible development of depression, but that diagnosis would require additional symptoms, and medication should not be prescribed without a diagnosis. Sadness and other symptoms that may be similar to depression are considered a normal part of bereavement. Evaluation for depression should be considered if the symptoms last longer than 2 months and interfere with the patient's mood or functioning.

13. **The correct answer is D.** The patient has symptoms consistent with several diagnoses, but after ruling out other causes (such as meningitis) the drug reaction to consider would be serotonin syndrome caused by the interaction of his selective serotonin reuptake inhibitor (SSRI; fluoxetine) with over-the-counter dextromethorphan. Patients often assume that any over-the-counter medication is "safe" and can be taken in virtually unlimited amounts, but even at prescribed levels there is a potential for serotonin syndrome with any SSRI and dextromethorphan. Dextromethorphan is a common over-the-counter cough suppressant included in many cold medications. With many patients now taking SSRIs, this interaction has become more common. Other medications that may be involved in serotonin syndrome include tricyclic antidepressants (seldom used for depression but still used for sleep), monoamine oxidase inhibitors (MAOIs; rarely used for depression because of the many interactions with other drugs and with foods), other antidepressants (bupropion, trazodone, nefazodone, venlafaxine), pain medications (codeine, fentanyl, meperidine, tramadol), and even some antibiotics/antivirals (linezolid, ritonavir). In addition, St. John's wort, a common herbal remedy for depression, is a potential cause.

14. **The correct answer is A.** A patient is oriented if she can identify who she is, where she is, and the date with the approximate time of day. In addition, a fully oriented patient should be able to give an explanation of the situation in which she finds herself, for example, "I'm at my doctor's office because my daughter thinks I'm slipping mentally." However, it is relatively uncommon to see a notation that a patient is "oriented × 4." The Mini-Mental State Exam, a commonly used measure of cognitive functioning, asks patients where they are and requires the name of the building, floor, city, state, and country for place and year, season, month, date, and day of the week for time. It does not ask the person's name, but this may be a worthwhile question for patients who have gone by different names; a regressed woman may give her maiden name, for example. The Mini-Mental State Exam does not attempt to assess orientation to situation.

15. **The correct answer is B.** Sleep problems can be broadly sorted into two types, trouble with onset and trouble with sleep maintenance. Problems with sleep onset may respond to sleep-hygiene interventions, such as avoiding caffeine and other stimulants (e.g., prescribed steroids) late in the day, avoiding activities such as television watching while in bed, and so on. Problems with maintenance of sleep, particularly with waking early and feeling worried or depressed, may be a sign of psychiatric disorder. In particular, depression may be characterized by this pattern of waking early and depressed but then feeling better as the day goes on. Patients with sleep problems without apparent cause should be questioned further in an attempt to determine whether poor habits or an underlying disorder (depression, chronic pain) may cause the problem. The patient is not reporting symptoms of mania, although some patients with depression obviously have a history of mania and may have bipolar disorder rather than unipolar depression. This patient would be assessed first for depression because that is the presentation. Traumatic brain injury may disrupt sleep patterns, but it would be a less common presentation than depression. Multiple sclerosis is well known for presenting with a variety of symptoms, but again, depression would be a more common explanation for this presentation.

16. **The correct answer is D.** Although there are a number of anecdotal reports by patients that "going cold turkey"—or stopping tobacco use all at once without external support—is effective, evidence supports the use of medication and behavioral intervention, especially a combination of these, as being more effective. Nicotine-replacement products (gum, patches, nasal sprays, inhaler, and lozenges) are effective. They are available over the counter, but patients are more likely to benefit if they are advised about how to use these products appropriately. For example, nicotine gum should be used on a regular schedule to prevent withdrawal symptoms, rather than waiting for a severe craving and then trying to use the gum rather than a cigarette for relief. Several prescription drugs

(e.g., bupropion, varenicline, buspirone) are indicated to help with smoking cessation. These may be associated with less weight gain, and certainly have less potential for a substitute addiction, in comparison with nicotine-replacement products. A nicotine vaccine is in development. Behavioral interventions, typically available as psychoeducational group programs, have been shown to increase an individual's chance of smoking cessation. The best advice would be to use a medication along with a smoking cessation program of some type. These may be available through local hospitals, health clubs, or the local lung or heart association.

17. **The correct answer is A.** Benzodiazepines (e.g., alprazolam, diazepam) provide quick symptom relief in anxiety disorders and can be prescribed on an as-needed basis. The primary risk is dependence. Antidepressants may afford long-term relief, but they can take several weeks for maximum benefit and it may be necessary to try more than one medication to find the one that is effective for a particular patient. Antipsychotics occasionally are used off-label for treatment of anxiety, but the side-effect profile makes them a poor choice. Beta blockers are effective for some patients in managing the physiologic symptoms of anxiety, but this use is off-label and the onset of action is not as rapid as with benzodiazepines.

18. **The correct answer is D.** Factitious disorder is diagnosed when the patient deliberately feigns symptoms of a physical or psychological illness or injury. Examples include self-injection with fecal material to induce fever; deliberate self-injury, such as inserting a sharp object to cause rectal bleeding; or describing suicidal feelings that the patient does not have. The motivation is to assume the patient role. The behavior is *not* classified as factitious disorder if there are obvious external incentives, such as disability payments or avoidance of a final exam. The goal of gaining hospital admission or attention from professionals is considered part of the motivation to play the patient role. Despite the fact that the patient may receive the "privilege" of staying in the hospital, this is not classified as an external incentive, because it is part of the patient role. Some cases can be difficult to classify. For example, a patient who has a bona fide psychiatric disorder may routinely decompensate toward the end of each month when his disability check runs out, thus receiving "free" food and shelter at the hospital until it is time to pick up his next check at the post office.

19. **The correct answer is A.** Depression and anxiety commonly coexist, and a patient with either disorder probably should be screened for the other. Fortunately, many antidepressant medications also have anxiolytic effects, including the commonly used selective serotonin reuptake inhibitors (SSRIs). Tricyclic antidepressants (TCAs) also have anxiolytic as well as antidepressant effects, but are less commonly used because of their potential side effects. Bulimia patients often have coexisting depression, but bulimia is less common than anxiety as a comorbidity with depression. Confusion and dissociative disorder were just put there to trick the unwary. Symptoms of depression include vague aches and pains, sleep disturbance, and fatigue, as well as sadness, lack of interest or enjoyment in usual activities, trouble thinking or making decisions (but not frank confusion), inappropriate guilt, and hopelessness. Symptoms of generalized anxiety disorder include excessive worry over many different things combined with an inability to control worrying; physical restlessness and irritability; trouble relaxing and "turning off" anxious thoughts; unrealistic fear that something terrible is about to happen; and simply feeling anxious much of the time.

20. **The correct answer is D.** Narcissistic personality disorder is fairly common, occurring perhaps in 1% in the general population, and it may occur disproportionately in males. It is characterized by self-centered arrogance and a feeling of entitlement (usually unwarranted), as well as a lack of concern for the feelings or needs of others. Although the person with narcissistic personality disorder has underlying low self-esteem, this might

not be apparent in primary care encounters. Depersonalization disorder is characterized by the patient feeling separate from himself in either mind or body, or both, as if viewing himself from the outside. Dysthymia is a depressive disorder characterized by relatively long-term depressed mood not severe enough to qualify as major depression. Passive-aggressive is a description of a behavior rather than a personality disorder diagnosis. It would not be an appropriate description of this directly aggressive patient. A passive-aggressive individual attacks others indirectly and sometimes in subtle ways, for example, by being consistently late for appointments. Such an individual is less likely to make direct demands or complaints.

21. **The correct answer is D.** The following medications can cause depression: progesterone–estrogen birth control devices; benzodiazepines and some other antianxiety drugs; some anti–Parkinson drugs, such as levodopa or amantadine; and some of the antihypertensives, with beta blockers most often being implicated. The triptans, including sumatriptan, can cause cardiovascular side effects. Lisinopril is an ACE inhibitor; the most common side effects of this class of drugs are hypotension and headache. St. John's wort is an herbal remedy with demonstrated effectiveness for mild to moderate depression if dosed correctly. Side effects include possible sun sensitivity and interaction with prescribed medications, including antidepressants and oral contraceptives. However, the drug itself is not a likely cause of depression. Any patient taking an estrogen–progestin preparation, whether orally or through another route, may have side effects including depression or hypertension. Therefore, this patient's birth control method should be reviewed because of both her depression and her hypertension.

22. **The correct answer is A.** The signs and symptoms best fit methamphetamine abuse. Patients with hysterical personality disorder may have flamboyant presentation and exaggerated emotional reactions, but typically are not paranoid or neglectful of self-care. A personality disorder would not cause an ammonia-like body odor, which is common in methamphetamine abusers. The scabbed lesions on the arms are not likely to be related to hysterical personality, but rather to methamphetamine abuse. Generalized anxiety disorder (GAD) typically presents as a patient with anxious appearance who may readily admit to anxiety, worry, and related concerns. However, none of the other symptoms is typical of GAD. Marijuana abusers may become paranoid, but the use of marijuana alone does not typically lead to severe self-neglect, agitation, or ammonia-like body odor. Patients abusing methamphetamines may be difficult to distinguish from patients with paranoid schizophrenia because of their paranoid behavior and agitation. Both groups often neglect self-care, and some schizophrenics also engage in self-abusive behaviors. However, methamphetamine abusers often scratch their arms, hands, or faces because of a feeling that bugs are under the skin. They have poor personal hygiene and self-care because of their continual search for and use of the drug. Because of their preoccupation with the drug, they may lose weight despite a craving for sweets. The frequent use of sugary foods and poor dental hygiene lead to tooth decay. An ammonia-like body odor is common in methamphetamine abusers but not in marijuana abusers or patients with generalized anxiety disorder (GAD), personality disorder, or schizophrenia.

23. **The correct answer is C.** Fibromyalgia is classified as a rheumatologic disorder, although depression is a common comorbidity. Antidepressant medication may be helpful for some patients in alleviating symptoms of both depression and pain. The pain typically is in soft tissue rather than bones or joints, thus an orthopedic consultation is not typically helpful. Sleep disturbance is common, and an antidepressant medication may be chosen with this in mind. Although the treatment of fibromyalgia is challenging, and may be frustrating for both the clinician and the patient, it is important to accept the patient's diagnosis as valid and avoid viewing it as a factitious or psychosomatic disorder. It is important to explain to the patient that, although psychological symptoms such as depression are often a part of the disorder, the problem is not "all in the patient's head."

24. The correct answer is D. Positive symptoms of psychosis are abnormal behaviors added to the repertoire of the patient's usual behaviors during psychotic episodes. These vary considerably and may include hearing voices. Visual hallucinations are much less common and should prompt a search for organic causes of the symptom. Thought broadcasting is the belief that others can read one's thoughts or the belief that things heard on the radio or television are directed specifically to the patient. Clang associations are the compulsive and nonsensical rhyming of words; for example, if a patient is told to "get in the car" she may respond with "car, far, bar, har-har." Of course, many individuals may occasionally think these types of things, but most control the impulse to say them aloud. Negative symptoms represent a decrease in normal, desirable behaviors due to psychosis. For example, the patient may quit attending to personal hygiene, fail to buy groceries or prepare meals, or fail to attend work or school. Typical antipsychotic medications are effective in the treatment of positive symptoms of psychosis, regardless of the cause, but are far less effective in the treatment of negative symptoms. Some of the newer antipsychotics (atypical antipsychotics) are potentially effective in treating negative symptoms as well.

25. The correct answer is B. Delirium is differentiated from dementia by its relatively abrupt onset, variable rather than progressively downward course, and particularly by the presence of a likely cause. The delirium may have more than one cause, and a patient with dementia may qualify for an additional diagnosis of delirium at times. Common causes of delirium include illegal drug use, withdrawal from alcohol or drugs, and side effects of appropriately used medications in susceptible individuals. Disease-related causes, such as hyponatremia or urinary tract infection, especially in elderly individuals, also are common. Antipsychotic medications, such as haloperidol may be useful, but the use would be off-label. The delirious patient may become violent, but this is not required for diagnosis.

26. The correct answer is A. Bulimia is a syndrome of habitual binge eating often followed by purging and is associated with maintenance of relatively normal body weight. Patients usually binge on easy-to-eat, high-calorie foods, such as ice cream. They may purge by vomiting, taking laxatives, or both. Binge eating is required for a diagnosis of bulimia. Some patients do not purge, and thus may become obese, but most bulimics maintain a relatively normal weight. If weight is not maintained at a level of at least 85% of ideal body weight, anorexia rather than bulimia is diagnosed. Problems associated with purging include metabolic disorder or electrolyte imbalance due to purging, laxative dependence, dehydration, and erosion of tooth enamel.

27. The correct answer is D. About 20% of patients who have taken an antidepressant (of any type) for more than about 6 weeks will experience at least some symptoms of discontinuation syndrome if they quit the medication abruptly. Symptoms usually are mild but may include flulike symptoms, trouble sleeping, hyperarousal, dizziness, headache, and gastrointestinal upset. The patient may feel anxious or depressed, but this typically is not severe.

28. The correct answer is B. In many domestic violence situations, the cycle of violence, contrition, and repeated violence is typical. The best predictor of future behavior is a look at past behavior, and abusive domestic partners usually require outside assistance to change. Although reporting of child abuse and elder abuse is mandatory, reporting of intimate partner violence is not, and state agencies are not empowered to intervene unless children are known to be at risk. Advising the patient to obtain a weapon would be unwise. Most communities now have resources available for victims of domestic violence. However, many patients leave an abusive partner and then return home more than once before finally freeing themselves from the situation. Intimate partner violence is an important health concern, but one that is seldom easily solved.

29. **The correct answer is C.** Down syndrome, or trisomy 21, is the most common genetic cause of mental retardation, occurring in about 1 of 1,000 births. Most of these patients live to adulthood and require all the usual medical care given to other adults, in addition to attention to some concerns specific to Down syndrome. Patients with Down syndrome have a shorter life expectancy than average (mid-50s) and develop Alzheimer's disease earlier and at a higher rate than the general population. Cardiac valve dysfunction can develop at any time in an individual with Down syndrome, even without the presence of other cardiac disease. Mitral valve prolapse occurs in up to 57% of adults with Down syndrome, and up to 17% develop valvular regurgitation that requires endocarditis prophylaxis. Other medical problems occurring more commonly in adults with Down syndrome include hypo- or hyperthyroidism, depression, obstructive sleep apnea, cataracts, and testicular cancer.

30. **The correct answer is B.** Of the statements given as possible answers, only one is an "I" statement, which shows an effort to understand the patient by saying what the clinician heard and asking for feedback. This demonstrates an attempt to improve communication. The other answers are all "you" statements about the patient or blaming the patient for the problem. Answer A may well be a correct statement of fact, but it sounds as if the patient and clinician are battling (which may be the case). Answer C sounds superficially like an "I" statement, because it is an admission of the clinician's feelings, but it blames the patient for these feelings ("You make me feel . . ."). Answer D also may be a correct statement of fact, but when phrased this way it is likely to be seen as a rejection by a difficult patient. A potentially more helpful way to approach a difficult patient in need of referral might be, "What would you think of seeing a specialist about this?" This leaves the door open for the patient to express her feelings in the matter and either accept or reject the referral (which is, in fact, her right).

31. **The correct answer is D.** Posttraumatic stress disorder (PTSD) can occur after any traumatic event, even if it is not life-threatening. Symptoms can include avoidance of situations that remind the patient of the event, hyperarousal, sleep disorders, impulsivity, intrusive thoughts, trouble concentrating, anxiety, depression, and substance abuse in an attempt to self-medicate. The precipitating event may be recent or remote. Self-mutilation is not typically a part of PTSD. It would more likely be a symptom of psychosis or personality disorder. The differential diagnosis should include adjustment disorder, anxiety, depression, and personality disorders. Treatment includes psychotherapy, substance abuse therapy, when appropriate; anxiolytics; antidepressants; and sometimes medications such as beta blockers to decrease anxiety or antiseizure medications to help with impulsivity.

32. **The correct answer is D.** All the alternatives are classified as anxiety disorders, but only generalized anxiety disorder (GAD) best fits the symptoms described. Obsessive-compulsive disorder involves obsessions (such as constant worry about bird flu) and compulsions (such as washing the hands repeatedly after coming in from outdoors, where bird droppings might be encountered). In contrast, GAD lacks these specific concerns and behaviors and is characterized by a more free-floating anxiety. Phobic disorder involves irrational fear of a specific object or situation, such as fear of heights. Panic disorder is very similar to GAD, but involves discrete episodes of sudden-onset fear, anxiety, and panic, often without apparent precipitant. In addition, the episodes occur in a more circumscribed period of time than is GAD. GAD is the most common anxiety disorder in primary care, with a lifetime prevalence of about 5% in the population. Symptoms of GAD include excessive worry over many different things combined with an inability to control worrying; physical restlessness and irritability; trouble relaxing and "turning off" anxious thoughts; unrealistic fear that something terrible is about to happen; and simply feeling anxious much of the time. In addition, patients usually have physiologic symptoms of anxiety, which may include cardiac symptoms, such as

elevated blood pressure and tachycardia; gastrointestinal symptoms, such as abdominal pain or dyspepsia; and neurologic symptoms, such as feeling faint, tingling in the limbs, and headache. The most common associated medical cause of GAD is hyperthyroidism, which should always be ruled out before diagnosing GAD. Treatment for GAD may include anxiolytic medications or antidepressants with anxiolytic properties (selective serotonin reuptake inhibitors, tricyclic antidepressants, and venlafaxine). Gabapentin is sometimes used (off label) for GAD, as are beta blockers. Relaxation training and cognitive behavior therapy have been shown to be effective, but often patients who have obtained immediate relief from minor tranquillizers are reluctant to give them up in favor of self-management techniques. Patients with GAD may attempt to self-medicate with alcohol or illicit drugs, particularly if they have not been correctly diagnosed and adequately treated. GAD is often associated with several chronic medical conditions, including chronic obstructive pulmonary disease (COPD), Graves' disease, diabetes, and cardiovascular disease.

33. **The correct answer is B.** The presence of secondary gain, of which disability payment is one of the most obvious examples, can be a significant contributor to the maintenance of chronic pain as well as other chronic disease. It is futile to try to determine how "real" the pain is. There are no reliable objective measures of pain, particularly in humans. Pain is real to the individual patient, even if a similar degree of injury would be less painful to another patient, and even if the pain is clearly out of proportion to the demonstrated injury. Psychosocial support is an important part of treating any chronic illness, but married versus single is not, by itself, as important a part of maintaining pain behavior as are secondary gains such as disability. Any part of the support system, including a spouse, may or may not be a source of secondary gain. For example, a single individual with chronic pain may have moved back in with his parents and thus been relieved of considerable responsibility. Topical creams should, of course, be included in a thorough survey of the patient's medications, but are not the most important factor listed.

34. **The correct answer is A.** Most erectile dysfunction is due to physiologic factors, which can include medication side effects; chronic health problems, such as cardiovascular disease or diabetes; or spinal cord injury. Before medical intervention was available for erectile dysfunction, psychological therapies were more often used. Psychological causes still occur, but some of the latest research indicates that they are less common and are a rule-out diagnosis. As always, we advise the clinician to read current evidence-based studies, to discuss with the appropriate referent individuals, and to draw the most appropriate conclusions. Undoubtedly social and cultural factors affect sexual function for both males and females, but they are seldom the focus of diagnosis and treatment.

35. **The correct answer is D.** Schizoid personality may be present in as much as 7% of the general population. It can cause distress or occupational dysfunction in some persons. Such individuals are seen by others as "loners," because they do not desire social relationships. No real treatment is available for the disorder, and, in any case, such individuals seldom seek treatment. The relatively flat affect on presentation and lack of social relationships may lead the clinician to believe that the patient must be depressed, but the feelings of hopelessness and extreme sadness characteristic of depression are not present. Schizophrenia involves thought disorder, as well as bizarre behavior. The individual with schizoid personality does not have the odd thoughts and behavior typical of the individual with schizophrenia. Bipolar disorder involves both mania and depression, neither of which is present in this patient. Antisocial personality is characterized by exploitive relationships, self-centeredness, and impulsive behavior without adequate consideration of the consequences. There is little regard for the feelings or needs of others, but the individual himself does display a range of affect and usually seeks out relationships. Frequent illegal behavior often leads to criminal prosecution.

36. **The correct answer is C.** Gastroenterology should be the first workup for this history. Physical causes of a medical problem almost always should be ruled out before considering psychiatric causes, even in a patient with a psychiatric history. Anorexia is unlikely because of the age of onset and because the patient is aware that her weight loss is inappropriate and is concerned about it. Bulimia would not be diagnosed because the patient is less than 85% of her ideal body weight and, again, because she is aware that she is too thin. An oncology consultation would be a consideration for any such unexplained weight loss, but gastroenterology would come first.

37. **The correct answer is A.** The usual age of onset for schizophrenia is the 20s, and it typically presents earlier in men than in women. Although it is diagnosed more often in people of lower socioeconomic status, a first break is not uncommon in college students. Symptoms of schizophrenia vary considerably, but may include odd behavior and speech, poor attention to hygiene, and social withdrawal. Thought broadcasting, or feeling that public messages are instead directed specifically to the patient, is a fairly common symptom. Schizophrenia must be differentiated from drug intoxication, although the use of any of several illegal substances can trigger a psychotic episode that lasts long after the substance is no longer detectable in the body or can be the initial event in a lifelong pattern of psychosis. In fact, psychosis, not otherwise specified, probably might be the provisional diagnosis until a pattern has been established in this situation, but schizophrenia is the best choice among the options provided. Symptoms of generalized anxiety disorder (GAD) include excessive worry over many different things combined with an inability to control worrying; physical restlessness and irritability; trouble relaxing and "turning off" anxious thoughts; unrealistic fear that something terrible is about to happen; and simply feeling anxious much of the time. In addition, patients usually have physiologic symptoms of anxiety, which may include cardiac symptoms, such as elevated blood pressure and tachycardia; gastrointestinal symptoms, such as abdominal pain or dyspepsia; and neurologic symptoms, such as feeling faint, tingling in the limbs, and headache. Patients may avoid social situations, but they do not have the odd behaviors or thoughts characteristic of psychosis. Obsessive-compulsive personality disorder is characterized by unusual behavior, but it is not as bizarre as in psychosis, and there is no thought broadcasting. Self-care rarely deteriorates, and, as with all personality disorders, symptoms would be of long duration, almost always from childhood. Antisocial personality disorder is typical of individuals with legal problems involving exploitation of others; the symptoms are not similar to those described here.

38. **The correct answer is C.** As with most mental disorders, alcohol abuse must interfere with an individual's social or occupational functioning or cause other medical problems or personal distress to be diagnosed as a problem. For men under age 65, consumption of more than 14 drinks per week or more than 4 drinks per occasion is considered high risk, but is not diagnosed as abuse if it causes no social, medical, or occupational problems. The type of alcohol, whether beer, wine, liquor with mixer, or liquor "straight," is not a consideration. Time of day is a social/cultural factor, with some segments of Western society considering consumption of alcohol early in the day to be a problem. The only medical issue here would be consumption of alcohol early in the morning to self-treat symptoms of withdrawal, but the patient in answer D has only one drink a day, so this is not a problem even if that drink is prior to 3:00 P.M. The only option indicating a problem with functioning is the arrest for driving under the influence. This is objective evidence of potential harm to both the patient and others from his drinking.

39. **The correct answer is D.** Overconsumption of alcohol significantly complicates the treatment of depression, and alcohol abuse is often overlooked in medical care. Although the other dietary habits mentioned likely are detrimental to the patient's health, alcohol is a central nervous system depressant and is directly linked to depression in some individuals. An alcohol use (and other substance use) history should be taken in all patients with psychiatric complaints, including depression.

40. The correct answer is B. Antidepressants may take up to 8 weeks to have their full effect and may not begin to have clinically significant effects for 2 to 4 weeks. However, the side effects usually begin almost immediately. Because of this, adherence to treatment is an important consideration, as is duration of treatment. Dosage may need to be adjusted upward in stepwise fashion to reach a beneficial level while minimizing side effects. One of the most common reasons for failure of antidepressant medication is inadequate dosing, either due to failure to prescribe adequate dosage or due to non-compliance. Antidepressant medication is not dosed by body weight, and rest periods during which medication is not taken are not advised. There is no evidence for the use of vitamins to relieve depression.

41. The correct answer is A. Monoamine oxidase inhibitors (MAOIs) have potentially fatal interactions with many common foods containing tyramines including most cheeses, many alcoholic drinks, and cured meats, among others; these must be avoided entirely by individuals taking MAOIs. In addition, other common foods, including yogurt, and caffeine-containing food and drinks, including chocolate, must be limited. MAOIs also interact with sympathomimetic medications, including some over-the-counter medications, such as pseudoephedrine. They are, however, relatively inexpensive, widely available in the United States, and FDA approved for treatment of depression.

42. The correct answer is D. Tardive dyskinesia can occur with any use of antipsychotic medications, although usually it occurs only after years of use. Early symptoms may include wormlike movements of the tongue and jaw movements. With continued use, the patient often develops constant chewing motions and lip smacking or other involuntary repetitive movements of the facial muscles. The patient also may develop involuntary movements of the rest of the body. These symptoms often are nonreversible, even with discontinuation of the drug, and occur in up to 20% of patients with long-term use. Prevention, by using the lowest dose possible and withdrawing the drug gradually if symptoms occur, is preferable. The other drug classes mentioned do not cause tardive dyskinesia.

43. The correct answer is C. The behavior suggests that the patient is now manic, and the history of depression about a year ago from which he has "gradually recovered without treatment" suggests that he may have bipolar disorder. The hyperactivity and inappropriate financial activities are typical of mania, which is associated with disinhibited behavior. Psychosis involves thought disorder, often bizarre, which also may occur during mania. However, this patient does not demonstrate thought disorder. Major depression might fit the patient's prior episode of depression, but he was not evaluated at the time, and individuals who have major depression are diagnosed with bipolar disorder rather than major depression if they have even one manic episode. Posttraumatic stress disorder is an anxiety disorder that may include depression but does not typically include manic behavior.

44. The correct answer is B. Symptoms of caffeine withdrawal usually include headache and may include irritability, lethargy, or nausea. Caffeine is widely used and is present in many soft drinks (even non-cola drinks), coffee, tea, chocolate, and even some herbal teas. It is present in some prescription and over-the-counter medication, particularly analgesics. Consumption of as little as 250 mg a day (about three cups of coffee) can lead to withdrawal symptoms if it is stopped abruptly. Symptoms usually resolve without treatment.

45. The correct answer is D. Malingering is deliberately faking the symptoms of an illness for secondary gain, such as a disability income, a civil suit, or to avoid military service. In factitious disorder, the patient also deliberately feigns symptoms of a physical or psychological illness or injury and frequently also produces symptoms, for example, self-injecting fecal material to produce a fever. However, the only goal is to assume the sick role; creating an illness for secondary gain (such as a disability claim) rules out factitious disorder. In somatoform disorder, the illness is not deliberately produced, although signs and symptoms are present without an identifiable medical cause. The patient must have multiple complaints that are not related to identifiable medical illness to qualify for the diagnosis. Fibromyalgia often is frustrating for both the patient and the clinician, and there has been a tendency to classify it as one of the other answer choices because the symptoms may not seem to "make sense." However, fibromyalgia is classified as a rheumatologic disorder. Although the treatment of fibromyalgia is challenging, it is important to accept the patient's diagnosis as valid and avoid viewing it as a factitious or psychosomatic disorder. It is important to explain to the patient that, although psychological symptoms such as depression are often a part of the disorder, the problem is not "all in the patient's head."

46. **The correct answer is A.** Common side effects of tricyclic antidepressants (TCAs) include anticholinergic effects, such as dry mouth and urinary retention, which may occur even at low doses. Other possible side effects include cardiotoxicity, sedation (which in this use is desirable), weight gain (at higher doses), and impotence. TCAs do not generally cause the other side effects listed.

47. **The correct answer is A.** Antidepressants and antiepileptics are commonly used in the treatment of chronic pain syndromes. Both have analgesic effects in some individuals, and antidepressants may have analgesic effects even at doses lower than would be used for depression. In addition, depression is a frequent comorbidity with chronic pain, making antidepressant medications an excellent choice. The other medications are not indicated for chronic pain. Although patients with chronic pain do sometimes have comorbid anxiety, chronic use of benzodiazepines has been shown to diminish cognitive functioning and there is a risk of addiction with benzodiazepines. If anxiety is a problem, an antidepressant with anxiolytic properties would be a better choice.

48. **The correct answer is D.** Cognitive behavior therapy and interpersonal therapy have been shown to help patients with depression. Exercise also has been shown to improve depression. Most patients benefit maximally from a combination of medication and therapy. Any therapy undertaken should be linked to clear goals and should be time limited.

REFERENCES

Colyar, M. R. (2006). "Methamphetamine abuse in the primary care patient." *Clinician Reviews*. 16: (3). Available at http://www.clinicianreviews.com/index.asp?page=8_215.xml. Accessed August 31, 2008.

Compton, P. K. (2006). "Factitious disorder." *Advance for Physician Assistants*, 14(10): 45. Available at http://physician-assistant.advanceweb.com/Editorial/Search/AViewer.aspx?AN=PA_06oct1_pap45.html&AD=10-01-2006. Accessed August 31, 2008.

Frances, C., Bent, S., and Saint, S. (2000). *Saint-Frances guide to outpatient medicine*. Lippincott Williams & Wilkins, Philadelphia, PA.

Geldmacher, D. S., and Whitehouse, P. J. (1996). "Evaluation of dementia." *New England Journal of Medicine*, 335(5): 330–336.

Haas, L. J., Leiser, J. P., Maginn, M. K., and Sanyer, O. N. (2005). "Management of the difficult patient." *American Family Physician*, 72(10): 2063–2068.

Kenreigh, C. A., and Wagner, L. T. (2005). "Medication adherence: A literature review." *Medscape Pharmacists*, 6(2). Available at http://www.medscape.com/viewarticle/514164_print. Accessed August 31, 2008.

Marcus, D. A. (2000). "Treatment of nonmalignant chronic pain." *American Family Physician*, 61(3): 1331–1338, 1345–1346.

Maseeh, A., and Kwatra, G. (2005). "A review of smoking cessation interventions." *Medscape General Medicine*, 7(2): 24.

Millea, P. J., and Holloway, R. L. (2000). "Treating fibromyalgia." *American Family Physician*, 62(7): 1575–1582, 1587.

Murphy, M. J., and Cowan, R. L. (2007). *Blueprints: Psychiatry*, 4th ed. Lippincott Williams & Wilkins, Philadelphia, PA.

National Institutes of Health. (2008). St. John's wort, a health fact sheet from the National Center for Complementary and Alternative Medicine of the National Institutes of Health. (Online). Available at http://nccam.nih.gov/health/stjohnswort. Accessed August 2008.

Olson, J. (2001). *Clinical pharmacology made ridiculously simple*. MedMaster, Miami, FL.

Prator, B. C. (2006). "Serotonin syndrome." *Journal of Neuroscience Nursing*, 38(2): 102–105.

Preston, J., and Johnson, J. (2003). *Clinical psychopharmacology made ridiculously simple*. MedMaster, Miami, FL.

Shannon, M. T., Wilson, B. A., and Stang, C. L. (2002). *Health professional's drug guide 2002*. Prentice Hall, Upper Saddle River, NJ.

Smith, D. S. (2001). "Health care management of adults with Down syndrome." *American Family Physician*, 64(9): 1031–1038, 1039–1040.

Terebelo, S. (2006). "Practical approaches to screening for domestic violence." *Journal of the American Academy of Physician Assistants*, 18(9): 30–35.

Tierney, L. M., McPhee, S. J., and Papadakis, M. A. (eds.). (2004). *Current medical diagnosis and treatment 2004*. Lange Medical Books/McGraw-Hill, New York.

Wittchen, H. U., Hoyer, J., and Friis, R. (2006). "Generalized anxiety disorder: a risk factor for depression?" *International Journal of Methods in Psychiatric Research*, 10(1): 52–57.

Warner, C. H., Bobo, W., Warner, C., Reid, S., and Rachal, J. (2006). "Antidepressant discontinuation syndrome." *American Family Physician*, 74(8): 449–456, 457.

CHAPTER 26

Geriatrics

John A. Batsis, MD
Paul Y. Takahashi, MD, FACP, AGSF

1. Which of the following is *not* a basic activity of daily living?
   - **A.** Taking medications
   - **B.** Bathing
   - **C.** Walking
   - **D.** Transferring from bed to chair
2. Which of the following is *not* an instrumental activity of daily living?
   - **A.** Using the telephone
   - **B.** Reading the newspaper
   - **C.** Going shopping
   - **D.** Taking your medications
3. Which of the following is the most common cause of long-term nursing home placement in the elderly population?
   - **A.** Dementia
   - **B.** Depression
   - **C.** Poor family support
   - **D.** Congestive heart failure
4. Which antibiotic class is most likely to be associated with *Clostridium difficile* infection?
   - **A.** Cephalosporins
   - **B.** Ampicillin
   - **C.** Clindamycin
   - **D.** Amoxicillin
5. Which of the following statements about *Clostridium difficile* infections in the nursing home is typically correct?
   - **A.** Patients who are initially infected require treatment with a 10-day course of intravenous vancomycin.
   - **B.** Patients who have received antibiotic therapy more than 60 days ago are at very high risk of infection.
   - **C.** Successfully treated patients require screening upon completion of their therapy.
   - **D.** Recently hospitalized patients who develop diarrhea should be screened for *Clostridium difficile*.
6. Which of the following patients do *not* usually contract health-care–associated methicillin-resistant *Staphylococcus aureus* (MRSA) infections?
   - **A.** Patients have attended a dialysis clinic in the 30 days before infection.
   - **B.** Patients have received wound care at home within the previous 30 days.
   - **C.** Long-term care patients in a nursing home are likely to develop a MRSA infection.
   - **D.** Patients receive home IV antibiotic therapy for 30 days after treatment completion.

7. Which of the following is *not* a typical measure to reduce the risk of falls in nursing home residents?

   A. Bed and chair alarms
   B. Adequate lighting in the bed and bathrooms
   C. Use of physical restraints
   D. Routine medication review by the practitioner

8. An 84-year-old male who is a long-term care resident with moderate Alzheimer's dementia is reliant on others for the majority of his activities of daily living. He appears sexually disinhibited, displaying poor judgment and making inappropriate sexual impulses toward the female residents. The family members of these female residents raise this issue with you. Which of the following statements is *false*?

   A. The practitioner should take a collaborative history of the patient's behavior, either from other residents or from caregivers, and adequately document it in the medical record.
   B. The practitioner should perform a physical examination to rule out a secondary cause of delirium.
   C. Wandering into other residents' bedrooms can, at times, face an erroneous description as sexual disinhibition, even if no sexual intent is sought.
   D. Antiandrogens may be appropriate to impair sexual function and behaviors.

9. You are examining a 77-year-old female nursing home resident with end-stage dementia. Over the course of the last year, she has lost 15 pounds. Her family is concerned, as is the nursing staff. She otherwise has diagnoses of coronary artery disease, hypothyroidism, and gastroesophageal reflux disease. She has a remote history of spontaneous pulmonary embolism. Her medications include aspirin, metoprolol, losartan, levothyroxine, and omeprazole. Her thyroid function tests are within normal limits. Which of the following is appropriate as an initial measure to induce weight gain in this patient?

   A. Megestrol acetate can increase a patient's appetite and weight and may be appropriate in this patient.
   B. A trial of an antidepressant may be worthwhile because the patient may have an untreated underlying depression.
   C. Antipsychotics such as quetiapine and risperidone are useful adjuncts to promote weight gain and are safe for long-term use.
   D. A family discussion regarding institution of a percutaneous endoscopic gastrostomy (PEG) tube may be appropriate, because they promote weight gain and improve survival and quality of life in this patient population.

10. Which of the following medications is a relative contraindication for patients with Lewy body disease?

   A. Fluoxetine
   B. Donepezil
   C. Haloperidol
   D. Clonazepam

11. Patients with Alzheimer's disease are thought to have a primary neurochemical disturbance with which of the following neurotransmitters?

   A. Acetylcholine
   B. Dopamine
   C. Serotonin
   D. Norepinephrine

12. A 66-year-old female presents with fluctuating cognitive impairment over the last year, leading her to forget names of people, telephone numbers, and appointments. During the interview, her husband describes that she acts out in her dreams and often inadvertently hits him. She has also developed a resting tremor, a shuffling gait, and masked facies in the past month. Which of the following is the most likely diagnosis?

A. Parkinson's disease
B. Alzheimer's disease
C. Lewy body dementia
D. Frontotemporal lobe dementia

13. Which of the following would you not expect to be a usual presenting feature in a patient with frontotemporal lobe dementia?

A. Schizophrenic symptoms
B. Memory problems
C. Expressive aphasia
D. Difficulty in planning their activities or day

14. Which of the following statements is usually *false* regarding the cholinesterase inhibitors donepezil and rivastigmine?

A. They can probably improve cognitive status in some patients.
B. They can likely improve a patient's activities of daily living.
C. They definitely prevent nursing home placement.
D. They are appropriate in select patients to limit behavioral disturbances.

15. Which of the following medications usually presents the *least* risk of increased falls in the elderly?

A. Citalopram
B. Diphenhydramine
C. Metoprolol
D. Ibuprofen

16. A 78-year-old female with a history of early onset Alzheimer's disease has a history of stress incontinence. Her Mini-Mental State Exam (MMSE) score has been progressively declining over the course of the last year. She had been on metoprolol and hydrochlorothiazide since her early 40s. She is on citalopram for depression and oxybutynin for mild urinary incontinence. She started on a course of donepezil within the last year to help improve her cognition. Her caregivers are somewhat concerned. Which of the following is the most appropriate treatment?

A. Discontinue oxybutynin.
B. Discontinue donepezil.
C. Add memantine.
D. Change citalopram to amitriptyline.

17. Which of the following is *not* a common osteoporotic fracture?

A. Femoral neck
B. Skull
C. Distal radial fracture
D. Vertebral compression fracture

18. Which of the following is *not* typically a secondary cause of osteoporosis?

A. Chronic steroid use
B. Hypoparathyroidism
C. Hyperthyroidism
D. Sun deprivation

19. A 66-year-old postmenopausal female presents with a vertebral compression fracture. She had a total abdominal hysterectomy with bilateral salpingo-oopherectomy at age 46 because of fibroids. The results of a bone density scan were as follows: T score of −2.8 at the hip, T score of −1.8 in the lumbar spine, and a Z score of 1.0. Based on these results, which of the following statements applies?

   A. The patient has documented osteopenia.
   B. You should only prescribe the patient 600 mg of elemental calcium daily, with a minimum of 400 IU of vitamin D daily.
   C. As her provider, you should inquire whether the patient has had any significant gastroesophageal reflux disease or esophageal problems in the past.
   D. The high likelihood exists that the patient has a secondary cause of osteoporosis; therefore, you recommend a secondary osteoporosis workup.

20. Which of the following is the most common cause of death from injury in elderly patients (>65 years old) living at home?

   A. Fire/burns
   B. Falls
   C. Traffic accidents
   D. Exposure to heat/cold

21. You admit a 68-year-old male to the intensive care unit following an exacerbation of chronic obstructive pulmonary disease. He has a history of coronary artery disease, congestive heart failure, and type 2 diabetes mellitus. He conveys that he is not a "doctor" person, has no immediate family, and his last contact with a medical provider was 3 years earlier for a myocardial infarction. His "roommate" assists him at home with many of his basic and instrumental activities of daily living. He allows her to live in his house in return for some assistance at home. His roommate also works part time at a separate job. The patient mentions to the practitioner that he has not seen his roommate for a few days, although he knows she's been home because the mail has been accumulating on the kitchen table. Which of the following statements is typically *false* concerning this patient?

   A. This patient is likely a vulnerable adult because he has significant impairments and disabilities that prevent him from performing his basic needs and protecting himself from maltreatment.
   B. There is a mandate for the caring providers to report this case to the local social worker. Failure to report this case makes them liable for any harm/damages he might suffer from maltreatment.
   C. This demonstrates a case of financial exploitation by the "roommate." She lives in the patient's house in return for providing requested services even though she does not receive cash payment.
   D. Law enforcement is not obligated under federal or state law to protect the vulnerable adult, even if requested by the patient to do so, until the investigation is complete.

22. Which of the following is usually the most common reason for erectile dysfunction in elderly males?

   A. Medication
   B. Neurologic causes, including stroke and multiple sclerosis
   C. Diabetes mellitus
   D. Psychogenic

23. Which of the following would *not* be a common presenting feature in a patient with benign prostatic hyperplasia?

   A. Urgency
   B. Hematuria
   C. Nocturia
   D. Urinary frequency

24. A 77-year-old male presents for a routine physical. He has no medical issues other than hypertension, for which he is taking hydrochlorothiazide. Recent blood work was significant for a prostate specific antigen (PSA) of 15 ng/ml. A transrectal biopsy was consistent with a Gleason 2+2, T3N0M0 cancer, with three of six biopsy specimens positive for cancer. Which of the following would be the *least* appropriate management for this patient?

A. Watchful waiting
B. Radical retropubic prostatectomy
C. Brachytherapy, with or without external beam radiation therapy
D. Androgen deprivation alone

25. A 79-year-old male with a history of prostate cancer T3N3M1 treated with radiation therapy 4 years earlier presents with a 3-day history of increasing back pain, lower extremity weakness, and difficulty in initiating his urinary stream, often feeling quite "full." In the last 24 hours, he has also complained of some fecal incontinence. Unfortunately, he has not received regular medical follow-up since his treatment 4 years ago. He tells you that he thinks his prostate is "acting up" and wishes to get a medication to "fix" this. Which of the following is the most appropriate course of action?

A. Obtain an emergent MRI of the lumbosacral spine.
B. Refer the patient to a neurologist.
C. Provide a prescription for tamsulosin and follow-up in 1 month
D. Provide reassurance and follow-up in 2 weeks time.

26. Medicare guidelines recommend that which of the following be performed or administered on a yearly basis in all patients who do not have any comorbid conditions?

A. Pneumonia vaccine
B. Digital rectal examination
C. Bone mineral density scan
D. Lipid screen

27. A 68-year-old male presents for a general physical. He is in generally good health, with a life expectancy of greater than 10 years, but he has not had a complete physical since his 62nd birthday. He had smoked a pack per day for 30 years, but quit after his wife died of lung cancer 15 years ago. Which of the following tests are *inappropriate* to order for screening purposes?

A. Abdominal aortic ultrasound
B. Lipid panel
C. Chest radiograph
D. Screening colonoscopy

28. Which of the following is typically the most appropriate treatment for neuropsychiatric symptoms in dementia patients, once you rule out delirium?

A. Quetiapine
B. Olanzapine
C. Donepezil
D. No medications are an appropriate first treatment. Redirection techniques are often helpful initially.

29. A 71-year-old male presents with his son for a 6-month history of weight loss. His wife died approximately 2 years ago, after being married for over 52 years. He has had a difficult time in coping with these events. The patient describes to you that his appetite is poor, and he has been unable to sleep at night. He does not smoke. The medical workup has been unremarkable. Which of the following medications would be most appropriate in this patient?

A. Amitriptyline
B. Bupropion
C. Citalopram
D. Trazodone

30. Which of the following is *not* an independent risk factor for depression in the elderly?

   A. Death of a spouse and isolation

   B. Multiple medical conditions

   C. Declining functional status

   D. Frequent practitioner follow-up

31. Which of the following is typically an appropriate management strategy in maintenance treatment of depression in the elderly?

   A. Tricyclic antidepressants (amitriptyline and nortriptyline are useful first-line agents because they not only improve symptoms of depression, but can also improve cognition).

   B. In elderly patients with major depression who responded to initial therapy, maintenance therapy should continue for at least 2 years, if not longer.

   C. Psychotherapy is as useful as pharmacologic therapy regarding maintenance of these patients.

   D. The goal of therapy is only to promote recovery of symptoms.

32. A 78-year-old male with congestive heart failure (ejection fraction 38%) secondary to a long-standing history of hypertension, chronic renal insufficiency, and severe asthma presents to the emergency department with palpitations over the past 7 days that have gotten progressively worse. He denies any chest pain, shortness of breath, or any other symptoms. He otherwise lives with his wife, who has moderate dementia. He has difficulty with most of his instrumental activities of daily living and uses a walker to mobilize. He rarely gets out of the house. He states that he is somewhat unstable on his feet and has had recurrent falls. He also has a history of two subdural hematomas, one of which needed evacuation a year earlier. His vital signs are as follows: blood pressure, 145/82 mmHg; heart rate, 178 beats per minute, irregular; respiratory rate, 20 breaths per minute, with SpO$_2$ of 97% on room air. His electrocardiogram is shown below. Which of the following is the most appropriate management of this patient?

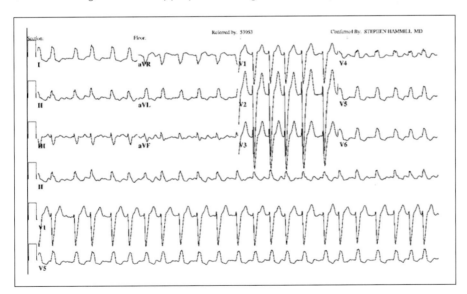

   A. The patient should be anticoagulated with heparin and started on warfarin therapy.

   B. The patient should be referred for immediate pacemaker implantation

   C. The patient requires immediate stress testing.

   D. Digoxin might be an appropriate medication to use to control the patient's rate.

33. You admit a 67-year-old female with lung carcinoma for shortness of breath. She has known metastatic disease to the bone and liver, and surgery is not a viable option. After you admit the patient, she asks you, "Can you tell me what kind of options I have to keep me comfortable in my dying days? I don't want to suffocate." Which of the following would *not* be an immediate and appropriate palliative therapy for dyspnea in this particular patient?

A. Nebulized morphine 0.5 mg/ml, as required
B. Lorazepam 0.5–1.0 mg orally or IV, as required
C. Duragesic patch 25 mcg/hr, change every 3 days
D. Oxygen therapy, titrate to patient comfort level

34. An 87-year-old male with severe aortic stenosis—Class IV New York Heart Association heart failure—presents functionally impaired. He is not a candidate for surgery. He and his family are interested in palliative measures. Which of the following statements regarding palliative care is typically *false*?

A. It improves quality of life for patients with advanced illnesses.
B. Its only aim is to relieve suffering.
C. The clinician should discuss advanced directives with the patient and family.
D. The clinician should discuss goals of care with the patient and his or her family at the beginning of treatment.

35. Which of the following statements is usually true regarding hospice services in the United States?

A. Patients receiving hospice should have a life expectancy of 3 months or less.
B. Medicare does not provide hospice benefits.
C. Hospice services typically exclude those wishing life-prolonging measures, such as salvage chemotherapy, from receiving hospice benefits.
D. Dementia patients do not fulfill the criteria for hospice benefits.

36. Which of the following is *not* an appropriate investigation/intervention in an 84-year-old nursing home patient with a history of end-stage dementia who has stopped eating and has recently become more somnolent?

A. Urinalysis with culture
B. Chest radiograph
C. CT scan of the head
D. Basic laboratory studies

37. Clinicians at your hospital admitted a 91-year-old male nursing home resident for a stroke yesterday. First thing in the morning, the staff found him on the ground, where they discovered an inadvertent left femoral neck fracture. He has a background history of moderate Alzheimer's disease; a ventricular tachycardia with an automatic implantable cardioverter defibrillator (AICD) in place; hypertension; diabetes; seizure disorder; and chronic obstructive pulmonary disease (COPD). He was not a candidate for reperfusion therapy, and his family decided that because of his poor quality of life surgical repair of the hip was not an option. Although they did not want any life-prolonging measures, they did want full medical treatment at this time. You are called to his bedside because his oxygen saturations have dropped; he has spiked a fever, as per the nursing staff; and he has become increasingly agitated. Which of the following interventions is inappropriate at this time?

A. Broad-spectrum antibiotics for possible aspiration pneumonia
B. Haloperidol for agitation
C. Restraints for his agitation
D. CT angiogram for a pulmonary embolism

38. An 83-year-old male presents with delirium that requires hospitalization. He had been doing very well at home, but has become increasingly confused, prompting his family to bring him to the emergency department. You take a collateral history and examine the patient. Although the patient is pleasant and not agitated, he is clearly confused. Which of the following should generally be encouraged?

    A. Ask his family to bring in his eyeglasses and hearing aids from home.
    B. Keep him in a lively and noisy room.
    C. Encourage the nursing staff to keep the blinds shut and dim the lights.
    D. Once his family leaves, leave him alone without any supervision.

39. An 87-year-old woman with end-stage dementia in the nursing home decreases her food intake and is less interactive. Which of the following would be an inappropriate question to pose to the nursing staff in order to determine the specific etiology?

    A. When was the last time the patient had a bowel movement?
    B. Is the patient coughing?
    C. Is the patient's moisture control garment wet?
    D. Has the patient stopped talking?

40. A 67-year-old presents with his spouse to your office. His wife has noticed a progressive decline in his gait, worsening of memory, and some urinary incontinence. She is quite worried, because these symptoms have progressed over the past few months to a point where she is unsure if she can care for him at home. Cerebellar signs are present on examination. You obtained a basic laboratory workup, which was noncontributory along with head imaging. Which of the following is the most likely diagnosis?

    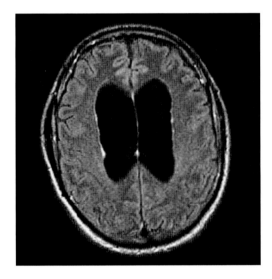

    A. Alzheimer's disease
    B. Normal pressure hydrocephalus
    C. Vestibular dysfunction
    D. Parkinson's disease

41. Which of the following is a suitable gait aid for a patient whose upper extremities do not exhibit any weakness and are not required for balance or weight bearing, but has difficulty walking due to a left lower extremity hemiparesis?

    A. Cane
    B. Hemi-walker
    C. Standard four-legged walker
    D. Front-wheel walker

42. A 74-year-old woman presents with a recurrent history of falls. Her daughter expresses concern that she may have some balance problems. The patient's history is notable for osteoporosis based on last bone mineral density scan. Her medication list is as follows: hydrochlorothiazide for hypertension; glyburide for diabetes; aspirin; and zolpidem for sleep. Her blood pressure is 125/75 mmHg, sitting, but she gets somewhat lightheaded when she sits up quickly and her blood pressure drops to 105/70 mmHg. Which of the following statements is *inappropriate* concerning this patient?

A. Discontinuation of the hydrochlorothiazide is appropriate because it can lead to orthostasis, and it is not the first-line agent for her diabetes.
B. Switch from glyburide to a non-insulin-secreting medication, such as metformin.
C. Benzodiazepines, if used appropriately, causes a very slight, but insignificant, risk of increased falls.
D. The clinician should prescribe calcium, vitamin D, and bisphosphonate.

43. A 75-year-old male patient who has had an open reduction and internal fixation (ORIF) of a femoral fracture presents for evaluation of a stage III pressure ulcer. The pressure ulcer likely developed from lying on his back for 5 hours before discovery. He is otherwise healthy, with a BMI of 23. The ulcer is clean without exudates; however, it is deep and fits criteria for a stage III ulcer. He is currently only toe-touch weight bearing. The nursing staff is turning him every 2 hours. Which of the following would be the most useful surface for his bed at the nursing home?

A. Standard mattress
B. Egg crate mattress
C. Low-air-loss mattress
D. Air fluidized bed

44. An 84-year-old female resident of a long-term care facility develops a new stage I pressure ulcer. She has moderate dementia; however, she has been ambulatory with a walker. Her weight has remained stable at 121 pounds (BMI of 20). Which of the following lab tests is most appropriate?

A. Albumin
B. Complete blood count
C. Erythrocyte sedimentation rate
D. Creatinine

45. A 74-year-old male smoker with a history of diabetes presents with a worsening ulcer on the bottom of his right foot. He reports that he has been having fevers over the last 24 hours and has a decrease in appetite. His diabetes has been under only moderate control for the last 5 years. Physical examination reveals a 3-cm ulcer on the metatarsal heads with bone showing. There is an obvious odor. There are decreased posterior tibial and dorsalis pedis pulses. Which evaluation would be *least* useful for this patient initially?

A. Pedal radiographs
B. Erythrocyte sedimentation rate
C. MRI
D. Probing the ulcer with a sterile instrument

46. An 84-year-old female presents with worsening sleep problems. She lives independently in her home and currently takes diuretics, a beta blocker, aspirin, and a multivitamin. Which of the following would be the most appropriate initial approach to help this patient with her sleep?

A. Acetaminophen, with diphenhydramine on schedule for 2 weeks
B. Lorazepam, as needed
C. Lifestyle modifications
D. Zolpidem, as needed

47. A 72-year-old resident of an assisted living center has been having worsening hypertension. His blood pressure is 174/72 mmHg. He has been feeling more fatigued recently and has been napping in his easy chair. His BMI is 37. Which of the following is the most appropriate next step in the evaluation of his worsening hypertension?

   A. Overnight oximetry
   B. Ultrasound of the renal arteries
   C. Urinary metanephrines
   D. AM cortisol

48. Which of the following describes what typically happens with calcium metabolism in aging patients?

   A. There are typically no changes in parathyroid hormone levels, vitamin D levels, or calcium levels.
   B. Parathyroid levels increase, vitamin D stays the same, and calcium increases.
   C. Parathyroid levels increase, vitamin D levels decrease, and calcium levels decrease.
   D. Parathyroid levels decrease, vitamin D stays the same, and calcium levels increase.

49. Which of the following statements is usually *false* regarding the genetic changes of aging?

   A. The number of telomere sequences increases.
   B. The number of DNA cross-strands increases.
   C. Chromosomal abnormalities increase.
   D. DNA methylation declines.

50. Which of the following describes how the sex hormones change as men age?

   A. Total testosterone stays the same, free testosterone stays the same, and sex-hormone-binding globulin stays the same.
   B. Total testosterone decreases, free testosterone decreases, sex-hormone-binding globulin increases.
   C. Total testosterone decreases, free testosterone decreases, sex-hormone-binding globulin decreases.
   D. Total testosterone decreases, free testosterone stays the same, sex-hormone-binding globulin stays the same.

51. A healthy 84-year-old male presents with slightly worsening constipation. Essentially, he had regular bowel movements prior to the last few years. He currently has a bowel movement every other day and must occasionally strain. He is otherwise healthy, and only takes metoprolol for hypertension and aspirin. A colonoscopy 5 years ago was negative for polyps or abnormalities. Which of the following is the most appropriate recommendation(s)?

   A. Lactulose 15 cc twice a day
   B. Docusate sodium 100 mg daily
   C. Senna one tablet daily at night
   D. Fiber and increased water intake

52. An 89-year-old female with end-stage Parkinson's disease who has been living in long-term care for 3 years has been having worsening problems with urinary incontinence. She currently wears incontinence pads. She has encountered numerous yeast infections in the groin because of the incontinence. The staff at the facility is asking for help with the incontinence. Which of the following is the most appropriate recommendation?

   A. Start oxybutynin 10 mg orally three times a day.
   B. Prescribe long-acting oxybutynin 10 mg daily.
   C. Institute timed toileting for urination every 2 hours while awake.
   D. Prescribe nortriptyline 10 mg daily.

53. A 67-year-old female presents to the outpatient clinic with worsening incontinence. She experiences incontinence with coughing, sneezing, or bearing down. Initially, she was able to use a light pad; however, the urinary incontinence has since worsened, requiring her to wear a full-thickness pad. Which of the following is the best first step for treatment of this patient's problem?

A. Tolterodine 1 mg daily
B. Pelvic floor exercises
C. Collagen injection at the urethral opening
D. Surgical intervention

ANSWERS

1. **The correct answer is A.** Basic activities of daily living typically include toileting, feeding, dressing, grooming, ambulation, and bathing.

2. **The correct answer is B.** Instrumental activities of daily living include using the telephone, shopping, preparing food, housekeeping, laundry, transportation, managing medications, and handling one's finances.

3. **The correct answer is A.** All of the answers are predictors of nursing home placement. However, dementia is the most common cause. In one study, within 5 years of diagnosis, 90% of all patients become institutionalized. All of the other causes can lead to nursing home placement; however, dementia is by far the most common cause.

4. **The correct answer is A.** Any antibiotic class can cause a *Clostridium difficile* infection. In the 1970s, clindamycin followed by ampicillin and amoxicillin were the prime culprits of this infection. Recently, cephalosporins and fluoroquinolones have been major causes of the disease, due to their overuse. Furthermore, recent strains are more virulent than previous ones.

5. **The correct answer is D.** Initial treatment recommendations for *Clostridium difficile* infection include treatment with oral vancomycin or oral metronidazole. The latter is often used initially due to its ease of use and low cost. Intravenous vancomycin is ineffective; thus answer A is incorrect. The Infectious Disease Society of America practice guidelines state that clinicians should suspect *C. difficile* in patients who have received systemic antimicrobial therapy in the previous 30 days and who are experiencing at least three watery or unformed stools within the last 24 hours. Successfully treated patients do not require retesting, as per guidelines. All recently hospitalized patients developing diarrhea require testing for *C. difficile*.

6. **The correct answer is D.** Health-care-associated and nosocomial-associated methicillin-resistant *Staphylococcus aureus* (MRSA) infections are strains of *S. aureus* that are resistant to oxacillin. Initially, MRSA was predominantly nosocomial in nature, but it has emerged as a community-based pathogen, too. According to the Centers for Disease Control and Prevention (CDC), patients hospitalized within the last year, or who live or attend nursing homes or dialysis centers are at much higher risks for health-care-associated MRSA. Furthermore, patients who have been in direct contact with health care workers may be at risk, including patients requiring home IV antibiotics or wound care. Normally, such patients are limited to a 30-day period whereby their classification is one of a health-care-associated MRSA.

7. **The correct answer is C.** Generally, early research showed that reducing restraints increases the incidence of falls; furthermore, if a patient is restrained, the likelihood of a fall is reduced. Providers typically use such restraints on patients who are more frail and susceptible to sustaining falls. However, research now suggests that reducing restraints,

especially in this population, would not *reduce* susceptibility for falls—to the contrary, it would *increase* the susceptibility of falls due to a variety of factors, including, but not limited to, the patient's inability to position appropriately or when restraints take the place of proper patient monitoring. Bed and chair alarms, lighting, environmental modifications, gait assessment, medication changes, assistive device evaluations, and exercise programs all reduce falls.

8. **The correct answer is C.** Because the patient is likely an unreliable historian due to his degree of dementia, a collaborative history by his caregivers is of vital importance. Any nursing home patient with a change of behavior needs full evaluation for reversible causes of delirium. All of the following are signs of hypersexual behavior: sexual comments, inappropriate touching, preoccupation with sex, touching oneself, and attempts at undressing oneself or another for sexual pleasure. Wandering into another resident's bedroom is only considered a sexual advance if the purpose is to chase a resident for sexual purposes. Antiandrogens have been used successfully and are indicated to control such behaviors.

9. **The correct answer is B.** Malnutrition is common in nursing home patients, especially in those with dementia. Adverse drug effects and depression are the most common reversible causes of weight loss, which therefore require the practitioner's primary attention. Of the answers listed, answer B would be most appropriate. Although antipsychotics do promote weight gain, they are not primarily used for weight gain. In addition, their use is associated with increased cardiovascular morbidity and mortality. Feeding tubes, although used in the past for nutrition, have limited evidence to support their use in end-stage dementia patients and do not improve survival. Megestrol acetate improves weight through appetite stimulation. However, it does carry a higher incidence of thromboembolic events. Because this patient has a history of a thromboembolic event and is currently immobile, megestrol would be inappropriate.

10. **The correct answer is C.** Patients with Lewy body dementia often have a hypodopaminergic state. Haloperidol is a typical antipsychotic; it is predominantly a dopamine antagonist. Administration of such a medication will often exacerbate symptoms and occasionally lead to an irreversible dystonic reaction. Because there is also a cholinergic deficiency in such patients, donepezil is most appropriate in patients with forgetfulness, apathy, or hallucinations. Fluoxetine is a selective serotonin reuptake inhibitor often used to control behavioral disturbances in these patients. Clonazepam has an indication for patients with Lewy body disease who also have a REM-related sleep disorder.

11. **The correct answer is A.** Patients with Alzheimer's disease have a neurochemical imbalance that leads to a reduction in acetylcholine secretion in the neuronal synapses. Medications indicated for this disease such as donepezil or rivastigmine, inhibit the enzyme acetylcholinesterase, which degrades acetylcholine in the synaptic cleft. Inhibition of this enzyme leads to relatively higher amounts of acetylcholine, with the hope that this will stimulate neuronal transport in these patients. Although other neurotransmitters are affected, acetylcholine is the primary neurotransmitter affected in patients with Alzheimer's disease.

12. **The correct answer is C.** Patients with frontotemporal lobe dementia often are young and present with frontal lobe symptoms, such as language disturbances, behavioral abnormalities, and psychiatric symptoms. Although this patient forgets people's names, telephone numbers, and appointments, she does have fluctuating cognitive impairment and sleep-related disturbances, which are uncommon clinical features of Alzheimer's disease. She does exhibit symptoms of Parkinson's disease—resting tremor, shuffling gait, and masked facies. However, the onset of these symptoms followed the onset of her dream-enactment sleep disorder and her fluctuating cognitive impairment, suggesting that this is Lewy body dementia rather than Parkinson's disease. Clinically, Parkinson's

disease with dementia resembles Lewy body dementia; however, the Parkinsonian features precede any of the other abnormalities by at least 1 year.

13. **The correct answer is B.** Patients with frontotemporal lobe dementia are younger patients who often are thought to have behavioral disturbances. Often, the diagnosis of schizophrenia is ascribed to these patients prior to the involvement of other cognitive domains. These patients can present with language difficulties, in particular an expressive aphasia. This entity is termed primary progressive aphasia. The clinician should rule out vascular etiologies, such as a stroke. Executive function often is impaired, leading to difficulties in planning. There is relative preservation of memory in the early course of the disease.

14. **The correct answer is C.** Most patients with cognitive impairment who take cholinesterase inhibitors have a small improvement in cognition and activities of daily living, thus the statements in answers A and B are true. Whether they prevent nursing home placement is not clear, because evidence is conflicting. Hence, clinicians should counsel patients and their families regarding the lack of evidence to support these statements. This makes answer C the correct answer to the question. Finally, some studies support the use of cholinesterase inhibitors for behavioral abnormalities in dementia patients.

15. **The correct answer is D.** The modified Beers criteria list medications considered hazardous in the elderly because they can predispose geriatric patients to falls. Of the medications listed, diphenhydramine highly predisposes to falls. However, in a meta-analysis by Leipzig et al. (1999), all of the indicated medications could possibly increase the risk. Of the choices presented, however, ibuprofen affords the least risk.

16. **The correct answer is A.** The patient has documented cognitive impairment and is initially on donepezil. Such patients should undergo a complete medication review to reduce the number of anticholinergic medications. Oxybutynin has significant anticholinergic effects, and one could consider discontinuing this medication because her symptoms are presently mild. Furthermore, such agents are ineffective for stress incontinence. They are indicated for overactive bladder or urge incontinence. Because the patient is still functional, discontinuing her cholinesterase inhibitor might not be the best option. Whether to continue this medication following nursing home placement is an area of controversy, though. Addition of another agent, such as memantine, may be of some benefit, especially in patients who are progressing quickly or who exhibit moderate to severe dementia. However, although this may be a suitable choice, it would be more important to eliminate unnecessary or confounding medications, such as the oxybutynin, prior to adding another medication. Switching her citalopram to amitriptyline would worsen her cognitive function because amitriptyline has significant anticholinergic effects.

17. **The correct answer is B.** Skull fractures are not typically associated with osteoporosis. The most common osteoporotic fractures are vertebral, accounting for 50% of all such fractures. Another 20% of osteoporotic fractures affect the hip and wrist. Colles' fractures are fractures of the distal radius.

18. **The correct answer is B.** All of the choices listed are secondary causes of osteoporosis with the exception of hypoparathyroidism. In fact, patients with hyperparathyroidism will have increased bone turnover, predisposing them to osteoporosis. If one suspects a secondary cause of osteoporosis, then a workup for hyperparathyroidism is appropriate.

19. **The correct answer is C.** The patient is at risk for osteoporosis because she had a bilateral premenopausal oopherectomy. In looking at her bone mineral density results, one looks at the T score at the posterior-anterior lumbar spine, femoral neck, or total hip. The T score helps make the diagnosis of osteoporosis, and one would identify the

lowest T score reported. The patient's T score of −2.8 at the hip is consistent with osteoporosis. The Z score is useful in identifying secondary causes of osteoporosis when it is less than −1.0. The recommendations are for this patient to consume a minimum of 1,500 mg of elemental calcium and a minimum of 600–800 IU a day of vitamin D. Patients with a history of significant gastroesophageal reflux may not be candidates for oral bisphosphonates. Therefore, practitioners should rule out this symptom at the time of evaluation. Because the patient's Z score was not abnormal, a workup of secondary causes of osteoporosis is unnecessary.

20. **The correct answer is B.** Injury to the elderly is a serious public health concern. Falls are the leading cause of death from injury, with more than 13,000 dying from fall-related injuries in 2003. The elderly accounted for 141,000 injuries in traffic accidents in 2004, accounting for 12% of all traffic deaths. Fire, burns, and exposure to heat or cold are less common causes of death.

21. **The correct answer is D.** Each jurisdiction has its own definitions of what constitutes a vulnerable adult. In all cases, three basic kinds of maltreatment can be present: abuse (physical, emotional, or sexual); neglect (caregiver neglect or self-neglect); or financial exploitation. In this case, the false statement is answer D. The patient allowed this "roommate" to live with him in exchange for assistance. This person has neglected to perform prior agreed-upon duties. This strongly supports the suspicion of financial exploitation. Furthermore, the patient has too many comorbidities. Additionally, this patient had been minimally functional to protect himself and was relying on this roommate to assist him. Generally in these situations, the law protects all health care providers without any liability, but they must report this incident to the local social worker. Social workers, in turn, usually investigate and involve additional authorities, as necessary. Statutes vary from state to state; however, the basic tenets hold true throughout the United States.

22. **The correct answer is A.** All of the following are possible etiologies of erectile dysfunction: medication, neurologic cause, psychological cause, and diabetes. In one study, medication accounted for up to 25% of cases of erectile dysfunction (including selective serotonin reuptake inhibitors, antihypertensive agents, and antipsychotics); neurologic causes accounted for 7% of cases; psychogenic causes, 14% of cases; and diabetes mellitus, 9% of cases.

23. **The correct answer is B.** The clinical manifestations of benign prostatic hyperplasia (BPH) are lower urinary tract symptoms, which include urinary frequency, hesitancy, nocturia, urgency, and a weak stream. It is important to note that these symptoms are not specific for BPH; therefore, the practitioner should correlate these findings with prostatic enlargement on examination or by ultrasound. Patients presenting with hematuria often need to have further workup for urothelial cancer, infection, or bladder calculi and, if appropriate, screening for sexually transmitted diseases.

24. **The correct answer is D.** The patient described in the vignette is a healthy patient whose prostate specific antigen was elevated and has a biopsy-proven prostatic adenocarcinoma. Unfortunately, research has not definitively determined which treatment is best—watchful waiting, surgery, radiotherapy, or androgen deprivation. Watchful waiting is useful in patients with a low risk of dying of prostate cancer within 20 years of follow-up; hence this approach is acceptable in our patient. Radical prostatectomy could also be useful in this patient, because it reduces the risk of metastatic and local disease spread, but it is associated with a higher risk of urinary and sexual dysfunction. Brachytherapy involves the implantation under anesthesia of small radioactive pellets that emit a low dose of radiation over a period of a few weeks to months into the prostate. It is appropriate as a primary therapy alone or in combination with external beam radiation or with androgen-deprivation therapy. Finally, androgen-deprivation therapy is rarely used as a primary treatment in a low-risk patient. However, it can be appropriate

in patients with intermediate and high-risk localized cancer or used as an adjuvant to external beam radiation therapy. Whether survival is affected is unknown. As such, this latter approach is not used alone.

25. **The correct answer is A.** This patient has had a known malignancy, which, based on the TNM classification system, was metastatic at presentation. Although successfully treated, such patients need monitoring for risk of recurrence. This patient presents with neurologic signs and cauda equina symptoms (difficulty with stream, incontinence, and weakness). Clinically, the patient has a spinal cord compression until proven otherwise. Danger signs or symptoms in patients with back pain include lower extremity weakness with neurologic signs, urinary retention, fecal incontinence or obstipation, fevers, chills, or a history of cancer. Such patients need emergent evaluation to rule out spinal cord compression. Referral to a neurologist is appropriate. However, the timely manner in which this occurs is often variable and if spinal cord compression is in the differential and confirmed on imaging, neurosurgical evaluation would be more appropriate. Because the patient has these "danger" signs, prescribing agents for benign prostatic hyperplasia are inappropriate at this time. Furthermore, reassurance would not be the optimal management at this time.

26. **The correct answer is B.** Medicare covers colorectal cancer screening with a digital rectal examination once every 12 months, making answer B the correct screening choice. After age 65 years or prior to that in those who suffer cardiopulmonary disease, all patients should receive the pneumonia vaccination once, regardless of age. All female patients, unless they have had one previously, should have a bone mineral density scan to evaluate for osteoporosis at a maximum of every 2 years. Medicare patients can receive assessment of blood lipid levels once every 5 years or yearly if they have significant vascular risk factors. This patient has no comorbidities, thus answer D is incorrect. A screening colonoscopy should be performed at 10-year intervals on all low-risk patients over the age of 50. As of January 1, 2007, all patients who have a family history of an abdominal aortic aneurysm or those patients who have smoked at least 100 cigarettes who are between the ages of 65 and 75 years are eligible for a one-time screen for an abdominal aortic aneurysm. There is no current recommendation for a screening chest radiograph.

27. **The correct answer is C.** See the explanation for question 26.

28. **The correct answer is D.** Increasing evidence indicates that nonpharmacologic measures, including redirection and behavioral methods, can be effective in dementia patients. This is the preferred method, because it avoids the high rate of adverse events associated with medication usage. Both quetiapine and risperidone are appropriate medications to treat neuropsychiatric symptoms, although there is increased monitoring of the use of such agents because of their side effects. They have been associated with increased mortality, therefore the practitioner should discuss the risk of using such medications with the patient's family. Cholinesterase inhibitors have some modest effects on cognition and some benefit for neuropsychiatric symptoms and have been given a Grade 2A recommendation for their use.

29. **The correct answer if C.** The patient described in the vignette demonstrates some signs of depression—weight loss, difficulty coping, poor appetite, and sleep disturbances. It is appropriate to consider treating this patient with a pharmacologic agent. Although amitriptyline may be appropriate in the treatment of depression, tricyclic antidepressants are now second-line agents. They are less favorable choices due to the larger number of side effects. Bupropion is often used either as an augmenting agent or as a first-line agent in patients who smoke. Citalopram is an often-used first-line selective serotonin reuptake inhibitor, making this the best choice. It has uses with neuropathic pain, panic disorder, or obsessive-compulsive disorder. Finally, trazodone can help with the patient's sleep, but it is a less potent agent for depression and it has no impact on appetite.

30. **The correct answer is D.** There is an estimated 1% to 4% prevalence of major depression in the elderly. Major risk factors for depression include physical illness, disability, cognitive deficits, declining functional status, social network losses and low social support, and negative life events. Although health care resource utilization is increased, those patients who see their clinicians more regularly often develop a relationship with their providers, causing them to feel more secure and lowering their risk for depression.

31. **The correct answer is B.** Selective serotonin reuptake inhibitors (SSRIs) are first-line agents in the management of depression. Tricyclic antidepressants are inappropriate first-line agents because they have anticholinergic activity, which can actually worsen cognition. A recent report published in 2006 suggests that maintenance therapy should continue for at least 2 years. Again, based on the results of this study and others, psychotherapy alone is not useful as monotherapy in maintenance treatment of depression. Finally, therapeutic goals include recovery of symptoms, but more important, as with most geriatric syndromes, improvement of quality of life.

32. **The correct answer is D.** In reviewing the electrocardiogram, it appears that the patient has an atrial fibrillation with a rapid ventricular response. Although rate control and anticoagulation with either heparin or low-molecular-weight heparin typically have use in the initial setting, this patient has moderate dementia and difficulty with most of the instrumental activities of daily living. Therefore, this patient is a high fall risk because he is unsteady on his feet and his history demonstrates recurrent falls. Anticoagulation with heparin and initiation of warfarin is not entirely appropriate. Furthermore, a history of subdural hematomas requiring evacuation would be a relative contraindication to anticoagulation. While a chemistry panel can provide important information, especially regarding the patient's electrolyte status, the presence of his atrial fibrillation changes the need as to which lab test is more important. Any patient with atrial fibrillation should have thyroid function tests performed because hyperthyroidism is a treatable cause of this arrhythmia. A stress test may provide evidence of cardiac insufficiency, however this patient has congestive heart failure. An echocardiogram would be useful because it can reevaluate the patient's cardiac function and left atrial size. If a transesophageal echocardiogram is performed, the clinician can evaluate for a left atrial thrombus, which may have developed if the patient has had symptoms for the past week. Rate-controlling agents that could be used include beta blockers, calcium-channel blockers, and digoxin. Because the patient has a history of severe asthma, beta blockers would be contraindicated. Calcium-channel blockers are a reasonable alternative. Digoxin might be an appropriate agent, although not first line, because it not only provides rate control, but also a slight inotropy to the patient who has congestive heart failure. Difficulties with digoxin would be with respect to his renal insufficiency to ensure that the levels do not exceed the narrow therapeutic index. While this patient may indeed require a pacemaker, it would be inappropriate as a first-line management.

33. **The correct answer is C.** All of the choices are suitable options to alleviate dyspnea except answer C, the fentanyl patch. This medication's effects are seen approximately 12 hours after application; therefore, it would not be recommended as an immediate measure to palliate dyspnea.

34. **The correct answer is B.** All of the choices, except answer B, are correct and form the foundation of palliative care. Although one of the aims of palliative care is to relieve suffering, it is not the only aim. It provides a multidisciplinary approach to patient care, including physical, mental, emotional, family, and spiritual support.

35. **The correct answer is C.** Patients in hospice normally have a life expectancy of 6 months or less. Medicare often covers hospice benefits, primarily at home. Dementia patients may receive secondary coverage under hospice, again, if deemed to have a life expectancy of less than 6 months. Salvage chemotherapy is a life-prolonging measure, which often

is not in line with the goals and principles of hospice care. However, treatment of these patients often means the use of surgical or medical measures. An example would be someone with a pancreatic lesion causing recurrent hepatobiliary obstruction. Pancreatic stent placement will be a covered procedure, because the primary indication for the procedure would be palliative in nature. The intent is palliative, not curative.

36. **The correct answer is C.** Elderly patients with dementia often have atypical presentations of systemic or local illnesses. The symptoms that this patient presents with are consistent with signs of delirium. Simple measures, such as urinalysis, chest radiograph, and basic laboratory studies often can be obtained with ease at nursing homes, contrary to a CT scan. Although a CT scan is indicated in some patients—requiring transport to the local emergency department—basic studies should be performed prior to the more expensive ones.

37. **The correct answer is C.** This patient just admitted for a stroke, is likely at risk for aspiration; hence, aspiration pneumonia is on the differential. Empiric antibiotics may be a reasonable choice in this situation because the patient may have an infection. Due to the prolonged immobility following a hip fracture, pulmonary embolism is common. Such patients can present with hypoxia and tachycardia, and a CT angiogram to rule out a pulmonary embolism is appropriate. Haloperidol should be avoided if possible, but can be used in situations where agitation is excessive. Restraints would be the least likely intervention in this patient scenario because the other choices are more appropriate first-line measures. Certainly, if the clinician performs all these measures to identify and treat the underlying cause of the delirium and the patient has not improved, one can consider restraints; however, this should always be discussed with the family for obvious reasons.

38. **The correct answer is A.** Nonpharmacologic methods to treat delirium should be encouraged, including the use of eyeglasses, hearing aids, and interpreters, if necessary. Furthermore, proven methods to improve confusion include keeping the patient in a quiet room with low-level lighting at night but normalizing sleep–wake cycles by discouraging naps and keeping lights on during the daytime. Finally, all such patients should be encouraged to use nurse aids or family for reorientation and patient protection.

39. **The correct answer is D.** The first three answer choices are important clues to the etiology of the patient's decreased responsiveness. Constipation (answer A) is often a subtle sign of altered mental status. Coughing in a patient with end-stage dementia may be an indication of aspiration pneumonia. If the patient has incontinence (as end-stage dementia patients often do), a moist adult garment is indicative of adequate hydration. However, if the garment is completely dry, this might indicate dehydration, again, a common sign of altered mental status. Stopping conversing would only give you an indication that something else may be going on, as opposed to a possible specific etiology, making this choice the least acceptable.

40. **The correct answer is B.** The patient has symptoms consistent with normal-pressure hydrocephalus, which includes the triad of gait instability, cognitive dysfunction, and urinary incontinence. The MRI is consistent with this diagnosis. Although these features can occur in Alzheimer's patients, the progression of symptoms is not consistent with this diagnosis. And although an MRI might show some hydrocephalus, it would not be as pronounced as that seen in the image. The sulci often visualize prominently as well. This patient does not have any other features suggestive of Parkinson's disease. Patients with vestibular dysfunction may present with gait abnormalities, but would not have cognitive difficulties or urinary incontinence.

41. **The correct answer is B.** This patient has lower extremity weakness on one side, but has excellent upper extremity strength that is not needed for balance or weight-bearing. A hemi-walker is the most appropriate aid because it provides compensation for their

lower extremity. Walkers are intended for patients who require assistance with weight-bearing. Canes are used primarily in patients who require slight assistance with balance and/or stability, rather than full weight-bearing.

42. **The correct answer is C.** The patient is at high risk for an osteoporotic fracture due to her osteoporosis. She is on numerous medications. Answer A may be appropriate. She currently is only on hydrochlorothiazide for her hypertension. First-line agents for hypertensive diabetics include angiotensin-converting enzyme inhibitors or angiotensin-receptor blockers. It may be appropriate to change glyburide, because it is an insulin-secreting medication, to metformin, which sensitizes the peripheral tissues to insulin and does not cause hypoglycemia. Benzodiazepines are high-risk medications for falls, as described by the modified Beers criteria. Clinicians should consider administration of calcium and vitamin D supplementation and a bisphosphonate to all patients with osteoporosis, as per the guidelines.

43. **The correct answer is C.** Standard mattresses are acceptable for patients or residents without a risk of pressure ulcers and do not possess an ulcer. Egg crate mattresses present a static environment for pressure reduction and are not as conducive for healing a stage 3 ulcer. The air-fluidized bed is the most aggressive option; however, it is costly and its primary use is for ulcers with marked exudates or in patients who are incontinent. Low air mattresses are effective in healing pressure ulcers over conventional care. Obviously, community standards of care, costs, and other factors figure in when treating patients. We advise the clinician to stay aware of these standards.

44. **The correct answer is A.** Obtaining an albumin would be an appropriate initial step. Malnutrition is a common challenge that can occur in residents with moderate to severe dementia. A low albumin level might indicate the development of malnutrition, which can addressed. A complete blood count (CBC) is an important test to rule out infection; however, the risks for infection with an intact ulcer would be low. The sedimentation rate assists with the evaluation of possible osteomyelitis, which is a low risk in this scenario. Creatinine may play a role, but not directly.

45. **The correct answer is C.** This 74-year-old patient has clear evidence of a neuropathic ulcer in the foot. In diabetics, neuropathic ulcers in the feet are often called "diabetic foot ulcers"; however, these ulcers can occur with any cause of peripheral neuropathy. Neuropathic ulcers often present with underlying infection, and this scenario would be worrisome for underlying osteomyelitis. Initial probing of the ulcer with a sterile instrument can be useful for potentially confirming osteomyelitis. An appropriate radiograph of the foot and a sedimentation rate are quick to obtain and assist with the diagnosis of osteomyelitis. An MRI, although very useful for this diagnosis, is often reserved for secondary evaluations if initial tests prove inconclusive.

46. **The correct answer is C.** Sleep agents can potentially cause falls in the elderly. Sedative medications such as lorazepam and diphenhydramine are particularly problematic. Zolpidem may be a better choice; however, it still has some risks. All patients with insomnia should have lifestyle modifications as a component of their treatment. This includes appropriate sleep habits (avoiding naps), stress reduction, and maintaining good sleep architecture.

47. **The correct answer is A.** Overnight oximetry would be an excellent next step for the evaluation of the resident's hypertension. Obstructive sleep apnea (OSA) is a common, yet underrecognized, illness in many older patients. It can dramatically affect blood pressure, alertness, and energy levels during the day. Appropriate treatment through surgery or a continuous positive airway pressure (CPAP) machine can dramatically improve both quality and quantity of life. Secondary evaluation for hypertension using urinary metanephrines, AM cortisol, and ultrasound of the renal arteries is appropriate in certain contexts; however, the fatigue points to possible OSA.

48. **The correct answer is C.** As individuals age, vitamin D levels start to decrease, with a concurrent slight decrease in calcium levels and a concurrent increase in parathyroid hormone (PTH) levels. The primary reason for these changes includes changes in dietary intake of calcium and decreased time in the sun for production of vitamin D.

49. **The correct answer is A.** Theories on aging have centered on many different hypotheses. Many involve changes in cellular genetics that occur with aging. As people age, they develop an increasing number of genetic abnormalities and have decreased capability of dealing with mistakes. DNA cross-stranding increases, as do chromosomal abnormalities. The number of telomere sequences decreases rather than increases with age. DNA methylation does decline with aging.

50. **The correct answer is B.** In men, total testosterone decreases with age. The proportion of bioactive testosterone in free testosterone decreases as well. This decrease in free testosterone is a result of multiple defects in the hypophysis (hypopituitary), pituitary, and testicular axis. Sex-hormone-binding globulin (SHBG) increases as men age; thus, the decrease in total testosterone may be partially masked by the changes in SHBG.

51. **The correct answer is D.** Lifestyle and dietary modification would probably be the first step for this healthy man. Fiber and adequate fluid intake may help eliminate his constipation. Medications such as calcium-channel blockers, diuretics, and calcium are common causes for constipation and certainly are changeable if needed. Stool softeners such as colace are often used next, with laxatives such as senna and lactulose used as the next option.

52. **The correct answer is C.** Functional incontinence is a very common source of incontinence in long-term-care settings. Residents with significant debility who cannot physically go to the commode or toilet often experience incontinence because they cannot get to the toilet in a timely manner. Offering or placing the resident on the commode or toilet in a scheduled manner may reduce functional incontinence and reduce the sequela from incontinence. Oxybutynin in short- or long-acting formulations is an effective medication for urge incontinence. Nortriptyline, likewise, has uses for urge and, sometimes, stress incontinence. Both might help; however, both medications have potential side effects for the resident.

53. **The correct answer is B.** This type of incontinence is a very common form of stress incontinence. Stress incontinence occurs with weakening of the pelvic floor muscles with age and often with multiple childbirths. Women initially treat the symptoms with pads or absorptive devices. Pelvic floor exercises (Kegel) exercises can be effective in younger women and may provide support with milder forms of stress incontinence. Surgical repair and collagen injection typically occur after lifestyle changes and strengthening exercises have proven ineffective. Tolterodine has a primary usage in urge incontinence and may not be particularly useful for stress incontinence.

REFERENCES

Alkhalil, C., Tanvir, F., Alkhalil, B., and Lowenthal, D. T. (2004). "Treatment of sexual disinhibition in dementia: Case reports and review of the literature." *American Journal of Therapeutics*, 11(3): 231–235.

American Geriatric Society. (2002). AGS position statement—Restraint use. (Online). Available at www.americangeriatrics.org/products/positionpapers/restraintsupdatePF.shtml. Accessed February 28, 2007.

Association of State and Territorial Health Officials. (2006). Injury prevention fact sheet. (Online). Available at www.astho.org/pubs/elderlyfactsheet.pdf. Accessed February 28, 2007.

Ayalon, L., Gum, A. M., Feliciano, L., and Arean, P. A. (2006). "Effectiveness of nonpharmacological interventions for the management of neuropsychiatric symptoms in patients with dementia: A systematic review." *Archives of Internal Medicine*, 166(20): 2182–2188.

Bartlett, J. G. (2006). "Narrative review: The new epidemic of *Clostridium difficile*-associated enteric disease." *Annals of Internal Medicine*, 145(10): 758–764.

Beckman, T. J., and Mandrekar, J. N. (2005). "Evaluation and medical management of benign prostatic hyperplasia." *Mayo Clinic Proceedings*, 80(10): 1356–1362.

Bentley, D. W., Bradley, S., High, K., Schoenbaum, S., Taler, G., and Yoshikawa, T. T. (2000). "Practice guideline for evaluation of fever and infection in long-term care facilities." *Clinical Infectious Diseases*, 31(30): 640–653.

Berlowitz, D. R., and Wilking, S. V. (1989). "Risk factors for pressure sores. A comparison of cross-sectional and cohort-derived data." *Journal of the American Geriatric Society*, 37(11): 1043–1050.

Boeve, B. (2004). "Dementia with Lewy bodies." *Continuum*, 10(1): 7–243.

Chervin, R. D. (2000). "Sleepiness, fatigue, tiredness, and lack of energy in obstructive sleep apnea." *Chest*, 118(2): 372–379.

Clark, C. M., and Karlawish, J. H. (2003). "Alzheimer disease: Current concepts and emerging diagnostic and therapeutic strategies." *Annals of Internal Medicine*, 138(5): 400–410.

Corey-Bloom, J. (2004). "Alzheimer's disease." *Continuum*, 10(1): 7–243.

Cummings, J. L. (2003). "Use of cholinesterase inhibitors in clinical practice: Evidence-based recommendations." *American Journal of Geriatric Psychology*, 11(2): 131–145.

Edmonds, M. E., and Foster, A. V. (2006). "Diabetic foot ulcers." *British Medical Journal*, 332(7538): 407–410.

Ell, K. (2006). "Depression care for the elderly: Reducing barriers to evidence-based practice." *Home Health Care Services Quarterly*, 25(1–2): 115–148.

Fantl, J. A., Wyman, J. F., and McClish, D. K. (1991). "Efficacy of bladder training in older women with urinary incontinence." *JAMA*, 265(5): 609–613.

Ferrell, B. A., Osterweil, D., and Christenson, P. (1993). "A randomized trial of low-air-loss beds for treatment of pressure ulcers." *JAMA*, 269(4): 494–497.

Finucane, T. E., Christmas, C., and Travis, K. (1999). "Tube feeding in patients with advanced Dementia." *JAMA*, 282(14): 1365–1370.

Gourlay, G. K. (2001). "Treatment of cancer pain with transdermal fentanyl." *Lancet Oncology*, 2(3): 165–172.

Graff-Radford, N., and Woodruff, B. (2004). "Frontotemporal dementia." *Continuum*, 10(1): 7–243.

Guerrant, R. L., Gilder, T. S., and Steiner, T. L. (2001). "Practice guidelines for the management of infectious diarrhea." *Clinical Infectious Diseases*, 32(3): 331–350.

Harman, S. M., Metter, E. J., Tobin, J. D., Pearson, J., and Blackman, M. R. (2001). "Longitudinal effects of aging on serum total and free testosterone levels in healthy men: Baltimore Longitudinal Study of Aging." *Journal of Clinical Endocrinology & Metabolism*, 86(2): 724–731.

Inouye, S. K. (2006). "Delirium in older persons." *New England Journal of Medicine*, 354(1116): 1157–1165.

Johnson, S., and Gerding, D. N. (1998). "*Clostridium difficile*–associated diarrhea." *Clinical Infectious Diseases*, 26(5): 1027–1036.

Kirkland, J. L. (2002). "The biology of senescence: Potential for prevention of disease." *Clinical Geriatric Medicine*, 18(3): 383–405.

Leib, E. S., Lewiecki, E. M., Binkley, N., and Hamdy, R. C. (2004). "International Society for Clinical Densitometry. Official positions of the International Society for Clinical Densitometry." *Journal of Clinical Densitometry*, 7(1): 1–6.

Leipzig, R. M., Cumming, R. G., and Tinetti, M. E. (1999). "Drugs and falls in older people: A systematic review and meta-analysis: I. Psychotropic drugs." *Journal of the American Geriatric Society*, 47(1): 30–39.

Locke, G. R. III, Pemberton, J. H., and Phillips, S. F. (2000). "AGA technical review on constipation." *Gastroenterology*, 119(6): 1761–1766.

Medicare Learning Network. (2004). MMA—Initial preventive physical examination. (Online). Available at www.cms.hhs.gov/mlnmattersarticles/downloads/mm3638.pdf. Accessed February 27, 2007.

Morley, J. E., and Silver, A. J. (1995). "Nutritional issues in nursing home care." *Annals of Internal Medicine*, 123(11): 850–859.

Morrison, R. S., and Meier, D. E. (2004). "Palliative care." *New England Journal of Medicine*, 350(25): 2582–2590.

National Osteoporosis Foundation. (n.d.) Osteoporosis Disease Statistics: Fast Facts. (Online). Available at www.nof.org/osteoporosis/diseasesfacts.htm. Accessed March 13, 2007.

Quang Vu, M., Weintraub, N., and Rubenstein, L. Z. (2006). "Falls in the nursing home: Are they preventable?" *Journal of the American Medical Directors Association*, 7(3, S1): S53–S58.

Reuban, D. B., Herr, K. A., Pacala, J. T., Pollack, B. G., Potter, J. F., and Semla, T. P. (2008). Geriatrics at your fingertips, online edition, 10th ed. (Online). Available at www.geriatricsatyourfingertips.org. Accessed August 2007.

Sherman, S. S., Hollis, B. W., and Tobin, J. D. (1990). "Vitamin D status and related parameters in a healthy population: The effects of age, sex, and season." *Journal of Clinical Endocrinology & Metabolism*, 71(2): 405–413.

Sink, K. M., Holden, K. F., and Yaffe, K. (2005). "Pharmacological treatment of neuropsychiatric symptoms of dementia: A review of the evidence." *JAMA*, 293(5): 596–608.

Smith, G. E., Kokmen, E., and O'Brien, P. C. (2000). "Risk factors for nursing home placement in a population-based dementia cohort." *Journal of the American Geriatric Society*, 48(5): 519–525.

Spinazze, S., Caraceni, A., and Schrijvers, D. (2005). "Epidural spinal cord compression." *Critical Reviews in Oncology/Hematology*, 56(3): 397–406.

Van Hook, F. W., Demonbreun, D., and Weiss, B. D. (2003). "Ambulatory Devices for Chronic Gait Disorders in the Elderly." *American Family Physician*, 67(8): 1717–1724.

Whooley, M. A., and Simon, G. E. (2000). "Managing depression in medical outpatients." *New England Journal of Medicine*, 343(26): 1942–1950.

Wilt, T. J., and Thompson, I. M. (2006). "Clinically localized prostate cancer." *British Medical Journal*, 333(47): 1102–1106.

Figure Captions

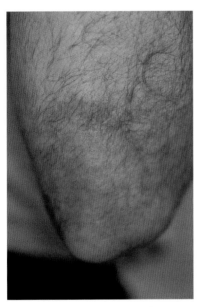

Figure 1-1   Granuloma Annulare

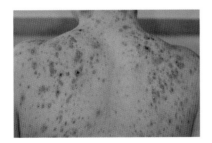

Figure 1-2   Cystic Acne

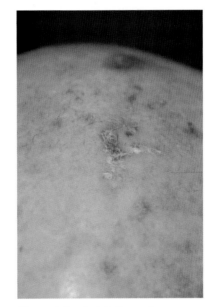

Figure 1-3   Actinic Keratosis

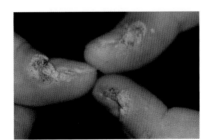

Figure 1-4   Verruca Vulgaris

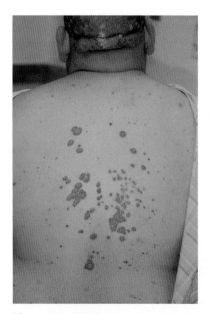

Figure 1-5 Psoriasis

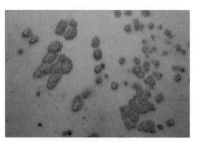

Figure 1-6 Psoriasis

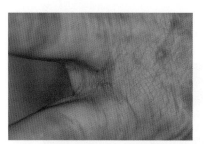

Figure 1-7 Scabies

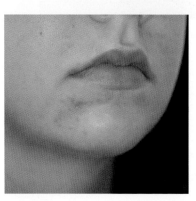

Figure 1-8 Perioral Dermatitis

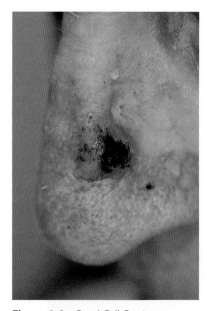

Figure 1-9 Basal Cell Carcinoma

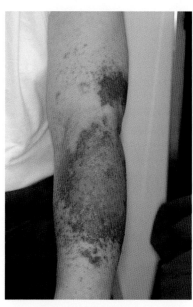

Figure 1-10 Atopic Dermatitis

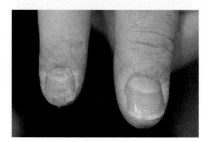

Figure 1-11 Paronychia

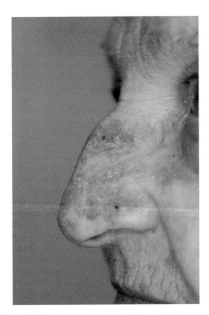

Figure 1-12 Actinic Keratosis

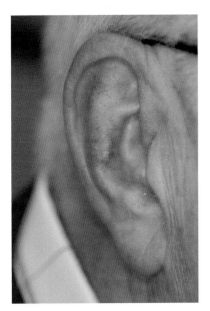

Figure 1-13 Chondrodermatitis Nodularis Chronica Helicis

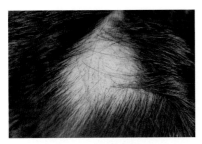

Figure 1-14 Alopecia Areata

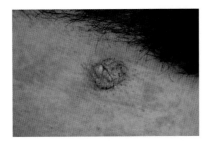

Figure 1-15 Verruca Vulgaris

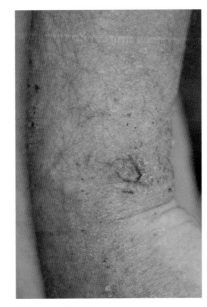

Figure 1-16 Eczema

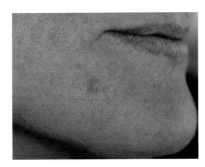

Figure 1-17 Pilar Nevus

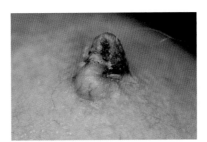

Figure 1-18 Actinic Keratosis

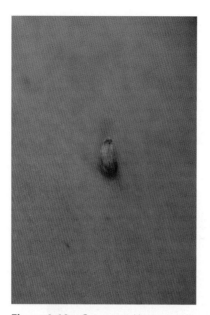

Figure 1-19   Cutaneous Horn

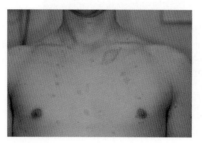

Figure 1-20   Pityriasis Rosea

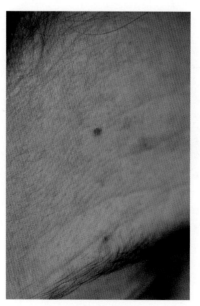

Figure 1-21   Cherry Angioma

Figure 1-22   Tinea Cruris

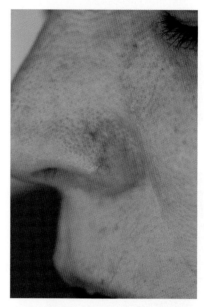

Figure 1-23   Spider Hemangioma

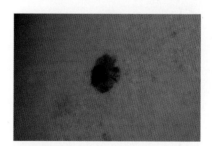

Figure 1-24   Malignant Melanoma

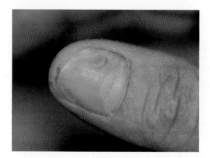

Figure 1-25   Onychomycosis

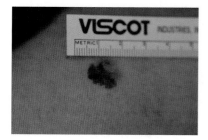

Figure 1-26 Malignant Melanoma
Prognostics

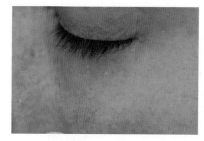

Figure 1-31 Syringoma

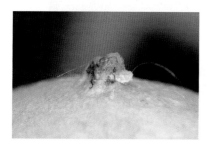

Figure 1-27 Cutaneous Horn

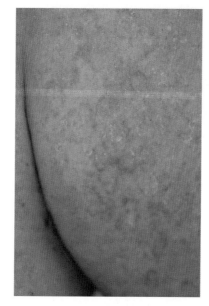

Figure 1-32 Tinea Corporis

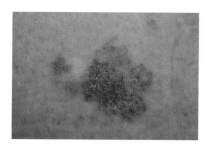

Figure 1-28 Bowen's Disease

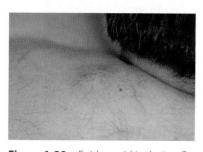

Figure 1-29 Epidermoid Inclusion Cyst

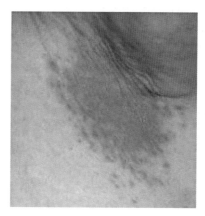

Figure 1-33 *Candida* dermatitis

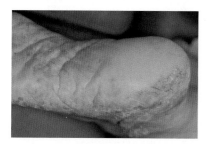

Figure 1-30 Palmoplantar Pustular Psoriasis

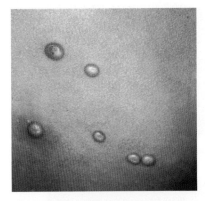

Figure 1-34   Molluscum Contagiosum

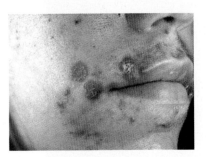

Figure 1-35   Impetigo

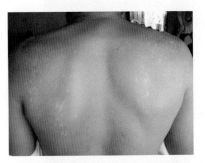

Figure 1-36   Tinea Versicolor

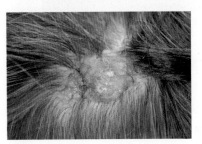

Figure 1-37   Nevus Sebaceous

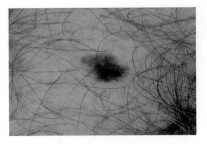

Figure 1-38   Malignant Melanoma ABCD

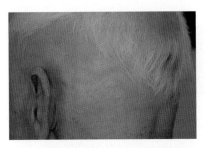

Figure 1-39   Alopecia Universalis

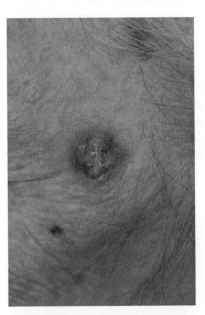

Figure 1-40   Basal Cell Carcinoma

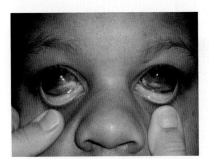

Figure 2-1   Bilateral Conjuctival Hemorrhages

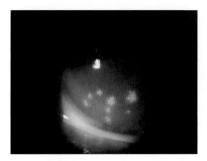

Figure 2-2   Herpes Simplex Keratitis

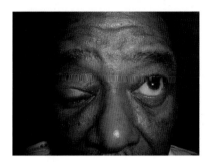

Figure 2-3   Preseptal Cellulitis

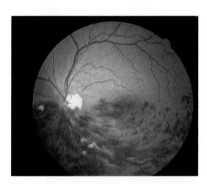

Figure 2-4   Central Retinal Artery Occlusion

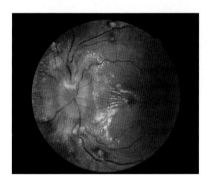

Figure 2-5   Malignant Hypertension

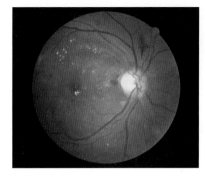

Figure 2-6   Hypertensive Retinopathy with Roth Spots

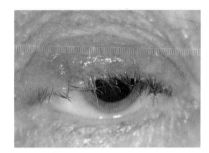

Figure 2-7   Blepharitis

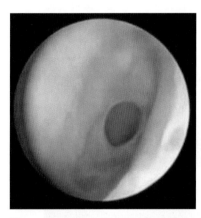

Figure 3-1   Otitis Media with Perforation

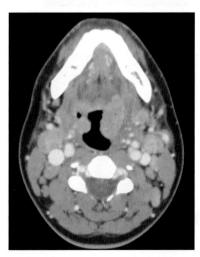

Figure 3-2   Peritonsillar Abscess

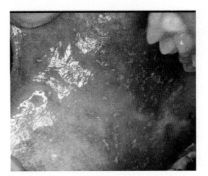

Figure 3-3   Koplik's Spots

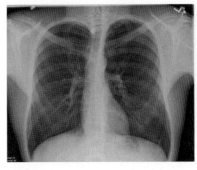

Figure 4-1   Left Pneumothorax

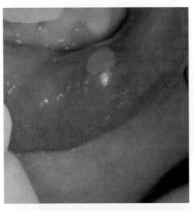

Figure 3-4   Apthous Ulcers

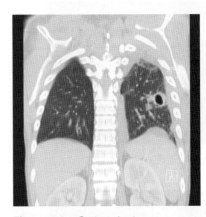

Figure 4-2   Cavitary Lesion

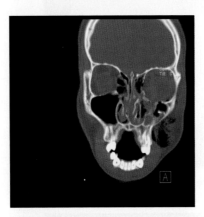

Figure 3-5   Blowout Fracture

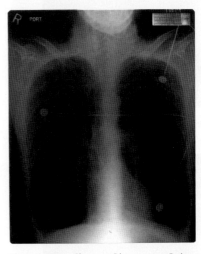

Figure 4-3   Chronic Obstructive Pulmonary Disease

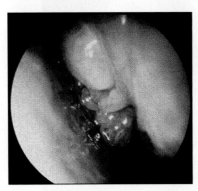

Figure 3-6   Nasal Polyps

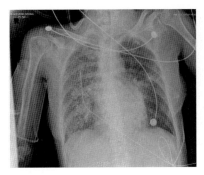

Figure 4-4   Miliary Tuberculosis

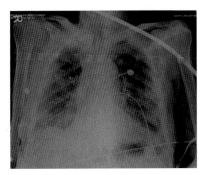

Figure 4-5   Asbestosis, Right Base Mass

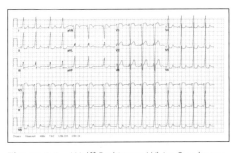

Figure 5-1   Wolff-Parkinson-White Syndrome

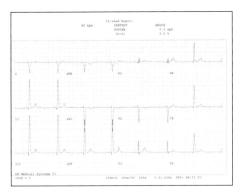

Figure 5-2   Stress Baseline

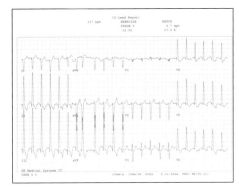

Figure 5-3   Stress Peak

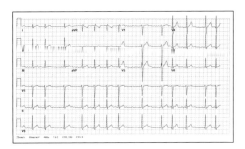

Figure 5-4   Atrial Fibrillation

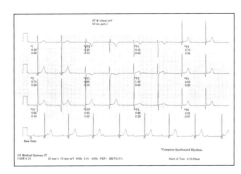

Figure 5-5   Complete Heart Block

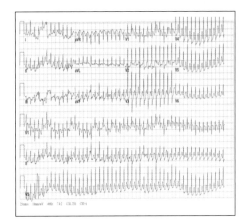

Figure 5-6   Supraventricular Tachycardia

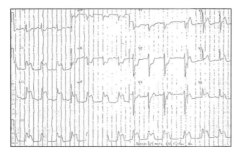

Figure 5-7   Inferior Wall Myocardial Infarction

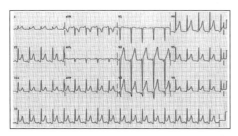

Figure 5-8   Pericarditis

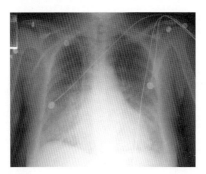

Figure 5-9   Kerley B-Lines

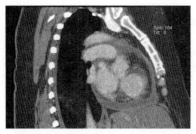

Figure 5-10   CT Scan Showing Pericardial Tamponade

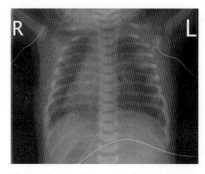

Figure 5-11   Dextrocardia with Situs Inversus

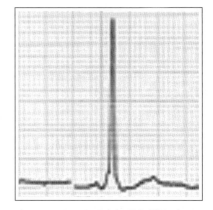

Figure 5-12   Individual Wolff-Parkinson-White Answers

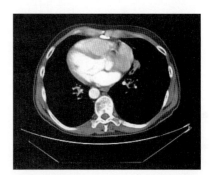

Figure 5-13   CT Scan Showing Situs Inversus

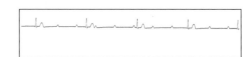

Figure 6-1   Complete Heart Block

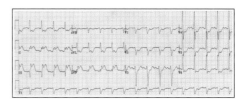

Figure 6-2   Inferior Wall Injury

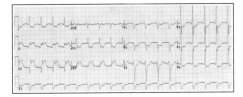

Figure 6-3   Inferior Wall

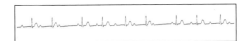

Figure 6-4   Second-Degree Heart Block Type I

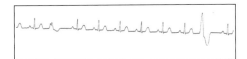

Figure 6-5   Multifocal Premature Ventricular Complexes

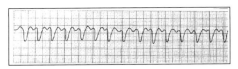

Figure 6-6   Ventricular Tachycardia

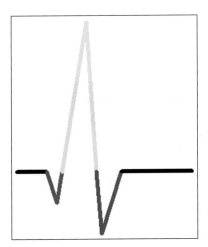

Figure 6-7   QRS + Deflection

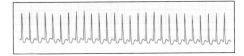

Figure 6-8   Supraventricular Tachycardia

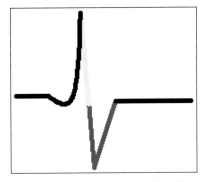

Figure 6-9   Swooping QRS of Wolff-Parkinson-White Syndrome

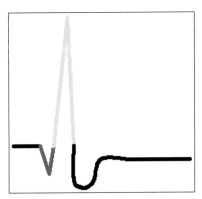

Figure 6-10   ST Depression

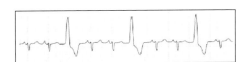

Figure 6-11   Trigeminy

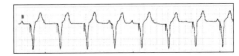

Figure 6-12   Ventricular Pacemaker

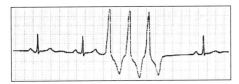

Figure 6-13   Run of Ventricular Tachycardia

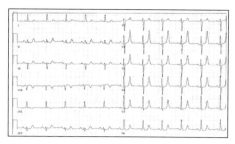

Figure 6-14   Hyperkalemia and Left Axis Shift

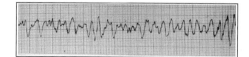

Figure 6-20   Ventricular Fibrillation

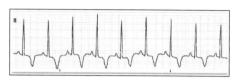

Figure 6-15   Ischemia

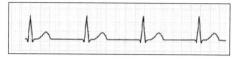

Figure 6-21   Junctional Rhythm

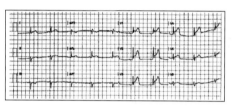

Figure 6-16   Anterior Wall Injury

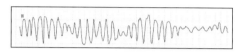

Figure 6-22   Torsades de Pointes

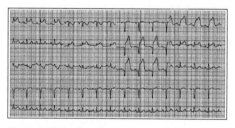

Figure 6-17   Significant Antero-lateral Infarction

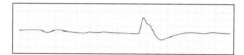

Figure 6-23   Agonal Beat

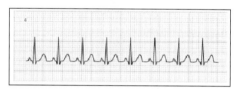

Figure 6-24   Pulseless Electrical Activity

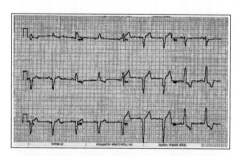

Figure 6-18   Left Bundle Branch Block

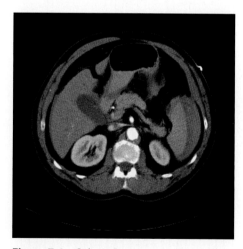

Figure 7-1   Splenic Rupture

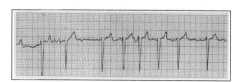

Figure 6-19   Sinus Artifact

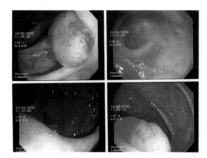

Figure 7-2 Colonic Polyposis

Courtesy of Christina Czyrko, MD

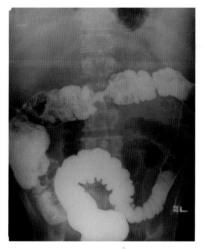

Figure 7-3 Apple-Core Lesion

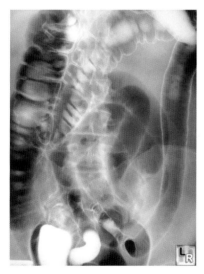

Figure 7-4 Ulcerative Colitis

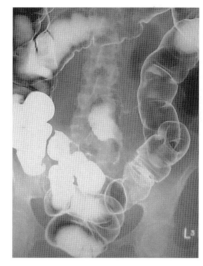

Figure 7-5 Crohn's Disease

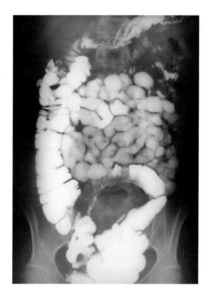

Figure 7-6 Crohn's Disease

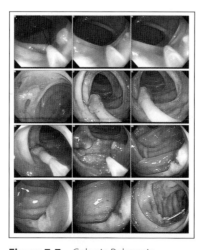

Figure 7-7 Colonic Polyposis

Courtesy of Christina Czyrko, MD

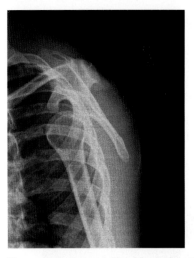

Figure 8-1   Anterior Shoulder Dislocation

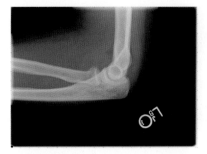

Figure 8-5   Radial Head Fracture

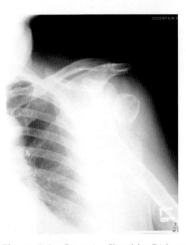

Figure 8-2   Posterior Shoulder Dislocation

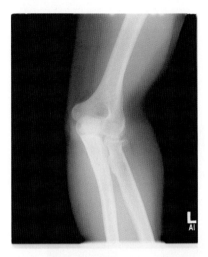

Figure 8-6   Radial Head Fracture

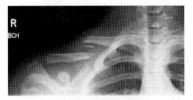

Figure 8-3   Clavicular Fracture

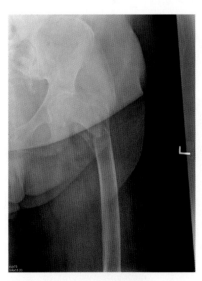

Figure 8-7   Left Hip Fracture

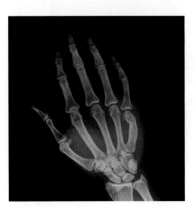

Figure 8-4   Boxer's Fracture

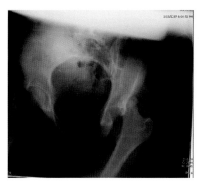

Figure 8-8   Posterior Hip Dislocation

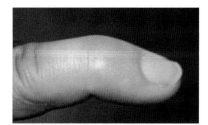

Figure 8-9   Mallet Finger

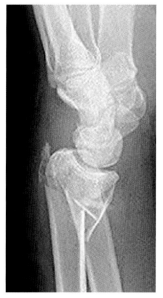

Figure 8-10   Smith's Fracture

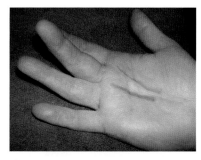

Figure 8-11   Dupuytren's Contracture

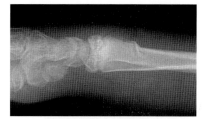

Figure 8-12   Torus Fracture

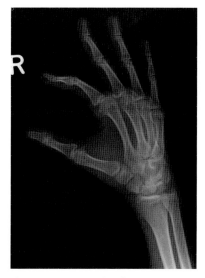

Figure 8-13   Scaphoid Fracture

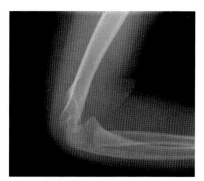

Figure 8-14   Normal Pediatric Elbow

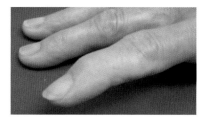

Figure 8-15   Heberden's Nodes

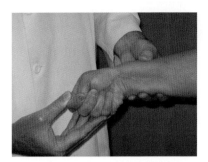

Figure 8-16   Finkelstein's Test

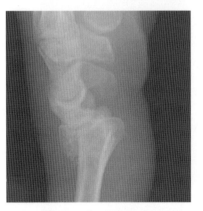

Figure 8-17   Colles' Fracture

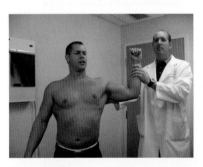

Figure 8-18   Apprehension Test

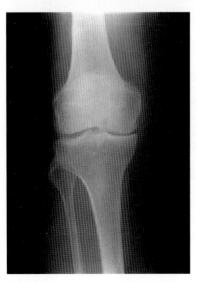

Figure 9-1   Osteoarthritis

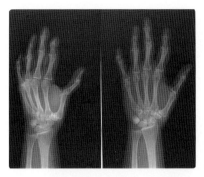

Figure 9-2   Osteoarthritis in Hands

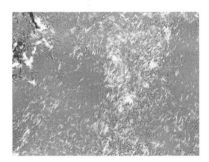

Figure 9-3   Uric Acid Crystals

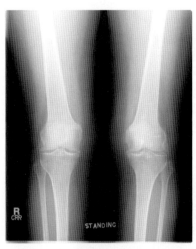

Figure 9-4   Calcium Pyrophosphate Dihydrate Deposition

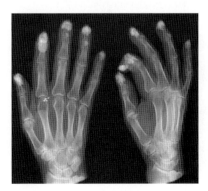

Figure 9-5   Chronic Tophaceous Gout

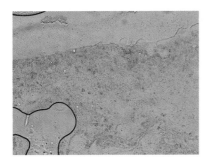

Figure 9-6 Pseudogout

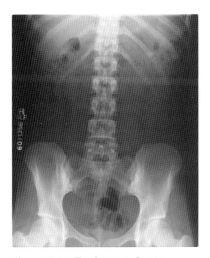

Figure 9-7 Trochanteric Bursitis

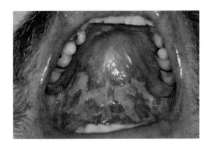

Figure 9-8 Canker Sores

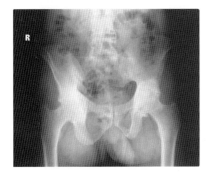

Figure 9-9 Arthritides

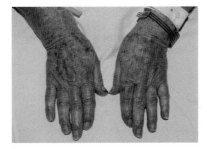

Figure 9-10 Psoriatic Arthritis

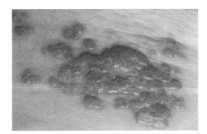

Figure 10-1 Herpes Zoster

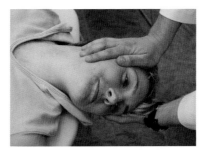

Figure 10-2 Dix-Hallpike Maneuver

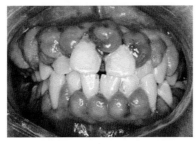

Figure 10-3 Gingival Hyperplasia

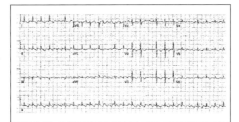

Figure 11-1 Atrial Flutter

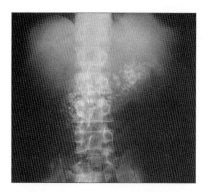

Figure 11-2 Abdominal Calcification

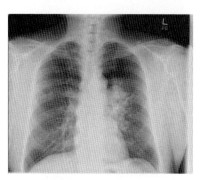

Figure 11-3 Pneumonia

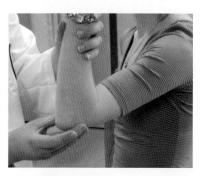

Figure 14-1 Palpation of Lateral Epicondyle

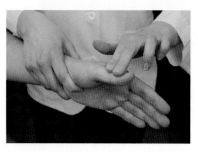

Figure 14-2 Abduction of Left Thumb Against Resistance

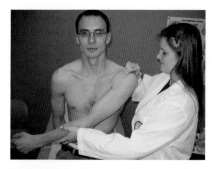

Figure 14-3 Crossover Test

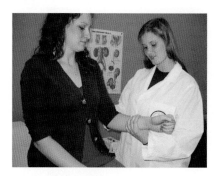

Figure 14-4 Medial Rotation of Left Arm Against Resistance

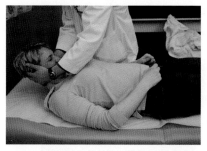

Figure 14-5 Brudzinski's Sign

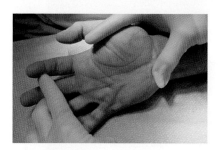

Figure 14-6 Right Dupuytren's Contracture

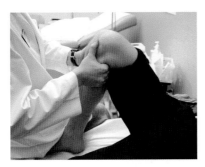

Figure 14-7 Anterior Drawer

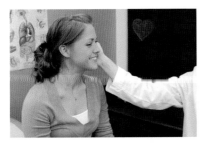

Figure 14-8 Turning Head Against Resistance

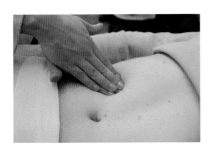

Figure 14-9 Murphy's Sign 1

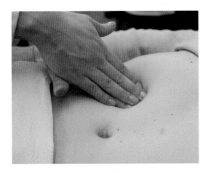

Figure 14-10 Murphy's Sign 2

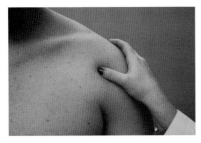

Figure 14-11 Bicipital Tendonitis

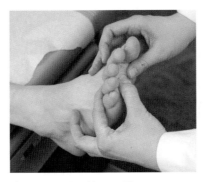

Figure 14-12 Morton Neuroma

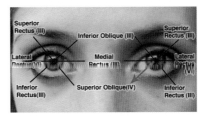

Figure 14-13 Extraocular Muscle, Arrow

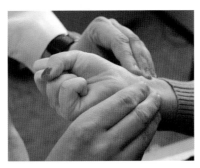

Figure 14-14 Allen's Test 1

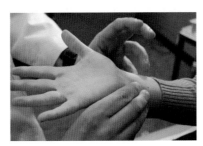

Figure 14-15 Allen's Test 2

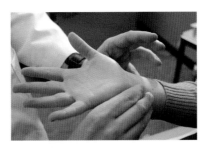

Figure 14-16 Allen's Test 3

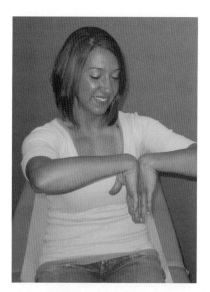

Figure 14-17   Phalen's Test

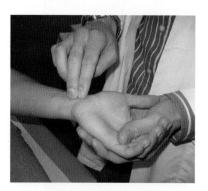

Figure 14-18   Tinel's Test

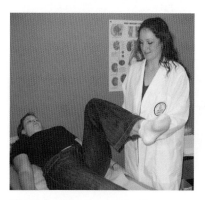

Figure 14-19   Kernig's Test 1

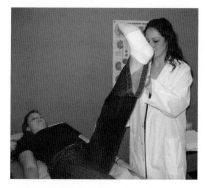

Figure 14-20   Kernig's Test 2

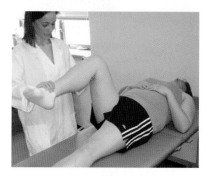

Figure 14-21   Thomas' Test

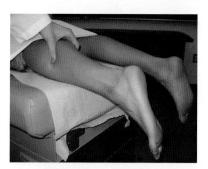

Figure 14-22   Thompson's Test

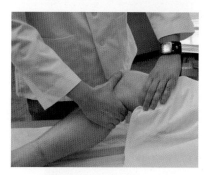

Figure 14-23   Lachman's Sign

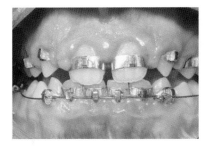

Figure 14-24 Gingival Hyperplasia

Courtesy of Dr. Joel Jaspan

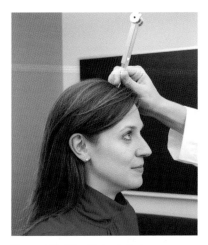

Figure 14-25 Weber's Test

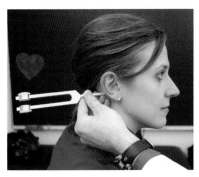

Figure 14-26 Rinne's Test 1

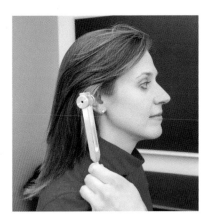

Figure 14-27 Rinne's Test 2

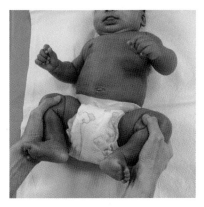

Figure 14-28 Ortolani Sign

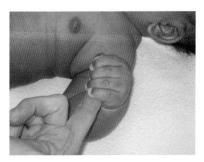

Figure 14-29 Palmar Grasp Reflex

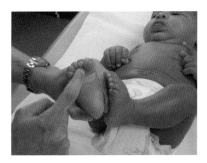

Figure 14-30 Plantar Grasp Reflex

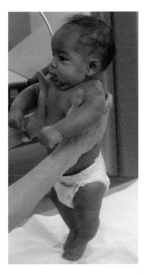

Figure 14-31 Stepping Reflex

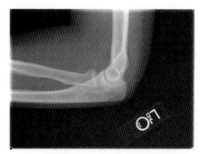

Figure 15-1   Colles' Fracture

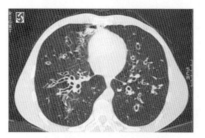

Figure 15-2   Bronchitis

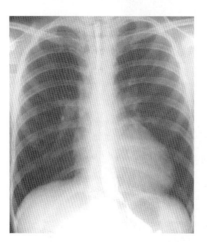

Figure 15-3   Rib-Notching

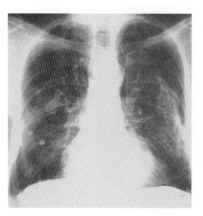

Figure 15-4   Cavitary Lesions

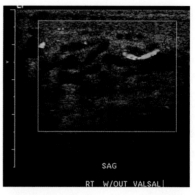

Figure 15-5   Varicocele

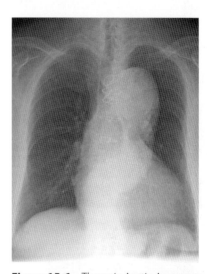

Figure 15-6   Thoracic Aortic Aneurysm

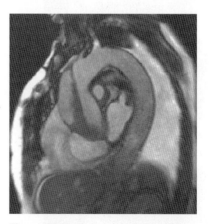

Figure 15-7   Ascending Aortic Aneurysm

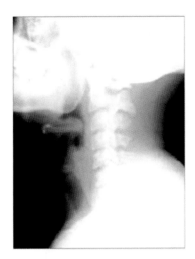

Figure 15-8 Epiglottitis

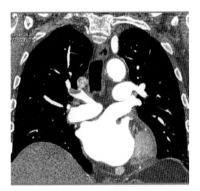

Figure 15-9 Pulmonary Embolism

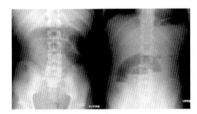

Figure 15-10 Small-Bowel Obstruction

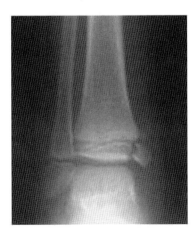

Figure 15-11 Salter IV

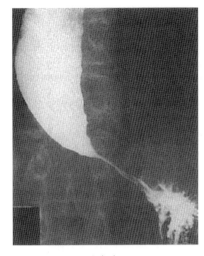

Figure 15-12 Achalasia

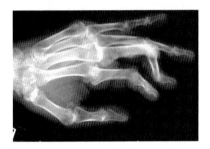

Figure 15-13 Rheumatoid Arthritis

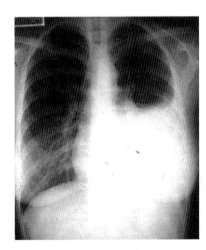

Figure 15-14 Pleural Effusion

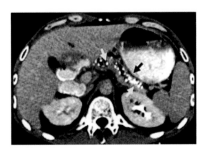

Figure 15-15 Chronic Pancreatitis

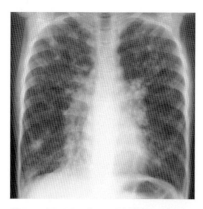

Figure 15-16 Cystic Fibrosis

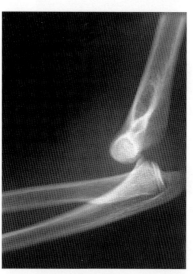

Figure 15-17 Elbow Dislocation

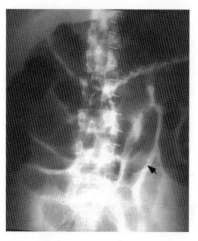

Figure 15-18 Acute Mesenteric Ischemia

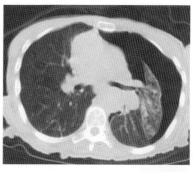

Figure 15-19 Tension Pneumothorax

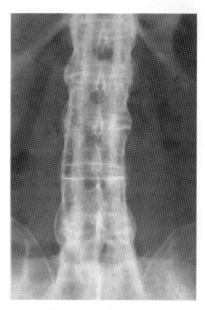

Figure 15-20 Ankylosing Spondylitis

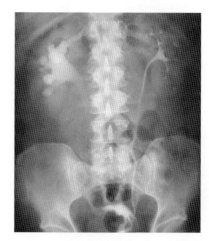

Figure 15-21 Hydronephrosis-Pyelonephritis

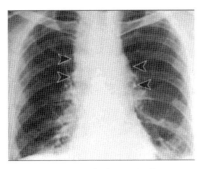

Figure 15-22   Inhalation Anthrax

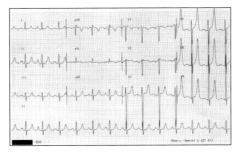

Figure 16-4   Electrocardiogram with Peaked T Waves

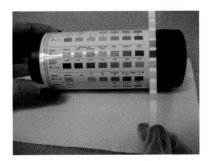

Figure 16-1   Urine Dipstick for Blood

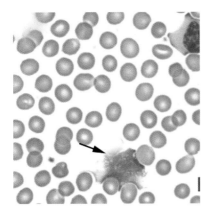

Figure 16-2   Smudge Cells

Permission granted by Donald Innes, MD, Department of Pathology, University of Virginia Health Sciences Center

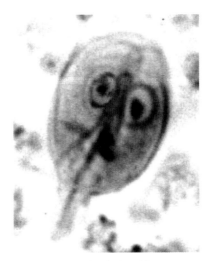

Figure 16-5   *Giardia Lamblia*

Copyright © 1999-2005 (Steve J. Upton). Used with permission.

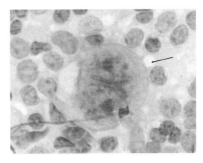

Figure 16-6   Reed-Sternberg Cell

© 2007 Rector and Visitors of the University of Virginia; Charles E. Hess, MD and Lindsey Krstic, BA

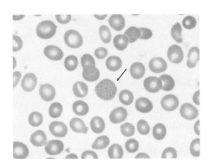

Figure 16-3   Basophilic Stippling

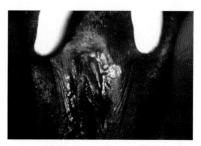

Figure 17-1 Primary Chancre of Syphilis
Courtesy of CDC

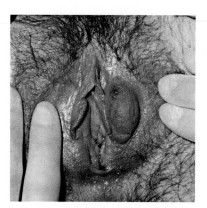

Figure 17-2 Bartholin Gland Abscess
© Wellcome Trust Library/Custom Medical Stock Photo

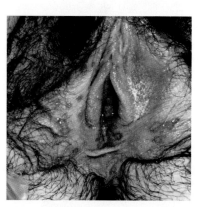

Figure 17-3 Genital Herpes
© Wellcome Trust Library/Custom Medical Stock Photo

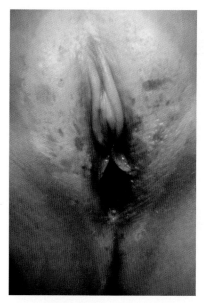

Figure 17-4 Lichen Sclerosis
Courtesy of Joe Miller/CDC

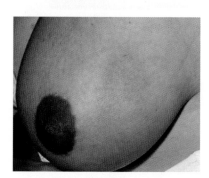

Figure 17-5 Mastitis
© SPL/Custom Medical Stock Photo

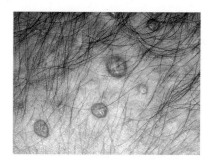

Figure 17-6 Molluscum Contagiosum
© Medical-on-Line/Alamy Images

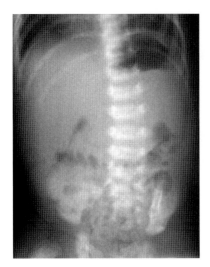

Figure 18-1   Pyloric Stenosis

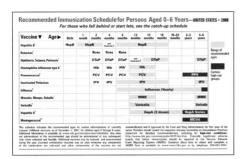

Figure 18-2   Catch-up Schedule

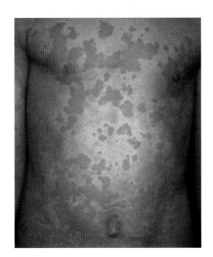

Figure 21-1   Urticaria

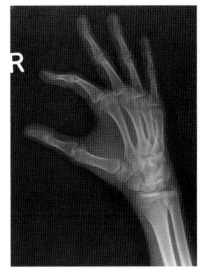

Figure 21-2   Navicular Fracture

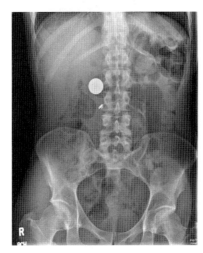

Figure 21-3   Radiograph of Coin in Stomach

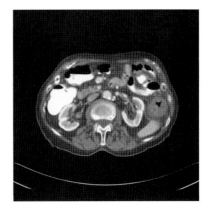

Figure 21-4   Colonic Thickening

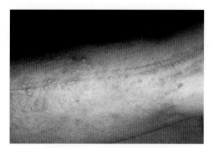

Figure 21-5 *Toxicodendron* dermatitis
Courtesy of CDC

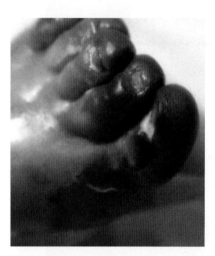

Figure 21-6 Frostbite

Glucose 560 mg/dL	Urine + for glucose, ketones
Potassium 3.6mEq/L	Serum ketones are positive
CO2 11 mEq/L	ABG with a pH 7.15
Anion gap 16	Amylase, lipase are both normal

Table 22-1 Lab Values

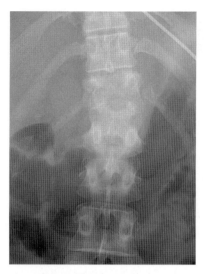

Figure 22-1 Thoracic Fracture

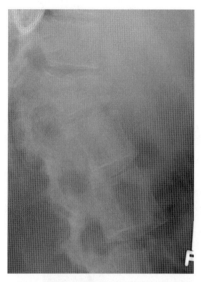

Figure 22-2 Thoracic Fracture, Lateral

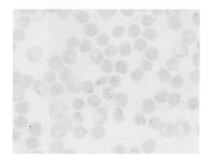

Figure 23-1 Heinz Bodies
© 2007 Rector and Visitors of the University of Virginia; Charles E. Hess, MD and Lindsey Krstic, BA

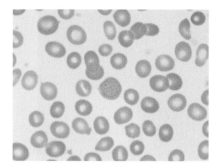

Figure 23-2 Basophilic Stippling

© 2007 Rector and Visitors of the University of Virginia;
Charles E. Hess, MD and Lindsey Krstic, BA

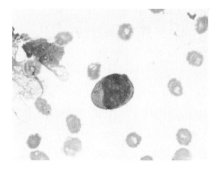

Figure 23-5 Auer Rod

© 2007 Rector and Visitors of the University of Virginia;
Charles E. Hess, MD and Lindsey Krstic, BA

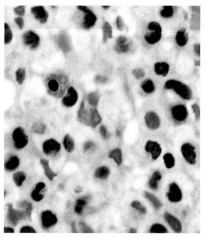

Figure 23-3 Bone Marrow Biopsy of Hairy
Cell Leukemia

© 2007 Rector and Visitors of the University of Virginia;
Charles E. Hess, MD and Lindsey Krstic, BA

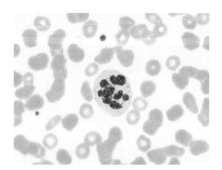

Figure 23-6 Hypersegmented Neutrophil

© 2007 Rector and Visitors of the University of Virginia;
Charles E. Hess, MD and Lindsey Krstic, BA

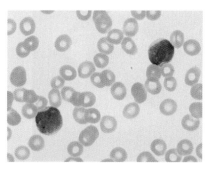

Figure 23-7 Acute Lymphoblastic Leukemia
Peripheral Smear

© 2007 Rector and Visitors of the University of Virginia;
Charles E. Hess, MD and Lindsey Krstic, BA

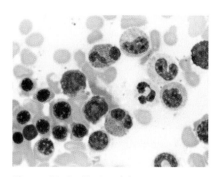

Figure 23-4 Eosinophil

© 2007 Rector and Visitors of the University of Virginia;
Charles E. Hess, MD and Lindsey Krstic, BA

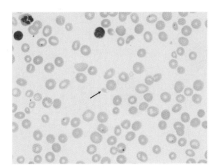

Figure 23-8 Schistocyte

© 2007 Rector and Visitors of the University of Virginia;
Charles E. Hess, MD and Lindsey Krstic, BA

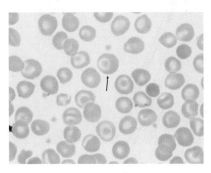

Figure 23-9 Target Cell

© 2007 Rector and Visitors of the University of Virginia;
Charles E. Hess, MD and Lindsey Krstic, BA

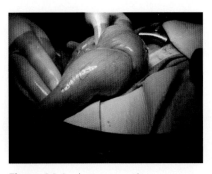

Figure 24-1 Intussusception

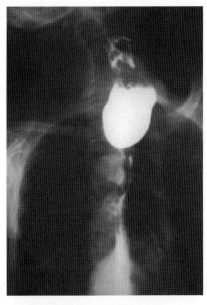

Figure 24-2 Zenker's Diverticulum

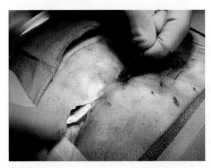

Figure 24-3 Pilonidal Cyst

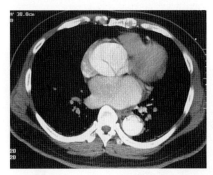

Figure 24-4 Aortic Dissection

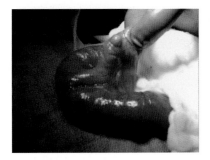

Figure 24-5   Meckel's Diverticulum

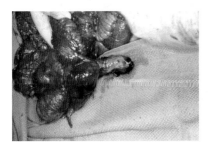

Figure 24-6   Necrotic Appendix

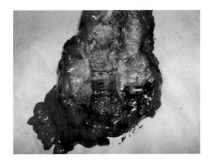

Figure 24-7   Diverticulitis

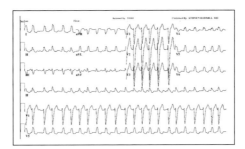

Figure 26-1   Atrial Fibrillation

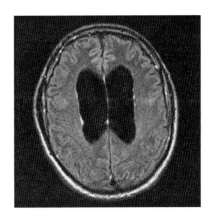

Figure 26-2   Normal Pressure Hydrocephalus